THE BENGAL DISPENSATORY AND COMPANION TO THE PHARMACOPOEIA

S. DAS

GYAN

Published by

Gyan Publishing House
5, Ansari Road
Daryaganj, New Delhi-110002
Phone: 011-47034999, 9811692060
E-mail: books@gyanbooks.com

Distribution Network
gyanbooks.com
India, USA, Canada, UK, Australia

ISBN: 978-93-7225-177-7 (PB)

First Published, 1929

2nd Impression 2026

Printed at: Gyan Press, Delhi.

THE BENGAL DISPENSATORY AND COMPANION TO THE PHARMACOPOEIA

Author: S. DAS

THE BENGAL DISPENSATORY AND COMPANION TO THE PHARMACOPOEIA

THE BENGAL

DISPENSATORY AND PHARMACOPŒI

Chiefly compiled from the Works of

ROXBURGH,
WALLICH,
AINSLIE,
WIGHT AND ARNOT,
ROYLE,

PEREIRA,
LINDLEY,
RICHARD,
AND
FEÉ;

And including the results of numerous special experiments.

PROFESSOR OF CHEMISTRY AND MATERIA MEDICA IN THE MEDICAL COLLEGE, CALCUTTA.

Vol. I.—The Dispensatory.

Introduction.

Four years have now elapsed since the appointment of a Committee,* to examine and report upon the state of the Honorable Company's Dispensary, and the possibility of substituting indigenous remedies for some which are only procurable from other countries, at prices which place their use beyond the means of the mass of the community. The question of the publication of an Indian Pharmacopœia was also submitted to this Committee for their opinion.

Death, ill-health, and the casualties of the service, scattered the Committee long before its members could accomplish the important labours they each most zealously undertook. To the Editor of this work was entrusted by the Committee the task of reporting on the subject of the proposed Pharmacopœia. In the Report he drew up, his colleagues generally concurred, while such differences as existed, were on matters of not very material importance. The subjoined and ample

* Consisting of Dr. W. Jackson, officiating Apothecary-General, since retired from the service.

Dr. J. Ranken, officiating Secretary to the Medical Board, soon after appointed Post Master General in the North-Western Provinces.

Mr. Bramley, Principal of the Medical College, since dead.

Dr. Pearson, Deputy Apothecary-General, soon after appointed Civil Surgeon to Juanpore.

Mr. James Prinsep, Assay Master to the Mint, soon after went to England, where he died.

Dr. W. B. O'Shaughnessy, Professor of Chemistry in the Medical College, Editor of the present work.

extracts from the document in question, will explain the views it set forth, and which were subsequently carried into effect, as far as practicable, on the recommendation of the Medical Board in their support.

FIRST REPORT

From the Committee appointed by the Right Honorable the Governor General in Council, to inquire into various subjects connected with the state of the Materia Medica of British India, &c. &c. ON the expediency of compiling a Pharmacopœia for Bengal and Upper India.

In obedience to the instructions received from the Right Honorable the Governor General, we beg leave to offer for his Lordship's consideration the following Memoranda on the expediency and advantages of compiling a special Pharmacopœia for the Bengal Presidency, and on the practicability, and utility of reforming the nomenclature connected with the prescription of medicines in this country.

In the subsequent memoranda we shall follow the subjoined outline. We shall first consider the nature and uses of Pharmacopœiæ generally—secondly, give a summary exposition of the causes which have led to the compilation of the numerous works of this kind in Europe and America—thirdly, we shall review the leading arguments for the preparation of a Pharmacopœia for Bengal, and notice some of the circumstances requisite to render it of the widest and readiest utility. Lastly, we shall give a sketch of the character and extent of investigation which must indispensably precede the compilation; and we shall develope in sufficient detail the subjects which this should embrace.

The numerous official Pharmacopœiæ at present in existence, have been issued at the public cost, under the sanction of Collegiate, Academic, or other official medical institutions. In connection with our inquiry, the following statistical statement may not be devoid of interest.

In Great Britain and Ireland there are three Pharmacopœiæ—one for each kingdom, and edited by the Colleges of Physicians in London, Edinburgh, and Dublin—in France one, edited by the Parisian Faculty of Medicine;—in the Russian Empire five; one for general use, one for the Army, one for the Navy, one for Poland, and the fifth published in Abo, for Finland. Denmark, Sweden, Holland, and Belgium, each possesses one. In the German States there are twenty-two; in Switzerland three; in Italy eleven; in Spain four; in Portugal one; in America there is but one, edited conjointly however by all the Medical Colleges and Societies of the United States.*

In all these works the same great objects are evidently held in view. No substance finds a place in any department of these volumes, the natural history of which has not been investigated, or the medicinal uses of which, rest on dubious or unauthenticated testimony. The public is thus presented with a catalogue of remedies as ample as science can supply. When danger co-exists with medicinal virtue, the precautions are usually specified under which the administration of the substance should be conducted. A few simple characters are frequently given to guide the purchaser of each article.

In all these works, again, we find simple directions, which enable an Apothecary, though possessed but of mediocre attainments, to collect, preserve, and manage officinal vegetables, so as to turn their products to the best account. The making of extracts, tinctures, in-

* The whole of these works have been published in one collection by Frederick Fleischer of Leipzic, in 1827, under the title of "Codex Medicamentarius Europæus."

fusions, &c. is provided for, and practical directions are given for the manipulations of Pharmaceutical Chemistry.

This is a most important fact. When these directions were first used, the class of men for whom they were deemed sufficient by the most eminent Colleges of Physicians in the world, was altogether uneducated in the principles of Chemical science. The Colleges anticipated, and justly, that no difficulty would arise in the practical fulfilment of their directions. We have thus the recorded opinions of a host of the best authorities on this subject, that in the preparation of numerous remedies to meet the demands of medical practice, neither profound chemical knowledge, nor large* manufacturing operations are at all essential. We shall have to return to this fact again, for it is fraught with important inferences, bearing forcibly on many points of the inquiry committed to our charge.

Such are a few of the objects and uses of Pharmacopœiæ generally. The causes of the existence of the very numerous local works of this kind do not altogether lie on the surface of the subject. That they have not originated in the difference of language in different countries, is sufficiently shewn by the fact, that of the 64 above mentioned, 49 are in the Latin, and but 15 in the vernacular languages. Varieties of climate, customs, and natural productions have given origin to the majority; academic and political rivalry have created a few. Tracing however the broad distinctions established by nature, observing the widely different effects of the same remedies on different races of mankind, and including in our glance the remarkable varieties of the material from which in different countries one and

* For instance, to make Tartar Emetic 1 lb. of each of the materials to be boiled in 1 gallon of water; to make Calomel 4 lbs. of Mercury, 30 ounces of sulphuric acid. To make sulphuric ether, 32 ounces of acid, and the same quantity of alcohol. To make the spirit of ammonia, ounce proportions of all the substances used. To make Lunar Caustic, 1 ounce of each article used. To make all the tinctures, ounce proportions of each ingredient to pints of spirit.

the same medicinal agent has to be prepared, we cannot but admit the wisdom of preparing Pharmacopœiæ to meet local circumstances and wants by sources of local supply.

We have alluded to varieties in raw material for medicinal preparations, as one of the causes for so many Pharmacopœiæ having been compiled. As the reason is an urgent one, and bearing strongly on our views, with reference to the necessity for such a work for Bengal, we feel it desirable to place this subject in a clearer light, and we may best accomplish this by illustrations selected from medicinal articles of known utility.

Take Potash and its compounds for example—obtained in Canada by the burning of the forest timber; in Ireland from the Fern; in France, Italy, and along the Rhenish wine-districts, from Cream of Tartar; in India with most economy from Nitre,—in each case a totally different process is required for its extraction, purification, and adaptation to medicinal use. Soda gives us another and a striking instance.—The Spaniard obtains it most easily from Barilla by mere washing; the Scot from Kelp by a much more laborious and unproductive process; in France, and latterly in England, it is prepared from common salt (Muriate of Soda) which is first decomposed by sulphuric acid, and then the resulting sulphate of Soda subjected to another process, which changes it into the Carbonate. In Bengal and Mysore, again, the soil, in many places, is so impregnated with the alkali, that incineration and washing extract from 35 to 50 per cent of fine soda.

The study of the reactions of several vegetable substances of one kind of medicinal power (for instance, of different purgatives, bitters, tonics, &c.) on other vegetable or mineral substances which it may be desirable to prescribe at the same time for the same individual, is also an imperative reason for the compilation of local Pharmacopœiæ. Thus the *Quassia Amara* of Jamaica, and *Menyanthes trifoliata* of Ireland, the *Gentiana lutea* of the Alps and Appenines, the *Agathotes Chirayta* and *Goluncha* of Bengal, all agree in being intensely bitter, and in possessing at least powerful tonic properties; but infusions of these vegetables act so differently on the preparations of iron, of magnesia, and other substances, that a different form of prescription is perhaps essential in each case. We might extend these illustrations almost indefinitely. Turn where we may to any standard work on Materia Medica, similar facts present themselves in every page. Admitting then that even in Europe there are good and adequate reasons for the existence of a majority of the Pharmacopœiæ we have enumerated, let us next consider, specially, the necessity and probable degree of utility of compiling such a work for Bengal.

Were we to confine our speculations to the necessities of the services, Military and Civil, we should meet but little comparative difficulty in discussing this subject. The extremely low wholesale prices of drugs in the English markets, with the favourable rates of freight the Government can command, the facilities for the purification and preparation of articles of local produce afforded by the present Dispensary establishment in Calcutta, or which might be secured by some modifications in the arrangement of that institution; all these circumstances would enable us to adapt the British Pharmacopœiæ to all the wants of the services. No printed work would be required, no reform in the nomenclature essential. But we have to deal with a subject of far greater moment and difficulty. We have to consider the wants of an immense, an ignorant, and poor population, among whom medical science is but beginning to establish itself; among whom were we at this moment to distribute a full proportion of well educated practitioners, whether European or Native, their acquirements must be all but useless, owing to an obstacle we shall notice in due detail, and which we have, providentially, the means of removing placed within our reach.

We allude to the high prices of all medicinal preparations sold by the private European establishments in Calcutta, Cawnpore, and Meerut,—the only localities in Bengal or Upper India where European Apothecaries have settled. Little competition existing, the prices of the most indispensable articles of medicine are fixed at such a rate that rich natives will not, the humbler cannot, avail themselves of the remedies which medical science has pointed out. Scarce a day passes that we do not meet with striking, and often tragic proofs of the operation of this evil. Pupils of the Medical College have brought to our knowledge cases in which their own relatives, labouring under dangerous, nay fatal maladies, deterred by the high prices alluded to, abandoned themselves to the cheap poisons of the bazar, to preparations such as the Bish Booree, and the like; compounds of the most deadly ingredients, administered by utterly ignorant empirics.

We are prepared to shew, that in the hands of well, nay highly, educated Natives, medicines of every kind may be retailed in Calcutta, and throughout India, at lower prices than even those of the London general practitioners, who charge at least 200 per cent. less than their Calcutta brethren, and give the patient the benefit of their attendance besides.

We have spoken freely and unreservedly on this subject, because we cannot but feel, that until this evil is fully remedied, every attempt to diffuse the inestimable blessings of medical science among the natives of India must prove entirely abortive.

The remedy for this serious evil is two-fold. We must supply the country with competent practitioners and druggists, and we must again furnish these individuals with instructions by which they may successfully perform all the operations and processes which pharmacy requires. The first of these objects is already in course of satisfactory fulfilment. The second, presents minor difficulties; but at the same time demands our serious consideration.

The first question which naturally suggests itself, is whether for the purposes required, we can adopt any of the English Pharmacopœiæ, or whether one should be compiled specially for Bengal. We can have no hesitation in recommending the latter alternative, when we take into consideration the subjoined reasons.

1. The British Pharmacopœiæ contain a great number of indigenous plants, which do not grow in India, or the limitrophe countries, but for which Indian substitutes may be found.

2. The British Pharmacopœiæ do not contain numerous plants indigenous in India, of proved utility as remedial agents.

3. The pharmaceutical processes in the British Pharmacopœiæ, especially with reference to distillation, evaporation, making of tinctures and alcoholic extracts, and many other articles, such as ethers, are modified so as to meet the dearness of labour, and spirit, and the operation of excise laws in Great Britain; restrictions which need not affect us here.

Here alcohol of the pharmaceutical strength (sp. gr. 835) may be had for 2*s*. 8*d*. the gallon of four imperial quarts—a circumstance which affords immense facility to a multitude of processes the druggist must carry on. The cheapness of spirit may moreover enable the Editors of the Pharmacopœia to effect decided practical improvements in the preparation of vegetable proximate principles, such as Quinine, and Morphine—as well as the extracts and tinctures, &c. It will enable them also to give efficient directions, and shew ready plans for prosecuting analytical researches after new vegetable remedies. Much will thus be done towards reducing the prices of a great number of medicines essential in clinical practice.

4. In the chemical preparations, especially those of the alkaline and metallic salts, perfectly new directions would be essentially necessary in many instances.

Continuing our sketch of the prominent features in which the Bengal Pharmacopœia in its chemical department must differ from the British, we may allude to the well known and valuable medicines of which Magnesia is the base. Sulphate of Magnesia being an abundant natural product in England, and sold wholesale at 2*d*. per pound, the other products, viz. the calcined magnesia, carbonate of magnesia, &c. are manufactured from that article. In India however our native druggists should receive instruction how to produce magnesia, from the residue after the preparation of common salt, from the magnesian limestone of Sylhet and the Himalayas, and from the magnesite of Madras.

To the modifications relative to the medicinal preparations of Potash and Soda we have already alluded,—Ammonia and its compounds would also require considerable alteration. Processes would be necessary for the reduction of several mercurial compounds from the Chinese Cinnabar, and the crude chloride, or Ruskapoor, of the Bazars. With reference to the antimonial preparations, methods should be pointed out of distinguishing between the sulphuret of lead and sulphuret of antimony,—two substances common and cheap in the Bazars, and resembling each other so strongly that they are constantly confounded even by the drug-dealers themselves.

It is unnecessary to go more minutely into these details. The facts we mention are brought forward but as illustrations, and constitute but an insignificant fraction of the mass we are prepared to adduce whenever the occasion arises.

5. Another and important reason for our recommendation, is the urgent necessity which exists for alteration of the nomenclature of the British Pharmacopœia to meet the circumstances and degree of education of the natives of this country. In a territory like this, where not one native understands the Latin language, where indeed the foundations of modern knowledge are but being laid at this moment, it would be monstrous pedantry were we to retain exclusively the Latin names of the present Pharmacopœiæ to the extent, or in the rank they occupy at present. Of the vegetable articles of the Materia Medica nine-tenths are of eastern origin, and have familiar names in the Bengali, Hindoostani, or English tongues. With their scientific appellations the natives of this country require no intimate acquaintance. As our object in the first place is to do the utmost benefit to the people of India, we should use the only terms they can comprehend. But as we are also bound to consult the interests of science, and the preservation of the universal language which enables scientific men of every country to commune in a general tongue, and as the Materia Medica of the East will doubtless be scanned with avidity by the studious in every land, we would recommend that each vegetable, animal, and mineral substance of the Pharmacopœia should in the descriptive part of the work be arranged in the following order,—the Bengali or Hindostani name to lead, followed by the English, and lastly by the Latin.

Where no native name exists, the English term should be introduced as a new word, and placed in the first column.

In cases of compound names not known in the eastern languages alluded to, and where, as often happens, two English designations exist for the same substance, the more scientific term should be adopted in an English form; thus, Acetate of Lead should be preferred to Sugar of Lead; Chloride of Antimony, to Butter of Antimony, &c. &c.

In the formulary these principles should be strictly adopted, the Latin term being never inserted in prescription where either a Bengali, Hindostani, or English term could be found. Common sense is at length banishing the Latin recipe system even from England, where that language is generally understood. It would scarcely be wise to preserve the system here, where Latin is almost unknown. The necessity for a vernacular formulary is indeed practically acknowledged in India by the most distinguished members of our medical establishment.

It would be a measure of great utility however to prefix to the Pharmacopœia a glossary of the conventional terms employed in the work; thus, "Chlorine," "Chloride," "Iodine," "Iodide," "Sulphate," "Nitrate," "Tincture," "Extract," &c. might with great advantage be explained in this manner.

The preceding reasons seem to us sufficient to warrant our recommendation of the compilation of an original Pharmacopœia for Bengal and Upper India, in preference to the adoption of any of the British official volumes. Other and perhaps much more powerful arguments are presented by circumstances we have still to detail in connection with the next head of the inquiry; namely, the extent, and character of investigation which must precede the publication of an Indian Pharmacopœia.

This investigation should, in the first instance, be directed to the careful scrutiny of the *claims* to medical repute of the native vegetable remedies hitherto described. This inquiry must comprehend—1st. the botanical identification of each plant; secondly, its accurate chemical analysis; thirdly, the preparation of its pharmaceutical products, viz. its tincture, extract, &c. on a sufficiently large scale for clinical researches; fourthly, its experimental use or trial in Hospital practice. Without this regular sequence of inquiry, no Pharmacopœia can be constructed on which the slightest reliance can, or ought to be reposed; and each step we have enumerated seems to us as essential as the others. An inspection of the best work yet published on Indian Materia, namely the 2nd vol. of Ainslie's Materia Indica, will convince any competent reader of the truth of our assertion. We find in that elaborate, and highly creditable production, a catalogue of several hundred plants, the products of which are used in medical practice by Native physicians. The majority are highly celebrated for their medicinal virtues. A great number have been identified and named, but scarcely one has been subjected to analysis, and very few have been made the object of clinical investigation. The work is hence valuable but as a key to ulterior researches, though immeasurably superior to the Ulfaz-Ul-Udwieh of Gladwin, and indeed to every other book yet written on this subject. Dr. Ainslie himself, with all the candour of a philosophic mind, anticipates the view we have taken of his labours.

The next step—the chemical analysis—is one of equal importance, and by the common consent of all physicians deemed essential to the pharmaçeutical history of every vegetable as well as mineral substance. To this branch of knowledge is it that mankind is indebted for the discovery of the inestimable *Sulphate of Quinine*, of strychnine, morphine, and a multitude of other powerful and valuable remedial agents.

On the analysis of each plant being completed a sufficient quantity of its powder, extract, tincture, proximate crystalline principles, (if any discovered,) &c. should be prepared in the H. C. Dispensary, and issued, under the sanction and orders of the Medical Board, to the chief Hospitals in the country, (European, Regimental, and Zillah,) for clinical trial, to be reported on by the Medical Officers of these institutions.

On the clinical reports being received, all the documents, botanical, chemical, and clinical, should be referred to a Committee composed of at least one Botanist, one Chemist, one experienced European, and one trust-worthy Native practitioner, to decide on the introduction or rejection of the plant or vegetable product, in question, and to draw up the Formulæ according to which it should be prescribed.

The same Committee should decide on the articles solely of foreign produce indispensable in medical practice, and which should be introduced into the Indian Pharmacopœia.

The modified chemical processes alluded to should be drawn up by some competent person, their practicability and superior economy demonstrated to the Committee, who, when satisfied on these points, should sanction the adoption of the process.

Lastly, the whole of the accumulated facts should be committed to some competent individual to arrange and publish; and a translation, made in Bengali and Hindostani, in the Native character, should also be issued. The work should be more comprehensive than a mere Pharmacopœia, but much less voluminous than the Dispensatories of Drs. Thomson or Duncan.

The annexed division of its subjects, and the mode of treating these, we would venture to recommend.

1st.—An explanatory glossary of technical terms.

2nd.—Concise and clear directions for conducting the primary pharmaceutical operations, such as distilling, subliming, &c. with Lithographic drawings of utensils, and instructions for their cheap construction, &c.

3rd.—The Vegetable Materia Medica arranged alphabetically. A sketch of the history of each individual to be given, its physical description, place of growth, average market price, medicinal uses, and the doses and preparations in which it should be used.

4th.—The chemical preparations, Alkaline, Earthy, and Metallic, in alphabetical order, with lithographs of utensils, cost of raw material, properties and uses in medicine and the arts.

5th.—Alcohol and the ethers similarly treated.

6th.—A Formulary, preparatory and prescriptive, for pills, tinctures, extracts, &c. with manufacturing details, and lists of prices, &c.

7th.—Tables of weights and measures, Indian and English, weights of given volumes of medicinal liquids, &c. &c.

It now only remains for us to point out briefly the benefits which we believe will accrue to the Native and European communities, and to the Government itself, from the execution of the proposed measure. Let us suppose this Pharmacopœia to contain sufficient instruction for the Native druggist. To educate any intelligent native, speaking English, Hindostani, or Bengali, so as to make him perfect master of its contents, would be a work but of trivial labour and expense. To profit by this instruction, there would be abundant candidates from every quarter. They would crowd to learn a trade, which they already know would confer a monopoly on its craftsmen, and which their experience in the complicated, though rude chemistry of their forefathers, has taught them requires no capital for its commencement beyond what any respectable native can command.

Let us again imagine one or more of these druggists established in any of the great Indian cities, where either an European or well-educated Native practitioner is stationed. An ample supply of excellent remedies is at once provided, at prices far below what even a London Apothecary would charge. Need we expatiate on the blessings which would be thus bestowed on the Native community; and on the European population not entitled to gratuitous supply at the public cost. The period too would rapidly come round, when the existence of a numerous class of individuals of this description would render the Government almost independent of importation or manufacture for its own emergencies. The Native druggists would gladly compete for the custom of the Government establishments in every locality. We can feel but little doubt, that a respectable and intelligent manufacturing druggist might thus be provided for every Zillah in our Empire, and that much of the demand for Military use, might, and would, be provided for in the cantonments themselves.

(Signed by the Committee.)

Several months after this Report was presented, the orders of Government were received for its suggestions being carried into effect, and a Committee* of supervision was appointed.

The Editor commenced his duties, by examining, both by chemical and clinical experiment, several articles of indigenous production, of reputation for their medicinal virtues. As quickly as any fact indicated a valuable result, he reported

* S. Nicolson, Esq. Surgeon to the General Hospital.
Dr. Wallich, Professor of Botany to the Medical College.
Mr. Egerton, Professor of Surgery to the College.
Mr. Strong, Surgeon to the Mysore Princes.
Dr. O'Shaughnessy, Professor of Chemistry, Medical College, Secretary to the Committee, and Editor of the Pharmacopœia.

its details to the Committee. The febrifuge powers of Narcotine,* the purgative Kaladana, the emetic Crinum, the extraordinary stimulant and narcotic Gunjah, with many other substances, were thus successively examined; materials, in short, were being collected, which in due time would have grown into a rich catalogue, when the Editor received new orders from the Medical Board of the day, which compelled him to relinquish much of his experimental researches, and devote himself to the task of compiling not only a Pharmacopœia, but a Dispensatory of general Materia Medica.

It would be highly presumptuous in the Editor to question the wisdom of this decision; he is well aware that its chief fault consisted in entrusting the task to one so imperfectly qualified as himself for its satisfactory performance. He attempted it however with the feeling, that if unsuccessful in the full development of the plan, the resulting work would at all events prove a useful class-book of Materia Medica for the instruction of his native pupils, and serve as the outline of one which, in a subsequent edition, more leisurely researches and opportunity might complete to his own satisfaction.

The volume now published constitutes the Dispensatory. It embraces instructions on pharmaceutical manipulations; on the mode of taking specific gravities; of making ordinary meteorological observations, (explanatory details being given under each head); an outline of Chemistry for the guidance of

* Or *Anarcotine*, as we subsequently ventured to term it, from its remarkable want of all narcotic properties.

the teachers of native apothecaries; a grammar of botany, constituting a systematized glossary of the terms used in botanical descriptions; a brief account of the mode of action of the several therapeutical classes of remedial agents; lastly, the Vegetable Materia Medica, arranged in the natural system.

In an appendix are inserted papers drawn up by the Editor, on the manufacture of an improved pottery in Bengal; on the investigation and treatment of poisoning; with meteorological tables and notices of miscellaneous subjects.

In his plan the Editor has followed, and he trusts in some respects improved on, those of Duncan and Thomson in their invaluable Dispensatories. He has limited his attention strictly to points of practical utility, and omitted all that merely bore on the literature or controversies of the subject. He was often tempted to wander into these more pleasing fields of inquiry, but as frequently recalled to the dry path assigned him, by the peculiar wants and circumstances of his pupils, and the restriction of the work to a volume of 800 pages.

Before dismissing the subject of the Dispensatory, the Editor wishes distinctly to state that it does not profess to be more than a compilation, for which the works specified on the title-page have afforded the chief materials, which he has re-arranged, commented upon, and added to, to the best of his ability.

The 2nd volume, the Pharmacopœia, now in the press, may be regarded either as a separate work, as the sequel, or companion of the Dispensatory. The following outline of its contents will suffice for the present information of the reader.

1.—A Conspectus of the Materia Medica in the natural system, with a short account of the medicinal properties of each article, being an epitome of the contents of the Dispensatory. This table serves as a catalogue of the medicinal plants in the Botanical Garden of Calcutta; as a guide to the introducer of new articles, and the inquirer after local substitutes.

2.—A table of Materia Medica, arranged according to the medicinal effects, giving the English and Latin scientific names, the familiar native name, the locality, part used, active principle, and a list of references to the works of Royle, Ainslie, Lindley, and other authorities, for fuller details.

3.—The Pharmacopœia list, embracing only those articles considered to be necessary as the stock of the druggist, excluding those doubtful or superfluous, giving brief descriptions of the proofs of genuineness and purity of several articles. This list is given alphabetically; and upheld by the high authority of the last edition of the Edinburgh Pharmacopœia; a nomenclature has been adopted, founded on utility and safety, exclusively, and without reference to more elevated scientific views. Thus the term *Calomel* is used instead of Protochloride of Mercury, *Tartar emetic*, for the Potassio-tartrate of antimony, &c.

4.—The preparations and compositions of the articles in list No. 2. Under this head it is the Editor's duty to remark, that while many processes are new, the majority are taken or imitated from the London and Edinburgh Pharmacopœiæ, the latter especially. The edition of this work, published in 1840, is now the best pharmaceutical guide of all the European Pharmacopœiæ. Its excellence is due to the unrivalled ability and skill of Dr. Christison, who for an adequate period devoted himself to the preparation of this edition.

All the processes of the Bengal Pharmacopœia have been repeated by the Editor; and whether they be original or imitated, he trusts their applicability will be recognized by those who conduct them for themselves.

5.—Lists of remedies, in the native character, and in the Sanscrita, Persian, Bengalli, and Urdu languages.

6.—Tables of the drugs imported for the use of the Honorable Company's establishments in Bengal, with prices—also of local articles, with their bazar rates.

It is necessary to observe, that the printing of the MS. of the Pharmacopœia from the third article still awaits the fiat and revision of the Committee; and owing to the ill-health, and unavoidable departure of the Editor, will devolve on the management of another individual, who is however fully acquitted of every error it may contain, for which its first Editor is alone responsible.

It remains for the Editor to express the warmest gratitude for the zealous co-operation afforded to him by his valued friend Dr. Wallich in the preparation of this work; while the Editor prepared all the MS. in the first instance, Dr. Wallich undertook the labour of revising the proofs, and correcting the errors he encountered; nor did his kindness stop here; for he added from his inexhaustible stores of *useful* botanical knowledge, illustrations of many subjects which the Editor could not have supplied. It is especially in the first table of the Conspectus that Dr. Wallich's aid has been conspicuous, rendering that part of the Pharmacopœia a guide to the Botanic Garden, of the highest practical value.

To Mr. Siddons, my zealous assistant at the Medical College, and my clinical clerks Messrs. Wambeck and Ludovice, (students from Ceylon,) I owe my cordial thanks for their most useful aid; and there are other friends who forbid me to include them in this catalogue, but without whose cooperation, scanty as these volumes are, they must have been still more imperfect.

The plates* require a word of comment. They have, with one exception, been lithographed by Mr. Ballin, who had to contend with insuperable difficulty in their preparation. They must be regarded as mere tracings, intended for the subjects for wood-engravings, with which I propose to illustrate a second edition, as soon as my health and circumstances permit me to undertake it.

Lastly; it would be discreditable were I to close this notice without an humble tribute to the anxiety, indulgence, and extraordinary practical knowledge of the subject with which the Earl of Auckland has watched the progress of these volumes. Deeply do I feel how unworthy they are of his Lordship's approbation, but in contemplating their final improvement, I am upheld by the views his Lordship has expressed

* One of the stomach-pump it has been found necessary to omit altogether.

in the following terms, in which, by his gracious permission, I offer the Dispensatory and Pharmacopœia to the *students of the Medical College,* the only class for whom I presume to consider them a fitting guide.

"With regard to the publication of the Indian Pharmacopœia, I am far from disposed to press you with undue impatience; and would readily, within limits, give you the time which you may think necessary in making the work creditable and useful, and for testing, with some approach to certainty, the experiments in which you may be engaged; but I would not have you ambitious to produce any but a very imperfect work; every work upon natural history must be so, and will be so to the end of time; and in a first essay of this kind you cannot expect to do more than to detail what is already known; to explain the results of your own experiments and speculations; to produce a good frame upon which new information may be recorded; and to give a general impulse to the researches of others."

W. B. O'SHAUGHNESSY, M. D.

Assistant Surgeon.

MEDICAL COLLEGE, CALCUTTA,

20*th October,* 1841.

THE

BENGAL DISPENSATORY

AND

PHARMACOPŒIA.

WEIGHTS AND MEASURES.

To ensure perfect uniformity in the preparation and doses of medicines, and at the same time to provide a standard universally and easily obtainable, we have adopted as the basis of our system, both of weights and measures, *the Honorable East-India Company's New Rupee.*

By numerous experiments it has been ascertained that the new Rupee, or tola, as found in circulation, is exactly equal to English Pharmaceutical grains... } 180

The ½ rupee and ¼ rupee (silver) of the new currency are equal to 90 and 45 grains each.

The new copper pice is equal to 100 grains.

The ¼ rupee (silver) we divide into 45 equal parts, each termed one grain.

This is readily done by taking an equal weight of wire, and cutting it into three equal lengths; each length is further subdivided three times, whereby five grain weights are obtained; each five grain wire divided into five equal parts, gives the units required.

Of these units or grains, (gr.)

		English Pharmacopœia wts.
20	are equal to	one scruple ℈
60	"	one drachm ʒi
480	"	one ounce ℥i

Twelve English Pharmacopœia or Troy ounces make one pound, (℔ i.)

The Avoirdupois pound is divided into 16 ounces (each 437·5 grains) each ounce into 16 drachms—each drachm is 27·34 grains.

	Grains.
1 Troy pound contains	5760
1 Avoirdupois pound	7000

In wholesale purchases, or sales of drugs, for example in large consignments imported from Europe, the avoirdupois pound is employed.

The measure of liquids we employ is derived from the rupee, but is equal to the legal standard of Great Britain.

A column of liquid of a base equal to the silver quarter rupee, and in length equal to $3\frac{3}{4}$ inches, measures exactly—

1 Pharmaceutical fluid ounce... f℥i
20 Fluid ounces are one pint ... Oi
8 Pints, are one gallon Ci

For measures of liquids less than the fluid ounce, we take a column of liquid having a circular base equal in diameter to the semidiameter of the $\frac{1}{4}$ rupee, and in length equal to one inch and eight-tenths, which measure is one fluid drachm, or sixty minims; of these fluid drachms there are eight in one ounce.

A fluid drachm of pure water at 76° Fahr. weighs fifty-eight troy grains.

The minim, is expressed by the mark ♏.

As liquids expand and contract by changes of temperature and atmospheric pressure, the bulks of the preceding measures are estimated at the standard of 62° of Fahrenheit's thermometer and 30° barometer. All measuring vessels should be graduated at such seasons as permit these circumstances to be observed.

The cubical inch of distilled water at this temperature weighs 252·458 grs.

The diameter of the new rupee is 1·20 English inch, or if divided into 12 equal parts, each is $\frac{1}{10}$th of an inch.

The diameter of the silver quarter rupee is $\frac{7}{8}$ of an inch.

The diameter of the new copper pice is precisely an English inch.

The preceding measures are best made of glass, silver, or pure tin. A uniform tube of the necessary dimensions is easily prepared by hammering the silver or tin round an iron rod of the required size. The tube should be soldered on the outside, and closed below by a perfectly flat piece also soldered from the outside.

For the construction of weights we recommend silver or pure tin, beat out into uniform thin plates; brass or copper rusts rapidly, and weights made of these metals soon become deceptive. A set of weights should comprise the rupee or tola, half and quarter rupee, a drachm, a half drachm, a scruple, a half scruple, and a series of small weights from six grains to half a grain. The pharmaceutical character, and the number, should be stamped on each weight.

For quantities above the tola weight, it is sufficient to recollect that the Troy pound contains 96 drachms, equal to 32 of the Company's new rupees.*

* For a table of Indian Weights and Measures, see the Appendix.

PHARMACEUTICAL MANIPULATIONS.

§ 1. WEIGHING.

The instrument used to shew the weight of a body is called a Balance. That in general use is formed of a beam, or solid inflexible bar, placed horizontally; to the extremities of this are attached strings or wires, supporting the pans or scales. The beam is supported by suspension from its centre on a prop.

If the pans be equally loaded, and the balance well constructed, neither preponderates; but if there be a greater quantity of matter in either pan, this inclines towards the earth.

Weighing is a simple application of the principle of the lever—the beam is the lever; both arms should be of equal length; the point of suspension is the fulcrum; the weight in one pan the resistance, the substance in the opposite pan, the power. Were one arm double the length of the other, half the quantity of matter would be sufficient to produce equilibrium with the resistance of the weight on the short arm. The Chinese first applied this principle to their balances, and they make one weight counterbalance various proportions of matter.

Spiral springs are also used for ascertaining weight, either by the elongation they experience on a body being suspended to them, or the degree of their compression when the body is placed upon them.

The practical apothecary should be provided with at least two balances, one for large, one for small, weighments.

The larger balance should be sufficiently delicate to be turned by ten grains, the smaller by half of one grain.

Brass pans may be generally adopted, but for cleanliness we recommend each pan to be provided with a slip of talc or window glass, one or two inches square, on which powders and other substances should be weighed. Care must be taken to adjust the talc or glasses so as to be of equal weight.

The pans or glasses must be most attentively cleaned after each weighment.

A balance is proved to be in good order by weighing a substance in one pan against its exact counterpoise in the other, and then changing these from one pan to the other. When the scales remain in equilibriô the balance is good; if not, the balance cannot be used until the fault is discovered and rectified. For the purposes of the practical druggist a balance of which one of the arms preponderates may be corrected by placing a small quantity of sand, shot, or other such substance, in the pan of the opposite arm till equilibrium is restored.

The centre of gravity of a balance must be always placed below its axis of suspension. The centre of gravity is the point of the balance through which the resultant of the weight of its elements passes, and on which the attraction of the earth is concentrated.

Unless the centre of gravity be in the same vertical line with the axis of suspension, the arms of the beam cannot be in equilibrium.

If the centre of gravity coincides with the point of suspension, the arms will remain in whatever position they may be placed.

If the centre of gravity be above the point of suspension, the balance is what the French expressively call "folle," or giddy. In such a balance the slightest additional weight in either scale causes it to set or to fall rapidly and give erroneous indications.

When the centre of gravity is below the axis of suspension and in the same vertical line, the arms oscillate like the pendulum when disturbed from the horizontal position.

The nearer the centre of gravity is to the axis of suspension, the more delicate the balance becomes, but the slower are its oscillations. In Kater's balance, and several others, the centre of gravity can be made to vary by a ball and screw.

The centre of gravity of a small solid body is easily found by suspending it freely from a cord, and drawing a line through the body in continuation of its line of suspension.

The centre of gravity is somewhere in this line.

Suspend the body freely once more from any other point, and again prolong the line of suspension; the centre of gravity is where the two lines intersect.

§ 2. MECHANICAL OPERATIONS.

These are chiefly pulverizing or powdering, trituration or rubbing, bruising, rasping, grinding, filtering, washing, and expression.

Pulverization.

Powdering may be performed by the mill, the pestle and mortar, the slab and muller, or by heat.

Hard seeds, barks, roots, &c. are best reduced to powder in the mill, as cubeb seeds, rhubarb root, the seed of the kaladana, the kernel of the kutkulegi, &c. Very oily seeds, such as the til-seed, mustard seed, the ground-nut, and others, are beaten in a mortar, and the oil expressed before they can be readily powdered.* The kuchila-nut (nux vomica) should be rasped with a coarse file, or heated in contact with steam, and then bruised.

Mortars may be of iron, steel, brass, agate, wood, porcelain, glass, marble, stone, or earthenware. The white mortars from England are called Wedgewood, from the name of their inventor, and are of great utility, being very strong and but little acted upon by chemical agents.

In *Plate* 1, *fig.* 1, is shewn a mortar *a*, with its *pestle* or bruiser, *b*. This shape is preferable to that of the mortars generally used.

Mercurial preparations must not be made in metal mortars; acids must be mixed in glass or porcelain vessels; many of the metallic salts, such as those of copper, are decomposed by the contact of iron; stone, earthen, or marble mortars must be used in such cases.

Porphyrization.

This term is applied to the process of powdering by means of a slab of very hard stone, such as porphyry or corundum, on which a heavy cone of the same material, called a *muller*, is moved about.

The glass of antimony, sulphuret of antimony, calomel, tartar emetic, and sulphate of potash, are thus reduced to fine powder, called *impalpable*, because its separate particles are not evident to the touch.

Levigation and Elutriation.

This consists in agitating a powder in water; the heavy coarse grains speedily subside, the finer remain buoyed up by the fluid, and may be poured off to another vessel in which they slowly settle. Powdered chalk, sulphuret of antimony, and vermillion are thus treated (see the section on *Washing*.)

The process is inapplicable to substances soluble in water.

Intermediate Pulverization.

This term is applied to the following processes:—

Melted phosphorus stirred under water or spirit, cools into a fine powder.

Calomel vapor sublimed in contact with steam—sulphur sublimed and its vapor suddenly cooled.

Precipitation by chemical interchange of elements, as in the formation of precipitated chalk from nitrate of lime by carbonate of soda.

Colocynth pulp if mixed with a solution of gum tragacanth, and the mixture dried, is then readily powdered.

Camphor is powdered by the addition of a little alcohol.

Vanilla is mixed with sugar—and the emulsive seeds, such as almonds, or ground-nuts, are also thus easily powdered.

The ductile metals (gold, silver, tin) may be powdered by triturating the leaf metal with honey, salt, or sugar, and then washing with boiling water.

Tin and zinc are readily powdered by pouring the melted metal into a wooden box rubbed on the inside with chalk, and agitating the box briskly till the metal solidifies. Zinc may also be powdered by pouring it while fluid into a hot iron mortar, and stirring it with a hot iron rod till cool. All these metallic powders are then sifted through silk.

Substances to be powdered must generally be perfectly dried, especially if organic tissues, because while moist they are soft, elastic, and ductile.

If of compact tissue, such as jalap, colombo, orris root and turmeric, they are first dried before the sun, or in a stove, and then bruised, or pounded. If of ligneous structure, such as guaiacum, sassafras root, quassia, or sandal, they are rasped. If very fibrous, such as liquorice, sarsaparilla, or hemidesmus, they are sliced by a knife, or chopped small with a hatchet.

To separate earthy matters, roots are well shaken, brushed, or sometimes washed.

Salep is steeped in cold water for twelve hours, then peeled and stove-dried—its horny consistence is thus softened. Nux vomica seeds and St. Ignatius' bean are first exposed to steam, and then rasped or ground.

During powdering it is necessary to guard against the escape of dust, which will either cause loss, or prove prejudicial to the operator, as would occur with cantharides, euphorbium, nux-vomica bark, viscum leaf, jalap, ipecacuanha, aconite, &c. A cone of leather should in these cases be tied by the base to the mortar, its apex tied round the pestle *(see Plate* 1, *fig.* 2*)*.

In powdering leaves and roots, the woody parts are the last to yield, and are generally rejected.

Sifting,

or the separating of solid particles of different sizes, is effected by means of sieves, or vessels with bottoms perforated with holes of particular sizes, or fitted with wire cloth with apertures of different dimensions—or lined with calico, muslin, cloth, or silk.

Making of Pills.

Pills are small globular masses made from materials of a soft ductile consistence. The weight should not exceed five grains each.

The materials for pills are kneaded into a consistent mass with a broad knife called a spatula, on a slab of porcelain or stone. The mass is rolled into a cylindrical shape, and subdivided according to the weight desired.

A machine is sometimes employed for this subdivision, but its use leads to inaccurate doses of medicines, and ought to be discouraged, at least among retail druggists.

Pills are sometimes coated with silver, gold, or tin foil. This is accomplished by moistening the pill with a strong solution of gum, placing the foil in a large pill box, dropping in the pills, and shaking all well together.

Pills are generally covered with magnesia, or very finely powdered liquorice; a portion of these powders should be placed in the box with each pill; the object of the process is to render the pills less adhesive to each other, to the mouth and throat, and less disagreeable to the taste.

Filtration and Expression.

Solids are separated from fluids by filtration, decantation, by the use of the syphon, and by pressure.

Filtration means the passage of the fluid through some porous material which arrests the solid matters.

Filters are made of paper, cloth, cotton, or wool, either raw or woven, of porous earthenware, sand, or powdered glass.

For delicate experiments Serampore white paper unsized and well washed is to be used (for instance in testing saltpetre and separating the silver precipitate); where the deposit is bulky the paper made in Nipal is the best substance, as it is very strong, and allows rapid filtration and subsequent expression.

The paper should be cut square *(a)*, then folded in a triangle *(b)*, this repeated *(c)*, and lastly it is to be opened so that three folds of paper may be at one side, and but one fold at the opposite side *(d)*. The dotted line at *c* shews the course followed in cutting off the corners of the filter so as to make it circular. *(Plate 1, figs. 3, 4, 5, 6)*.

The paper filter is supported in a funnel *(fig. 7)*, a conical vessel of glass, porcelain, or tinned iron, ending in a tube.

A slip of wood or a glass rod is very advantageously placed between the paper and the funnel, by which means the filtration takes place with great rapidity. *(fig. 8)*.

Sometimes with small quantities of liquids the funnel may be dispensed with, a small cone of paper placed on a narrow test glass with a slender rod of wood or glass intervening, being found sufficient. *(fig. 9)*.

More complicated forms are recommended for filters in chemical researches and delicate experiments, but in practical pharmacy the simple filter above described is quite sufficient for all occasions in which paper is available.

Cloth filters (of calico, flannel, or other woollen fabric) are often very useful, especially in vegetable analysis, and in numerous processes in pharmacy. These filters are stretched on a frame, and by proper management the same cloth may be very frequently used. An illustration of the use of cloth filters will be found under the head of Anarcotine.

Woollen filters are used for syrups and jellies; they are made of flannel cloth, and are usually sewed up in the form of a cone.

The orifice is strengthened by a wooden collar.

In filtering through woollen fabrics, alkalies must be carefully avoided, as they corrode the cloth.

Essential oils are filtered through a funnel having the throat slightly obstructed with a little loose raw cotton.

Water for drinking is frequently filtered through porous sandstone or earthenware. Mechanical or solid impurities remain on the upper surface of the stone, which must be carefully cleaned from time to time; but the finer particles entering the interstices of the stone so soon obstruct it as to deprive it of value.

Pounded charcoal is very much employed. Besides being a good mechanical separator, it acts chemically upon numerous liquids, which it bleaches, or frees from unpleasant odours. Calcined animal matters afford the best charcoal for this purpose, and the finer the state of division of its particles, the greater will be the bleaching or disinfecting power.

Filtration through sand or broken glass is practised with some strongly corrosive liquids, such as the mineral acids. The throat of the funnel is first loosely obstructed with a pebble or piece of thick glass, smaller pieces are then added layer by layer, and the powdered glass or sand on the surface.

Before use the sand-filter must be washed with strong muriatic acid and the acid subsequently removed by water.

Filtration, may be accelerated by particular contrivances.

Thus in Mawe's filter (so called from the maker's name) the funnel is placed over a vessel which can be deprived of its air by a pump. On thus exhausting the lower vessel, the surface of the liquid is pressed on by the atmosphere with a force equal to 15lbs. on each superficial inch, and the rapidity of filtration is proportionally increased. (*Plate* 1, *fig*. 10.)

In filtering some solutions it is necessary to exclude atmospherical air—for example, with solutions of caustic, potash, soda, or lime. Dr. Andrew Duncan contrived for this purpose a very simple and effectual apparatus.

This consists of a funnel with the wide end ground so as to fit exactly to a plate of glass, a tube ½ an inch in diameter is introduced into the axis of the funnel, leaving a space about ¼ of an inch all round. This space is obstructed by fragments of glass and coarse sand, and the whole is then inserted into the neck of a common bottle, and secured air-tight by a cork. (*Fig.* 11.)

Here as the fluid filters through the sand the air it displaces rises through the central tube, so that the materials come in contact only with the quantity of air contained originally in the apparatus.

Riouffe's apparatus consists of a funnel with an air-tight lid and a bent tube, fitting into a glass, earthenware, or metallic, vessel, provided with two necks. From the lateral neck a bent tube proceeds and enters the lid of the funnel. A stop-cock below permits the fluid to be drawn off at pleasure. This apparatus is especially useful in filtering etherial and alcoholic solutions, as it prevents great waste by the evaporation of these valuable liquids.

For large operations two barrels may be easily adjusted to each other so as to form an apparatus of this kind. We recommend such an arrangement, for example, in the manufacture of Anarcotine.

See fig. 12.—*a* and *b* are two barrels placed one above the other, and connected by the central pipe *d* and lateral pipe *e*;—*f* shews a replenishing funnel with stop-cock, and *g* a cloth filter in the upper barrel supported on a circular wooden ledge.

In the section on the Pharmaceutical operation of making tinctures, the new and valuable mode of filtering by *displacement* is described.

Washing.

Washing, or *edulcoration*, is a very useful mechanical process.

Mixtures of solids and liquids may be separated to a great degree by the modes previously described, but the solid on the filter always contains in its interstices a quantity of the original fluid.

Where pressure can be employed, this is the best mode of forcing out the fluid from the kind of sponge in which it is retained, but pressure in the majority of cases cannot be used, and washing is then had recourse to.

Washing may be performed with water, or spirits, or other

solvents, according to circumstances, varying in each case. The fluid employed may also be at different temperatures.

In edulcoration, washing is performed without the use of a filter. The solid substance to be washed is agitated by means of a glass, earthenware, or wooden rod, in a vessel with a narrow orifice and wide bottom; on ceasing the agitation the solid particles subside, and the fluid may be removed in various ways—

a. By the sucking tube, (only fit for small operations.)

b. By the syphon (see that head.)

c. Through an opening in the side of the vessel above the layer of solid matter.

d. By a vessel with a bent tube proceeding from below upwards. *(Fig. 13.)*

To wash a precipitate or deposit on a filter with a cold fluid, there are several contrivances:—

a. The dropping tube or pipette. This is a long slender tube, with a bulb in the middle, and open at each end. *(Fig. 14.)*

It is filled by sucking into it with the mouth, then closed by the lip or fore-finger. By removing the finger the fluid gushes out in a full stream, and may be directed against the object to be washed, so as most effectually to separate all the soluble parts.

b. The washing funnel. This is simply a funnel with the throat obstructed by a piece of paper or clean cloth, so as to permit a frequent dropping of the fluid from above. These drops are permitted to fall from some height on the deposit to be washed. *(Fig. 15.)*

c. The washing bottle. A very simple and effective contrivance. A flask of common bazar shape, with a flat bottom, is fitted with a perforated cork into which a glass tube or jet is introduced. *(Fig. 16, 17.)*

By blowing into the tube the air inside is condensed, and on inverting the bottle a stream of fluid flows out for a considerable time; or the fluid may be brought to boil by holding the bottle over a lamp, and then by inverting it, it may be used as before without breathing into the bottle. A ring of thick worsted cloth, or a wooden handle, is adjusted to the neck of the bottle when the contents are to be warmed, to permit of its being handled without inconvenience.

In acting on very small quantities of materials, superfluous fluids may be removed by touching the edge of the mixture with a roll of filtering paper. The fluid rises in this by capillary attraction. By tearing off the moistened parts more may be removed, till nothing but the dry substance remains.

In washing precipitates it is more economical and speedy

of execution, to divide the total quantity of fluid into several parts, than to use the whole at once. In washing saltpetre earth in the manufacture of *nitre*, this process is very advantageously resorted to.

To economise the labour of constantly renewing the liquid several self-regulating pieces of apparatus have been contrived :—

a. The syphon washer. (For a description of this syphon see the section on "*Atmospheric pressure*.")

This maintains the same level of liquid constantly in the funnel.

b. The German washing tube. (*Fig.* 18.)

A tube of this form is inserted by a cork through which the end *c* passes into a flask nearly filled with water, and inverted. No water escapes from *a*, the capillary resistance of the opening being greater than the difference between the gravitating force of the water and the pressure of the atmosphere. By immersing *a* in a fluid on a filter, for example, the capillary resistance is overcome, and if the level *a* subsides, fresh water issues from the tube to preserve the level constant, bubbles of air being admitted through *b* as the air in the flask becomes rarified by the escape of water from within.

Expression.

This operation is very often had recourse to in Pharmacy—as in the expression of the juice of lemons; of various precipitates, such as Anarcotine; and of oil seeds of different kinds, &c.

The screw press is so well known all over India that there is no need of describing it. We insert in the Appendix an account of a very efficient apparatus, described in Hebert's Cyclopedia. We use it in experiments on oil seeds, and find it very powerful, cheap, and convenient. (*See Hebert's Cyclopedia*, vol. ii. p. 322—4.)

Under the section on Heat, a description will be found of the *supports* which we recommend for funnels, and other pieces of apparatus which require to be held in particular positions.

§ 3—SPECIFIC GRAVITY.

By the *specific gravity* of a solid or liquid is meant the comparative weight of an equal bulk of the substance in question, and of distilled water at the same temperature.

By the weight of a body, is meant the result of the force with which it tends to fall towards the centre of the earth, and which can be estimated by the common balance.

If a solid substance be introduced into a liquid it will displace a portion of the liquid exactly equal to its own bulk, and its tendency to fall towards the centre of the earth will be resisted in all directions by a force equal to the weight of the liquid displaced.

If we weigh a heavy solid in air, and afterwards weigh it in water, oil, spirit, acid, or any other liquid, we will find it to lose weight. The loss is the exact weight of its own bulk of the liquid in question.

Thus by weighing a piece of glass in air and then in water, we ascertain the specific gravity of the glass by dividing its weight in air by the weight it has lost in water. And then by weighing the glass successively in spirit, acids, oils, alkaline solutions, or other liquids, we ascertain exactly the different weights of equal bulks of these fluids.

Various instruments are employed to ascertain specific gravities. All act on the principle above described.

The Hydrostatic Balance,

is a pair of scales, one of which is arranged so that it can play over a vessel containing water; this scale is provided with a hook by which the substance under examination can be suspended. *(Fig. 19.)*

The substance is first weighed in air, its weight noted, then it is placed in water and weights removed from the opposite scale till the balance is restored; the loss is the weight of the bulk of water it has displaced. When its weight in air is divided by this, the quotient gives the specific gravity.

Example.

A piece of bell-metal weighed in air,...	...	2815 grains.
——————————— in water,	...	2500
Loss,		315

being the weight of the same bulk of water as the piece of metal.

As 315 : 2,815 : 1,000 = 8,936.

If the substance be lighter than water, for example, cork or wood, it is to be attached to a piece of glass or metal heavy enough to sink it. Each is to be previously weighed separately in air, then the specific gravity of the heavy body is to be ascertained; finally, both are to be weighed together in water. The difference between the loss of weight of the bodies when weighed together, and of the loss of weight of the heavy body separately weighed in water, shews the weight of the bulk of water equal to the lighter body.

Example.

Bell metal, wt. in air, ...	2815 grains.
Cork	47
Total,	2,862
Both in water,...	2,158
Loss,	704

704 being equal to wt. of water equal to the bulk of both. Deduct 315 the bulk of water, equal to metal, ... 704
... ... 315

The weight of water equal in bulk to the cork, is therefore ... ... } 389

As 389 : 47 : 1000 = 0,121

A very convenient instrument for ascertaining the specific gravities of solids of small size, is a glass tube graduated into 100ths of a cubical inch.

First, weigh the tube, then introduce half a cubic inch of water, then introduce the solid to be examined, and note the increase of weight, and the parts of a cubic inch of water displaced.

The weight of the water displaced divided into the weight of the solid body, gives the specific gravity.

Hydrometer and Gravimeter.

These instruments are constructed of metal or glass, and are so adjusted as to sink to a certain depth in liquids of particular density. They are comparatively limited in their scale of indications, and hence separate instruments are used for almost every variety of fluid.

Under the head of alcohol, the excise or abkaree hydrometer will be described in due detail.

The hydrometer acts by displacement of the fluid—the lighter the fluid is, the deeper the instrument sinks. It should be remembered, that the hydrometer sinks to that point precisely at which the weight of the fluid displaced is equal to that of the whole instrument, of the part immersed as well as of that above the fluid. Thus, if the hydrometer in air weigh 1000 grains, it will sink in distilled water till 1000 grains of water shall be displaced. This may be proved experimentally by means of a jar graduated into cubical inches. Weigh the hydrometer, then observe the bulk of inches of water displaced, and they will be found to correspond exactly.

An instrument on this principle is much used by chemists for ascertaining the specific gravity, and thereby the strength, of the mineral acids. The instrument consists of two similar tubes, one graduated from 1000 to 1500, and the second from 1501 to 1850. The degree to which the stem sinks (and which is marked off on a scale enclosed in the stem) indicates exactly the density and strength of the acid. *(Fig. 20.)*

The *specific gravity* bottle however is the simplest and best of all contrivances to ascertain the density of liquids.

Take a phial with a narrow neck, and ascertain its weight exactly. Then weigh into it any quantity of distilled water (at 62° of Fahrenheit's thermometer), say 100, 500, or 1000 grains, and mark the level of the liquid exactly. To ascertain the specific gravity of any other fluid, clean and dry the phial, and fill it with the liquid to the same level. The result shews at once the relative weights of equal bulks of the two liquids.

Thus, if the phial contains 1000 grains of distilled water, it will hold 1850 grains of concentrated sulphuric acid, and 835 of alcohol of the standard pharmaceutical strength.

Beads or bulbs of glass have been made and so adjusted as to shew the density of a fluid by their sinking or floating. If too heavy, they sink. If too light, they float on the surface. If of the same density, the bead remains wherever placed in the fluid. A number engraved on the stem of the bead shews the specific gravity compared with that of water.

The beads are of the size shewn in *fig.* 21, and their relative positions in experiments are indicated in *fig.* 22.

Many other modes of ascertaining specific gravities have been described and recommended. The balance and specific-gravity bottle, however, are the only instruments which the practical apothecary absolutely requires.

ATMOSPHERICAL CIRCUMSTANCES INFLUENCING PHARMACEUTICAL OPERATIONS.

There are several circumstances connected with the state of the atmosphere, a knowledge of which is essential to the proper management of numerous pharmaceutical processes. The density, temperature, and state of dryness of the air, chiefly demand attention.

§ 1. PRESSURE OF THE ATMOSPHERE.

This is a subject which we deem of much importance to the practical pharmaceutical chemist, and we wish to place it before him in the plainest possible light.

The air we breathe, and which surrounds this globe, is possessed of weight. This we prove by weighing a flask full of air, and then by pumping out the air we observe a loss of weight which is restored on re-admission of the air. Accurate experiments fix the weight of 100 cubic inches of air at the level of the sea, and at the freezing point of water, to be 31·0117 grains.

Astronomical observations further shew that the atmosphere of this earth is between 45 and 50 miles in height. Since all matter, in obedience to the attraction of gravitation, presses towards the centre of the earth, the pressure of the atmosphere on the surface of the globe is so great as to give rise to many most important circumstances, the nature of which has only been revealed since the discoveries made by Galileo in the year 1640 of the Christian era.

This pressure is proved, by conclusive experiments, to be equal to nearly 15 pounds on each superficial inch at the level of the sea. We are not sensible, by ordinary observation, of the existence of the pressure even on the surface of our bodies, because the solid and fluid matters contained therein are pressed on equally on all sides, and by their elasticity or natural firmness counteract, without effort, the weight of the load of air; but if this resistance be in any way removed, the pressure of the air becomes immediately obvious.

As our knowledge of the phenomena of evaporation, boiling, and distilling, the preparation of extracts, the action of pumps, syringes, cupping glasses, and syphons, the management of airs and gases, and several very important modifications of pharmaceutical operations at different elevations—depends on correct ideas of this subject, we deem it necessary to explain it at some length.

The Air-Pump.

The nature and effects of atmospheric pressure are rendered most obvious by the instrument called the air-pump.

The essential part of the air-pump is a cylinder fitted with a piston, and closed at one end, the closed end being provided with a valve which opens inwards. In the piston is a valve opening in the same direction. *(Fig. 23.)*

When the piston rod is drawn up, the lower valve is opened, air enters, while the upper valve closes and prevents the entrance of air from above.

If the piston be depressed the lower valve is shut, while any air between it and the piston is forced upwards through the upper valve, and escapes through the open end of the cylinder.

In the air-pump two such cylinders are connected, and the pistons worked by a cogged wheel playing in teeth cut in the piston rods. *(Fig. 24.)*

A tube leads from each cylinder to a connecting pipe, terminating in a broad brass plate, carefully ground and polished. On this plate are placed glasses, jars, and other articles for experiment.

By this pump the air-may be very nearly removed from the glass vessel, which can be exhausted so as not to retain more than $\frac{1}{100}$th part of its original volume of air.

We can with this instrument prove the pressure of the atmosphere by many experiments.

If we place a glass cylinder with open neck on the plate, and cover the neck with the palm of the hand, on pumping the air from beneath, we find that the hand is pressed down so forcibly that it cannot be withdrawn.

If a membrane be tightly tied on the aperture, on removing the air from beneath the membrane, it is pressed down until it bursts.

This shews what takes place with the cupping glasses of the surgeon.

The cupping glass is a small glass vessel with a wide mouth, into the neck of which a brass syringe is screwed for the purpose of exhausting the air. On placing the mouth of the glass on the body and drawing up the rod, the glass will adhere forcibly, and by pumping for some time a large swelling of the part takes place. *(Fig. 25.)*

Or, without a syringe, the air may be expanded in a common glass by introducing within it a match of cotton dipped in spirits and lighted. By dexterously placing the mouth of the glass on the part, the same phenomena are observed on the cooling and contraction of the air, as were described in speaking of the more complicated syringe apparatus.

The cupping glass is used to draw blood to any part from which it is desirable to remove that fluid—to prevent the absorption of snake and other poisons from wounds,—to draw milk from the breasts,—and for many other purposes.

The Barometer.

The amount of the pressure of the atmosphere differs at different elevations, and may be accurately measured by the length of the column of water or mercury which a pump can lift, or by the instrument termed the barometer.

If a tube, 40 feet vertical length, be immersed in water at its lower extremity, then connected with the plate of the air-pump by its upper aperture, on pumping out the air, water will rise in obedience to the pressure of the atmosphere till it reaches 34 feet, at this height the column of water is of exactly the same weight as that of a column of the entire atmosphere of equal base. The pump can elevate the water no further, because the water is lifted only by the piston of the pump causing a vacuum above the water, and enabling the atmosphere to press on it from beneath.

A column of mercury can be elevated by a pump to a height of 30 inches at the level of the sea, because columns of that metal 30 inches long, of water 34 feet long, and of air the entire depth of the atmosphere, if of equal base, are of the same weight.

Consequently if a glass tube more than 30 inches long, closed at one extremity, be filled with mercury and placed vertically with the open end in a cup containing the same metal, the metal will subside in the tube till it stands at 30 inches—a true vacuum, or empty space, existing above that level.

This tube is termed a Barometer, or measurer of the weight of the atmosphere, and the empty space has been named the Torricellian vacuum, in honour of its discoverer Torricelli.

If the mercurial Barometer be carried down into a deep mine, as it is then pressed on by a deeper and heavier column of air, the mercury stands higher than 30 inches. If it be taken to the top of a lofty building, or a mountain, as the liquid is then pressed on by less of the atmosphere, the mercury sinks, and stands at an elevation exactly proportionate to the height of the place where the experiment is performed.

The following table shews the mean altitude of the Barometer at some remarkable places and elevations.

Places.	Feet in height above the sea level.	Barometer mean.
Level of the sea,...	... 000.00	... 30.00
Calcutta, (*Chandpal ghatá,*)......	... 15	... 29.893
Titalya, ...	... 275	... 29.570
Benares, ...	... 300	... 29.464
Saharunpore, ...	... 1013	... 28.766
Seringapatam, ...	... 2412	... 27.568
Chira Punji, ...	... 5000	... 26.900
Nepal Residency, ...	... 4400	... 25.330
	... 5000	... 24.797
Dargeeling, ...	... 6957	... 23.408
Ootacamund, Nilgiris	... 7221	... 23.054
	... 10,000	... 20.499
2 miles, ...	... .	... 20.290
	... 15,000	... 16.941
3 miles, ...	... .	... 16.680
	... 20,000	... 14.000
4 miles, ...	... .	... 13.720
5 ditto, ...	... .	... 11.280
10 ditto, ...	... .	... 4.240
15 ditto, ...	... .	... 1.600
20 ditto, ...	... .	... 0.950

Thus within 5000 feet the fall of one inch of mercury corresponds nearly to 1000 feet of elevation. Although the barometer is generally employed so as to give the most accurate information as to the altitude of mountains, the working of the problem is attended with many difficulties.

The air is not of the same density at all elevations. As air, in common with all fluids, transmits pressure exactly in all directions, and is moreover very elastic, being pressed on less in the higher regions in proportion to the quantity of the atmosphere below, it diminishes in density as we ascend; thus 100 cubic inches at the level of the sea weigh 31 grains; at about 15,000 feet the mercury in the barometer stands at 15 inches; one half of the atmosphere is thus left below; the air is expanded to twice its bulk at the level of the sea, and consequently 100 cubic inches weigh but 15 grains and a fraction.

Neither does the density of the air diminish in an arithmetical progression. The pressures are inversely as the squares of the distances from the surface of the earth;—for example,

At 15,000 feet the density is,	=	$\frac{1}{2}$
30,000	„	$\frac{1}{4}$
45,000	„	$\frac{1}{8}$
60,000	„	$\frac{1}{16}$

The indication of the barometer has also to be corrected according to the temperature of the air,—the temperature of the mercury,—the quantity of moisture in the air, and the expansion of the glass tube in which the mercury is contained.

The effect of heat in expanding mercury and glass being constant, and accurately known, tables are constructed which at once supply the necessary correction. The data necessary for ascertaining the influence of moisture are supplied by an observation of the dew point.

The barometer, moreover, is known to undergo daily in the same place a variation in its altitude, supposed to depend on the flow and ebb of tides in the atmosphere. Thus in Calcutta, the barometer stands highest at 10 A. M., subsides again until 4 P. M., rises once more till 10 P. M., and again falls until sun-rise.

The mean results of three years' observations give thus—

Sun-rise,	10 A. M.	Noon,	$2\frac{1}{4}$ P. M.	4 P. M.	Sun-set.
29·778,	29·818,	29·783,	29·734,	29·710,	29·727.

In consideration of this fact, it is necessary to record the hour of the day when the observation is made.

To enable us to measure minute fractional differences in the altitude of the barometrical column, a small sliding scale, termed a "vernier", is affixed to the instrument. The inches on the principal scale are subdivided into tenths. The vernier, or moveable scale, is equal to eleven of these, but is divided into 10 parts, each of which is thus equal to eleven-hundredths of an inch, and is respectively one-hundredth of an inch longer than a tenth subdivision of the principal scale.

The vernier is made to slide on the principal scale by a screw. When an observation is made, the top of the vernier should be made level with the mercurial column. It will be found then that some one of the divisions of the principal scale coincides with one on the vernier. Thus, suppose the mercury be at $29\frac{6}{10}$ths and a fraction, and that the scales coincide at 4 of the vernier, the result will be 29·64.

The last precaution to be observed in making a correct barometrical observation is, that the instrument should stand *vertically*. This may be accomplished by suspending it from a hook or frame, or the branch of a tree. Some instruments are provided with a tripod and moveable joints, by which the perpendicular position is assumed by the instrument itself.

Two places of figures are quite sufficient for useful observations.

On each observation being made, if the barometer has to be removed, the mercury should be made to ascend in the tube by gently turning the regulating screw at the base of the frame. This prevents agitation and concussion of the mercury during travelling, and tends much to the preservation of the instrument.

The barometer is much used by navigators in consequence of its, in almost every instance, falling remarkably before the occurrence of storms. Thus during the great gale on the 21st May, 1832, the mercury fell at Saugor from 29·09 at 8 A.M. to 26·30 at 11 A.M. In October, 1838, the day previous to the gale at the Sandheads, during which the melancholy wreck of the "Protector" took place, the mercury fell nearly one inch. The same event has been remarked before earthquakes. The cause of the descent of the column on these occasions is not yet clearly understood.

By careful attention to the directions now given, the apothecaries, for whose instruction this work is drawn up, can make accurate observations of the pressure of the atmosphere, and these, together with a register of the quantity of rain and degree of dryness, kept by instruments subsequently described, should be transmitted annually to the Medical Board, to the Surveyor General's Office, or to the Medical College.

As we proceed with the consideration of the subjects of boiling, distilling, and making extracts, we shall perceive important practical applications of the foregoing principles and experiments.

The Sympiesometer.

This is a very simple, and beautiful instrument, invented by Adie of Edinburgh, and which indicates with great precision the changes in the pressure of the atmosphere. (*Fig.* 25.)

It consists essentially of a tube closed above, and terminating in an open cistern. The cistern is filled with olive oil. The upper part of the tube contains hydrogen gas, which is introduced perfectly dry, and at the temperature of 32° Faht. the freezing point of water, and when the barometer stands at 30 inches.

The gas inclosed within the bulb and part of the tube changes its bulk, or occupies more or less space according to the pressure of the atmosphere upon the surface of the oil.

But the gas also expands or contracts according to change of temperature. In constructing the instrument, the scale of expansion from 32° to 120° is found experimentally, while the pressure indicated by the barometer is constant, and equal to 30 inches.

We are thus enabled to understand how far the expansion or contraction depends upon changes of temperature, and how far on changes of pressure. A thermometer attached to the scale shews the temperature of the air. A sliding scale is adjusted to an engraved table so as when the index is placed at the number expressing the temperature the pressure is read off in inches, tenths, or hundredths, as in the mercurial barometer.

The instrument is very portable, prompt in its indications, and exceedingly accurate when carefully managed. It is highly valued by nautical men, as it gives warning of approaching storms much sooner than the mercurial column.

To use the instrument the inventor gives the following directions.

"Suppose the temperature to be 52·4, slide the scale until the pointer is at 52·4 on the fixed scale at the right hand side. The number on the sliding scale which is on a level with the top of the column of oil shews the pressure in inches and fractions corresponding to the mercurial barometer."

A modification of the instrument has been constructed for measuring heights, and has been found to give very correct indications.

The Baroscope.

This is an instrument recently devised by Mr. Cooper, of London, which indicates atmospheric pressure by the observation of the quantity of water displaced by a given volume of air under a constant temperature. The apparatus is described in the *London and Edinburgh Philosophical Journal for May*, 1839. p. 36.

§ 2. TEMPERATURE OF THE ATMOSPHERE.

The degree of sensible heat of any substance is ascertained by the instrument named the Thermometer, or Measurer of Heat.

The construction of this instrument depends on these facts,—1st, that within certain limits all bodies expand uniformly by equal additions of heat; 2nd, that at the level of the sea, in usual states of the atmosphere, water boils always at the same degree of heat, and a mixture of ice and water also observes a uniform temperature so long as any ice remains unmelted in the mixture.

The thermometer of Fahrenheit is a small glass bulb filled with pure mercury, and connected with a long narrow stem. The mercury being heated totally fills the tube, the end of which is then sealed by fusion. On cooling, the mercury contracts, leaving an empty space or vacuum at the top of the tube; when quite cold the bulb is immersed in a mixture of ice and salt, the mercury sinks in the stem, and when it becomes stationary the point is marked. The bulb is now allowed to regain its natural temperature, and then introduced into water, which is heated till it boils briskly. The level of the expanded mercury is again taken. The first is called zero, and the interval to the point of boiling water is divided into 212° equal parts. At 32° of these parts above zero water freezes.

A better division is from melting ice to boiling water, 180°, because a mixture of ice and salt may become much colder than 0° in extremely cold weather.

Thermometers on the same plan are used to indicate very high temperatures, such as those of boiling oil or mercury. In some of these instruments the stem of the thermometer is left open above.

To denote very low temperatures, thermometers filled with coloured spirit are employed, because spirit cannot be frozen at any temperature we have the means of producing.

In France, the interval between the temperature of freezing and that of boiling water is divided into 100 parts, and the instrument is called "Centigrade." Reaumur's thermometer, still much used on the continent of Europe, reckons only 80 divisions in the same scale. De Lisle's, now obsolete, is divided into 150 parts.

The Register Thermometer

consists of two thermometers, one mercurial, the second of spirit. The stems are placed horizontally. In that of the mercurial thermometer there is contained in advance of the mercury a small piece of iron. As the mercury expands by heat it pushes the iron before it, and on cooling again the iron remains stationary, the end next the mercury thus shewing the maximum temperature attained. In the spirit thermometer a little piece of ivory is substituted for the iron. The spirit on expanding passes by the ivory; but if contraction ensue from cold, as the spirit returns the ivory follows it by adhesive attraction, and thus the minimum temperature is shewn.

The temperature of the atmosphere is ascertained by placing a thermometer in a shady situation free from contact with other bodies.*

To convert the degrees of different scales into each other, the rule of common proportion suffices; thus,—

What is 80 Cent: on Fahrenheit's scale?

As 100 : 180 : : 80 : 144 + 32 = 176—†.

What is 70 Reaumur on the centigrade scale?

R. Cent.

As 80 : 100 : : 70 : 87-5.

The Pyrometer

is an instrument intended for the measurement of very intense degrees of heat, viz. beyond the boiling point of mercury or of oil. The expansion of a bar of platinum or of a globule of air, or the fusion of alloys of gold and silver, or gold and platinum, are severally used for this purpose.

§ 3. TO ASCERTAIN THE DEGREE OF MOISTURE IN THE ATMOSPHERE.—HYGROMETRY.

For this purpose the instruments called Hygrometers, or Measurers of Moisture are employed. The varieties of these contrivances are numerous, and some are very beautiful, especially that invented by Professor Daniell. But for purposes of practical utility, a simpler apparatus is requisite in India.

The hygrometer we recommend, is one of great accuracy and simplicity, and depends on the fact that moisture is deposited in a perceptible ring or dew, on all bodies colder than the atmosphere, when the temperature is reduced to a degree proportionate to the quantity of moisture present.

Thus if a piece of ice, or some saltpetre, or sal-ammoniac, be dissolved in water, in a thin metal cup, gilt and polished, we soon find dew depositing on the cup. If we examine with the thermometer we find during wet weather that the slightest depression of temperature causes the deposit; in dry weather, on the contrary, the thermometer sinks several degrees before the dew is observed. The degree at which the mercury stands at this moment is called the "dew point," and from the difference between this point and the temperature of the atmosphere, with the aid of Daniell's tables, the degree of moisture of the air is calculated. These tables are given in the Appendix.

* For valuable tables of the mean temperature of the seasons, we are indebted to Dr. Wise of Calcutta; the tables are inserted in the Appendix.

† 32 degrees are added here because Fahrenheit's scale commences 32 degrees below the freezing point of water from which the Centigrade begins.

Daniell's Hygrometer.

This very elegant instrument (of which we give a cut, copied from that in *Graham's Elements of Chemistry*, p. 81) consists of a tube bent at two right angles, having a bulb at each end, and containing a little ether in contact with etherial vapour, all the air having been expelled from the tube during its construction before its being sealed. In the long leg a small thermometer is contained. (*Fig.* 26.)

Use.—Incline the instrument until all the ether flows into the bulb of the long leg, then drop sulphuric ether on, or apply ice to the bulb *a*. The vapour within is thereby condensed, and the ether in the first bulb evaporates rapidly, causing great cold. The thermometer in the tube sinks very quickly, and as soon as it reaches the dew point, a ring of moisture is observed to form on the bulb *b*. The temperature indicated at that moment by the included thermometer is the dew point, and the difference between this and the temperature of the air, shewn by the thermometer on the brass pillar, gives the data required for using the tables quoted in the Appendix.

Saussure's Hygrometer.

This instrument consists of a hair, perfectly dried and connected with an index. Hair, wool, and similar bodies, readily attract moisture, and thereby lengthen, contracting again on drying. The change of the length of the hair thus serves as a measure of the moisture of the atmosphere. In very practiced hands this instrument affords valuable results, but it is not calculated for general use.

Leslie's Hygrometer

consists of his differential thermometer, one bulb of which is kept constantly moistened with water, the evaporation of which causing cold, and consequent contraction of the air in the bulb, the ascent of the liquid indicates the degree of moisture of the atmosphere. Dr. Butter, of the Bengal Medical Service, has pointed out a remarkable error in the graduation of this instrument, by which it is rendered unfit for the accurate determination of the air's dryness. The error is in the use of the arithmetical instead of the geometrical division of the scale. Thus 140° of Fahrenheit is laid down instead of 128°.*

* Butter's Outlines of the Topography, and Statistics of Oude, p. 16.

The wet-bulb Hygrometer

more commonly used, consists of two mercurial thermometers (*fig.* 27,) the bulb of one of which, *a*, is kept constantly moistened with water, the bulb of the other, *b*, remaining dry. If the air is saturated with moisture no depression occurs in *a*. The less moisture the air contains, the more rapid will be the evaporation, and the greater the depression in *a*. The difference between the temperature indicated by the stationary depression and that by the other thermometer, affords the elements for calculating the desired result.

On the Rain-gauge, or Pluviometer.

The quantity of rain which falls at different seasons, is an important feature in the history of various climates, and bears so strongly on the health of the population, that all those who have the opportunity should make and record their observations on the subject.

To construct a pluviometer for practical use, take a funnel of tin plate, copper, or glass—measure its diameter, take half of this as the radius in inches, and multiply by 3·1416.

The result is the superficial measurement of the area of the funnel in inches, and decimals.

Multiply this by 252·458, the weight in grains of a cubic inch of distilled water at 62°, the product gives the weight of water corresponding to one inch in depth of the area of the funnel.

Weigh this quantity of water into the receiving glass vessel, and having levelled this by the spirit level, mark the level on the vessel with a file on three different points. Repeat the operation for each inch the vessel will contain.

Fractional parts of an inch may most readily be ascertained by weighing the receiving vessel.

A correction may be applied, according to the temperature of the water, to reduce it to inches at 62°. But as the total increase of volume of water, when heated from zero to 212° is no more than 0·012th, this may be safely neglected in practice.

Prinsep's Evaporometer.

Mr. James Prinsep's instrument consists of a tube provided with an open cup, and fitted with a sliding rod and piston. The ratios of the area of the basin and length of the tube may be such, that each degree on the latter may equal ·01, or ·001 inch depth of evaporation from the former.

The instrument is charged by drawing the piston rod down to zero, and filling the tube with distilled water to a mark in the narrow neck at top. The water is then passed upwards into the cup, and the diminution ascertained by drawing down the piston until the neck level is adjusted, and reading off the degrees as marked by the piston's upper edge.

To graduate the tubes used in the construction of these instruments, a cubical inch measure is supplied by taking a glass tube containing 252·458 grains weight of water cooled to 62° of Fahrenheit's thermometer.

With a diamond, crystal of corundum, or a file, we mark on the tube the fractions of the cubical inch, ascertained by the requisite proportions of water.

We would propose to modify Mr. Prinsep's apparatus by taking a circular metallic vessel of one inch in depth, ascertaining its area, and its weight when nearly filled with water. The loss of weight in a given time divided by the area, shows the evaporation per superficial inch.

APPLICATION AND MANAGEMENT OF HEAT.

Under this head we propose to give such instructions only as are practically required by the preparer or manufacturer of medicinal products.

Heat may be communicated in various modes.

SOLAR HEAT.

The heat of the sun may be very economically and readily applied in this country so as to effect drying, crystallization, concentration of extracts, nay, even boiling, as we will subsequently point out.

The sun's rays are capable of elevating the temperature of liquid or solid objects to 170° of Fahrenheit's thermometer.

At the Ishapore Government Powder Works the gunpowder is dried by exposure to the sun, on terraces. In November, 1838, it was ascertained by the editor that the temperature of the powder was 135°.

Vast quantities of salt are annually prepared near Calcutta, at the Bengal Salt Works, by evaporating brine on brickwork terraces. The temperature of the brine rises as high as 117° Fahr.

Sulphate of soda, carbonate of soda, and saltpetre, are frequently crystallized in the same manner.

A very fine and efficient extract of Hyosciamus is prepared at Agra by solar evaporation, according to a process contrived by Mr. Superintending Surgeon Ludlow, and now introduced into this Pharmacopœia.

A mode of distillation of water, spirits, &c. by solar heat, aided by a barometric vacuum, has been successfully adopted by the editor, and is noticed under the head of distillation.

FUEL.

Of the various kinds of fuel used by the chemist, we may specify,

Coal and oil gas.
Spirit.
Oil, tallow, and wax.
Charcoal, and wood.
Coal, and coke.

Coal and Oil Gases.

These gases, which consist of carburets of hydrogen in various states of admixture, are easily prepared on a small scale, and are strongly recommended to the practical apothecary. Coal gas, however, contains sulphuretted hydrogen, a very deleterious substance, from which it requires to be carefully purified. Oil gas is preferable in this country, on account of the great cheapness of the material from which it is made; it also gives more light and heat, and containing no sulphur, does not require purification.

We subjoin a description of the oil gas apparatus at the Medical College.

This apparatus consists of, 1 an iron retort, in which the oil is decomposed; 2, a reservoir for supplying fresh quantities of oil; 3, a furnace in which the retort is heated; 4, a delivering pipe; 5, the gasometer; 6, pipes by which the gas is distributed; and, lastly, the jets in which it is burned.

Retort. The retort consists of an iron bottle (one of those in which mercury is imported) 12 inches long, by 5 in diameter, and having the usual orifice firmly closed by a screw, as shewn in the drawing. (*Plate 2, fig.* 28).

Into the upper surface of this bottle two gun-barrels are firmly welded, one being five inches shorter than the other.

The latter barrel has the end recurved, as shewn in the drawing, where the feeding cistern is also represented. This cistern is a box of sheet iron, twelve inches square and six deep, air tight. The gun-barrels perforate it from below. Two apertures also exist above, one for a funnel with stopcock, by which oil is poured in, the second for the delivery pipe, by which the gas is permitted to escape.

The furnace is built of common bricks lined with firebricks, the fire-place being nearly of the shape of the retort, but six inches distant from it in every direction. In the College laboratory it is connected with a very tall chimney, but ten feet of chimney are amply sufficient.

The *retort* is prepared by introducing some pieces of broken bricks or tiles, in order to extend the hot surface on which the oil is to drop. The reservoir is charged with oil (of castor, poppy, or sesamum) so as to be about two inches above the level of the orifice of the bent gun-barrel.

When the retort is at a low red heat, oil is allowed to drop in very gently by turning the cock in the gun-barrel. The gas produced rises through the bent tube, and any undecomposed oil reunites with the oil in the reservoir, the gas thus undergoing the only purification it requires. It now passes freely to the gasometer along the delivering tube.

The gasometer is a hollow vessel of sheet iron, well rivetted and varnished, 4 feet long, by 4 broad and 4 deep, being thus equal to 64 cubic feet. The gasometer is suspended on a frame by a chain and weight of 100 lbs. in a masonry tank of corresponding dimensions filled with water, and provided with pipes, as seen in the drawing, *fig*. 29.

When the gasometer is filled, the cock is closed in the tube between it and the furnace; on opening the cock in the delivering tube, the gas passes freely along the branch tubes to the burners.

The burners are either single, rose-head, or circular, or formed of pieces of wire gauze; each burner fits by a screw on a stop-cock, by turning which the consumption of gas is regulated.

The single jet is used where a concentrated flame is required; the rose-burner, *b*, for heating small crucibles; the concentric, *c c*, for boiling. The best mode of using gas for boiling, however, is by allowing it to enter a small chamber from the branch tube, the chamber being covered with a piece of wire gauze; on kindling the gas it burns with a diffused, equable, but very powerful flame.

Spirit.

Alcohol rectified to the density of 835 affords excellent materials for applying heat in all small operations. The spirit burns without smoke, and with a pale flame, and may be made to give heat sufficient even for the fusion of fine platinum wire.

Spirit Lamps.

In *fig*. 30 are shewn, 1, the ordinary glass spirit lamp; 2, a substitute, very easily constructed with a common stoppered phial, a brass burner, and cotton wick. When the lamp is not in use, the burner is taken out, the wick pressed dry, and both placed in a small box.

Prout's spirit lamp for heating long tubes is shewn in *fig.* 31.

It consists of two brass reservoirs capable of holding about two ounces of spirit, and connected by a brass tube provided with tube burners, as shewn in the drawing.

The *circular wick spirit lamp* of brass, for fusing salts in small crucibles, and other operations in which a very high temperature is required, is shewn in the drawing, *fig.* 32; the description in the note is taken from *Griffin's Chemical Recreations*, pp. 19, 20*.

Oil Lamps.

The lamp with circular wick, if supplied with oil instead of spirit affords a very ready, convenient, and manageable source of heat for pharmaceutical operations.

Furnaces.

The variety of furnaces is very great, but for pharmaceutical purposes, the following will be found best suited.

The Draught, or Melting Furnace.

The body of the furnace is built of masonry lined with fire-brick. The walls are 14 inches thick. The hollow space of square shape, 48 inches deep, 18 inches square. A grate, of square ¾ inch iron bars, with an angle upwards, and half inch interval, is placed 28 inches from the top of the furnace. It is supported on strong hinges built into the back wall, and by a moveable bar which can be withdrawn at pleasure, so as to let the fire fall into the ash pit. The flue is 9 inches square, and runs horizontally for a distance of four feet, where it joins a vertical flue, either of iron or masonry, and of variable height, according to the situation or object of the laboratory. For pharmaceutical operations 20 feet, for chemical researches 40 feet height of chimney may be allowed.

* Experiments which require a great degree of heat, such as the ignition of refractory substances, and the decomposition of minerals by fusion with alkaline carbonates, demand the assistance of the spirit lamp with circular wick, or double current of air. This is one of the most indispensable instruments of the analytical chemist, for there are many accurate experiments which cannot be performed without it. This lamp is represented in a complete state in the lithographed figure. It is commonly made of brass, but sometimes of japanned tin plate. Its most important parts are as follows:—

The wick *c* passes between two cylinders which are connected below by a horizontal plate, and it can be raised or depressed by means of the toothed wheel *e*, and the toothed bar *g*. The lower end of the latter is connected with a cross

The space below the grate is the ash-pit. It communicates with the external air by a sliding iron door, which may be opened to any desired height.

In front of the furnace are two apertures, one commencing eight inches above the grate, terminating within nine inches of the top, and closed by an iron plate, or piece of fire-brick, which can be withdrawn at pleasure. A second and similar aperture commences four inches below the grate, and reaches to the ground; this also is provided with an iron plate or brick door.

In the side walls of the furnace, and exactly in the middle of the space above the grate, are two opposite holes two inches square, through which gun-barrels, or other tubes, may be passed.

The superior aperture of the furnace is fitted with a moveable iron pot five inches deep, to contain sand, and is also provided with a lid of thick wrought iron, lined with fire clay for about two inches in depth.

The horizontal flue is covered with a similar iron plate which drops in between the side walls, and is covered with a layer of sand, about three inches deep.

bar *o*, upon the end of which a ring is fastened, on which ring the wick is stuck. The cross-bar and toothed rod work up and down in the box *b*. In some lamps the wheel and bar *e g* are omitted, the wick holder being constructed like those of sinumbra lamps. The box *b* does not form part of the spirit holder *a a*, as it does in common lamps, but is separated from it by the open spaces *t t*, or at any rate by a partition on each side. The spirit passes from *a a* into *b* through the pipe *k*, which forms the only communication between the spirit holder and the box which holds the wick. The object of this contrivance is to prevent the explosion which frequently takes place when the common spirit lamps are inflamed, and which is owing to the inflammation of the mixture of atmospheric air and vapour of alcohol which forms in the spirit holder *a a*. At *m* is an opening by which the spirit is poured into the lamp. This is afterwards closed by a cork, or a screw. A piece of glass is cemented in the front of the lamp, at *s*, to afford an opportunity of readily ascertaining how much spirit the spirit holder *a* contains. The lamp is provided with an iron chimney, *l*. By raising or depressing the wick, the flame is increased or diminished. The air is brought to the spirit, externally by the side, and internally by the canal *i*. The wick must be cut quite level, and must never remain in a charred state. When a lamp is constructed in this manner, and according to the following scale:

———————————————— 1 Foot.

it affords heat sufficient to fuse 380 grains of carbonate of soda in about fifteen minutes, supposing the salt to be contained in a platinum crucible of the weight of from 300 to 380 grains, and large enough to contain an equal weight of water. A lamp which is incapable of effecting the fusion of at least 180 grains of carbonate of soda, though useful in a great many experiments, is not powerful enough to be generally employed in the analysis of minerals. The experimental chemist ought to possess two lamps of this description; one for fusing, and another for other experiments. In the latter case, the rods which support the lamp may be strong, but for the fusing lamp, the rods must be made as thin as possible, in order that they may not carry away too much of the heat.

Some improvements have recently been made upon this lamp, which are not shown in the above figures. The first is a hinge for the chimney, upon which it is fixed in such a manner as to be readily turned *upon* or *from* the flame. The second is a hinged door, which closes the mouth of the wick holder when the flame is extinguished. The third improvement consists in the application of a sort of dome or jacket, to protect a heated crucible from the free air.

The fuel employed in this furnace is coal or coke. Coke is coal previously heated to redness and freed from all its volatile matters. It consists of carbon and earthy matter alone. The heat it produces is very intense and uniform. Being free from volatile matters it burns without flame. Coke is much used in furnace operations in the arts. To light it, introduce a layer of chips or dry brush wood, with a few pieces of charcoal; close the upper orifice, open the ash-pit door, and light the chips from below with a match. A very powerful fire is obtained in a few minutes.

The fire is regulated by closing or opening the ash-pit door, and by a plate of iron called a "Register," which slides across the chimney, and is supported by a chain and pulley.

The drawings at *fig.* 33 shew the points to be attended to in the erection of this furnace.

The uses and applications of this furnace are very numerous, and will be specified under the head of the particular operations we describe.

The Blast, or Bellows Furnace.

In a few operations an exceedingly powerful heat is required in a smaller space than we can conveniently reduce the former furnace to act in. The blast furnace described by Griffin is that which we have found most efficient, and which we recommend for adoption. (*See Griffin's Recreations*, p. 33.*)

* Blast Furnace.—The highest degree of heat is produced in a furnace into the middle of which air is forcibly blown from many different points at once. Such a furnace is best formed of two iron cylinders, placed one within the other, as shown in the cut, fig. 34, where *c c c* represent the outer cylinder, and the inner is shown lined with, *g*, a thick mass of fire clay. Both cylinders are provided with a bottom, and are fixed together at the top, air-tight, and in such a manner as to leave an equal space between their bottoms and sides. This is exhibited in the figure. The smaller cylinder and its lining of fire clay, is pierced near the middle of the sides with eight holes, all pointing towards the centre of the furnace. The crucible to be heated, is placed upon stones in the middle of the furnace. The air is blown in at the opening *a*, which is connected with the bellows; it is thus compressed in the space *b*, and thence driven through the holes *o o* into the middle of the furnace. The heat thus produced is very intense. In a furnace, proportioned as above, and measuring 27 inches from *c* to *c*, half a pound of feldspar can be completely melted in half an hour. Iron and other substances of difficult fusion melt in it with ease. The fuel used for this furnace requires to be very uniform in size, to be all, for example, of the bulk of a cubic inch. This uniformity is gained by breaking the fuel to nearly the size required, and then sifting it through two sieves, one of which retains all the pieces that are too large, and the other lets through all that are too small. If coke is used, it must be of a sort that gives very little ashes. The crucibles that answer best are the Hessian; but neither these, nor those of plumbago withstand entirely the melting power of this furnace.

The Apothecaries Furnace.

For purposes in which but a low degree of heat is requisite, such as boiling, preparation of extracts, distilling water and essential oils, we have found the following arrangement extremely useful.

A range of five fire-places is erected in a mass of brick work, 7 feet long, 4 feet broad, and 2 feet 3 inches high. The central fire-place is 12 inches square, and 12 deep to the grate. The fire-places next the centre are each 8 inches square, the depth in all being the same.

From each fire-place there runs a separate flue provided with an iron throttle, which can be lifted out at pleasure. All these flues terminate in a common flue, led to a chimney 15 feet high.

By this arrangement five fire-places can be used at once, and the work of a large compounding establishment very easily transacted. The fire-places are covered with tiles, and provided with sand and water-baths for use when required.

Crucibles.

Crucibles are vessels in which we subject various substances to the operation of intense heat. They are either metallic, or mixtures of different non-metallic or earthy ingredients.

Metallic crucibles are for common purposes made of *iron, silver, or platinum.*

Cast-iron crucibles are made of various sizes and forms, and are sometimes provided with lids; they are much used in operations on the precious metals. These vessels fuse at a comparatively moderate temperature. In pharmacy they are used in the reduction of the ores of antimony and lead, and in the calcination of the bitartrate of potash, preparation of black flux, &c. &c.

Silver crucibles are employed in fusing the fixed alkalies, potash and soda. They bear a low red heat without danger, but melt if the temperature be suddenly raised above that point. They should not be heated in direct contact with the fire, but be placed in another crucible of some earthy material. Silver crucibles are destroyed by melted lead, antimony, or zinc, by mercury, by the mineral acids, and by several salts.

Platinum crucibles. These very expensive vessels are of corresponding value in numerous experimental processes, especially in analyses of soils, and operations on several saline bodies.

Their especial uses will be afterwards pointed out. They may be regarded as altogether infusible by any temperature we can command.

The high price of these vessels requires us to point out clearly the precautions to be observed in their use. They must not be exposed to free chlorine; saltpetre and the alkalies must not be fused, nor metals reduced in them; nor compounds of phosphorus so treated as to set that substance free. Oxides of lead, bismuth, copper, cobalt, zinc, and antimony, if heated intensely, render the inner surface rough and porous. Platinum crucibles should, in all furnace operations, be protected from the immediate contact of the fuel, by being placed in a Hessian or other earthen vessel.

Earthen Crucibles.

The paste of crucibles is usually formed of crude clay and of a cement made by burning clay at a red heat, and then reducing this to powder, which is sifted. Three parts of the calcined clay are then well mixed with one of the crude paste. This prevents the cracking of the vessel during the subsequent drying or heating. ***Hessian or porous crucibles*** are composed of clay and sand in such proportions that according to Berthier's analysis they consist of

Silica, ...	709
Alumina, ...	248
Oxide of iron,	38
Magnesia a trace,	
	995

They are prepared from a mixture of a rich aluminous clay and quartzose sand; they are very refractory, and will stand sudden alternations of temperature without breaking. But the great proportion of silica they contain renders them liable to corrosion by litharge and other fusible metallic oxides. Their coarse grain too renders them so porous that fused saline matters readily escape through them.

Beaufaye's French crucibles, which are highly esteemed on the Continent, contain,

Silica, ...	646
Alumina, ...	344
Oxide of Iron,	10
	1000

They are made with clay simply, mixed with a cement of the same material without sand, and they are coated with a thin layer of simple clay, which renders the surface smooth and level. They are very refractory, little liable to fracture from changes of temperature, and superior to the Hessian crucible in resisting the action of fused metallic oxides.

Fragments of coke, sifted sand, or the powder of used crucibles, are often employed as the cement.

Plumbago answers well, and very good crucibles may be made by grinding stoneware vessels to coarse powder, using this as the cement.

The crucibles are readily moulded on a block of wood, previously sprinkled with road dust. When partly dry, they are gently beaten on the mould with a wooden mallet to render the paste more compact; the drying is then slowly carried on, and they are lastly heated to redness in a potter's furnace.

Porcelain crucibles are very useful in many chemical operations. If they are well annealed and glazed with porcelain, they resist very sudden alternations of temperature, are quite infusible, and impermeable to melted bodies. They answer extremely well for fusing the nitrates of silver and potash, boracic acid, fusible metal, &c. and for instructive experiments on the reduction of metallic oxides.

Blue pots (or, as they are absurdly called, black lead crucibles), are composed of carburet of iron, (plumbago) and clay. The plumbago found lately in Darjeeling answers very well. The best proportions are, plumbago three parts, clay one part.

These crucibles are destroyed by saline substances, but resist sudden changes of temperature. In India during the rainy season they absorb moisture very rapidly, and if placed in the furnace without being previously dried, fly to pieces with a loud report, in consequence of the sudden extrication of steam.

The bazar goldsmiths' crucibles are useful and cheap vessels, but fusible at a high heat.

Colgong Clay-pots.

Three parts of the white clay called *Khari*, found abundantly near Colgong, with one part of the fuller's earth called Saboon Mati, from the same place, if well mixed with water and baked at a red heat, give crucibles, which are, in many respects, far superior to those brought from Europe. They are perfectly infusible, impermeable to melted metals or saline matters, and bear sudden heating and cooling without fracture.

[INTERMEDIATE APPLICATION OF HEAT.]

The Water-Bath.

Water at 30° barom. boils at 212°, of Fahr's. thermometer. If, over a vessel of boiling water a second vessel be placed, as shewn in *fig.* 34, any temperature not exceeding 212° can be communicated to the latter. This is especially valuable in drying various vegetable and animal matters, and some chemical products, which would be either decomposed, or would occasion explosion if heated beyond that temperature.

The water-bath shewn in the figure, consists of two capsules of porcelain, tinned copper, or iron, the lower containing water kept boiling by the lamp, the upper containing the substance under experiment.

Solutions of saline matters in water will communicate a higher temperature than 212°. A saturated solution of

Bitartrate of Potassa boils at	214°
Alum, ...	220°
Borax, ...	222°
Common salt, ...	224°
Tartrate of Potassa, ...	234°
Muriate of Ammonia,...	236°
Nitre, ...	234°
Rochelle salt, ...	280°

Metal-Baths.

An alloy composed of eight parts of bismuth, five of lead, and three of tin, fused together, melts below 212°, and will bear a red heat without giving off vapors.

Tin melts at	441°
Lead, ...	609°

By fusing these metals in an iron pan, well supported, the temperature will not rise as long as any of the metal remains solid, so that by throwing in lumps from time to time the heat may be kept constant.

Oil-Baths.

Linseed oil bears a temperature of 640° Fahr. and may consequently, with the assistance of a thermometer, be used to give any temperature desired below that point, but owing to the vapours being very inflammable, great caution is necessary in using these baths.

Steam-Bath.

The vapour of water, boiling at 212°, will communicate that degree of heat to other bodies, and is a most convenient source of heat for many chemical operations. We recommend the following simple apparatus for this very important object:—

For large experiments, provide a double copper vessel with two apertures, of the shape shewn at *fig.* 35, resembling indeed very closely the hot water plates commonly used in India. The vessel has two apertures, to one of which is attached the end of a pipe connected with a kettle, or other small boiler, in which the steam is generated. The other aperture serves for the discharge of the steam, and by connecting it with a cooling apparatus distilled water may be collected at the same time.

This is an excellent apparatus for innumerable experiments in vegetable chemistry, as we will subsequently point out.

Hot-Air Stove.

It is sometimes desirable to dry vegetable substances slowly, at a temperature not exceeding 160° Fahr. For this the hot-air stove is the best apparatus.

The following very simple method is adopted for this purpose in the Medical College:—

Over a pan of heated charcoal is placed a double cylindrical cap of sheet iron; the sides one inch apart, and with two tubes two inches in diameter, opening into the outer case, as shewn in *fig.* 36. (The outer case is best made of tin plate.) A tin plate box with a door is fitted on the upper tube, and has a draught pipe of equal dimensions, provided with a slide at top to regulate the current of air.

The combustion of the charcoal is maintained by air led through a tube of sheet iron, passing below the case, while the smoke and carbonic acid escape through a similar tube in the upper part, as shewn in the drawing.

In the preparation of anarcotine, morphine, quinine, and other vegetable principles, this stove is used with great advantage.

PHARMACEUTICAL EFFECTS OF THE APPLICATION AND SUBSTRACTION OF HEAT.

This is a very important subject, as it comprehends vaporization, evaporation, boiling, subliming, distilling, the preparation of extracts, and other practical operations.

VAPORIZATION.

Vaporization is defined by Dr. Duncan to be the conversion of a solid or fluid into vapour, by the agency of heat.

Some solids, such as ice, camphor, and carbonic acid are capable of passing into vapour directly, without previous liquefaction. Generally, however, the solid first liquefies, and then evaporates.

Vaporization is impeded by increase of pressure, and facilitated by its removal. Thus under the pressure of the entire atmosphere = to 14.9 lbs. per superficial square inch or = to 30 inches of mercury, water boils at 212°.

The boiling point of water is therefore an index of the altitude of the place where the experiment is performed. A thermometrical barometer has been constructed on this principle.

The subjoined Table shews the boiling points of distilled water at different elevations, up to 17,455 feet:—

Thermometer. Degrees.		*Elevation.* Feet.	*Thermometer.* Degrees.		*Elevation.* Feet.
212	=	0	195	=	8953
211	=	0509	194	=	9502
210	=	1021	193	=	10,053
209	=	1534	192	=	10,606
208	=	2049	191	=	11,161
207	=	2566	190	=	11,719
206	=	3085	189	=	12,280
205	=	3607	188	=	12,843
204	=	4131	187	=	13,408
203	=	4675	186	=	13,977
202	=	5185	185	=	14,543
201	=	5718	184	=	15,124
200	=	6250	183	=	15,702
199	=	6786	182	=	16,234
198	=	7324	181	=	16,868
197	=	7864	180	=	17,455
196	=	8407			

Thus a fall of one degree in the boiling point, corresponds to about 530 feet of elevation within certain limits, and one inch fall of the barometer is equivalent to about 1·76 degrees of thermometrical depression of the boiling point.

Spirit of wine at common pressure, boils at 173; in vacuô, at 33°. Sulphuric ether at common pressure, boils at 100°; in vacuô it boils at a temperature far below that of freezing water. So that, by surrounding a tube containing water with sulphuric ether, and removing pressure by the air-pump, the water is rapidly frozen, while the ether boils. Liquids boil in vacuô at about 140 degrees below the boiling point in air.

Practical applications of these facts will be immediately pointed out.

Evaporation.

Evaporation in pharmacy denotes the expulsion of liquid from solutions, in a state of vapour, the liquid not being collected.

Spontaneous evaporation is where this change occurs without boiling, or at common temperatures, as in he manufacture of salt from brine by solar heat; in the inspissation of opium by mere exposure to the air, &c.

Spontaneous evaporation occurs most rapidly during the dry season, and during the prevalence of easterly winds. A current of air passed over the evaporating surface greatly accelerates the process.

Partial evaporation is termed in pharmacy *concentration*, or *inspissation*, the former being applied to saline, the latter to animal or vegetable solutions; the latter operation must generally be performed by a steam or water bath. Exsiccation means the total drying of the solution or mixture, as in the preparation of Mr. Ludlow's extract of Hyoscyamus; of the tyre, or Indian dried milk, &c. &c.

Ebullition.

Ebullition, or boiling, occurs when the vapour is disengaged in bubbles, which burst on the surface of the liquid. The bubbles are sometimes so large as to endanger the loss of the materials, or breaking of the vessel. A coil of platinum or gold wire placed in the fluid entirely prevents this commotion. This is practically seen in the boiling of sulphuric acid in glass vessels.

Some salts, such as borax, sulphate of soda, and sulphate of zinc, containing much water of crystallization, liquefy when heated, then boil, and finally concrete into a dry mass. This operation is called the *watery fusion*.

Torrefaction and Incineration.

When the volatile or fixed matters undergo decomposition, new compounds being formed, the process is named torrefaction, roasting, or incineration.

Roasting, or *torrefaction*, is performed on seeds, such as coffee, kaladana, arachis root, rhubarb, or succory;—on the impure acetates of potash and soda, preliminary to their conversion into acetic acid. The substance is put in a shallow iron vessel over a fire, and stirred continually, or in a cylinder of iron, kept constantly turning on its axis. By this process several volatile matters are expelled, mucilage dried, coloring matters decomposed, or rendered insoluble in water.

Charring is torrefaction carried to the extent of totally expelling the gaseous elements of the substance, while the carbon remains behind.

Incineration is performed when the substance is heated to redness with the free contact of atmospheric air, so that all the carbon is converted into carbonic acid by the oxygen of the air.

Distillation.

When the volatile products are collected, the process is called *distillation* if the products be liquid, as water, spirit, &c., *sublimation* if solid, as camphor, benzoic acid, or calomel.

Distillation is of several kinds; *dry*, when solid matters are operated on, as wood for production of acetic acid, bones for animal charcoal and ammonia, sulphate of iron and saltpetre for the preparation of nitric acid; *humid*, when fluids are distilled, as spirit, water, volatile oil, water of ammonia, &c.

Distillation again varies according to the *pressure* at which it is performed, and may be conveniently considered as distillation under common, and distillation under diminished pressure.

The distilling vessels consist essentially of two parts—1st. the vessel in which the vapors are formed; 2nd, in which these are condensed.

We shall describe the varieties of distilling vessels most useful to the practical druggist.

a. The *Cold Still.*

This apparatus consists of two parts, the still-pot and the capital. The still-pot is most advantageously shaped like the common copper cooking vessels, only having an upright neck, into which the capital fits securely and closely.

The capital is shewn in *fig.* 34. It has an inverted

edge within, and a hollow reservoir above, for containing water. A tube leads from the space immediately above the inverted edge to a receiver, in which the distilled products are collected. When the water above becomes too hot it is drawn off by the cock, and cold water renewed.

This very useful apparatus is employed in our pharmacopœia in the distillation of gurgun oil.

b. The *Still* and *Worm.*

The body of this still is too familiarly known to need description. The *worm* is a spiral coil of pewter or tin tube quite water-tight, and immersed in a tub containing water, as shewn in the drawing, *fig.* 35.

In some processes the liquid in the tub is kept at a low temperature by dissolving in it saltpetre or glauber salt. An instance of this occurs in the preparation of sulphuric ether.

The Double-cone Condenser.

Two truncated hollow cones of thin copper are placed one within the other, so as to be half an inch apart; they are soldered by a band above and below. The neck of the still enters above, the discharging pipe proceeds from below; the whole is placed in a bucket of water; a very large surface is thus exposed to the action of cold, and condensation proceeds with great rapidity.

The body of the still above described, is made of copper or iron, coated with tin,—the head, of copper lined with lead or tin. For manufacturing sulphuric ether a leaden still is employed, which we shall describe in treating of that article.

The Still and straight Condenser.

After distilling highly scented materials, such as volatile oils, rose water, &c. unless the condenser be thoroughly cleaned the flavour of the article next operated on is apt to be altered or injured. It being very difficult to clean worm-condensers, a very simple and useful arrangement has been devised for this kind of Distillation.

The straight condenser consists of a long tin, pewter, or leaden tube, open at both ends, and surrounded by an external tube of copper, as shewn in *fig.* 36. One end of the internal tube is connected with the body of the still, the other end introduced into a receiver; cold water is allowed to flow into the copper tube at its lower end, and to escape in a constant stream from above. Perfect condensation thus takes place.

Retorts and Receivers.

For several distillations glass vessels are employed. Those usually employed are termed *retorts*, and are now commonly made in many parts of India.

Retorts are either plain, or stoppered, of white or green glass, the two first varieties are seen in *figs.* 37, 38.

Excellent green glass retorts are sold in the Machua Bazar, Calcutta, at from four to eight annas each. Those should be selected which are free from air globules in the sides and bottom, and are of uniform and moderate thickness.

These retorts are made of broken French bottles, and stand high heat much better than the neater looking English white glass.

Retorts may be heated over charcoal, by spirit lamps, the sand, water, steam, saline, oil, or metal baths. They will bear a low red heat, without danger of breakage or fusion. If it is intended to subject them to a very high temperature, they should be previously coated with a little clay made into a paste with water, and carefully dried.

Receivers are employed to collect the products of the distillation.

Receivers are plain, stoppered, or quilled.

A common flask answers well for a receiver.

Tubulated receivers are of various kinds, as shewn in *figs.* 39, 40. The appropriate uses of these vessels will be subsequently described.

Quilled receivers are of much use in several operations. Their form and mode of arrangement is shewn in *fig.* 40.

Adopters are long tubular glass vessels, employed as intermediate connectors between retorts and receivers.

Retorts are supported on brass or iron stands with moveable rings, as shewn at *fig.* 40.

The *Receivers* are kept cool when requisite by immersion in water, which may be brought to a low temperature by ice, saltpetre, or sulphate of soda; or folds of cloth or paper may be placed on the receiver, and kept cool by water allowed to drop from a reservoir above.

Kedgeree pots, fitted with tin or leaden covers make good distilling vessels in many processes, especially in the preparation of water of ammonia.

Safety Tubes.

When plain retorts and receivers are used, they must not be joined air-tight, as the generation of vapour might burst the apparatus.

But there are many contrivances which enable us to prevent the accumulation of the vapour, so that all danger of this kind is obviated. These expedients are available only with the tubulated instruments above described.

The first kind of safety tube is shewn in *fig.* 40. It is introduced so as to dip just beneath the surface of the fluid in the retort, and mercury or water is poured into the bent part, so that if undue expansion takes place within, the vapours press the mercury or water into the funnel. Should contraction ensue, air enters in the reverse manner.

A series of receivers are sometimes connected together. The best apparatus of the kind is called "Woolfe's bottles". These consist of bottles provided with three necks, and are arranged thus, as shewn in the same figure.

From the first receiver a long bent tube proceeds to the triple-necked bottle, No. 1. In the centre neck is a straight tube, open at each end, the lower end just dipping beneath the surface of the fluid. From the third neck proceeds a bent tube to No. 2, and so through a series of any number. The last bottle generally terminates in a very long tube, under water or mercury.

Should too great expansion occur in these bottles, the fluid rises a little in the middle tube, and then the contained vapour escapes until equilibrium is restored;—or if condensation takes place within, the reverse occurs and air enters.

These connecting tubes are readily broken by lateral movement. To prevent this, flexible joints of Indian rubber have been constructed, and the tubes act as shewn in the drawing.

These caoutchouc joints are easily made of the thin sheets of Indian rubber now prepared in Assam, by cutting them with a very sharp scissors into long strips half an inch broad, and coiling these strips spirally round a cylinder of wood of the required diameter; the recently cut edges adhere firmly, and an air-tight tube is formed.

To prevent the tube adhering to the wood, this should be sprinkled with flour or powdered chalk.

An improvement has recently been made in Woolfe's bottles, which renders these joints needless, and at the same time obviates the danger of fracture by lateral motion.

A very wide tube is fitted by grinding into one neck of each bottle, and the usual narrow tube, bent twice at a right angle, proceeds from the other neck. The bottles are adjusted together by passing the latter tube down the former, so that the lower lip of the narrow tube projects beyond the side of the wide one. (*Fig.* 41.)

The wide tube here acts as a safety tube, and effectually

prevents any mischief to the apparatus by expansion or condensation.

A very convenient substitute for Woolfe's expensive apparatus may be made with wide-mouthed bottles, closely fitted with wooden covers, and provided with the requisite tubes. Leaden tubes may be used in many cases, are very useful, and are easily secured and adjusted.

Distillation under diminished pressure.

The advantages of this process are, first, economy of fuel; secondly, the preventing of the article under the process from being injured by excessive heat.

The pressure of the atmosphere may be removed,

a. By an air pump attached to the receiver.

b. By expelling the air from the space between the surface of the liquid to be distilled and the receiver, introducing steam, and then condensing the steam by the affusion of cold water from without. (*Fig.* 42.)

The first of these vessels represents the still, the second the receiver, which can be filled with steam from boiling water in the third vessel. When all the air is expelled and the central vessel filled with steam, the communication is cut off from the third vessel, and water poured on No. 2, from the reservoir. Condensation occurs, and a vacuum is formed. Communication being opened between No. 1 and No. 2, distillation goes on rapidly at about forty degrees less than the ordinary boiling point of the liquid.

This method of distillation was applied with extraordinary success by Howard to the refining of sugar, and by Barry to the preparation of medicinal extracts.

The Editor has erected an apparatus at the Medical College for rectifying spirit in vacuô, on a principle first suggested by Dr. Andrew Duncan, but now for the first time put in practical operation.

The College apparatus is erected on a platform on the roof, and consists, 1, of an air tight iron vessel for containing the spirit; 2, a leaden pipe, 50 feet long, terminating in a stop cock immersed in a small cistern; the pipe at ten feet from the top, enters a condensing worm, from the lower end of which it proceeds again, as shewn in *fig.* 43.

To prepare Alcohol, sp. gr. 835, in this apparatus, the still is filled with proof rum, and the lower cock of the barometer pipe being shut, the pipe is filled with alcohol, sp. gr. 835.

Of this spirit, a column one inch square and 41 feet high, weighs 14·9 lb. and is consequently equal to the pressure of the atmosphere.

Hence on opening the lower cock, all being air-tight above, all the spirit in the still above the upper orifice of the tube, and 9 feet of that within the tube, escapes into the cistern, leaving a column 41 feet long in equilibrium with the atmosphere, and a vacuum in the tube and iron vessel above that height.

On exposing the still to the sun's rays, the spirit now boils freely. The vapour entering the cooling worm, which is kept cold by saltpetre, is condensed into spirit. Whatever quantity is condensed at the summit of the column, an equal portion descends through the cock into the reservoir below.

This still, without any consumption of fuel, and by the attention of one servant, affords alcohol at 835° of far superior quality to that obtainable where fire is used.

This process can be adopted on any scale in tropical climates, and it is thought will supersede most other modes of distilling spirit. It is equally applicable to the raw washes of sugar or malt, and in hilly districts the barometric column required will be short in proportion to the elevation of the station, while the solar heat in all cases will be more than sufficient.

Sublimation

is essentially the same as distillation, excepting that solid products are obtained.

The substance to be sublimed is placed in a vessel capable of resisting a high temperature, having a receiver luted to the top.

Subliming vessels may be of glass, earthenware, or metal. The *figure* 45 shews one formerly very much used, but expensive, and easily broken.

The vessel is heated in sand; the solid matter collects in the capital; and any liquid which may be formed passes off by the narrow tube.

Two glass flasks, placed as shewn in *fig.* 46, make a good subliming apparatus.

Soda water bottles, small Kedgeree pots, and similar common vessels, may be employed successfully in many sublimations.

On the small scale, glass tubes afford us very manageable and excellent vessels. They may be heated in the spirit lamp flame.

Some of the mercurial compounds, calomel for example, are heated in iron retorts, and the products received in vessels containing the vapour of boiling water.

In connexion with this head, it is necessary to define or explain some terms much used in the description of pharmaceutical processes.

Cohobation is the distilling of the same fluid product repeatedly from the original substance operated on, as in the distillation of some essential oils.

Rectification is the repeated distillation of a product to free it from impurity. Thus spirit distilled from sugar is called rum, is of sp. gr. 0.920, and contains 50 per cent of water. Rum distilled once to one-third yields alcohol sp. gr. 825° containing 92 parts of water per cent.

This alcohol mixed with quick lime, carbonate of potash, or dried muriate of lime, and distilled, gives absolute alcohol sp. gr. 0.793, and is as free from water as it can be procured.

This process is also called by the older writers *dephlegmation*, a term now no longer employed.

Lutes.

Different lutes or pastes are required for the adjustment of the joints in distilling apparatus.

For distilling spirits and volatile oils, a paste of flour and water is smeared over the junction between the body of the still and its head, and between this and the commencement of the condenser.

Plaster of Paris (sulphate of lime made into a thin paste with water,) makes also an excellent joint.

Moistened bladder, cut in slips, may be rolled round the joints of tubes, and tied on with dry twine.

Quicklime in fine powder, mixed with white of eggs and instantly applied, hardens almost instantly, and forms an excellent lute, especially in distilling ether.

Quicklime and one-sixth part of common salt, or moistened clay, form a strong lute.

In distilling ammonia, the latter lute is especially useful.

Besides the apparatus above described, the practical apothecary ought to be provided with funnels with very long and narrow necks, for pouring fluids into plain vessels without soiling their necks.

ABSTRACTION OF HEAT.

Some methods of artificial cooling have been already noticed. We subjoin tables of various mixtures for effecting this object.

Cooling mixtures without Ice.

	Parts.	Degree of cold produced.
Nitrate of ammonia, water, ... each	1	46
Nitrate of ammonia, carbonate of soda, water, each	1	57
Phosphate of soda, ...	9	62
Sulphuric acid, ...	4	
Sulphate of soda, ...	8	50
Muriatic acid, ...	5	
Sulphate of soda, ...	5	47
Dilute sulphuric acid, ...	4	
Phosphate of soda, ...	9	47
Nitrate of ammonia, ...	6	
Dilute sulphuric acid, ...	4	

The fall of the thermometer is here calculated from 50°, and the full effect is not produced, unless the materials employed, and the substance acted upon, be previously cooled to that point.

Cooling mixtures with Ice.

	Parts.	
Pounded ice or snow, ...	2	From any temperature to—5°
Common salt, ...	1	
Snow or pounded ice, ...	12	Ditto, ... —25°
Common salt, ...	5	
Nitrate of ammonia, ...	5	
Snow, ...	3	From ... ... 32° to—23°
Dilute sulphuric acid, ...	2	
Snow, ...	8	Ditto, ... —27°
Muriatic acid,...	5	
Snow, ...	7	Ditto, ... —30°
Diluted nitric acid, ...	4	
Snow, ...	4	Ditto, ... —40°
Muriate of lime, ...	5	
Snow, ...	2	Ditto, ... —50°
Cryst. muriate of lime, ...	3	
Snow, ...	1	From ... ... 0° to—60°
Cryst. muriate of lime, ...	2	
Snow, ...	1	From ... ... 40° to—73°
Cryst. muriate of lime, ...	3	
Snow, ...	8	From ... ... 68° to—98°
Diluted sulphuric acid,...	10	

Cold produced by Evaporation.

Wollaston's Cryophorus, is an instrument which shews very beautifully the production of cold by evaporation.

It consists of two glass bulbs with an intervening tube, one bulb containing water. In making the instrument it is sealed while full of steam, all the air having been carefully expelled. If the bulb *b* be placed in a mixture of ice and salt the vapour within being rapidly condensed, *boiling* occurs in *b* and the cold thereby occasioned very soon causes the *boiling water* to freeze!

Liquid carbonic acid, when allowed to escape suddenly through a very small orifice against a shallow metallic cup, evaporates so rapidly that one-third becomes congealed into a solid substance like snow. This solid carbonic acid mixed with ether, produces, by its gradual evaporation, the most intense cold which has been obtained, namely 137° below the zero of Fahrenheit's scale.

Cold produced by Radiation.

Cold is also occasioned by heat leaving bodies by *radiation.*

Thus a hot body, placed in the centre of a room, parts with heat in rays proceeding in all directions till an equilibrium of temperature is established with all surrounding bodies.

The upper regions of space being intensely cold, on cloudless nights terrestrial objects part with heat in this manner, and thus is explained the process for manufacturing ice in India, when the temperature of the air is far above the freezing point of water.

Shallow earthen pans, containing a few ounces of water, are disposed on the ground on dry straw, to prevent the heat of the earth passing by contact into the cup. Radiation taking place freely, the surface of the water soon becomes frozen.

PART II.

EPITOME OF PHARMACEUTICAL CHEMISTRY.

We have now described such processes and operations as can be carried on without any knowledge of the principles of chemistry. For the comprehension of the subsequent pages, some information of this kind is indispensable. Other works, it is true, exist, in which such knowledge may be gained, but it is our aim to supply in one volume all that the apothecary really requires.

In the subsequent epitome of chemistry, we will therefore only enlarge on those principles, and describe those substances, the knowledge of which is absolutely necessary for the pharmaceutical student; the rarer elements need only be known to the student of abstract chemistry, or of that science as applied to arts and manufactures.

PROPERTIES OF MATTER.

The properties of matter are of two kinds, general and secondary.

The general properties of matter are—weight, extension, impenetrability, porosity, and indestructibility.

The secondary properties of matter are—colour, form, taste, odour, figure, &c.

The ultimate particles of matter are indivisible, and are called atoms.

Matter is inert, or incapable of changing its state of motion or rest, excepting in obedience to external forces.

These forces are referable to two kinds, *attraction* and *repulsion*.

VARIETIES OF ATTRACTION.

1. The attraction of Gravitation—by which bodies are drawn towards the centre of the earth, by which the heavenly bodies are balanced in space, and which acts between substances at immense distances from each other.

2. The attraction of Electricity. If during dry weather a piece of glass be rubbed by silk, or wax be rubbed by flannel, or paper by Indian rubber, all these bodies are found capable of attracting towards them light substances, such as dust, feathers, thread, gold leaf.

3. The attraction of Magnetism. If two pieces of natural magnet stone (chemuk-pathar), be freely suspended near each other, it will be found that in certain positions they will attract each other. This power they communicate to steel

by simple friction. Two steel bars freely balanced will attract each other by two ends, and each bar by itself will turn and settle in a line passing through the North and South cardinal points of the compass.

This embraces also the electro-magnetic attraction, of which examples will be subsequently given.

4. Attraction of Cohesion. This is exemplified in the cohesion of the particles of all solid substances, such as stone, glass, &c.; of pieces of Indian rubber, the edges of which, if recently cut, reunite as before.

All the preceding varieties of attraction take place either at infinite, sensible, or imperceptible distances, and between masses as well as atoms of matter;—but neither the general nor secondary properties of the bodies attracted are thereby altered.

5. Chemical attraction, or *affinity*. This occurs only at imperceptible distances between the atoms, not the masses of matter, and the secondary properties thereof are often altered by the action.

Thus by virtue of chemical attraction, sulphur, a yellow solid, and mercury, a silver-like fluid, unite and form a *red* solid.

A chemical union cannot be subverted by mechanical means. We may reduce this red sulphuret of mercury to the finest powder, but each particle contains sulphur and mercury still.

Chemical union takes place between definite proportions of the attracting bodies; thus sulphur and mercury unite in the proportion of mercury 202, sulphur 16 parts—and if there be more of either ingredient combined, it will be found to be in a simple multiple of the first proportion, as mercury 202, sulphur 32 parts, or 2 proportions.

These proportions are termed "combining equivalents."

The particles into which a compound body may be mechanically reduced, are called its integrant particles, and are themselves compound.

The substances into which the integrant particles are decomposable by chemical means, are called *constituent* particles.

A substance which cannot be decomposed into two or more substances of different secondary properties, is termed a simple substance.

These simple substances are 54 in number, and of these, in various modes of union, the material world of which we have cognizance is composed.

Varieties of Chemical Attraction.

When two simple bodies unite and form a third of different secondary properties, the action is called single affinity; as in the case of sulphur and mercury.

Bodies composed of two simple elements are called ***Binary*** compounds.

If, of three substances, two unite, excluding the third, this is called single elective attraction. Thus if we heat iron filings with the compound of sulphur and mercury, the sulphur leaves the mercury and unites with the iron.

Double elective attraction is where two binary compounds mutually decompose each other, thus—

Sulphuretted Hydrogen.	Sulphur.*	Lead.*	Oxide of Lead.
	Hydrogen.†	Oxygen.†	

Form.

* * Sulphuret of lead.
† † Oxide of Hydrogen or Water.

The forces of attraction are modified by a counteracting power to which the name of Repulsion is given.

For example, two magnetic needles point North and South. If we mark the ends which point North, it will be found on bringing these together that they repel each other.

A strip of paper is attracted by rubbed wax and then immediately repelled by it. If it touch any metallic body in contact with the ground it is again attracted.

Chemical attraction is promoted by whatever tends to bring the particles of combining bodies into intimate contact with each other.

Thus, heat promotes chemical union in the case of mercury and sulphur, by melting the sulphur, and allowing its atoms to flow in free contact with those of the metal.

But heat may overcome chemical attraction by expanding the particles of one or more of the combining elements, so as to remove these beyond the sphere of action of the others, thus the oxide of mercury is decomposed by heat, and all its oxygen expelled.

Mechanical solidity interferes also with chemical action, by preventing the free contact of the ultimate particles of the bodies. Thus solution or powdering promotes affinity, and is generally had recourse to for this object.

ELEMENTS OR SIMPLE SUBSTANCES.

The simple substances are 54 in number, as shewn in the subjoined table. The substances marked with an asterisk are those to which the apothecary has to direct his chief attention.

They are either gases (or airs), non-metallic solids or liquids, and metals.

The elements have further been classified into those which are inflammable—and those which, on the contrary, cannot be burned themselves, but must be present to support the combustion of the first class.

Simple Gases or Airs.

Oxygen,*
Hydrogen,*
Nitrogen,*
Chlorine.*

Non-metallic Substances.

Sulphur,*	Boron,*
Selenium,	Fluorine,
Phosphorus,*	Iodine,*
Carbon,*	Bromine.*

Metals.—1st. Class.

(See page 68.)

Potassium,*	Silicium,*
Sodium,*	Aluminium,*
Lithium,	Thorinum,
Calcium,*	Glucinium,
Barium,*	Zirconium,
Strontium,	Ittrium.
Magnesium,*	

2nd. Class.

Manganese,*	Cadmium,
Iron,*	Cobalt,
Zinc,*	Nickel,
Tin,*	Uranium,
Copper,*	Titanium,
Lead,*	Cerium,
Antimony,*	

Bismuth,*	Tellurium,
Arsenic,*	Vanadium,
Molybdenum,	Tungsten,
Chromium,*	Columbium,
Mercury,*	Palladium,
Silver,*	Rhodium,
Gold,*	Osmium,
Platinum,*	Iridium.

COMPOUND BODIES.

All bodies with which we are acquainted, not mentioned in the preceding table, are compounds of elements therein named. Thus water is a compound of oxygen and hydrogen gases; air, of oxygen and nitrogen gases; red lead, of lead and oxygen; common salt, of chlorine and sodium; oil of vitriol, of sulphur and oxygen; brass, of zinc and copper. Animal and vegetable bodies consist essentially of carbon, oxygen, hydrogen, and often nitrogen.

Compounds are,

Binary,	if	composed	of	2	elements.
Ternary,	,,	,,	,,	3	,,
Quaternary,	,,	,,	,,	4	,,
Quinary,	,,	,,	,,	5	,,

Compounds of	*With*	*Are called*
Oxygen, ...	Metals and inflammables	Oxides.
Chlorine, ...	ditto,	Chlorides or chlorurets.
Iodine,...	ditto,	Iodides or iodurets.
Sulphur, ...	ditto,	Sulphurets.
Carbon,...	ditto,	Carburets.
Phosphorus,... ...	ditto,	Phosphurets.
Bromine, ...	ditto,	Bromides or bromurets.

According to the number of equivalents present the syllables Proto. (1) Bi. or Deuto. (2), Ter. (3), are prefixed; thus—*Proto*-Chloride—*Bi*-Carburet—*Ter*-Sulphuret, &c.

The oxides of the metals Potassium, Sodium, and Lithium, are called *alkalies*.

The oxides of Calcium, Barium, Magnesium, and Aluminium are called *earths*.

Sulphur, Chlorine, Nitrogen, Phosphorus, Iodine, Bromine, and several other bodies, form with oxygen and hydrogen compounds of very remarkable properties, which are termed *acids*.

These acids change many vegetable blues to red; they unite with the alkalies and oxides, and the resulting compound is termed a *salt*.

There are however many other compounds termed salts, in which neither acid nor alkali is present.

Sometimes the oxygen or hydrogen forms with one substance several compounds, differing only in the proportion of oxygen or hydrogen present. Thus nitrogen and oxygen form six compounds—of these three are acids.

In such a case the acid containing least oxygen is named by adding the syllable *ous*, to the name of the other principle—the acid containing most oxygen by adding the syllable *ic*. If there be several degrees of oxygenation the word *hypo* is often prefixed; thus,

Hypo-Nitr*ous* acid, ...	Nitrogen,	1.	,,	ox.	3.
Nitr*ous* acid, ...	Nitrogen,	1.	,,	ox.	4.
Nitr*ic* acid, ...	Nitrogen,	1.	,,	ox.	5.
Hypo-sulphur*ous* acid, ...	Sulphur,	2.	,,	ox.	3.
Sulphur*ous* acid, ...	Sulphur,	1.	,,	ox.	2.
Sulphur*ic* acid, ...	Sulphur,	1.	,,	ox.	3.

Salts, composed of acids and alkalies, are named from both; thus, if the acid end in *ic*, as sulphur*ic* acid, they are called sulphates; in *ous*, as sulphur*ous* acid, sulphites.

The maximum degree of combination is frequently designated *Per*, as per-oxide, per-chloride, per-salts.

Salts of protoxides, deutoxides, or per-oxides, are termed protosalts, deutosalts or persalts. *Sesqui* is the term for 1½ equivalent, as sesquinitrate, sesqui-oxide.

CRYSTALLIZATION.

Chemical as well as mechanical attraction very frequently causes the particles of a body to assume a definite molecular arrangement, so that various many-sided figures of great regularity result.

These figures are called crystals.

The preparation of crystals (crystallization), is of such great importance to the practical chemist and apothecary, that we deem it necessary to enter on the subject in some detail.

According to Mr. Brooke there are fifteen primary forms of crystallization.

1. The cube (*fig.* 47) bounded by six square planes.

2. The regular tetrahedron, bounded by four equilateral triangular planes.

3. The regular octohedron, or two four sided pyramids, united base to base. The common base being a square, and the planes equilateral triangles. *(Fig. 48)*

4. The rhombic dodecahedron, contained between twelve equal rhombic planes.

5. The octohedron with square base, contained within eight equal isosceles triangular figures.

6. The octohedron, with a rectangular base, its planes isosceles triangles, but not equal.

7. Octohedron with a rhombic base, contained within eight equal scalene triangular planes, all its dimensions being variable.

8. The right square prism. *(Fig. 49)*

9. Right rectangular prism, whose three edges are unequal.

10. Right rhombic prism.

11. Right rhomboidal prism.

12. Oblique rhombic prism.

13. Oblique rhomboidal prism.

14. Rhomboid, or rhombohedron.

15. The regular hexagonal prism.

Bodies of the same composition are generally of the same crystalline form.

But different bodies may have the same crystalline form, and are then called isomorphous.

Crystals are usually obtained from bodies in a state of fusion or solution. Thus sulphur, phosphorus, and spermaceti crystallize when cooling from the melted state; salt, nitre, &c., from watery, morphia, strychnia, &c. from acoholic solutions.

Examples of Crystals.

Common salt, ...	the cube.
Alum, ...	regular octohedron.
Sulphate of magnesia, ...	{ right prism with rhombic base. four sided prism.
Nitre, ...	six sided prism.
Sulphate of soda, ...	{ oblique rhombic prism. striated six sided prism.
Citric acid, ...	right rhombic prism.
Bi-tartrate of potash, ...	right rhombic prism.
Tartaric acid, ...	oblique rhombic prism.
Morphia, ...	right rhombic prism.
Nitrate of silver, ...	right rhombic prism.

Sulphate of iron, ...	oblique rhombic prism.
Bi-Chloride of mercury,	right rhombic prism.
Chloride of mercury, ...	square prism.
Acetate of lead, ...	right oblique angled prism.
Sulphate of potassa, ...	right rhombic prism.
Bi-sulphate of potassa. ...	right rhombic prism.
Tartrate of potash, ...	right oblique angled prism.
Carbonate of soda, ...	oblique rhombic prism.
Tartrate of potash & soda,	right rhombic prism.
Sulphate of lime, ...	right rhombic prism.

The student will find that the rhombic prism is the primary form of the majority of pharmaceutical crystals. The crystals themselves are frequently very irregular, but when split and dissected according to their natural cleavage, the primary form is evolved.

The angles of crystals are measured by goniometers, instruments but little used by the apothecary.

During crystallization the forms are liable to many modifications.

Crystals may be *truncated* or *bevelled* at their angles or edges, a portion being apparently cut off.

Some crystals *effloresce*, or lose their transparency, and fall to powder in the air, as sulphate of soda; others, such as tartrate of potash, attract moisture, and run into a liquid—this is called *deliquescence*. Many crystals contain definite quantities of water which is essential to their crystalline state, (water of crystallization) and when this is parted with, as by efflorescence or drying, they lose their crystalline shape. Crystals containing no water are called anhydrous. Some crackle or decrepitate like common salt, when thrown into the fire—an effect caused either by unequal expansion of the crystal, or the sudden conversion of its water into steam.

Regular and large crystals are best obtained by the slow, or even spontaneous evaporation of their solutions.

Crystallization often enables us to separate different salts from a mixed solution. Thus common salt crystallizes separately from a solution of nitrate of potash. But isomorphous salts, or salts of the same acid, or of analogous constitution, very often crystallize together.

Mr. Brande mentions a beautiful experiment in illustration of these facts. Dissolve two parts of saltpetre and three of sulphate of soda in five of warm water. Fill two bottles with the solution; in one place a crystal of nitre, in the other a crystal of sulphate of soda; place both bottles in ice-cold water; nitre only will crystallize in one, sulphate of soda in the other.

Solid particles, strings, &c. are introduced into crystallizing solutions, and are found to promote the process, and improve the size of the crystals. Thus threads are placed in solutions of sugar to obtain sugar-candy—bushes in saltpetre vats—sticks in solutions of verdigris, &c. &c.

Solutions of salts made in close vessels or in vacuô, may often be cooled to a very low degree, and no crystals form. A saturated solution of sulphate of soda boiled in a flask, and the vessel then corked closely, shoots into an apparently solid mass if, after cooling, the cork be suddenly removed. Agitation of the surface produces the like effect in many cases. Thus in northern climates in calm weather, water frequently becomes colder than its freezing point, and no congelation occurs till a breeze ripples the surface, when it becomes immediately frozen.

Crystals, like leaves, have a strong tendency to form or move towards the *light*. Some *vegetate*, or creep along the sides of the vessels in which they are formed.

The shape of crystals is further modified by the nature of the liquid from which they form. Common salt from solutions of urea assumes an octohedral instead of a cubic figure. Muriate of ammonia from the same liquid takes a cubic instead of an octohedral shape. Saltpetre if made to crystallize from lime-water, is deposited in unusually large crystals.

The liquid which remains after crystals have separated, forms a solution or mixture by manufacturers termed the *mother* liquor.

SIMPLE SUBSTANCES.

FIRST DIVISION—INORGANIC.

Simple Gases.

OXYGEN GAS.

This gas exists naturally in air, in water, in animal and vegetable matters, and in combination with many simple substances, in the state of oxide.

Air contains by measure 20 parts per 100 of this gas; water by weight, eight parts in every nine.

Oxygen is a colourless, inodorous, and tasteless air, slightly soluble in water. All burning bodies have their combustion increased very much by this element. Its presence in the air is essential to the support of ordinary flame. But its most remarkable property is, that it is indispensable to the maintenance of animal life, being consumed largely in the process of respiration.

100 Cubic inches weigh 34.19 grains. Its specific gravity, compared to atmospheric air, is 1,026.

Preparation.

Oxygen is obtained by heating chlorate of potash, (Chlorine 1. Potassium 1, Oxygen 6.) in a vessel of green glass; or by heating nitrate of potash, (Nitrogen 1, Potassium 1, Oxygen 6), in a large iron vessel—the gas thus obtained is however impure; or by heating peroxide of manganese, (Man. 1, oxygen 2,) in an iron retort to full redness—half a proportion of oxygen is expelled, and sesquioxide of manganese remains; or by boiling peroxide of manganese in a green glass retort with sulphuric acid—1 proportion of oxygen comes off, and proto-sulphate of manganese is formed. The third process is that generally employed.

The equivalent of oxygen is 8.

We append a few examples of the compounds formed by oxygen with other simple substances.

Oxygen with	1 Eq: Hydrogen—Forms water.	
„ „	4 times its Vol. of Nitrogen—Atmospherical air.	
5 Eq. „	1 Eq: Nitrogen—Nitric acid.	
Oxygen with	Metals, ———	Oxides and acids.
„ „	Carbon, ———	Carbonic oxide and acid.
„ „	Sulphur, ———	Several acids.
„ „	Carbon, Hydrogen and Nitrogen in various proportions, ———	Vegetable and animal structures.

It is necessary to notice here the vessels for collecting and examining this and other gases not soluble in water.

The Gas-holder. Any large air-tight vessel full of water may be used as a gas-holder.

The floating gasometer has already been described under the head of oil gas. See page 28.

Pepy's gasometer is an excellent instrument.*

* *Description of Pepy's Gasometer.* It is made of sheet-iron, tin, or copper, japanned or painted inside and outside. The figure No. 50 represents Mr. Pepys's gas-holder, the most convenient form of this apparatus hitherto contrived. A is the body of the gas-holder intended to contain the gas; B a trough supported on three pillars, resting on A; *c* a flexible tube conveying gas through an aperture that permits the water to escape as it enters; *b* a stopcock connected with a flexible tube through which the gas may be propelled after it has been collected; *e* another stop-cock connected with a tube open at both ends, and passing between A and B, through which the gas may be made to pass (when *b* is shut) into a jar full of water, placed in the trough B. A tube *(a)* open at both ends, passes through one of the pillars supporting B, and is continued to the bottom of A; *d d* a glass tube open at both ends, and cemented into the upper and lower part of A, to indicate the quantity of gas inside, the fluid in the tube being always at the same level with the fluid in it. When the gas-holder is to be used, the aperture at *c* is closed

Pneumatic Trough.

There are several instruments of this kind. One of the best is shewn in the cut. It is made of varnished sheet iron, is circular, 20 inches wide, has a channel in the middle 6 inches deep, the sides being but 2 inches deep. A moveable tray with holes, and a small inverted funnel complete the apparatus. *(Fig. 51.)*

Bottles or jars are used for holding the gas. They are filled with water, inverted, and the gas is introduced from below—when filled, the bottle or jar is closed below by a copper or glass plate, and then removed for experiment. *(Fig. 52.)*

Jars are often provided with brass stop-cocks, and graduated into cubic inches. These are vessels of great value to the scientific chemist, but are little used by the apothecary. *(Fig. 53.)*

HYDROGEN GAS.

This simple gas forms one-ninth by weight of water, is found in all animal and vegetable matters, and in combination with carbon is evolved abundantly in mines and marshes.

It is, when pure, colourless, transparent, tasteless, and inodorous, insoluble in water, exceedingly inflammable, though burning with a pale flame. The heat of its combustion is greater than that afforded by any other body. It is the lightest substance in nature, 100 cubic inches weighing only 2½ grains. Hence when large bags of varnished silk, (balloons) are inflated with this gas, the weight of the balloon and its contents being less than that of an equal volume of air, it rises in the atmosphere. Machines of this kind have risen to an elevation of 27,000 feet, and have buoyed up five men, with instruments, ballast, &c. weighing altogether several hundred pounds.

by a plug made to screw upon it; and water being poured into B, it passes down through *a* into the body of the gas-holder, the atmospheric air being forced through *b* (which is also opened) as the water rises in A. All the stop-cocks are shut when the gas-holder is full of water, and the plug which closes the aperture at *c* being unscrewed, the tube which conveys the gas may be introduced, which will rise through the water, as represented in the figure, while the latter flows out in a continued stream as long as any gas enters; great care must be taken not to open any of the stop-cocks while the plug at *c* is unscrewed, as the water would then be forced out with great violence by the pressure of the atmosphere, and the gas-holder filled with atmospheric air in a few seconds. When the gas-holder is full, the tube *c* is withdrawn, and the plug screwed on; the trough *b* is then filled with water, and on opening the stop-cock in the tube *a*, the water descends and presses upon the gas; but none escapes unless the stop-cocks at *b* or *a* are opened, through either of which it may be propelled by opening the one and shutting the other.

The stop-cocks alluded to are made of brass and very easily constructed according to the section and drawings given in the plate, *fig.* 54. The glass tube mentioned in the description may be left out without material inconvenience.

Two measures of hydrogen burned with one measure of oxygen, are changed into water. Water if decomposed by the galvanic battery, yields oxygen and hydrogen in the like proportions.

A mixture of these gases may be inflamed by a taper, a red hot wire, the electric spark, or by the presence of finely divided platinum.

Hydrogen gas is obtained from water by several processes. 1. The steam of boiling water passed over red hot iron is decomposed; its oxygen unites with the iron, and its hydrogen is set free. 2. Sulphuric acid and zinc, in contact with water decompose it; its hydrogen is evolved, its oxygen unites with the zinc, and the oxide of zinc with the sulphuric acid, forms the sulphate of zinc. 3. Iron may be substituted for zinc in the last experiment. 4. By the galvanic battery water yields both oxygen and hydrogen, separately, in large quantities, and in atomic proportions.

Hydrogen being the lightest body in nature, is taken as unity in the scale of combining equivalents.

The following are examples of some of the compounds into which it enters :—

Hydrogen forms with	Nitrogen,	Ammonia.
,, ,, ,,	Chlorine,	Muriatic acid.
,, ,, ,,	Oxygen,	Water.
,, ,, ,,	Carbon.	Oil and coal gases, &c.&c.
,, ,, ,,	Cyanogen,	Prussic acid.

NITROGEN, OR AZOTE.

This simple gas exists most abundantly in atmospheric air, which is composed of nitrogen four parts, oxygen one part by measure, with traces of substances afterwards described.

By burning hydrogen, phosphorus, sulphur, or potassium, in 100 measures of atmospheric air, twenty parts of oxygen combine with the inflammable body, and seventy-nine and a half parts of nitrogen remain. There are many other processes by which this gas can be obtained.

Properties. Inodorous, colourless, tasteless, slightly soluble in water. 100 cubic inches weigh 30.34 grains. Difficultly inflammable—devoid of the power of supporting respiration or combustion. With oxygen it forms several compounds of great importance; two compound gases—nitrous oxide and nitric oxide; and three acids—hyponitrous, nitrous, and nitric acid; with hydrogen it forms ammonia; with carbon it produces cyanogen, the basis of Prussian blue. Nitrogen combines in the proportion of 14 parts by weight.

CHLORINE.

Chlorine, or the green gas, was discovered by Scheele in 1774. It exists in nature, chiefly in combination with sodium, with which it forms common salt.

If common salt, (chloride of sodium) be mixed with sulphuric acid and water (oxygen and hydrogen) as shewn in the first column, the second column denotes the result of the decomposition.

Common salt,	Chlorine, Sodium,	Chlorine, Hydrogen,	*Hydrochloric*, or *Muriatic* acid.
Water,	Oxygen, Hydrogen,	Sodium, Oxygen,	Soda, or oxide of sodium.
Sulphuric acid.			*Sulphate of Soda.*

The acid and soda unite, and form sulphate of soda. Muriatic acid gas (a compound of hydrogen and chlorine) is set free.

If peroxide of manganese be mixed with the preceding ingredients, oxygen is evolved. This gas unites with the hydrogen of the muriatic acid, and chlorine is liberated.

Properties.—Greenish colour; smell and taste exceedingly acrid and suffocating; absorbed by cold water—hence it is collected in bottles filled with hot or with salt-water; a supporter of the combustion of some metals, such as copper, zinc, antimony. With hydrogen in equal volumes forms an explosive mixture which, when inflamed by a taper or by the electric spark, or by exposure to the sun's rays, unites chemically and forms hydrochloric or muriatic acid. It bleaches animal and vegetable colours, and destroys all odoriferous principles—hence it is used for purifying prisons and hospitals.

Combining proportion, 35—100 cubic inches weigh 76 grs. Spec. gravity 2.47. Chlorine forms several very important compounds.

Chlorine	with	Sodium forms	Common salt.
,,	,,	Lime, ...	Bleaching powder.
,,	1 eq.	Mercury, ...	Calomel.
,,	½ an eq.	Mercury, ...	Corrosive sublimate.
,,	1 eq.	Hydrogen, ...	Muriatic acid.
,,	5 eq.	Oxygen, ...	Chloric acid.
,,	1 eq.	Antimony, ...	Butter of antimony.

and several other interesting substances; for instance, the chloride of nitrogen—the most dangerous of all explosive compounds.

SIMPLE SUBSTANCES.

SECOND DIVISION.

Simple Non-metallic Solids and Liquids.

CARBON.

Carbon is the elementary basis of charcoal, and of earth-coal—exists in a state of perfect purity in the diamond—united with oxygen in carbonic acid or choke-damp—and with hydrogen as carburetted hydrogen (fire-damp) it occurs in abundance in many situations.

Pure mineral carbon, or the diamond, is crystalline, transparent, colourless, of exceeding hardness, and is combustible in oxygen gas, forming carbonic acid. Of impure mineral carbon, or pit-coal, there are many varieties, of which the anthracite of miners is the one most free from foreign matters.

Vegetable carbon, or charcoal, is obtained by heating wood in close vessels.

Animal charcoal is procured by the similar treatment of various animal matters.

Carbon is insoluble in water, little affected by acids or alkalies, and does not rot on exposure to air or moisture. When finely divided it absorbs and destroys several colouring and odorous principles, and on account of this property it is much used by manufacturing druggists.

With oxygen, carbon forms two gaseous compounds—carbonic acid, and carbonic oxide, and a compound of both these and water, named oxalic acid. All these are powerful poisons. With hydrogen, it forms several inflammable gases and vapours, of which coal and oil gases are the best examples.

Carbonic acid is generated during respiration; by the combustion of animal and vegetable matter; and by decomposition or fermentation. 10,000 parts of common air contain four parts of this gas. It is extremely poisonous, but has nevertheless many useful applications in medicine and the arts, as described in the sequel of this work.

The combining equivalent of carbon is 6,12.

SULPHUR.

Sulphur is a yellow brittle solid, sometimes crystalline in its structure—fusible and volatile by a moderate heat. Sp. gr. 1.99. Occurs in the simple state in Nepal, Java, Persia, and many other countries, and is purified by sublimation; exists chiefly in combination with metals, especially lead, zinc, arsenic, mercury, iron, and copper; is combustible in air and oxygen, with which last it forms sulphurous and sulphuric acids; unites with hydrogen, forming a very fetid acid gas, of great use in chemistry, but very fatal to animal life. Sulphur exists also in many plants, such as the mustard—and in some animal matters, such as blood and the white of eggs.

Parts.				
16	Sulphur with	16	Oxygen form	Sulphurous* acid.
16	... ...	24	... ...	Sulphuric* acid.
32	... ...	16	... ...	Hypo-Sulphurous acid.
32	... ...	40	... ...	Hypo-Sulphuric* acid.
16	... ...	1	Hydrogen	Sulphuretted hydrogen gas*
32	... ...	202	Mercury....	Vermillion.

Of these the compounds marked * are important in pharmacy, and are minutely described in another part of the work.

IODINE.

A solid simple substance, of steel gray colour, very volatile, its vapour of a rich violet colour; smell heavy, and like that of sea-water; strikes a deep blue colour with solutions of starch.

Exists in combination with potassium, sodium, and hydrogen, in marine plants and animals, and in the waters of some seas.

The preparation of iodine is described in the Pharmacopœia. Equivalent 126—its vapour so dense that 100 cubic inches weigh 270 grs.

Iodine	with	Hydrogen forms	Hydriodic acid.
,,	,,	Potassium... ...	Ioduret of potassium.
,,	,,	Sodium	Ioduret of sodium.
,,	,,	Oxygen	Iodic acid.
,,	,,	Lead	Ioduret of lead.
		Mercury	Ioduret of mercury.

When iodine is left in contact with ammonia it unites with its nitrogen, and forms an explosive compound, of very dangerous properties.

PHOSPHORUS.

Phosphorus is a pale yellow solid like wax, exceedingly inflammable, and luminous in the dark. Exists in combination with oxygen and lime, in the bones of animals; when bones are burned phosphate of lime remains. This acted on by

Sulphuric acid, yields to it part of its lime, so that Bi-Phosphate of Lime is procured. Bi-Phosphate of Lime, heated with carbon, yields to it the oxygen of the Phosphoric acid, and the simple element Phosphorus is liberated. The process is difficult, and rarely succeeds on a small scale.

Combining equivalent 15.7. Specific gravity 1.7.

Phosphorus forms with oxygen several compounds, of which the Phosphoric acid is the most important.

With hydrogen it forms a gas which possesses the singular property of inflaming spontaneously when it comes in contact with air. This gas occurs naturally in a fountain at Chittagong, and is often seen in burial places and swampy grounds.

BORON.

Borax (the tincal or sohaga of Thibet) is a compound of boron, oxygen, and sodium. To obtain the simple substance, boracic acid is decomposed by the galvanic battery, or by potassium.

Colour dark brown—inflammable, oxydized by nitric acid. Combining equivalent 10.9.

Boron with oxygen forms Boracic acid.

... ... oxygen and soda, Borax.

Both these substances are subsequently described in the Pharmacopœia.

SELENIUM.

Selenium exists in association with metals. It is a very rare substance, of a leaden colour, and possessed of no very remarkable or useful properties; not employed in Pharmacy.

BROMINE.

Bromine resembles chlorine and iodine in its sources and properties. It is a brown-coloured liquid, obtained from the mother-water of sea-salt. Its vapour is irrespirable.

Sp. gr. 3—equivalent 78. With hydrogen it forms Hydro-Bromic acid,—with potassium, Bromide of potassium—both of value in Pharmacy. (Vide Pharmacopœia.)

FLUORINE.

This principle exists in fluor-spar, a mineral composed of fluorine and calcium, the metallic base of lime. It is a gas of a yellowish colour and exceedingly corrosive. It is separated in combination with hydrogen, by pouring sulphuric acid on powdered fluor-spar.

Fluorine has a powerful affinity for silicon, the basis of flints and of glass. Hence we derive a useful process for marking bottles and other glass vessels.

Coat the vessel with a thin layer of wax, on this with a needle trace the intended marks, and pour on sulphuric acid. Lastly, add powdered fluor-spar, and in about a quarter of an hour marks are traced on the vessel as if by a graver.

SIMPLE SUBSTANCES.

THIRD DIVISION.

The Metals.

Metals are simple combustible substances. They occur either "native," that is uncombined—or "mineralized," being associated with sulphur, chlorine, iodine, oxygen, &c. or as "alloys," that is, combined with each other in different proportions.

All metallic bodies are opaque, shining, good conductors of heat and electricity. Many are crystalline, especially antimony, zinc, bismuth, iron, and arsenic.

We subjoin a table of the specific gravities of the most important metals.

Platinum,	21.00
Gold,	19.30
Mercury,	13.50
Lead,	11.35
Silver,	10.47
Bismuth,	9.80
Copper,	8.89
Iron,	7.78
Tin,	7.30
Zinc.	7.00
Manganese,	6.85
Antimony,	6.70
Arsenic,	5.80
Sodium,	0.972
Potassium,	0.865

Some metals are *malleable*, or may be beaten out into thin leaves. Others, on the contrary, are very brittle. The malleable metals in the above list are gold, silver, copper, tin, platinum, lead, heated zinc, iron, potassium, sodium, and frozen mercury. The malleable metals are *ductile*, or may be drawn into wires. A grain of gold may be drawn into 500 feet of wire; gold, silver, platinum, iron, copper, zinc, tin, and lead, have this property in the order in which they are named.

The tenacity of metals varies much, iron being the strongest, copper next, and lead least in the power of supporting weights. Antimony, arsenic, bismuth, and manganese can be reduced to powder.

Action of Heat on Pharmaceutical Metals.

Mercury is fluid to	—	39° below zero.
Potassium melts at	+	140° above zero.
Sodium, ...	...	200°
Tin, ...	...	450°
Lead, ...	...	600°
Zinc, ...	...	700°
Antimony, ...	...	800°
Silver, gold, and copper a reddish white heat.		
Iron, ...	...	white heat.
Platinum, ...	...	requires the oxy. hydrogen blowpipe, or voltaic battery.

Arsenic volatilizes without melting at 400°.

Action of Oxygen on the Pharmaceutical Metals.

Potassium, and sodium, barium, manganese, and some others unite with oxygen very rapidly at common temperatures—lead, iron, and copper slowly oxidise by exposure to cold air, but very rapidly when heated to melting or redness. Platinum, gold, and silver, will not combine with oxygen at any temperature by simple exposure, even to the pure gas itself.

Some metals can reduce the oxides of others to the metallic state; thus, iron decomposes the oxides of potassium, and of mercury; potassium, the oxides of manganese, aluminium, &c.

Solutions of metallic salts are frequently decomposed by the insertion of another metal; thus,

Solution of	*Is reduced to the metallic state by*
Sulphate of copper,	Iron.
Nitrate of silver, ...	Mercury, zinc, copper.
Acetate of lead, ...	By zinc.
Nitrate of mercury,	By copper, &c. &c.

In these experiments the metal is often deposited in very fine crystals.

Oxygen is communicated to metals—by exposure to air, as potassium and sodium; by the action of nitric acid, as silver, copper, tin, and bismuth, in which case nitric oxide is set free, and a nitrate of the metal is formed; by decomposition of water, as in the process for making hydrogen; by deflagation with saltpetre, &c.—by the joint action of air and acids, as in the case of lead and acetic acid.

The oxides of several metals are decomposed or reduced by heat, as the peroxide of mercury, gold, silver and platinum—by precipitation by an alkali, as gold and platinum—by other metals, as potassa by iron—by carbon or hydrogen, as the oxides of arsenic, tin, antimony, bismuth, copper, silver, &c.—by electrical action—or by the action of light, —by heat and combustible matter, &c.

Oxides may be soluble or insoluble in water; of every colour; possessed of acid, or alkaline, or neutral properties—when basic they unite with acids, and thus constitute the class of bodies termed oxy-salts.

Chlorides of Metals.

Chlorine has a very powerful attraction for many metals—copper, antimony, bismuth, and arsenic in leaf or powder at common temperatures; mercury and iron when warm, take fire on being introduced into this gas. Chlorine at a red heat can even decompose many oxides, such as lime, magnesia, potash, and soda, oxygen being evolved, and a chloride of the metallic base obtained.

Most of the chlorides are soluble in water, are volatile, fusible, and crystalline, and in their structure and general properties resemble salts. Many are decomposed by hydrogen gas at a red heat, muriatic acid being formed. Some chlorides are decomposed by heat alone, all by hydrous sulphuric acid, or by charcoal if aided by heat and moisture. Solutions of chlorides give with solutions of salts of silver a white precipitate, the chloride of this metal.

When watery solutions of the alkalies or alkaline earths are heated with chlorine, iodine, or bromine, the water undergoes decomposition, and owing to a new arrangement of its elements, important changes take place which deserve attentive study. Thus—

If potassa (oxide of potassium,) be heated with water and chlorine, part of the water is decomposed into oxygen and hydrogen; and chloric acid (chlorine 1 = oxygen 5 =) and muriatic acid (chlorine 1 = hydrogen 1 =) are formed. These acids unite with the alkali potassa, and chlorate and muriate of that base are formed.

Chlorine unites with some oxides, such as lime and soda, with which it forms compounds, much used for their bleaching powers.

Iodurets of Metals.

Iodine is inferior to oxygen and chlorine in affinity for metals; metallic iodurets are therefore decomposed by chlorine; nevertheless some metallic oxides, viz. those of potassium, sodium, lead, and bismuth, are decomposed by iodine at a red heat, oxygen being set free and an ioduret of the metal formed. All other known iodurets are decomposed by oxygen under the like circumstances. All yield iodine when acted on by chlorine, bromine, sulphuric and nitric acid.

Iodine, boiled in watery solutions of alkalies, by the decomposition of the water, forms the iodate and hydriodate of the particular base.

Bromides of Metals.

Bromine has less affinity for metals than oxygen and more than iodine; with alkalies it forms bleaching compounds.

Sulphurets of Metals.

Sulphur may be made to combine with metals by direct union, as by fusing together copper or iron filings and sulphur. The two bodies combine in definite proportions with the evolution of heat and light. Or the vapour of sulphur may be passed over the metal heated to redness in a porcelain tube.

Some metallic oxides are decomposed by sulphur. Several salts, such as sulphate of soda, are brought to the state of sulphuret by being ignited in contact with hydrogen gas or carbon. Several metallic salts in solution, especially those of arsenic, antimony, copper, bismuth, and lead, are decomposed by sulphuretted hydrogen gas, or by solutions of alkaline sulphurets—and an insoluble precipitate of the sulphuret of the metal is formed. These precipitates assume different colours, such as yellow, orange, white, brown, and black—hence sulphuretted hydrogen is much used for testing in analysis.

Sulphuretted hydrogen gas is prepared by acting on the sulphuret of iron by dilute sulphuric acid; a bottle and bent tube are the only apparatus required. The gas is intolerably fœtid, and very detrimental to the health; experiments with it should therefore be performed in a well ventilated place. Sulphuret of iron is made by igniting together in a glass flask, a crucible, or earthen vessel, four parts of iron filings and two of sulphur by weight.

Native sulphurets of metals are mostly opaque, brittle, and crystalline; some of metallic lustre; all fusible; and those of arsenic and mercury, easily sublimed. Sulphur combines with metals in several proportions; any excess above one equivalent is generally expelled by heat. All sulphurets are decomposed by oxygen gas or air, if aided by heat or moisture; a metallic oxide, or sulphate, or the reduced metal being left. Hydrogen gas decomposes some sulphurets, the metal being left; of this, the sulphurets of antimony, bismuth, and silver, are examples.

Sulphur very rarely combines directly with metallic oxides.

If sulphur be boiled with water and an alkali or alkaline earth, changes occur analogous to those described under the head of Chlorine.

The water yields
Oxygen, to Sulphur, & forms Sulphurous & sulphuric acids.
Hydrogen ,, Sulphur, ,, ,, Sulphuretted hydrogen.

These three acids lastly unite with the alkali or earth, to form sulphite, sulphate and hydro-sulphuret of the base.

Chlorides, iodides, and sulphurets of metals when dissolved in water may exist in simple solution—or by decomposing the water, the non-metallic element may form an acid with the hydrogen—the metal an oxide with the oxygen.

CLASSIFICATION OF METALS.

The pharmaceutical metals may be arranged thus in two classes:—

CLASS I. By oxidation, yield alkalies and earths.
CLASS II. Yield oxides, neither alkalies nor earths.

CLASS I. *Order* 1.—Metallic bases of the alkalies—potassium, and sodium. These decompose water or even ice, attract its oxygen, and the first in doing so bursts into a flame. The alkalies saturate acids powerfully, and restore the blue colour of litmus paper previously reddened by acids.

Order 2. Metallic bases of the alkaline earths, barium, calcium, magnesium.

Order 3. Metallic bases of the earths, among which aluminium is the only one of interest in pharmacy.

CLASS II. *Order* 1.—Metals which decompose water at a red heat, viz. manganese, zinc, iron, and tin.

Order 2. Metals which do not decompose water at any temperature, and the oxides of which are not reduced by heat alone—arsenic, chromium, antimony, bismuth, copper, and lead.

Order 3. Metals, oxides of which are reduced by a red heat—mercury, silver, gold, platinum, &c.

TESTS OF METALS.

The tests by which the metals may be distinguished from each other are given under each special head in the division of this work which treats of the metallic medicinal preparations.

Organic Chemistry.

Organic Chemistry relates to the substances which have at any time been endowed with life, or which have been found as the products of previously animated things.

The essential constituents of organic matter are carbon, hydrogen, and oxygen; nitrogen is frequently present, especially in animal matters. Traces of inorganic matters, such as earths, metals, &c. are usually associated with the above named principles.

The apparently infinite variety of animal and vegetable products are thus traceable to a very few *ultimate* elements.

Substances possessed of specific and distinct properties, but still susceptible of ulterior decomposition, are termed *proximate* principles, such as sugar, gelatine, albumen, resin, gum, oil, &c.

As several very important considerations are involved in the proper arrangement of organic matter, and as this arrangement can only be duly based on a correct knowledge of the analysis of the varieties of organic compounds, we deem it necessary to give some details respecting the mode in which organic analysis is conducted, and the results to which it has led.

To ascertain the proportion of oxygen, hydrogen, carbon, and nitrogen in an organic matter, it is exposed to heat in a green glass tube with the oxide of copper and shreds of this metal.

Oxide of copper is prepared by dissolving copper in nitric acid, evaporating to dryness, and then heating the residue to redness in a platinum crucible. Oxide of copper is of a deep black colour, and 39 grains contain 8 oxygen, 31 copper.

This substance may be heated by itself to any degree, without losing its oxygen, but if organic matters be present, the following changes occur—

The *carbon* of the organic matter takes oxygen from the oxide of copper, and becomes *carbonic acid.*

The *hydrogen* with oxygen from the same source forms *water*.

The *oxygen* of the substance under analysis is either consumed in forming water and carbonic acid, with its hydrogen and carbon—or else is given off in the simple state. The nitrogen is either obtained free, or combined with oxygen; from the oxide of copper it becomes prot-oxide or bin-oxide of nitrogen. But these gases meeting with metallic copper at a red heat are decomposed, yielding pure nitrogen while oxide of copper is reproduced.

The weights of the water, carbonic acid, azote, and oxygen obtained, compared with the loss of weight of the oxide of copper, and the original weight of the substance analysed, afford the data for calculating its composition.

The weight of the water produced is known by leading the gases, as fast as formed, through a tube containing a known weight of dry chloride of calcium. This substance attracts moisture with great force; the increase of weight indicates the quantity of water absorbed.

After passing through the chloride of calcium, the dried gases are led through bulbs containing a strong solution of potash. This absorbs the carbonic acid, and the increase of its weight shews the quantity formed.

Lastly, the nitrogen and oxygen not being absorbed by chloride of calcium, or solution of potash, pass on and are collected in a graduated jar over mercury.

The proportion of nitrogen to the oxygen may be ascertained in several ways, of which the following is the best.

Take one-tenth of a cubic inch of the mixture; introduce an excess of pure hydrogen, say two-tenths—pass the electric spark. If there be no diminution in volume, there can be no oxygen present. Should the hydrogen inflame, and diminution ensue, one-third of this denotes the proportion of oxygen present, for two volumes of hydrogen unite with one volume of oxygen to form water, which is condensed within the tube.

The sketch shews the whole arrangement; *a*, the tube containing the subject of analysis, the copper and its oxide; *b*, a charcoal furnace for heating the tube to redness; *c*, the tube containing the chloride of calcium; *d*, the bulbs containing potash; *e*, the jar for receiving the oxygen and azote. (*Fig.* 55.)

Although the theory of this process is exceedingly simple, its experimental details are the most difficult and complex in which the practical chemist can possibly engage.

PROXIMATE VEGETABLE PRINCIPLES.

We proceed to enumerate the principal proximate constituents of vegetable matters, describing their leading properties, but reserving minute details for the sequel of this work. The present outline will suffice to render many descriptions of such vegetable products as may occur in the Materia Medica, much more intelligible than they otherwise could be.

Gum.

Gum is a very abundant substance, which exudes from the barks of several trees, for example, the babul of India. Gum-Arabic is the best instance of this principle.

Mucilage is gum dissolved or suspended in water.

Gum, or mucilage, exudes in a semi-liquid state, hardens by exposure to air and heat, is transparent, colourless, or tinged of a reddish brown; soluble in water and acetic acid, insoluble in alcohol and ether; combines in definite proportions with the oxide of lead.

Composition,	Carbon, ...	41.4
	Hydrogen, ...	6.5
	Oxygen, ...	52.1
		100.0

Pectin.

Pectin is the principle of the jelly of fruits, such, for example, as that yielded by the corunda of Bengal, (carissa corundas,) the mango, and other fruits.

It is procured by adding alcohol to the expressed juice of the fruit, collecting and drying the gelatinous precipitate. This is very soluble in hot water, the solution thickens as it cools; insoluble in alcohol and ether; boiled with alkaline solutions, it assumes acid qualities, and a pectate of the base is formed.

Sugar.

Sugar is the sweet principle of the cane, the beet root, and of numerous fruits and vegetable juices.

There are many varieties of sugar. The pure chemical principle is white, crystalline, soluble in water and in alcohol. Sp. gr. 1.5; when the solution is mixed with some animal matters or with ferment it is decomposed, and alcohol and carbonic acid are formed. Sugar is changed into *gum* by alkalies; fusible by heat.

Crystallized sugar contains 1 eq. of water. Deducting this, sugar contains,

Carbon, ...	42.85
Oxygen, ...	50.80
Hydrogen, ...	6.35
	100.0

Starch.

Starch is contained in all the grains used as food, in many roots, (potatoes, onions, arrow-root) especially those of the tuberous form—in the stems of some palms (sago), in several lichens, as the Ceylon moss, &c. &c.

Pure starch is obtained by washing in water wheat-flour tied loosely in a muslin bag. The starch is washed through, and collects as a white powder.

Dried starch is white, pulverulent, crystalline, sp. gr. 1.5, insoluble in cold, very soluble in hot water, which retains it dissolved on cooling. Insoluble in alcohol and ether. The cold aqueous solution is turned blue by iodine. Starch may be, by several processes, converted into sugar.

Composition,	Oxygen, ...	50.85
	Carbon, ...	42.80
	Hydrogen, ...	6.35
		100.0

Gluten and Albumen.

Gluten is found in several seeds and vegetable juices. It is most readily obtained from wheat flour; in the process for making starch it remains within the cloth through which the starch passes.

Gluten is solid and opaque, not crystallizable, insoluble in water. While moist it is very ductile and tenacious,—it is soluble in boiling alcohol, and is also dissolved by some of the acids and alkalies. When dry it is transparent and brittle—moistened and rubbed with the resin of guaiacum it acquires a deep green colour. This principle is sometimes called *Gliadine.*

Vegetable albumen is associated with gluten in wheat, and many other substances. It is not dissolved by boiling alcohol. When contained in the natural juices of a plant it solidifies or coagulates when exposed to a heat of 180°. The coagulated albumen cannot be redissolved in water. The juice of the papaya fruit *(Carica papaya)* is very rich in this principle.

Composition,		
	Carbon, ...	55.7
	Hydrogen, ...	7.8
	Oxygen, ...	22.0
	Nitrogen, ...	14.5
		100.0

Owing to the presence of nitrogen, gluten is extremely nutritious. It is also very liable to rot, and during putrefaction evolves ammonia (hydrogen, nitrogen) cyanogen (nitrogen, carbon) and other gases of peculiarly offensive smell.

Lignin.

Lignin is the woody fibre of vegetables, and composes the bulk of woods of every kind.

After all other principles are separated from wood the residue constitutes this principle.

Composition,		
	Carbon, ...	49.80
	Hydrogen, ...	5.58
	Oxygen, ...	44.44

Equal to 3 = Carbon,
2 = Hydrogen,
2 = Oxygen,
or 3 Carbon and 2 water.

Vegetable Extractive.

This term applies most strictly to the brown matter extracted by water from peat and turf. It is also called gein, humine, or ulmin. It exists in many barks, and other vegetable substances, and is sometimes of an intensely bitter taste.

Bitter vegetable extractive is scarcely entitled to be considered a peculiar principle, and all its varieties very probably contain some more definite compound.

Colouring Principles.

Of these the most important are the reds, yellows, and blues.

Red Colouring Principles.

Madder, safflower, brazil, log-wood, and sapan wood, red saunders wood, alkanet, and litmus, are the most important varieties of the vegetable red. The cochineal and lac insects are the most valuable from the animal kingdom. All these articles have a place in the Pharmacopœia.

Yellow Colouring Principles.

Of these there are several varieties, of which we may notice the turmeric, saffron, annatto, barberry, and mishmeteeta, as occurring in the Pharmacopœia.

Blues.

The blue juices of the red cabbage, and the flower of the hibiscus (or shoe-flower) are very fugitive, being readily changed to red by the acids, and to green by the alkalies. Indigo is, on the contrary, a very permanent colour, and the most valuable of all vegetable dyes.

Details relative to several of these principles will be given in the body of the work.

Fixed oils.

These are ternary compounds of carbon, hydrogen, and oxygen, the two former principles much predominating. They are exceedingly combustible. Oils are fixed or volatile.

The fixed oils are obtained by expression, chiefly from seeds, as the almond, castor, croton, arachis, sesamum, &c. The sp. gravity varies from 0.918 to 0.936. They are all insoluble in water, and mostly in alcohol; some however dissolve in this fluid. All are dissolved by sulphuric ether.

Several oils are frozen at moderately low temperatures. If subjected to pressure in this state, a solid matter is obtained, termed *stearine*, and a fluid passes through termed *elaine*.

Several oils absorb oxygen from the air, and dry into a resinous substance; linseed, poppy, walnut, and hemp seed oil are of this kind, and are called drying oils.

The fixed oils cannot be volatilized without decomposition, which occurs at 600° Fahr.

The fixed alkalies convert these oils into soaps. By sulphuric and nitric acid, assisted by heat, they are altogether decomposed.

Exposed to a red heat they are all decomposed, and various inflammable gases, composed of carbon and hydrogen, are evolved in great abundance.

All oils differ in their composition, as well as in their secondary properties. The composition usually approaches the subjoined average,

Carbon, ...	77
Oxygen, ...	10
Hydrogen, ...	13
	100

Wax.

The berries of the ***Myrica cerifera*** afford this principle by boiling in water. It is best known however in the form of bees' wax, as collected by that animal, or secreted in its system.

Pure wax is white, insipid, and inodorous. Sp. gr. 96°, insoluble in water, fusible at 150°, and may be distilled nearly unchanged. Very inflammable. Partially soluble in boiling alcohol and ether, dissolved by all fixed and some volatile oils, with which it forms several medicinal ointments. It is but little acted upon by the mineral acids.

Wax contains,	Carbon, ...	81.784
	Hydrogen, ...	12.672
	Oxygen, ...	5.544
		100.000.

Volatile Oils.—Benzule.

Volatile oils exist in many vegetables; are obtained by distillation, or expression; they are generally of strong odour, very inflammable, very soluble in alcohol and ether, and but slightly in water; volatile about 212°.

Some volatile oils consist of carbon and hydrogen alone; for instance, the essential oils of turpentine, copaiba, of lemons, and of gurjun-balsam. These by combination with oxygen generate camphor.

The other essential oils are chiefly oxides of carbon and hydrogen, and are analogous in composition to solutions of camphor in liquid hydro-carbon.

The oil of bitter almonds rapidly absorbs oxygen, with which it forms benzoic acid. This oil is consequently inferred to be a compound of hydrogen and a principle named *benzule*.

Benzule unites with hydrogen, chlorine, oxygen, sulphur, bromine, iodine, &c. and forms very interesting compounds, which will be subsequently described.

Resins.

Resins are either natural exudations, or are obtained from some vegetable compounds by the aid of alcohol, in which they are freely soluble; in water they are altogether insoluble; they are brittle, tasteless, electric when rubbed, fusible at a moderate heat, soluble in the fixed and volatile oils, and some in the muriatic and acetic acids. They unite with alkalies, and with the oxides of some metals form insoluble compounds, several of which are much used as plasters.

Resin consists of carbon, hydrogen, and oxygen in variable proportions. Some resins are acid, and form definite crystallizable compounds with alkaline bases or oxides.

Dammer affords a good example of this class of bodies.

Caoutchouc.

Caoutchouc, or Indian rubber, is obtained from several South American and Indian trees.

It exudes as a milky juice which soon thickens into a dark, very elastic solid. It is insoluble in alcohol and water, but is softened and dissolved by ether, by naptha, pure oil of turpentine, gurjun-balsam, &c. Acids and alkalies affect it very little. It is very inflammable, and fuses at about 600°. On distillation it yields a liquid hydro-carbon called caoutchoucine, which dissolves caoutchouc, and many resins and varnishes.

Caoutchouc owing to its impermeability to moisture, its flexibility, and elasticity, and cheapness, and the ease with which it may be cut or spun into various forms and fabrics, is an article of the highest importance in several arts and manufactures.

VEGETABLE ACIDS.

The principal acids of vegetable origin are the acetic, tartaric, oxalic, citric, malic, benzoic, and hydrocyanic.

The tartaric acid exists chiefly in grapes and tamarinds; the oxalic acid in sorrel; the citric acid in lemons; the malic in apples; the benzoic in benjamin or loban; the hydrocyanic in the kernels of peaches, or bitter almonds, &c. &c.

The acetic acid, or vinegar acid, is minutely described in the Pharmacopœia.

Tannic and Gallic Acids.

These acids constitute the active principle of astringent vegetables, such as catechu, gall-nuts, babul bark, &c.

The process for preparing tannic acid is given under the head of "Nut-galls." Its properties require notice here. It is exceedingly astringent to the taste, reddens vegetable blues, decomposes alkaline carbonates with effervescence. In solutions of animal gelatine it forms an abundant precipitate, termed *tanno-gelatine*, the basis of leather; with the salts of the protoxide of iron it causes no precipitate; with the salts of the peroxide an abundant one of dark blue colour. It causes copious precipitates in solutions of the vegetable alkalies.

Tannic acid is composed of,

Carbon, ...	50.70
Hydrogen, ...	4,23
Oxygen, ...	45.07
	100.00

Gallic Acid.

Gallic acid generally co-exists with the tannic, or is formed by oxydation of the latter, when this is long exposed to air and moisture.

Gallic acid crystallizes in needles; is soluble in alcohol, ether, and water; does not precipitate solutions of gelatine. With per-sulphate of iron, it produces a dark blue precipitate.

Gallic acid is composed of,

Carbon, ...	49.4
Hydrogen,...	3.6
Oxygen, ...	47.0
	100

The gallic and tannic acid are of importance, in consequence of the frequency of their occurrence in vegetable analysis, and the numerous coloured precipitates they occasion in metallic solutions.

The other acids above named are fully described in the Pharmacopœia.

VEGETABLE ALKALIES.

This most important class of bodies possesses the common property of saturating acids, with which they form salts. They all contain nitrogen; nearly all are crystallizable; they are usually bitter, or form bitter salts. All their salts are decomposed by the mineral alkalies, by ammonia, and the alkaline earths. The most remarkable are,

Quinia, Cinchonia, Aricina,	obtained from,... ...	Peruvian bark.
Morphia, Anarcotina,	... ...	Opium.
Strychnia, Brucia,	... ...	Koochila nuts & bark.
Aconitina,	... ...	Aconite.
Nicotina,	... ...	Tobacco.
Atropia,	... ...	Deadly nightshade.
Daturia,	... ...	Stramonium.
Conia,	... ...	Hemlock.

NON-SALIFIABLE CRYSTALLINE BODIES.

Of these the most important are,

Salicine,	... ...obtained from	Willow bark.
Piperine,	... ...	Pepper.
Caffeine,	... ...	Coffee.
Plumbagine,	... ...	Lalchitra.
Cathartin,	... ...	Senna.
Colocynthin,	... ...	Colocynth.
Elatin,	... ...	Elaterium.
Rhein and Rhabarbarin,	... ...	Rhubarb.
Canellin,	... ...	Canella leaves.
Gentianin,	... ...	Gentian & chiretta.
Berberin,	... ...	Rasout.
Corydallin,	... ...	Corydalis goviniana.

Animal Matters.

Animal matters, whether solid or fluid, are chiefly composed of carbon, oxygen, hydrogen, and nitrogen, sometimes sulphur occurs, and there are variable proportions of metallic oxides and earthy salts.

The analysis of animal matter is carried on in the same manner as described with reference to vegetables.

The proximate principles of animal matter are few, and of but little importance to the practical druggist. The points, moreover, to which the attention of the medical student should be directed, are fully dwelt on in chemical treatises.

The Blood.

Human blood is a very complex fluid.

It consists according to Lecanu's statements, of the following ingredients—

Water,...	780.145
Fibrine,...	2.100
Colouring matter, ...	133.000
Albumen, ...	65.090
Fat, crystalline, ...	2.430
Ditto, oily, ...	1.310
Extractive, soluble in water and alcohol, ...	1.790
Albumen with soda, ...	1.265
Chlorides of sodium, with, Carbonates, Phosphates, Sulphates, of soda & potassa,	8.370
Carbonate of lime & magnesia, Phosphate of lime, magnesia, & iron, ... Peroxide of iron, ...	2.100
Loss, ...	2.400
	1000.000

Blood, as drawn from a vein in bleeding, is of a dark red colour and uniform liquid consistence; temperature 98°. Specific gravity from 1,050 to 1,070. Soon after being drawn the blood coagulates, and separates into two parts, one liquid and colourless, termed *serum*, the other red and solid, called *crassamentum*, or clot.

100 parts of *serum* consist of water 90, albumen 7.6, saline and albuminous matter 2.4. Its specific gravity is 1,130. Owing to its containing soda, it is alkaline to test papers.

The *crassamentum* consists of solidified fibrine, involving the colouring particles or *globules*, and holding also a large quantity of serum diffused through it like water in a sponge. The colouring particles being heavier than the serum, often subside through the clot, leaving its surface of a pale yellow colour. This appearance is called the "buffy coat," and is remarkably indicative of inflammatory action in the system.

The *serum* is solidified by the temperature of 180°, by several acids, by alcohol, corrosive sublimate, and prussiate of potash. These phenomena depend on the albumen of this fluid.

The *fibrine* is the spontaneously coagulable principle of the blood. Like albumen, once solidified it is not again soluble in water.

The *colouring matter* is a peculiar animal dye, and does not derive its colour from iron, as was long supposed.

Iron nevertheless may be detected in the blood by drying and burning that fluid, and acting on the ashes by dilute sulphuric acid, which dissolves the iron. With the tests of prussiate of potash and tannic acid the presence of this metal is shewn by the blue and black precipitates produced.

The blood is altered remarkably in some diseases;—thus in cholera its aqueous parts pass off, and it becomes thick. Much of its saline matter is also thrown off. The peculiar principle of the urine (urea) at the same time rapidly accumulates in the blood, and causes serious disturbance in the system.

In scurvy, on the contrary, the aqueous portions of the blood predominate, the solid being much deficient.

Blood differs in colour if drawn from an artery or vein; from the former it is of bright scarlet, from the latter of a deep crimson colour. Venous blood also contains carbonic acid, which has not yet been detected in arterial blood.

Blood when exposed to the air in thin layers at common temperatures, dries without coagulation, and may be detected on linen or iron by the following tests—

1. The stain washed with distilled water gives a blood red liquid, and leaves a fibrous whitish substance (fibrine).
2. The red fluid coagulates if heated to 180° (albumen).
3. Both the solid and fluid dried and reduced to ashes in a platinum crucible, give indications of iron with prussiate of potash and tannic acid.

Milk—Curd and Whey.

Milk varies slightly in composition, according to the animal from which it is procured, and even from the same animal, according to age, health, &c.

Milk is a white opaque fluid, sp. gr. 1,030, of sweet taste. It contains several substances, such as water, oil, butter, sugar, curd, mucus, and various salts.

The curd of milk, or caseum, resembles albumen in several of its properties. It is separated from milk by acids, in the solid state; it is not coagulable by heat unless aided by the action of an acid. Caseum is the basis of cheese, contains nitrogen, and is highly nutritious.

When the butter and caseum are removed from milk the residual liquor is termed *whey*. This fluid contains a crystalline substance, termed *sugar of milk*. Whey is an excellent drink for sick persons, and directions for its preparation will be found in the Pharmacopœia.

Milk readily absorbs oxygen from the air, and becomes sour in consequence of lactic acid being formed. Perfectly fresh milk dried below 120° retains its solubility in water, and constitutes an excellent article of food.

Bile—Gall-stones.

Bile is a greenish yellow, bitter, alkaline fluid, composed as follows,

Water, ...	90.44
Biliary matter, picromel, ...	8.00
Mucus, ...	0.30
Extractive, common salt, and lactate of soda, ...	0.74
Soda, ...	0.41
Phosphate of soda and lime and a substance insoluble in alcohol,	0.11
	100.00

Gall-stones are formed of the several ingredients of the bile, with a quantity of a fatty crystalline principle termed *cholesterine*. This principle is soluble in hot alcohol, from which it crystallizes on cooling.

Saliva.

Saliva is a very complex fluid, consisting of water, mucus, traces of albumen, and several saline matters. Its specific gravity is 1.004. It sometimes contains free acetic acid.

Gastric Juice.

The fluid of the stomach secreted during digestion is called gastric juice. It contains free muriatic acid and acetic acid, but its exact chemical nature is not clearly understood.

Pus.

Pus is the yellow fluid secreted by inflamed and ulcerated surfaces. Sp. gr. 1.030. It much resembles mucus and liquid albumen, from which it can scarcely be distinguished in mixed fluids.

Urine.—Urea.

Urine is composed of water, urea, uric acid, traces of albumen—phosphoric acid in excess, combined with lime, phosphates of soda, ammonia, and magnesia,—common salt, and sulphate of soda, mucus, colouring matter, &c. The density is very variable—from 1.000 to 1.040, but it is generally in healthy persons 1.029. Urine putrifies very rapidly, disengaging an abundance of ammoniacal products. 1000 parts contain water 933, urea 30.

Urea is a white crystalline organic principle, soluble in alcohol and water, and composed of, carbon 1, hydrogen 2, oxygen 1, nitrogen 1—equivalents. Two equivalents of urea contain the same ingredients, in the same proportion, as one eq. of hydrated cyanate of ammonia. Artificial cyanate of ammonia indeed possesses all the properties of pure urea.

In some diseases the urea is decomposed, and renders the urine exceedingly ammoniacal.

Uric Acid.—Diabetic Sugar.

This acid exists in small quantity, combined with soda in healthy urine. In the pure state it is insoluble in water; from its alkaline compounds it is precipitated by acids. When this occurs in the human bladder a stone or calculus is often formed, which lays the foundation of a formidable, and frequently fatal disease.

In inflammation of the kidneys, and in some dropsies, the urine contains so much albumen that it coagulates on being boiled.

In diabetes, urine contains a large quantity of sugar, which may be fermented, and will yield alcohol.

In cholera the urine is entirely suppressed, and its peculiar principle, urea, is formed in large quantity in the blood.

Several medicinal agents enter the circulation, and pass off by the urine either in the same state as they were taken, or decomposed into new combinations. For several interesting examples of this fact, the reader is referred to the section on Diureties.

Urinary Sand—Gravel—Stone.

Urinary sand is of two kinds, the *white* and *red.*

White sand consists of phosphate of lime, or phosphate of ammonia and magnesia, or mixtures of both these salts, and is soluble in acids.

Red sand is composed chiefly of the uric acid, and is soluble in alkalies.

Urinary gravel or stones are chiefly composed—

1. Of phosphate of lime—white, smooth, soluble in acids, infusible before the blowpipe.
2. Phosphate of ammonia, and magnesia—soluble in acids, gives off ammonia by alkalies, and before the blowpipe.
3. Carbonate of lime—soluble in some acids, of rare occurrence.
4. Uric acid—soluble in alkalies, destroyed by ignition.
5. Urate of ammonia, &c. &c.
6. Oxalate of lime—rough, brown, insoluble in acids or alkalies, changed by the blowpipe into carbonate of lime, and ultimately into caustic lime.
7. and 8. Cystic oxide and silica—very rare.

Gelatine.

Gelatine is the peculiar principle of animal jellies. See Isinglass, (*Pharmacopœia.*)

Animal Fat.

Animal fat and oils, in ultimate and proximate composition and in properties so closely resemble those of vegetable origin, that it is sufficient to name them in this place; their most important applications in pharmacy will be afterwards described.

Shell and Bone.

Shells are composed of carbonate of lime and gelatine.

Bones contain phosphate of lime, some carbonate of the same base, and gelatine.

By acting on bones with dilute muriatic acid the earthy matter is dissolved, and the gelatine remains.

Pearls and shell are identical in composition. The enamel of the teeth contains phosphate of lime 78, carbonate of lime 6, gelatine 16, in 100 parts.

When bones are distilled in close vessels, the decomposition of the gelatine leads to the production of ammonia, water, carbonic acid, and fetid oil—and charcoal and phosphate of lime remain in the state termed *ivory black*.

The foregoing Epitome of Chemistry, if practically studied and understood, is sufficient to prepare the pharmaceutical student to comprehend most of the chemical details in the ensuing pages.

We have next to give a brief sketch of the subject of Electricity in its various forms, in order to enable the student to understand some of the numerous applications of this extraordinary agent in the manipulations of Chemistry, and in the treatment of disease.

Electricity.

Electricity derives its name from the earliest phenomena of its nature having been observed in amber (electrum) which when rubbed with woollen cloth, was observed to acquire the power of attracting and repelling light particles of paper, dust, feathers, &c.

More intimate knowledge of the effects of this power enables us to cause it to produce vivid sparks, intense light and heat, to effect chemical decomposition, occasion violent commotions in the bodies of living or recently dead animals, to excite magnetism in steel and iron, and, to produce numerous and extraordinary movements in material substances.

These phenomena are exhibited by various means, and under different forms.

1. *Mechanical*—by the friction of glass, silk, resin, caoutchouc, amber, sulphur, &c.

2. *Chemical*—by chemical action upon metals and other substances.

3. *Magnetic*—by the action of natural or artificial magnets.

4. *Calorific*—by the influence of unequal temperature on metals and other solid bodies.

5. *Vital*—by various electrical animals, as the torpedo, electrical eel, &c. &c.

FRICTIONAL OR MECHANICAL ELECTRICITY.

A piece of glass, or a stick of lac or sealing-wax, or a roll of sulphur, if rubbed on woollen cloth or silk, immediately becomes capable of *attracting* light bodies, as before described.

The substance attracted is immediately repelled with equal force, and is not again attracted until it comes in contact with the earth, with moist air, with metallic bodies, animals, &c. when it is again attracted and repelled as before.

It is observed that the substance which is attracted by rubbed glass is repelled by the other bodies above mentioned if also excited by friction—namely by sulphur, resin, lac.

A feather suspended by a silk thread, will thus be alternately attracted and repelled between a plate of glass and a stick of wax, each excited by friction.

Two kinds of electricity, the glassy, and the resinous, are thus distinguished.

A large plate of glass or ball of resin strongly excited by friction retains its electrical activity for a very long time in dry air, provided it be suspended by silk, or supported on glass, resin, sulphur, very dry wood, &c. On the other hand, if it communicate with the ground by the human body, by metals, moist air, water, charcoal, and many other substances, the electrical excitement immediately ceases.

The former bodies are called insulators, or non-conductors; the latter, conductors of electricity.

We subjoin the most important of each class.

Non-Conductors.	*Conductors.*
Lac.	Metals.
Resins.	Animals.
Sulphur.	Acid and saline solutions.
Glass.	Water.
Silk.	Living vegetables.
Caoutchouc.	Damp air.
Dry wood.	Several flames.
Dry air.	

Electrical machines have been constructed which exhibit in a very striking manner the phenomena above described.

Two glass machines are chiefly used, the plate and cylinder, of which drawings are given. The plate or cylinder is turned by a winch, or multiplying wheel, and as it revolves is rubbed by a silken cushion slightly covered with an amalgam of mercury and tin; a bent brass bar, termed the "prime conductor," is adjusted to the stand on which the glass is mounted.

This prime conductor being insulated on glass receivers, retains the electricity of the glass plate or globe. It attracts and repels all light bodies, and if conductors be brought near it gives off a bright spark with a sharp snapping noise. If a pair of light sola balls be suspended by thread from the conductor they diverge widely. (*See figs.* 56, 57.)

Electrical Induction.

If a metallic bar be suspended by silk, and brought near the prime conductor at such a distance that no spark may pass, the bar shows signs of electrical excitement, as proved by the divergence of sola balls hung at each end. That the excitement is confined to the opposite ends is proved by the quiescence of the central balls.

If while in the excited state we bring an excited glass tube near the balls at the end furthest from the prime conductor, they are immediately repelled, shewing that their electricity is of the vitreous, or positive kind. If the glass rod be brought near the end next the conductor, the balls are attracted, shewing the electricity to be resinous or negative.

Electrical bodies are consequently when excited capable of *inducing* temporary excitement in adjacent good conductors—and the excitement is of two kinds, the surface next the primary exciter being in a different state of electricity, the surface distant from it being in the same state.

This is called electrical induction, and proceeds from the operation of the law, that similarly electrified bodies repel, and dissimilarly attract each other.

The Leyden Jar.

This extraordinary instrument was invented in Leyden, whence it derives its name. (*Fig.* 58)

It consists of a common glass jar, on both sides of which tinfoil is pasted to within two inches of the top. Through the cork passes a wire which comes in contact with the inner coating, and externally terminates in a metallic knob.

The *inner* coating being in contact with the prime conductor, participates in its excitement, and becomes highly charged with vitreous electricity.

The outer coating has two surfaces, one next, one furthest from the glass. Owing to the influence of *induction* through the glass, the electric excitement takes place in the whole of the outer metallic coating. As similar electricities repel each other, the positive state of the inner lining causes the *outer* surface of the outer coat to become *positive* also. Accordingly for every spark which passes from the prime conductor into the jar, one passes from the outer surface of the outer coat of the bottle to any conductor in its vicinity.

The charge on the inner coating accumulates and is retained, in consequence of the proximity of a surface of metal dissimilarly electrified and separated by a non-conductor of glass.

If in this state a conductor be interposed between the inner and outer coatings, the whole of the dissimilar electricities unite with a violent discharge, aloud detonation, and a brilliant flash. If this discharge be passed through animals they suffer violent shocks, or even life may be destroyed.

A series of such jars is called the Leyden Battery. By the discharge of a numerous series, metals are fused and dispersed, animals destroyed, and all the phenomena of miniature lightning exhibited.

That the electricity given off from the outer coating is of the same kind as that received by the inner from the prime conductor, is shewn by the following experiments.

Insulate the jar on a glass stand, pass sparks to its inner coating from the prime conductor, and let the corresponding sparks from the outer coating pass to the inner coating of a second jar. It will be found that the inner sides of both jars attract or repell the same objects, and are therefore in the same electrical state.

Several very beautiful experiments are exhibited by lecturers in demonstration of this principle.

Influence of Points, &c. in removing electrical excitement.

If a pointed wire or a lighted taper be held in the vicinity of the prime conductor, the whole of its excitement almost immediately disappears, and if the experiment be performed in darkness, a star or brush of flame is seen on the point.

On this principle it is that lightning conductors are attached to buildings. The electric clouds lose their excitement by the influence of the pointed metallic bars.

If the quantity or intensity of the electricity be too great, an explosive discharge may take place to the point, as is often seen in thunder storms, when the lightning strikes the conductors, although properly constructed.

Owing to the inductive influence of heated air and flame, lightning often strikes the chimnies of factories and even of private buildings.

Electrometers.

The intensity of electricity is estimated in various ways.

By the *quadrant electrometer*—consisting of a pith ball attached to a light stem of wood moving in the centre of a graduated arc. The ball participates in the electrical excitement of whatever it is attached to, is repelled, and the amount of repulsion is read off on the index. Thus in charging a jar the electrometer is inserted into the knob communicating with the inner coating, (*Fig.* 58.)

The *discharging electrometer* is a graduated metallic rod, supported on a bent glass stem. The distance through which the spark or explosion passes is taken as the index of its quantity.

The *balance electrometer* shews the amount of the electric accumulation by the distance through which a known weight is attracted. A very accurate instrument of this kind has been invented by Mr. Harris.

To pass shocks through a patient, the outer coating of a Leyden jar, of the size judged expedient, is brought into metallic connection with the part through which the discharge is to be directed. By leading a chain or wire from any adjacent part to the inner coating, the discharge passes in the interval.

In these experiments a discharging rod is sometimes used. The instrument consists of two brass rods, terminating in balls moving in a universal joint, and mounted on a glass handle. (*Fig.* 59.)

By placing a person on a stool mounted on glass legs, if he touches the prime conductor he participates in its excitement, his hair stands on end, he gives out sparks to any adjacent body, can charge the Leyden bottle, inflame combustible bodies, and exhibit many other surprizing phenomena. This arrangement is often had recourse to in the treatment of paralysis, and nervous diseases—sparks being drawn from the affected part.

The laws of the distribution of electricity, its effects in vacuô, &c. belong to general physics, and do not claim consideration in this work.

CHEMICAL ELECTRICAL EXCITEMENT.

Simple Galvanic or Voltaic Circle.

Chemical action on metals gives rise to electrical excitement of great power, and of many peculiar properties. To obtain experimental evidence of the existence of this state, two metals are employed, one *not* acted upon by the chemical agent.

The proofs of electrical excitement of the metals, are afforded by conductors attached to the metals. These conductors are found to be capable of affording sparks, effecting chemical decomposition, producing shocks, and deflecting the magnetic needle from its natural position of north and south.

The most convenient mode of exhibiting this excitement in its simplest form, is by the use of amalgamated zinc, platinum wire, and dilute sulphuric acid.

Amalgamated zinc is prepared by rubbing metallic mercury over zinc previously moistened with dilute sulphuric acid. Such zinc is not dissolved or corroded by any quantity of dilute sulphuric acid. But if a piece of platinum, gold, or copper be introduced into the acid mixture, and made to touch the zinc, water is immediately decomposed, hydrogen escapes in abundance, and sulphate of zinc is formed.

The same occurs if the metals do not touch in the acid, but are connected by a wire out of the acid, as shewn in *fig*. 60.

If the wire be divided, the extremities are found to be in opposite electrical states, corresponding to the vitreous (positive) and resinous (negative) excitement in frictional electricity. This arrangement is called a simple galvanic circle.

If the ends of the divided wire be dipped in a drop of a solution of ioduret of lead or hydrochloric acid, these substances are decomposed; chlorine and iodine appearing at the wire in connexion with the zinc; hydrogen and lead appearing at the wire in connexion with the platinum, gold, or copper.

If the connecting wire be made to pass in a straight direction N. and S. above and below a magnetic needle, the needle is deflected, and points east and west.

If instead of taking but one turn, the conducting wire be coated with silk or resin to prevent lateral escape of electricity, and then be made to turn repeatedly round the needle, the effects are very much increased in delicacy. Coils of such construction are separately made, and have each of the ends of the wire led into a little cup containing mercury, to form a metallic connexion. The detached instrument is called the galvanometer.

If the conducting wires *z. p.* be made to change directions with respect to the ends of the galvanometer—for example, if *z.* be led to the mercury cup, *a.* instead of *b.* and if *p.* be led to *b.* instead of *a*, the magnetic needle immediately turns in the opposite direction, and its north pole points to W. instead of E. *(Figs.* 61, 62.*)*

If the conducting wire covered by silk be wound into a close spiral (helix)—and if by drawing out into a straight line the middle turn of the helix the ends be bent down, as shewn in the drawing *fig.* 63—additional, and very interesting magnetic powers of the conductor are observable.

If a common needle be introduced into each helix with the points in the same direction, the needles immediately become magnets, but the point of one has a north, and the other a south pole. This polarity may be reversed by changing the connexions of the conducting wires, as before described.

If the helix be made to surround the legs of a bar of soft iron bent into a horse-shoe form, this instantly becomes a powerful magnet, and will support enormous weights so long as it is in connexion with the plates. The legs of the temporary magnet are respectively north and south in polarity. This may be changed by reversing the connexions, and the magnetism disappears when the contact with the plates is broken, and the iron between the legs of the magnet removed.

Magnets have been constructed on this principle capable of supporting two tons weight.

Lastly, a single pair of plates of very large dimensions has great heating powers, the connecting wires becoming ignited, and even fused.

Such are the leading effects a single pair of plates can produce. When several pairs are connected, the effects become more than proportionally enhanced, and that most magnificent of all instruments, the *Compound Galvanic Battery*, is formed.

Compound Galvanic Batteries.

We shall give a brief account of the chief varieties of this apparatus.

Volta's Pile is the earliest instrument, and is called after the illustrious discoverer of this species of electricity. It consists of a series of discs of zinc and copper soldered together. A piece of cloth soaked in dilute sulphuric acid, or in solution of common salt or sal-ammoniac, is placed between each pair of discs. The whole is arranged one above the other, so that all the zinc surfaces have the same aspect. A wire is attached to the last plate above, and to that below, and these form the conductors. (*Fig.* 64.)

The heavy line expresses the copper; the light line, zinc; the dotted line, the cloth; 50 or more such discs may be used.

The effects are slight and transitory. The conductors when touched, and again separated, give sparks. On being grasped, they communicate smart shocks. The chemical, magnetic, and igniting effects are very trivial.

Cruickshank's Trough Battery is constructed of rectangular plates of copper and zinc soldered together, the faces of the same metal being in the same direction; these plates are cemented into a wooden trough, and an interval of half an inch left between each pair.

Into the cells is poured a very dilute acid mixture—the best is 100 parts water, 4 sulphuric, 2 nitric acid, by measure.

The battery though more convenient to manage, is not for equal sizes more powerful than Volta's pile.

Wollaston's Battery is composed of zinc plates surrounded by copper at both sides. Each battery has 10 such couples. The zinc of each couple is soldered to the copper of the next. The whole is introduced into a porcelain vessel subdivided into ten cells. The battery is excited by dilute acid in the same proportions as that above mentioned. (*Fig.* 65.)

Such batteries are in every respect superior to those above described. With 50 such plates, 12 inches square, some magnificent experiments may be exhibited.

The best and cheapest instrument yet constructed is that invented by Mr. Mullins and Professor Daniell, and subsequently modified by the editor of this work.

Mullins' Constant Battery, consists of a series of copper cylinders covered with a bladder, and surrounded by a strip of sheet zinc. The whole is placed in an earthen jar. A strong solution of sulphate of copper is poured into the copper cylinder; a solution of sulphate of soda outside the membrane in contact with the zinc. A wire from the zinc leads to the mercury cup attached to the copper cylinder of the next couple. (*Fig.* 66.)

In *Daniell's Batteries* the zinc is within the copper cylinder. The membrane surrounds the zinc, and acid is employed in contact with the metal.

In the *Editor's* arrangement both these plans are combined, the copper cylinder having two zincs, one internal, one external. The internal zinc is covered with membrane. The copper is also covered. Solution of sulphate of copper is poured into the copper cylinder—of sulphate of soda within the internal zinc cylinder, and also outside the membrane surrounding the copper. Each set consists of ten such couples.

The Medical College of Calcutta possesses 500 such couples, arranged in 50 sets, the area of each copper cylinder being one superficial foot.

Another arrangement is effected thus:—copper cells are made of rectangular form, water-tight. Each cell is provided with a moveable zinc plate surrounded by a leather or pasteboard case. The College battery of this form is of 100 cells, each zinc 15 inches square. (*Fig.* 67.)

The College also possesses a series of 12 batteries on the same principle, each exposing 46 superficial feet of metallic surface.*

Effects of Compound Batteries.

The effects of compound batteries may be classified under the chemical, physiological, calorific, deflagrating, and magnetic.

Chemical Effects.

The *chemical effects* are measured by the quantity of a known compound decomposed in a given time. Water is usually employed as the standard.

The *Decomposing Bottle* is shewn in the drawing. It consists of a wide-mouthed glass jar, provided with an air-tight cover, furnished with a bent tube. The bottle contains two large platinum or gold plates; each provided with a thick wire terminating in a mercurial cup placed on the lid. (*Fig.* 68.)

The bent tube terminates under a graduated glass jar in the water bath. The bottle is charged with water mixed with $\frac{1}{8}$th its bulk of sulphuric acid.

On connecting this instrument with the conductors of a battery of eight double zinc cans (Mullins'), water is decomposed, and 20 cubic inches of oxygen and hydrogen gases are obtained in three minutes.

Every increase of surface produces corresponding increase in decomposing energy.

Six to eight cells constitute the most economical number in proportion to the effects produced.

* For a description of a superb battery of 50 gold cylinders, which the Editor has recently constructed, see Appendix.

Theory and Laws of the Chemical action of the Battery.

Each zinc plate is separated from the copper by a bladder or membrane, impermeable to fluids in its ordinary state.

In contact with the copper is a solution of sulphate of copper, in contact with the zinc a solution of sulphate of soda. So long as the battery is not in action these fluids do not mix, and do not act on the metals with which they are in contact.

When the battery is connected and at work, there is simultaneous decomposition in all the fluids. The water yields its oxygen and hydrogen,—the sulphate of copper its acid. The oxygen unites with zinc, the sulphuric acid with this oxide. The hydrogen acts on the oxide of copper which the sulphuric acid had abandoned, and reduces this oxide to the metallic state, fresh crystallized copper being deposited on the copper element.

If the plates of zinc and copper be weighed, and the gas from the decomposing bottle be collected, it will be found that for every equivalent—72 inches (8 grs. ox. 1 gr. hyd.) evolved from the bottle, 32 grains of zinc (1 eq.) are corroded from each zinc plate, and 31 grs. of copper (1 eq.) deposited on each copper cylinder.

This holds good whatever number of plates be in the battery; 1 eq. of zinc is dissolved from each for every equivalent of water decomposed.

By the chemical force of the galvanic battery a great number of compounds have been decomposed—and it is invariably found that hydrogen and the metals are separated at the copper side; oxygen, chlorine, bromine, iodine, fluorine, and the acids, at the zinc side of the battery.

Dr. Faraday has applied some new terms in his investigations into the laws of electricity, which it is necessary for the student to recollect.

A compound body decomposable by electricity is termed an *electrolyte*.

The decomposing plates are termed *electrodes*.

The *anode* corresponds to the positive pole or zinc side of the battery. The *cathode* to the negative pole, or copper side.

Physiological Effects.

Under this head we include the effects produced by the battery on living or recently dead animals.

A single pair of plates, however large, do not by simple contact with the body give the sensation termed a shock.

A series of ten plates however small, gives a perceptible shock, and this increases in proportion to the number of plates, and not to their size. Thus 12 plates 4 inches square give as great a shock as 12 plates each 46 feet square, the area of the great cell battery belonging to the Medical College.

Cruikshank's, Wollaston's and Mullins' arrangement when carried beyond 50 alternations, give disagreeable commotions. The shock of the College battery of 500 couples is altogether intolerable, and is moreover felt so long as the body is in contact with its poles.

The galvanic current, as it is termed, is made to flow through any part of the body by placing upon it the extremities of the conductors or poles provided with small sponges dipped in salt and water.

As it is only on making or breaking contact suddenly with the battery, that violent shocks are given, one of the conductors is, for medical purposes, provided with a forked end, by which the current can be gradually increased in power without shocks being given. One conductor remains constantly in connexion with one end of the battery. One branch of the forked end is brought near, and then by turning the forked extremity from plate to plate, the operator can proceed to the other end of the battery and back again without breaking contact or occasioning a sudden shock.

It is chiefly in paralysis, sciatica, and rheumatism that the galvanic current is applied, and often with decided success. It is also used in the attempts to resuscitate persons recently drowned, or labouring under asphyxia produced by noxious gases or narcotic poisons.

Igniting, Deflagrating, and Illuminating effects of large Compound Batteries.

A few alternations of plates of very large surface suffice to produce the most intense heat, which we can artificially command. The large 12 cell battery of the College has fused in one second, into small globules, 7 feet of thick platinum wire stretched between its poles. All the other metals it acts on still more powerfully.

When the number of alternations is increased the igniting effects cease, but are succeeded by still more brilliant phenomena, namely the deflagration or rapid combustion of the poles.

Thus 50 of Mullins' batteries with double zincs, cause the deflagration and dispersion of platinum, steel, copper, &c. with the most brilliant combustion that can be imagined.

If the poles be terminated by slips of box-wood charcoal, and these brought in contact, the charcoal ignites and sheds a light of such dazzling brilliancy that it transcends any other light but that of the sun itself.

If a very numerous series of Mullins' double cylinders (say 250) be employed, the charcoal poles may be slowly drawn asunder, but an arch of magnificent flame extends between them. This arch of flame is, moreover, a delicate magnet, and may be attracted and repelled by ordinary magnets at our pleasure.

Magnetic effects of Compound Batteries.

The magnetic effects of single pairs have been already pointed out, and notice taken of the phenomena of this kind which Volta's pile, Cruikshank's and Wollaston's arrangements can give rise to.

All these effects are extraordinarily increased by the use of the constant batteries, and in these the effects are proportionate to the number of plates, the extent of their surface, and the temperature of the apparatus.

The connecting wires of the great cell battery before alluded to, though made of copper $\frac{1}{4}$ of an inch thick, move towards each other by attraction whenever contact is made by the primary conductors. To soft iron this battery communicates, through a spiral conductor, magnetic power almost beyond estimation.

ELECTRICITY EXCITED BY HEAT.

Several years ago it was observed that antimony and bismuth bars if heated at one extremity while cooled at the other became sufficiently electric to cause the deflection of the magnetic needle. Recently such combinations have been made so powerful as to afford sparks, communicate shocks, and effect chemical decomposition.

The Medical College has a large battery of this kind. It consists of a series of bars of antimony and bismuth, each four inches long, and as thick as a pencil. The metals are placed alternately, in a spiral, commencing with bismuth in the centre. The first bismuth is soldered at the end by a wire to the first antimony, this to the second bismuth, and so on. To the first antimony and last bismuth, poles are soldered. The battery is excited by placing an iron heater below and pieces of ice above. It instantly becomes electric, gives sparks, effects decomposition of water, and gives sensible shocks. (*Fig* 69.)

MAGNETICAL ELECTRICITY.

As galvanic currents occasion magnetic phenomena in magnets, whether natural or artificial—permanent or temporary magnets conversely have the power of inducing electricity.

The natural magnet (chemuk-pathur) is an ore of iron, composed of oxide of iron, silica, and alumina. It occurs in shapeless masses, and is distinguished by its attracting small pieces of iron.

By contact with the natural magnet, as well as by other means, the same property is communicated to bars of steel. If these be supported freely, so as to move on a well balanced centre, one end always turns to the north cardinal point of the earth.

The extremities of magnets are termed north and south poles.

If the magnet be suspended so that it can only move vertically, one pole dips below the horizon. This dip varies in different latitudes, in Calcutta at present it is 26.39.4 N.

Poles of the same name repel; of different names attract each other.

A horse-shoe magnet is a piece of steel to which magnetism has been communicated after it has been cut in that form. (*Fig*. 70.)

The armature, or keeper, is a moveable piece of iron by which the poles of a magnet are connected.

When magnets attract iron they do so by inducing in it magnetic polarity, its poles being dissimilar to those by which the iron is attracted.

If an insulated spiral of copper wire be made to surround a piece of soft iron, and the ends be united—and if the soft iron be made by induction magnetic—by removing the inducing magnet the magnetism of the soft iron is destroyed, and on breaking contact in the wires at this moment a spark is observed.

The cut (*fig*. 71) shews the simplest form of this apparatus —*a*. a steel magnet, *b*. a soft iron armature with copper helix, *c*. a lever and handle by which the armature can suddenly be detached from the magnet, *d*. a cup of mercury in which the ends of the copper helix meet, and from which one rises at the moment the armature is lifted from the magnet. The spark is seen on the surface of the mercury.

The next figure gives a view of the splendid instrument constructed by Mr. Saxton, in which this principle is applied so as to produce the most brilliant results. (*Fig*. 72.)

1500 feet of thin insulated wire are wound in a spiral round a soft iron armature made to revolve on a mandril, moved by a multiplying wheel; one end of the spiral is soldered to the disc *a*, the other end to the arrow *b*, this quits the mercury in the cistern *d*, just as the armature loses its magnetism by rising at right angles to the steel magnet. This machine gives severe shocks, effects chemical decomposition, gives bright sparks, and deflects the magnetic needle.

The most powerful and beautiful arrangement of this kind, and at the same time the simplest and cheapest, is the electrical helix machine, of which the following is a description.

A coil of well insulated copper wire, 1-12th inch thick, is wound round a bobbin of wood, having a central aperture one inch in diameter. The ends of this coil are led through the sides of the bobbin. *(Fig. 73.)*

Over the first coil is wound a second, composed of 1500 feet of wire (insulated) 1-30th inch in diameter, and the ends of this wire are also exposed and connected with brass handles. *(Fig. 74.)*

If the ends *a*, *a*, of the primary thick coil, be connected with a small galvanic battery of one pair, on the handles of the secondary thin coil *b b* being grasped, no effect is perceptible—but on breaking contact with the battery by lifting out the wire *a*, a smart shock is perceived. This shock is increased by putting a solid iron bar in the core of the bobbin; still more so by a tube of sheet iron, and becomes absolutely overwhelming if a bundle of insulated iron wires be introduced.

To break contact more perfectly, a ratchet wheel and silver spring are interposed, and connected with one of the primary wires; on moving the ratchet by a multiplying wheel several hundred shocks can be given in a minute.

The whole machine is neatly fitted on a stand. It costs but 50 Rs., weighs about 3lbs., and affords to the physician the very best mode of applying electricity yet invented. We give a drawing of the machine. *(Fig 75.)*

The theory of its action is very simple; the primary coil becomes magnetic by connexion with the small battery, and thus induces electricity in the secondary coil, all the effects being multiplied by the insulated iron wires in the centre.

PART III.

OUTLINE OF STRUCTURAL BOTANY AND CLASSIFICATION.

Vegetable Anatomy.

To enable the student to understand the descriptions of medicinal plants given in subsequent parts of this work, we deem it indispensable to afford an outline of the structure of vegetables; to facilitate his inquiries after indigenous plants, a knowledge of classification is also essential—and this also we endeavour to supply the means of acquiring. In our outline we have adhered to the arrangement, and in many parts condensed the descriptions of M. Richard in his *Elemens de Botanique*. The examples have been however selected, as far as possible, from the familiar productions of Bengal. In our observations on classification we follow closely the excellent article by Professor Lindley in his *Introduction to Botany;* his table of Natural Arrangement we have adopted without change.

ELEMENTARY STRUCTURE.

There are two principal forms of vegetable structure—the *cellular* and *vascular*.

CELLULAR TISSUE.

The cellular, or areolar tissue is composed of cells in contact with each other, but having distinct sides. They are frequently of hexagonal form, but vary much in length, diameter, &c. They are generally inconceivably small; the largest scarcely equal 1-30th of an inch in diameter. The walls communicate probably by pores or slits. Lindley denies this, and considers the appearance of pores to depend on errors in the microscope employed, or on the presence of granular dots on the sides of the cells. In woody vegetables these cells are often elongated into tubes, generally parallel to each other; intervals may exist between these tubes, filled only with air, and are then in communication with pores in the epidermis, or outer bark.

These cells are easily torn; the space left by the destruction of cells is called a *lacuna*, and is usually filled with air.

Cellular tissue can absorb fluids, and is contractile.

The *figure* (76) is a section of the stem of the Aescynomene aspera, L. (Sholā) a well known plant in Bengal.

VASCULAR TISSUE.

Vascular, or tubular tissue is composed of plates rolled on themselves so as to form canals or tubes, with thick walls, and numerous apertures. These vessels are not continuous from end to end of the plant, but interwoven with each other.

Of these vessels there are seven principal kinds. 1. Beaded. 2. Porous. 3. Slit or streaked vessels. 4. Spiral. 5. Mixed. 6. Proper or peculiar. And, lastly, 7. Simple tubes.

The beaded vessels are by some considered merely modified cells. Slit vessels, or false tracheæ, are abundant in woods. The spiral vessels occur in most perfection in the leaves. The proper tubes are destitute of pores, and contain the peculiar juices of the plant, such as resin, oil, sugar, &c. The simple tubes are destitute of pores, and serve for the circulation of the sap.

Collected in bundles and united by cellular tissue, these varieties of tubes and vessels form the *fibres* of plants. The uniting or intermediate tissue is termed the *parenchyma*.

Medullary rays are composed of small horizontal tubes or cells placed transversely, and which always contain air.

Glands are cellular bodies, filled with oil, resin, or other principles, and placed in the substance of plants. There are many varieties in the form of these organs, which serve to secrete, and elaborate the peculiar fluid they contain.

Hairs occur chiefly on plants growing in dry situations. They are generally tubular, and often in connection with glands. Their forms, size, &c. are manifold—being simple, branched, soft, rigid, stinging, &c.; sometimes being solitary, sometimes grouped.

COMPOUND ORGANS OF VEGETABLES.

The compound organs of vegetables are,—

1. The root. 2. The stem. 3. The leaves. 4. The pistil, or female sexual organ. 5. The stamina, or male sexual organs. 6. The corolla or inner covering of the flower, generally coloured. 7. The calyx or outer covering of the flower, generally green. (The four last organs compose the flower.) 8. The seeds. 9. The pericarp, or envelope of the seeds. These two organs constitute the fruit.

Of the root, the stem, and leaves, we reserve the description for another place.

THE FLOWER.

The flower essentially consists of the sexual organs, stamen, and pistil, and the sheaths by which these are protected, (corolla, and calyx.)

A flower may be male, female, or hermaphrodite, but it must possess at least one sexual organ, or its rudiment. The corolla and calyx are often deficient.

The pistil, or female organ, occupies the centre of the flower, and consists of a hollow inferior part, the *ovary*, in which the seeds are formed; and the *style*, a tube which leads from the ovary, and terminates in a glandular expansion called the *stigma*. The style is often deficient, and the stigma is then termed *sessile*. The number of pistils varies from one to many. The stamina consist essentially of an *anther*, or membranous pouch, generally two-celled, containing a powder called *pollen*, the principle of fecundation. The anther is supported on a *filament* of variable length.

The corolla, or membranous expansion next the organs of generation, is composed of one or more pieces called *petals*. If there be but one petal, the corolla is *monopetalous*;—*polypetalous*, if composed of numerous distinct pieces.

The parts of the *calyx*, or outer membrane, are called *sepals*. If the calyx have but one, it is *monosepalous*, if more, *polysepalous*.

THE FRUIT.

The fruit consists of the pericarp and the seeds.

The *pericarp* is the enlarged ovary, and contains the *seeds*. It consists of three parts, the *epicarp*, or outer membrane, *endocarp*, or inner membrane, immediately in contact with the seed; and *sarcocarp*, or parenchyma, between both these membranes.

The *seed* is contained in the *pericarp*, and is attached to it by the *trophosperm*, or placenta, by which it is nourished. The part where the seed is attached is called the umbilicus, or navel. If the trophosperm partially or entirely covers the seed it is called an *arillus*.

The seed is covered by a proper skin, called *episperm*, within which the *kernel* is contained. The kernel consists of the *embryo*, or rudiment of the future plant, and of an adjacent substance called the *albumen*, or *perisperm*.

The embryo has three parts,—the *radicle* which produces the root; the *gemmule* which changes into the stem; and the *cotyledon*, or seed lobe, by which the embryo is nourished.

If there be but one seed lobe, the seed is called *monocotyledonous*—*dicotyledonous*, if two lobes be present. This distinction is so important, that all plants having sexual organs are divided into two classes, according to the number of cotyledons.

Plants having sexual organs are called *Phanerogamic* (θανεροσ apparent, γαμη marriage). Where these are deficient, or the mode of reproduction unknown, they are called *Cryptogamic* (χρυπτος concealed, γαμη marriage). These being destitute of seed lobes are also called *Acotyledones*, or *Inembryonate*.

ORGANS OF NUTRITION.

These are the roots, stem, buds, leaves, stipules, spines, prickles, and tendrils.

ROOTS.

The root is that part through which the plant derives its nourishment, and which is ordinarily concealed in the earth or water.

Roots are formed of a body, neck, and radicles, or thin fibres. In duration they either exist one year (annual), two years (biennial), or they are indeterminate (perennial). In form, size, direction, structure, &c. they vary exceedingly.

A bulbous root (improperly so called) is made up of a flat solid disc, which supports a bud formed of scales, or concentric coats.

Roots are woody, fleshy, vertical, oblique, horizontal, simple, branched, spindle-shaped, top-shaped, conical, rounded, tuberous; testiculate when composed of two tubers; palmate, or divided like fingers to the middle of the root; digitate, when divided like fingers to the base of the root—knotty, granulated, fasciculate, or bundled; articulate or jointed; contorted or twisted; capillar, or hair like; comose, resembling bushy hair &c., &c.

STEMS.

The stem resides in the air, is exposed to light, and supports the leaves, flowers, fruit, &c. It is sometimes, but very rarely, absent in dicotyledonous plants.

The varieties of the stem are the trunk, the stipe, the culm, the stock, and the *stem* properly so called.

The *trunk* is the stem of the dicotyledonous trees, and is formed internally of concentric layers.

The *stipe* is the stem of the monocotyledonous trees, such as the palms, is generally of uniform diameter, and is formed internally of irregular cells and fibres.

The *culm* is the stem of grasses, such as Dūrbā, (Panicum dactylon, L.) wheat, bamboo, sugar-cane, &c.; it is generally hollow and knotted.

The *stock*, or *rhizoma*, is a horizontal and subterranean stem, one end of which throws up the aerial stem, the other end dying as the new one advances.

Lastly, all aerial supports differing from the preceding, receive the common name of *stems*.

Qualities of Stems.

Herbaceous, or tender and green; semiligneous, or half woody; ligneous, or woody; solid, hollow, pithy, spongy; soft, firm, rigid, flexible, brittle; flleshy, or succulent; cylindrical, wandlike, compressed, two-edged, angular, triangular, quadrangular, pentagonal, or five-angled; hexagonal six-angled; knotty; jointed; bent like the knee or geniculate; sarmentaceous; climbing; twining—with respect to which it is to be observed that most plants twine to the right, exceedingly few to the left; slender, threadlike, simple, branched; dichotomous, or dividing in two limbs; trichotomous in three limbs; vertical or erect; prostrate, creeping or lying on the ground, and taking root its whole length; stoloniferous, sending off from the main stem small lateral stems called *stolons*, which take root, and form new plants.

Oblique, ascending, forming a curve at its base, with the concavity upwards, and then vertical.

Reclining; reflexed or bent back suddenly, tortuous or twisted, leaf-bearing, or leafless, scaly, winged, or having membranous leafy appendages. Smooth, glabrous, even, powdery, glaucous, the powder being of a dull green colour. Dotted, spotted, rough, or scabrous. Verrucose or warty, tuberous or knotty. Rimose or chinked, striated or streaked, sulcate, grooved or furrowed, downy, hairy, villous when the hairs are long, soft, close. Woolly, cottony, silky. Tomentose or velvety; ciliate, or fringed. Hispid, the hairs being placed on tubercles. Prickly or aculeate. Unarmed or destitute of thorns or prickles.

Structure of the Stem in the Dicotyledones.

The transverse section in the drawing (*fig.* 76) shews the structure of the stem to be formed of concentric rings or layers. These consist of the central or medullary tube containing the pith—the woody layers, and, lastly, or most externally the bark.

The Bark.

The bark consists of the *epidermis*, the *cellular tissue*, the *cortical layer*, or outer bark, and the *liber*, or inner bark.

The *epidermis* is a very thin layer of semitransparent tissue, and is analogous to the scarf skin in animals. It has numerous pores and glands. The use of the cortical pores is to allow the access of air to the internal parts of the stem.

The epidermis is sometimes studded with lenticular glands, from which roots occasionally spring. Sometimes silicious, as in grasses—sometimes it is cork-like, as in the Nirmullî *(Strychnos potatorum.)*

The *cellular tissue*, or herbaceous envelope, lies immediately under the epidermis, and external to the outer bark. It is generally of a green colour, and is a continuation of the green and cellular tissue of the leaves.

The respiration of trees and leafy plants, and the circulation of the sap, take place chiefly in this tissue, and in it again the peculiar secretions or juices are usually deposited.

The *cortical layers*, or *outer bark*, are sometimes absent, and generally difficultly distinguishable from the true bark.

The *liber*, or inner bark, is made up of layers separated by cellular tissue.

If the bark be partially removed from a healthy tree, an adhesive juice, called *cambium*, immediately issues from the surface of the wood, by which the liber is reproduced.

The Wood.

The wood consists of two parts—the *alburnum*, and the wood properly so called.

The *alburnum* is the youngest part of the wood, and external to the mature woody tissue.

The *wood* itself is composed of hardened alburnum, by which it is annually formed in a new ring, concentric to those of previous years.

The alburnum is destitute of vessels. The wood until of very great age contains tracheæ and porous vessels, through which the sap circulates.

The Medullary Canal.

The medullary canal is placed in the centre of the stem, and its sides are formed of long parallel vessels. This canal contains the *pith*.

The *pith* is a spongy, colourless, light substance, formed of cellular tissue. The pith is in some vegetables green and succulent at first, then becomes dry, and lastly disappears altogether, leaving a hollow stem.

The pith sends out rays to the cellular part of the bark. These are called the medullary rays.

The uses of the pith are still unknown, although many theoretical speculations have been advanced as to the office it performs in the vegetable economy.

Structure of the Stem in Monocotyledones.

The stem of this great division of plants is generally simple, and does not divide into branches.

The stem of Monocotyledones is destitute of concentric layers; its whole substance is occupied by modified pith, and loose bundles of woody tissue. The hardest parts are external; there is no bark, or one scarcely distinguishable from the inner structure. These peculiarities are strikingly seen in the section of a palm. *(Fig. 77.)*

In the manner of growth of Monocotyledones and Dicotyledones there is great difference; the latter increase *laterally*, or from without, by conversion of cambium into alburnum, and of this into wood, longitudinally, by annual shoots. The trunk is consequently formed by a series of concentric cones, of which the external is the youngest.

For example,—A stem of ten years growth has ten layers at its base, nine at the first shoot, eight at the second, and but one at the tenth.

The stem *stipe* of the Monocotyledons is formed, on the contrary, by a bud springing annually from the centre, expanding laterally, pressing outwards the last year's leaves, which fall off, and their dried bases form a solid ring. A series of these rings placed one above the other forms the stipe of this division.

Instead of being enlarged by the cambium, the stipe thus grows by a terminal bud, but the nourishing juices ascend from the common subterranean root, the stipe being perennial, the head of transitory duration.

Uses of Stems.

Stems supply wood and fibre for all its manifold uses. Some yield sugar; others colouring matter, such as sapan, log-wood, sandal-wood, &c.; astringent matter, such as the catechu tree, oak, &c.; some, lastly, yield most important medicinal substances, which we will subsequently describe.

BUDS.

Buds, are bodies which contain the rudiments of flowers, leaves, or both; and are the secondary agents in the continuation of the species of vegetables.

Buds are of several kinds—1. buds properly so called; 2. the turio, or subterranean bud; 3. the bulbus; 4. the tubercle; 5. the bulbil.

Buds properly so called.

These bodies vary in form and appearance, are generally scaly externally—sometimes naked—occurring on branches between leaves and stems, or at the extremities of twigs. In temperate or cold climates they are downy within. The external scales are generally imperfect leaves, or other abortive or modified organs. Buds are *leafy*, when scales are formed of abortive leaves; *petiolar*, the scales consisting of the bases of the *petioles* or leaf stalks. They may be also stipular or fulcraceous; terms which will be intelligible when stipulæ and fulcra are described.

Buds are further distinguished into leaf-buds, flower-buds, and mixed buds, according to the organs they contain.

The Turio.

The *Turio* is a subterranean bud, which produces annually a new stem; for example, the edible part of the asparagus.

The Bulb.

The bulb is generally the bud of Monocotyledonous plants.

Bulbs are either *solid*, *scaly*, or *tunicated*, as shewn in the drawing. (*Figs*. 78, 79, 80.)

Bulbs are round, oval, elongated, curved, simple, or multiple.

Tubercles

Are subterranean bulbs, simple, multiple, or compound.

Example—Simple tubercle, orchis or salep misree; multiple, the saxifrage; compound, the potatoe.

Bulbils.

Small solid or scaly bodies, growing on different parts of vegetables, and capable of reproducing the vegetable by

P

themselves. These occur frequently in cryptogamic plants, and are then called sporules.

OF THE LEAVES.

Leaves are enclosed in the buds prior to their development. In the buds they are variously situated, and the disposition is called *præfoliation* or *vernation*, a very important character in classification.

Præfoliation.

Within the bud the leaves may be folded—1. *Length-wise* in a single fold, the margins of each fold corresponding. 2. From above downwards. 3. *Longitudinally* like a fan. 4. Rolled *spirally*. 5. Margins rolled outwards or downwards. 6. Margins rolled inwards or upwards. 7. Like an architectural scroll.

After Development.

Leaves are membranous expansions, arising from the root, neck, stem, or branches, and formed by a series of vascular fibres issuing from the stem.

Leaves are *sessile* if attached without an intermediate or proper stem. The ordinary leaf stalk is called a *petiole*. The expansion of the leaf is named the *disk* or *limb*.

The subdivisions of the petiole on the lower surface of the leaf are termed *nerves*, one of which, in the same line as the petiole, is called the *midrib*, or middle nerve. The smaller and alternate branches of the nerves are called *veins*, and *venules*, terms exceedingly inconvenient and absurd, as these parts are in no wise analogous to the organs of the same name in the animal creation.

The situation and direction of the nerves are important in classification: parallel nerves with little subdivision characterise the Monocotyledonous—branching nerves the Dicotyledonous class.

Leaves are attached to the stem in different ways. 1. By an articulation or joint, and such leaves fall off early. 2. Permanently, by intermingled woody fibre. 3. The base of the leaf or petiole may entirely embrace the stem (amplexicaul), as the poppy; or half embrace it, (semi-amplexicaul), or *sheath* it, for a considerable distance, as in the grasses. In these plants a small membranous strap or *ligule* occurs at the neck, where the sheath and leaf join. Leaves if prolonged on the sides of the stem, produce what is called the *winged* stem. If the limb is apparently pierced by the stem, it is *perfoliate; connate,* if the bases of two leaves are joined, and the stem passes through the centre.

A *simple* leaf has no division in its disk or petiole. A compound leaf is made up of numerous leaflets attached to a common petiole, either being sessile upon it, or having partial leaf-stalks.

Intermediate varieties of leaves exist, such as the *toothed, lobed,* &c. &c.

Simple Leaves.

Simple leaves are called *seminal,* when formed by the development of the cotyledons; *primordial,* or the first which spring after the seminal; *radical,* when proceeding from the root; *cauline,* from the stem; *floral,* accompanying or at the base of the flowers—in which case if they differ from the common leaves they are called *bracteæ.*

Leaves may be opposite, alternate, scattered, or *whorled,* that is when more than two arise at the same place round the stem. Whorls are *ternate,* if of three leaves; *quaternate,* if of four; *quinate,* if of five; *senate,* if of six; and *octonate,* if of eight. Leaves may be *geminate* or in pairs; *distichous* or in two opposite ranks; *unilateral,* when all directed to the same side; distant, close; imbricated when placed over each other like tiles. Imbricated leaves are *biserial,* if in two rows; *triserial,* if in three; *quadriserial,* if in four. Tufted or fasciculate, crowning as in the papaw tree, rose-like, spreading, inflected, curled inwards or involute, curled outwards or evolute, pendent, inverted, *humifuse* when spread on the ground, floating, emersed, half under, half over water, &c. &c.

In outline, leaves are orbicular or nearly circular; oval, oboval, or an oval with broad end upwards; elliptical; oblong; lanceolate; linear; ribbon-like; awl-shaped or subulate; needle-shaped, or acerose; capillar, hair-like; filiform, thread-like; spatulate, or narrow below and broad outwards; cuneate, or wedge-shaped; parabolic; falcate, like a scythe; inequilateral, when the middle nerve divides the disk unequally.

According to the outline of the base, leaves may also be—*cordate,* or heart-shaped; *reniform,* or kidney-shaped; *lunulate,* or crescent-shaped; *sagittate,* arrow-like; hastate, spear-like.

According to their terminations at the summit, leaves are—acute; pungent if ending in a stiff point; *acuminate*, the tip being prolonged very much; *mucronate*, with a small slender point; *uncinate* or hooked; obtuse, *emarginate*, or notched; *retuse*, or notched at the summit; *obcordate*, inversely heart-shaped, or split at the summit into two equal segments; bilobate, if the divisions are separated by a blunt section; bipartite, when the divisions are very deep and sharp.

The outline of the leaf may be *rhomboidal*, having four angles, two of which are acute; *deltoid*, or triangular; *trapezoidal*, having four unequal sides; quadrangular, having four angles, &c. &c.

Simple leaves may be *trifid*, or having three deep lobes; *quadrifid*, having four; *quinquefid*, five; sexfid, six; *laciniate*, when the lobes are deep and unequal; palmate; pandurate, or approaching the form of a violin; *sinuate*, with rounded notches; pectinate, or divided like a comb; lyrate, lyre-shaped; runcinate, or having lateral lobes with sharp angles.

The margin of a leaf is entire; eroded, or having small unequal teeth; *crenate*, having small round projections separated by re-entering angles; *double-crenate*, when each rounded part is subdivided; *dentate*, or toothed; *serrate*, or saw-like; doubly serrate; spinous, with the nerves terminating in thorny points; *ciliated*, or provided with hairs like the eyelashes.

The membranous expansion or limb of the leaf may be flat; convex; concave; ensiform, or sword-shaped; striated, or streaked; *undulated* or waved; shining; even; glabrous, or smooth; *pertuse*, or marked with little holes; *canceilated* when the leaves have scarcely any cellular tissue, and are formed by a net-work of nerves; glandular; scabrous, or rough; glutinous; scarious, dry and thin; coriaceous, leathery; soft; rigid; fleshy; fistulous; long and hollow; green coloured; glaucous, or dull green; differently coloured, or having its two surfaces of different tints; spotted; hoary; or pure white.

Leaves may resemble various *solid* bodies, and are then called *ovate*, or egg-like; *obovate* when the narrow end is next the petiole; cylindrical; linguiform or tongue-shaped—triquetrous like a triangular prism; tetragonal, like a four-sided prism; compressed or thick; fleshy; laterally flattened, &c. &c.

A leaf is *peltate*, if the petiole is attached to the centre of its lower surface, and the nerves radiate from the attachment. The *petiole* has many modifications of form, the epithets applied to which are intelligible from the preceding glossary, in which we have marked in italics the words which occur most commonly in botanical descriptions.

Compound Leaves.

The compound leaf is formed of several leaflets on a common petiole. This petiole may be simple or ramified. When simple the leaf is termed *simply compound*—when ramified, the leaf is doubly compound, or decompound.

Simply compound leaves, when the leaflets all issue from the end of the petiole, are called *digitate*—when from the sides of the petiole they are *pinnate.*

Digitate leaves may vary in the number of their leaflets, and receive corresponding numerical names.

The leaflets of the pinnate leaf may be opposite; alternate; *uni-jugate,* when there is but one pair; bi-jugate, tri-jugate, &c. according to the numbers of pairs; *pari-pinnate,* when there is no terminating odd leaflet; *impari-pinnate,* an odd leaflet terminating the central petiole; interruptedly pinnate, when the leaflets are alternately large and small.

Decompound Leaves,

Or those on a branching *petiole,* may be digito-pinnate, when pinnate leaflets issue from the end of one petiole; bi-geminate, when each secondary petiole bears one pair of leaflets; bi-pinnate, when the secondary petioles are themselves pinnate leaves.

Supra-decompound leaves are formed by the secondary petioles giving off others also regularly subdivided.

In medicinal qualities, leaves may be emollient, bitter, stimulant, aromatic, narcotic, purgative, &c.

OF THE APPENDAGES TO THE LEAF.

The Stipules and Ochrea.

The *stipules* are small leafy appendages observed at the place where the leaf comes off from the stem or petiole.

The stipules are generally in pairs, and are either free or attached to the petiole.

The *ochrea* is by some botanists considered to be a membranous sheath formed by the union of two stipules. It is an important organ for purposes of classification.

The forms, situations, &c. of stipules, are expressed in terms corresponding to those by which leaves are described.

Of Tendrils or Cirrhi, Claspers, &c.

These are appendages on different parts of the plant, serving to support the stems and branches of climbers, by clasping or winding round solid bodies. They are abortive organs already described, such as flowers, stipulæ, leaves, or petioles, as may be recognized by their situation.

In plants which are at the same time sarmentaceous and climbers, the roots sent forth in the air are termed *claspers*. In *Tecoma radicans* the clasper has the form of a bird's foot.

Spines and Prickles.

Spines or thorns are sharp organs formed by prolongations of the internal tissue. *Aculei*, or prickles, are connected with the epidermis, or bark alone. *Spines* are often formed by the change or degeneration of large stipules, petioles, and other organs, and receive descriptive names from their shape, number, position, &c. which will be intelligible by reference to the nomenclature of leaves.

Examples of the Spine.—*Babul* (Acacia arabica). *Shij*, (Euphorbia antiquorum).

Examples of the Prickle.—The *Rose*. *Begun*, (Solanum Melongena.)

ORGANS OF REPRODUCTION.

The organs of reproduction are the sexual apparatus by which the species is renewed and preserved. These organs are composed of the *flower* and *fruit*.

We have already described the general anatomy of these organs; but more minute details are required. We shall first describe the supports and appendages of the *flower*.

Of Peduncles and Bracteas.

The *peduncle* is to the flower what the *petiole* is to the leaf. When branched, each division is named a *pedicel*. When the pedicel springs from an assemblage of root leaves, it is called a *scape*. If it springs from the surface of a leaf, it is called *epi-phyllous*. With respect to its form, situation, &c. consult the terms under the section on leaves.

Bracteas.

Bracteas are small leaves placed near a flower, and differing altogether from the leaves of the parent-plant. They are to the flower what the *stipule* is to the leaf. If the bracteas form an additional envelope to the flower, they are called an *involucre*, and when the peduncle is subdivided, and each pedicel has a similar appendage, it is termed an *involucel.*

Bracteas are sometimes made up of small scales surrounding the flower. When these remain after the fruit is ripened they are called a cupula or cup, which may even surround the entire fruit.

The Spathe.

The spathe is a leafy involucre, which in some plants covers the flowers until they expand and burst to allow these to protrude. The species of *Keora* (Pandanus) give a good instance of this appendage. The spathe has many forms, and every variety of colour and texture.

The Glume.

In *grasses* the corolla and calyx are deficient, and their place supplied by a variable number of scales, termed a *glume*.

OF THE INFLORESCENCE.

By inflorescence is meant the general disposition of the flower on its supports.

Flowers may be solitary, terminal, lateral, axillar, geminate, ternate, or fasciculate, terms already explained.

A *spike* is that form of inflorescence in which the flowers are sessile on a common simple stalk.

Example—Ispagul, (Plantago ispaghula). Gilla, (Entada pursaetha). Marua, (Eleugsine coracana).

A *raceme* is when the common peduncle bears flowers on short equal pedicels, (partial peduncles).

Example—Nimda, (Buddlea neemda). Sonali, (Cassia fistula).

A *thyrsus* is where the common peduncle is erect, the pedicels irregularly divided, and the whole flower of pyramidal shape.

Example—The Vine, (Vitis vinifera). Sterculia sillosa.

In the *panicle*, the peduncle is branched, the secondary divisions very irregularly and widely separated.

Example—Teak, (Tectona grandis). Mango, (Mangifera indica). Bhant, (Clerodendrum viscosum).

In the *corymb* the peduncles and pedicels spring from different points of the stem, but the surface of the flower is level.

Example—Bahuri, (Cordia myxa).

In the *cyme* the peduncles proceed from one point, but the pedicels subdivide irregularly, and raise the flowers to the same level.

Example—The Elder, (Sambucus nigra). Dhol shamudra, (Leea macrophylla). Harjora, (Vitis quadrangularis).

Flowers are *umbellate* when all the peduncles are equal, and the pedicels spring from the same point, and are also equal, and the general surface convex.

Example—The family of Umbelliferæ; Juvani, (Ptychotis ajowan). Panax ginseng.

A *whorl* or *verticil*, is that arrangement in which the flowers spring all round the stem at an equal height.

Example—Species of Tulsi, (Ocymum). Bengal Sage, (Meriandra bengalensis).

The *spadix* is that species in which a common peduncle is covered with flowers of one sex, destitute of calyx. It is peculiar to Monocotyledonous plants and to the peppers. The spadix is often enveloped in a spathe.

Example—Tal, (Lontarus domestica), and the Palms generally. Ol, (Arum campanulatum).

The *catkin*, or *amentum*, is a form in which flowers of one sex are inserted upon scales which serve as a peduncle.

Example—Pani jama (Salix tetrasperma). Geria (Excoecaria agallocha).

The *capitulum* is formed by a variable number of very small flowers, sessile on the enlarged summit of a peduncle; this enlargement is called phoranthium, and may be concave, convex, cylindrical, &c.

Example—Kadam, (Nauclea cadamba). Ach, (Morinda).

OF PRÆFLORATION OR ÆSTIVATION.

By these terms, which are analogous to vernation, we mean the mode in which the flower is disposed previous to its expansion; it is a most important subject in classification.

The petals before expansion may be *imbricated*, or disposed like the planks of a vessel, the edges slightly lapping over each other,—*plaited; spirally twisted; puckered;* or *corrugated;* simply in *contact* by their edges, &c. &c.

The *quincuncial* prœfloration is where there are five petals, two external, two internal, and one covering the two inner by one side—and on the other side covered itself by the two outer petals.

The calyx before flowering has the same modifications of disposition.

OF THE FLORAL ENVELOPES.

The *perianth* is the Linnæan term for the whole of the parts surrounding the sexual organs.

Of these the calyx and corolla are sometimes entirely deficient. A single perianth is named calyx, whatever be its colour; thus in all the Monocotyledonous plants the coloured flower is properly a calyx. When the perianth is double, the part next the sexual organs is the corolla.

The *perianth* of the Orchideous family has six divisions, three internal, three external. The latter are often joined to two of the former, and produce a helmet-like body over the sexual organs. The middle, and lower division of the inner part is of different colour to the rest, and is called the *lip* or *labellum*. The forms and aspect of this lip are sometimes very extraordinary. It is often provided with a hollow horn or spur, *calcar*.

Of the Calyx.

In the Monosepalous calyx there are distinguished—1. the tube or lower part; 2. the limb or upper expanded part; and, 3. the throat *(faux)*, or the line between the limb and the tube.

The forms of the calyx differ widely, and are described in the same terms as those previously explained.

The Monosepalous calyx may be *regular*, when all its incisions are equal to each other; *irregular*, when they differ in size and figure; turbinate, having the form of a top; urceolate, or bellied, swelled below, contracted at the throat and the limb dilated; *inflated*, when thin and membranous like a bladder; campanulate, when shaped like a bell; dipterous, having two lateral membranous appendages; tripterous, having three, &c.; *enlarged*, after floration, &c. &c.

The Polysepalous calyx presents similar modifications of form.

The calyx and corolla are often blended with each other.

Q

Of the Corolla.

For a general description of this organ, see page 100.

Each petal is composed of two parts—1. the *unguis*, or claw; 2. the *lamina*, or disk.

A regular corolla is that in which all the parts are equally arranged round a centre or axis. The corolla is irregular when there is more at one side than the other.

A Monopetalous corolla has three parts, the tube; the limb, or upper and expanded part; and the faux, or throat, a line between the tube and the limb.

Varieties of the regular Monopetalous Corolla.

The most remarkable varieties are the following.

Tubulate, Ex.: Bara manda (Loranthus bicolor), *(Fig. 81.)*

Campanulate, or Bell-shaped. Ex.: Bistaruka (Argyreia speciosa), ... *(Fig. 82.)*

Infundibuliform, or funnel-shaped. Ex.: the species of Datura, ... *(Fig. 83.)*

Hypocrateriform, or salver-shaped. Ex.: Rungun (Ixora bandhuca), ... *(Fig. 84.)*

Rotate, or wheel-shaped. Ex.: Begun (Solanum melongena), ... *(Fig. 85.)*

Urceolate, or pitcher-shaped. Ex.: Mahua (Bassia latifolia). ... ... *(Fig. 86.)*

Varieties of irregular Monopetalous Corolla.

This is two lipped, or bilabiate, when the limb is divided into two unequal lips. This form occurs in a whole family of plants called accordingly *Labiatæ*.

The corolla is *personate*, or mask-like, if the tube be elongated, throat very wide, and closed by the lips being in contact, so that the corolla resembles the mouth of a mask.

The limb, faux, and tube of the Monopetalous corolla have many varieties in colour, form, &c., the terms applied to which are the same as those already quoted under the head of leaves, stems, &c.

Polypetalous Corolla.

The petals in the Polypetalous corolla may be of various numbers, forms, dispositions, &c. corresponding to those described in speaking of other organs. Thus it may be regular or irregular, according to the position of its petals round the axis, &c. &c.

Regular Polypetalous Corolla.

Of this there are three principal varieties—

1. The *cruciform*, or cross-shaped, formed of four unguiculate petals, placed in opposite pairs, (mustard, &c.) *(Fig. 89.)*

2. *Rosaceous*—three to five petals, with very short claws, spreading like the single rose, almond-flower, &c. *(Fig. 90.)*

3. *Caryophylaceous*, or pink-like, formed of five petals, the claws being very long and covered by the calyx. *(Fig. 100.)*

Irregular Polypetalous Corolla.

Example—*Papilionaceous*, or butterfly-like, formed of five irregular petals, each of different form. In this, one petal is superior, two lateral, two inferior. The superior is called the standard or vexillum; the lateral the wings or alæ; the inferior, which are often united, the carina or keel.

Instances of this corolla are seen in the numerous sort of beans; Ex.: *Makun shim* (Canavalia gladiata); and indeed in almost all the great natural family of *Leguminosæ*. *(Fig. 101.)*

The petals may correspond in position to the sepals of the calyx, or may be alternate. There are other characters to which terms before explained are applied.

OF THE SEXUAL ORGANS.

For a general description of these organs, see page 100.

Flowers are either unisexual, or hermaphrodite. But distinct male and female flowers may be found in the same plant, when it is called Monoicious, (or inhabiting one dwelling) —if the separate sexes be on different plants, then they are named Dioicious or (having two dwellings) of which the date palm is a good example.

Where male, female, and hermaphrodite flowers co-exist, they are called *Polygamous*.

These three characteristics are important to be remembered, being adopted by Linnæus in his System of Classification.

OF THE MALE ORGAN, OR STAMEN.

This organ is composed of three parts—the anther, a membranous pouch, generally two-celled; 2. the pollen, a powder contained within the anther; 3. the filament on which the anther is supported. This last part is not essential, and is often deficient.

The number of stamina in each flower deserves much attention.

When a flower has		*It is called,*	*Example.*
1	Stamen,	Monandrous.	Turmeric tribe.
2	,,	Diandrous.	Jui pana, (Rhinacanthus communis).
3	,,	Triandrous.	Grasses.
4	,,	Tetrandrous.	Chandan, (Santalum album).
5	,,	Pentandrous.	Datura Stramonium.
6	,,	Hexandrous.	Bura kanur, (Crinum asiaticum).
7	,,	Heptandrous.	Asok, (Jonesia asoca).
8	,,	Octandrous.	Mendi, (Lawsonia inermis).
9	,,	Enneandrous.	Cinnamonum zeylanicum.
10	,,	Decandrous.	Nata, (Guilandina bonduc).
12 to 20	,,	Dodecandrous.	Canella alla.
More than 20	,,	Polyandrous.	Padma, (Nelumbium speciosum).
Two long and two short stamina,		Didynamous.	Species of Tulsi, (Ocymum).
Four long and two short stamina,		Tetradynamous.	Sursun, (Sinapis dichotoma).

The preceding distinctions constitute, along with the three of Monoicous, Dioicous, and Polygamous, already described, and with others to be subsequently noticed under the head of Filament and Androphorum, the chief classes in the Linnæan artificial arrangement.

Stamina are said to be included, when shorter than the corolla or calyx—exserted, or protruded, when they are longer.

Of the Filament and Androphorum.

The filament has many varieties in its shape, size, and disposition. If the filaments adhere so as to form one or more parcels, these are termed *Androphorum.*

When the Androphorum is single, it is called *Monadelphous.* If double, *Diadelphous.* If manifold, *Polyadelphous.* These three varieties afford as many Linnæan classes.

By the influence of cultivation, and other causes, the stamina frequently change into petals. The *double* flowers of gardeners are generally of this kind.

The Anther.

This body is shewn in the *figure* 102.

Each cell of an anther has generally a groove where it eventually opens. The grooved surface is called the *face*, the opposite surface the *back*.

The anther is generally divided internally into two cells by a membrane, and is then called bi-locular; if there be but one cell, it is uni-locular; if four, which is very rare, it is quadri-locular.

The anther is usually fixed to the summit of the filament. The attachment may be by the base, back, face, or apex. If the face of the anther be turned to the centre of the flower it is called introrse; if towards the circumference of the flower, extrorse.

The mode in which the anther opens is important to be noted, and is termed *dehiscence.*

Cells are longitudinally dehiscent when they open along the groove on the face—or they may be open by pores, valves, or slits.

The anthers may unite so as to form a tube, as in the *figure* 103.

This is called *syngeneseous*, and is the type of a Linnæan class. Sometimes the stamina are united with the pistil, this disposition is called *gynandrous*. The stamina are however never united with the ovary. The filaments and style form the common support of the anther and stigma.

The Pollen.

This substance is the fecundating principle contained within the anther.

It is of two kinds—powdery or viscous—of different colours. It may be coherent in one mass, or simply pulverulent. Before the microscope it is found to consist of membranous globules, which burst on contact of water, and allow the escape of a multitude of granules, or of long tubular bodies of extreme minuteness.

OF THE PISTIL, OR FEMALE SEXUAL ORGAN.

The pistil is composed of three parts—the *ovary*, the *style*, and the *stigma*. (*Fig.* 104).

When there is more than one pistil, they are often attached to a prolongation of the receptacle termed *gynophorum*.

When the base of the ovary is contracted, and thus elevates the pistil, this part is termed a *podogynum*. The gynophorum often becomes fleshy and edible, as in the strawberry and raspberry.

The Ovary.

The ovary is placed at the lowest part of the pistil. It contains cells in which the ovules or germs are situated—its form generally resembles an egg. Its base usually corresponds to the insertion of the corolla and stamina. Sometimes the ovary is situated *below* the insertion of these organs, and is united with the tube of the calyx; this is called *adherent* or INFERIOR; the former disposition is *free* or SUPERIOR. The position of the ovary in this respect is a most important natural character.

The *parietal* ovary is often confounded with the *inferior*. In this the pistils are attached to the walls of a calyx having a very narrow throat. This is seen in the rose, and similar flowers.

According to its position, the ovary is either sessile or supported. As to its cells (loculamenta) it may be unilocular, bilocular, trilocular, quadrilocular, multilocular.

The number of ovules or germs in each cell may vary in separate flowers from one to an indefinite number; and their position with respect to each other, offers many diversities.

Of the Style.

This organ has already been described, vide page 100. In number, position, &c. it presents many varieties.

Of the Stigma.

The stigma is composed of elongated utricles or little bladders, converging towards the style, and adhering by a mucilaginous cement. The observations relative to form, &c. in the last paragraph apply equally here.

The Nectary.

This term is only properly applicable to little glands on different parts of a plant, and which secrete a sweet juice, like honey. We quote it under the description of the flower, as many writers use the term to denote organs in the flower, not properly included under any of the preceding heads.

The Disk.

This is an accessory organ, not always present, but when found, of great importance for the construction of natural families of plants. It is a fleshy body placed beneath the ovary, upon its summit, or on the inner wall of the calyx.

The disk may be Hypogynous, Perigynous, or Epigynous.

The *Hypogynous* disk is placed beneath the ovary, which it lifts up from the bottom of the flower.

The *Perigynous* disk is a thick body lining the inner wall of the calyx.

The *Epigynous* disk is situated on the summit of an inferior ovary.

Of the Insertion of the Stamina.

The stamina are inserted beneath, around, or upon the ovary. When beneath, they are termed hypogynous; when inserted in the calyx, perigynous; when upon the top of the ovary, epigynous.

All these characters are of much value as guides to natural classification.

OF THE FRUIT.

The fruit is the fecundated and enlarged ovary, and consists of two parts—the *pericarp*, and the *seed*. See page 100.

The *pericarp* is the part of the fruit formed by the walls of the *ovary*, and containing the seed. It is never absent, though sometimes so thin as to be difficultly perceptible.

The pericarp (*see page* 100) consists of an external, middle, and internal body. The first is the epicarp; the second, the mesocarp or sarcocarp (flesh of the fruit); the third, the endocarp.

When the ovary is inferior, the epicarp is formed by the tube of the calyx, the parenchyma of which becomes the sarcocarp of the fruit.

When a part of the sarcocarp becomes hard and woody, surrounding the seed it is termed a *nut*.

If there be but one cavity within the fruit, it is termed unilocular, or one-celled; when the cavities are numerous, the partitions are called dissepiments; these partitions are formed by reflections of the endocarp. These layers of course enclose a plate of the sarcocarp. When the fruit dies it often happens that these layers separate from each other, presenting the appearance of additional cells. The true partitions always alternate with the stigmas.

There are *false partitions* in several fruits, for instance in the cucumber and poppy families; they are distinguished from the true dissepiments by their not being formed by the endocarp, and by their corresponding to the stigmas.

Partitions are either complete or defective, as they reach from end to end of the pericarp or not.

The point where the seed communicates with the pericarp is named the hilum, or navel. The body within the pericarp, on which the seeds are supported, is the *trophosperm*, or placenta. The trophosperm is in communication through the endocarp with the fleshy part (sarcocarp), which affords nourishment to the seed. The trophosperm sometimes offers little projections, or partial seed supports; these are called *podosperms*. When the trophosperm is prolonged over the seed, it is called an *arillus*. The arillus never occurs in plants having a monopetalous corolla.

Dissepiments are usually longitudinal, rarely transverse; the false are formed either by expansions of the trophosperm, or by inflexions of the pericarpial valves.

The pericarp is described as having a summit, base, and axis. When the axis is real, it is called a columella.

Pericarps which open to permit the escape of seeds, are called dehiscent; indehiscent when they fall off entire. The dehiscence may be—1. an irregular fracture (ruptile); 2. by holes at the upper part; 3. by indentation; 4. by valves. The edges of closed valves are called sutures, and the number of valves corresponds to the number of cells; according to the number of valves, the terms univalve, bivalve, trivalve, &c. are employed.

Appendages to the Pericarp.

Of these the pappus and the alæ (wings) are most deserving of notice.

The pappus is a hairy or feathery appendage, sometimes formed by the summit of the calyx. It is formed of simple or divided pairs, sometimes sessile, sometimes supported on a little stem or stipe. *Ex.* Dandelion, (Taraxacum densleonis). (*Fig.* 105.)

The alæ (wings) are membranous expansions of various forms.

These appendages serve to render seeds buoyant, and readily transported by the winds from place to place.

Ex. of winged fruit: The Wood-oil or Gurjun tree, (Dipterocarpus turbinatus.) Winged seeds: Mahogany, (Swietenia mahogani). Shona, (Bignonia indica).

OF THE SEED.

The seed is formed of two parts, the *episperm*, or external membrane, and the *kernel*.

The base of the seed is that part which corresponds to the hilum; its summit the opposite point. The face of a seed is that surface which is directed towards the axis of the pericarp.

The episperm is sometimes double, as in the castor oil seed. In this case the outer membrane is called the *testa*, and the inner the *tegmen*.

Before impregnation, the ovule is composed also of two membranes, and a kernel. The vessels of the pericarp enter at the hilum, and proceed within the testa nearly to its summit, forming an expansion termed a *chalaza*. The summit of the inner membrane has a small aperture through which vessels proceed to the kernel. This is cellular, and consists of two parts—the outer thick and fleshy, the *chorion;* the inner a cellular sac, the *amnios*, filled at first with fluid. Within this sac, after impregnation, the embryo is developed.

The Kernel.

The kernel is formed essentially of the embryo, besides which an endosperm is generally present.

The endosperm is formed of vascular tissue, containing starch, gum, or oil. It is placed beside, or around, the embryo, for the nourishment of which it is intended; its colour is usually white, its consistence viscous.

The Embryo.

The embryo is epispermic, when there is no endosperm; endospermic when this organ is present. If the embryo surrounds the endosperm, it is called *extrary;* if contained within it, *intrary*. It is composed of four parts—

1. The *radicle*, which subsequently gives rise to the root. When the radicle is external and exposed, the plants are called *exorhizous;* if covered by a sheath, this is named *coleorhiza*, and the plants are *endorhizous*. If the radicle is entirely incorporated with the endosperm, the plant is called *synorhizous*.

2. The *cotyledon*, see *fig*. 106. Plants having but one cotyledon in each seed are monocotyledonous; where two cotyledons exist, they are termed dicotyledonous. The cotyledons after germination often rise above ground, and are changed into *seminal* leaves. There are instances of several cotyledons being present.

3. The *gemmule*, (often named the plumule) is the ascending part of the embryo, and contains the rudiments of the stem, and of all other parts destined for exposure to the air.

4. The *caulicle* is the part which during germination forms a continuation between the radicle and gemmule, and on which the latter ascends.

The *Dicotyledonous embryo* has been already sufficiently described.

The *Monocotyledonous embryo* is that which before germination is entirely undivided.

Classification of Fruits.

Fruits are *simple* when they proceed from a single pistil contained in a flower; *multiple*, when from several pistils contained in the same flower ; *compound*, from several pistils placed near each other, but contained in different flowers.

Fruits, again, are dry or fleshy ; closed, or indehiscent ; valvular, or dehiscent ; monospermous ; dispermous, &c., according to the number of seeds.

The pericarp is sometimes so thin, that it is confounded with the substance of the fruit. These were erroneously deemed naked seeds, and are now called pseudosperms.

CLASS I.—§. SIMPLE FRUITS.

SECTION 1.—DRY FRUITS.

**Indehiscent Dry Fruits.*

These are generally olygospermous (few-seeded,) pericarp thin and adherent.

Species 1. *Cariopsis;* monospermous; pericarp confounded with the seed. Ex. Family of grasses, rice, &c.

——— 2. *Akenium;* monospermous, with distinct pericarp. Ex. Synanthereæ, sunflower, &c.

——— 3. *Polakenium ;* a simple fruit, when ripe dividing into akenia. Ex. Umbelliferæ, parsley, &c.

——— 4. *Samara ;* aligospermous, coriaceous, membranous, compressed, and often winged. Ex. Ventilago madraspatana.

——— 5. *Acorn* or *gland;* single celled, one seeded, proceeding from an inferior multilocular ovary; pericarp internately attached to the seed, partly contained in a scaly or leafy involucre. Ex. Oaks, hazel.

Species 6. *Carcerulus;* dry, many celled, many seeded. Ex. Sida, Malva.

——— 7. *Gymnobasic fruits*, are those in which the cells are separated so as to appear to form several distinct fruits. Ex. Fruits of Labiatæ and Boragineæ, Bengal sage, &c.

** *Dehiscent Dry Fruits.*

Generally polyspermous, and usually called capsular.

Species 1. *Follicle;* twin or solitary, membranous or celled, one valved, with longitudinal suture; Ex. The whole family of Asclepiadeæ, Akund, (Calotropis gigantea).

——— 2. *Siliqua;* dry, elongated, bivalve, trophosperm sutural and double; often divided into two cells by an expanded trophosperm. Ex. Cruciferæ, mustard, &c.

——— 3. *Silicula*, differs only from the former in being much shorter. Also seen in Cruciferæ.

——— 4. *Legume* or *pod;* two valved, trophosperm single and parallel to the suture, sometimes separated into cells by false dissepiments. Ex. Pea, Cassia fistula, &c.

——— 5. *Pyxydium;* generally globular, opening transversely into two hemispherical valves. Ex. Hyoscyamus, &c.

——— 6. *Elaterium;* a fruit separating longitudinally into many distinct parts or coccæ, usually connected by a central pillar. Ex. Euphorbiaceæ.

——— 7. *Capsule;* under this head is comprised any species not referrible to those above described.

SECTION 2.

Fleshy Fruits.

Indehiscent, pericarp thick and pulpy, number of seeds variable.

Species 1. The *Drupe;* a fleshy fruit containing a nucleus, formed by hardened endocarp. Ex. Peach, cherry, plum, mango.

——— 2. *The Nut.* Ex. Almond and walnut; sarcocarp being thinner than in the drupe.

——— 3. *Nuculanium;* a fleshy fruit rising from a free ovary. Ex. Ivy, elder, achras sapota.

——— 4. *Melonida;* fleshy fruit, formed of several juxtaparallel ovaries, attached to the tube of the calyx, which becomes enlarged and forms the fleshy part of the fruit. Ex. Pear, apple, &c.

Species 5. *Balausta;* many celled, many seeded, issuing from an inferior ovary, and crowned by the teeth of the calyx. Ex. Pomegranate and Myrteæ.

——— 6. *Peponidæ.* Ex. Cucumbers, gourds, colocynth. The cells are scattered in the pulp.

——— 7. *Hesperidium.* Ex. Orange and melon.

——— 8. *Berry* or *bacca*—all the fleshy fruits, destitute of nucleus, and not comprehended by preceding species. Ex. Grapes, &c.

CLASS II.—§. MULTIPLE FRUITS.

Multiple fruits result from the collection of several pistils contained in the flower. These are sometimes termed *Syncarpium.* Ex. Custard apple, fruit of raspberry, ranunculi, &c.

CLASS III.—§. AGGREGATE OR COMPOUND FRUITS.

Species 1. *The Cone;* composed of several membranous utricles concealed below large dry bracteas, disposed conically. Ex. Fruits of firs, pines, &c.

——— 2. *Sorosis;* several small fruits united by their fleshy floral envelopes. Ex. Mulberry, jack, pine-apple.

——— 3. *Synconium;* a monophyllous involucre, internally fleshy, flattish, or oval, containing numerous drupes. Ex. Figs, &c.

We have now described succinctly all the organs of phanerogamous plants, and cursorily alluded to the functions they perform. We have subsequently to shew how these plants are classified, and to explain the mode by which a student familiar with organization can identify unknown plants—or if previously known, can find their places in works of botanical reference.

It is necessary here briefly to allude to the great division of *flowerless* plants. These are divided into ten groups—1. Filices (ferns); 2. Lycopodiaceæ; 3. Marsiliaceæ; 4. Salviniaceæ; 5. Mosses; 6. Hepaticæ; 7. Characeæ; 8. Lichens; 9. Algæ; 10. Fungi.

As very few cryptogamic plants are included in the Pharmacopœia, a general description of all these groups would be misplaced, we shall therefore reserve a notice of them till treating of the individual articles.

General Classification.

There are two systems of classification in use among British botanists—the *artificial* and the *natural.*

The artificial system was invented by Linnæus, and is founded on the peculiarities of plants as to the number, form, and disposition of the stamina and pistils.

The natural system was devised by Jussieu, and depends on the resemblance or analogies of all the organs of which a plant is composed.

LINNÆAN SYSTEM.

ARTIFICIAL OR SEXUAL METHOD OF CLASSIFICATION.

This system comprises 24 classes, characterized by the number and disposition of the stamina ; and numerous orders known by the varieties in the female organ, and other peculiarities subsequently noticed. We append a table of the *classes.*

CLASSES.

1 Stamen	1,	Monandria.
2	2,	Diandria.
3	3,	Triandria.
4	4,	Tetrandria.
5	5,	Pentandria.
6	6,	Hexandria.
7	7,	Heptandria.
8	8,	Octandria.
9	9,	Enneandria.
10	10,	Decandria.
11	12 to 19,	Dodecandria.
12—20 or more inserted into calyx, ...		Icosandria.
13—20 or more into receptacle, ...		Polyandria.
14— 2 long and 2 short, ...		Didynamia.
15— 4 long and 2 short, ...		Tetradynamia.
16 Stamina united by filaments into a tube, ...		Monadelphia.
17 ———— into two tubes, ...		Diadelphia.
18 ———— into many tubes,		Polyadelphia.
19 ———— by anthers into a tube,		Syngenesia.
20 ———— with the pistils, ...		Gynandria.
21 Stamens and pistils in separate flowers on same plant, ...		Monœcia.
22 ———— on separate flowers and separate plants, ...		Diœcia.

23. Separate or united on same or different plants, ... } Polygamia.
24. No sexual organs known, ... Cryptogamia.

The characters of the orders depend on the number of stigmas for the first thirteen class.

ORDERS—*for* 13 *first classes.*

Style	1	... ...	Monogynia.
	2	... ...	Digynia.
	3	... ...	Trigynia.
	4	... ...	Tetragynia.
	5	... ...	Pentagynia.
	6	... ...	Hexagynia.
	7	... ...	Heptagynia.
	8	... ...	Octogynia.
	9	... ...	Enneagynia.
	10	... ...	Decagynia.
	12	... ...	Dodecagynia.
	More than 12	...	Polygynia.

In the 14th class, Didynamia, the orders depend on the character of the ovarium.

The first order is called Gymnospermia; the ovarium has four lobes, each of which contains a single seed. The second order is Angiospermia—the ovarium is not lobed, is usually two celled and many seeded.

In the 15th class, Tetradynamia, the orders are taken from the character of the fruit. Siliquosæ have a long pod; Siliculosæ a short one.

The orders of the 16th, 17th, and 18th classes are founded on the number of stamina, and are named as in the first 13 classes.

The orders in *Syngenesia* are complicated. They are taken from the arrangement of the flowers and sexes of the florets, thus—

CLASS SYNGENSIA.

1st Order, *Polygamia æqualis*—each floret is hermaphrodite, or has both male and female organs of generation.

2nd —— *Polygamia superflua*—florets of the disk hermaphrodite, of the ray female.

3rd —— *Polyg. frustranea*—florets of the disk hermaphrodite, of the ray sterile.

4th —— *Polyg. necessaria*—florets of the disk male, of the ray female.

5th —— *Polygamia segregata*—has several florets either

simple or compound, but with a proper calyx included with a common calyx.

The orders of the 20th, 21st, and 22nd, classes depend on the number of the stamens.

The orders of the 23rd class, Polygamia, depend on their being monoicious or dioicious.

The last class, Cryptogamia, is divided into orders specified at page 124; of which the most important are—1. Filices, or ferns; 2. Musci, or mosses; 3. Hepaticæ, or liverworts; 4. Algæ, or seaweeds; 5. Fungi, or mushrooms.

This system is very valuable to a student in a country the botany of which is known and described. It serves him as an index to any standard work, and enables him readily to obtain practical knowledge of the plants about him. Even in India it is of great utility, as several thousand plants have been arranged on this system and described by Dr. Roxburgh in his most valuable Flora Indica. Where a student has access to that great work, if he finds a plant he does not know, by the examination of its stamina and pistils according to the Linnæan key, he is guided to the class and order in Roxburgh. The form of the flower, stem, leaf, &c. will then supply more precise marks, until in many cases he is enabled to identify the specimen.

NATURAL SYSTEM.

In the natural system the botanist is not contented with the comparison of the parts of fructification alone, but all the organs are contrasted. This method is more difficult than the former, in exact proportion to the greater amount of knowledge of botanical structure it must require. It is of the highest value to the medical practitioner, especially in India; as experience has proved, that the same natural families of plants possess generally the same chemical and medicinal properties; and thus that an indigenous species may often be substituted for one not found in the country.

According to the natural system, there are two great *classes* of plants—

1. The *vascular*,—or flowering.
2. The *cellular*,—destitute of sexes, flowers, and of spiral vessels.

VASCULAR PLANTS.

The 1st class, or VASCULAR, is sub-divided into the following sub-classes:—

1. *Exogens*—plants with reticulated leaves, stem having wood, pith, bark, and medullary rays. Flowers with a five-fold division. Cotyledons, two or more opposite.

2. *Endogens*, or Monocotyledonous plants.

Leaves with parallel veins; stems without distinction of wood, bark, or pith; flowers with a triple division; cotyledon 1, or if 2 alternate.

The 1st sub-class, or Exogens, embraces two tribes—1. *Angiosperms*, or those having seeds enclosed in a pericarpium; 2. *Gymnosperms*, or seeds destitute of a pericarpium. The first of these comprehends the vast majority of all the medicinal plants. The pines and sago trees only are embraced by the second.

The Angiosperms, or pericarpial plants, are further divided into—*polypetalous*, those the flowers of which have distinct petals—*apetalous*, or those having no petals—*achlamydeous*, having neither calyx nor corolla—*monopetalous*, having but one petal.

Of these the POLYPETALOUS group is the most numerous, and requires further sub-division. It is accordingly separated into two sections—the *Thalamifloræ*, in which the stamens are hypogynous, or adhere to the sides of the ovarium; and 2. the *Calycifloræ*, in which the stamens are perigynous, or distinct from the corolla, when this is monopetalous. Lastly, both the thalamifloræ and calycifloræ are divided into—*Apocarpæ*, or those with distinct, sometimes solitary, carpella—and *Syncarpæ*, or those in which the carpella cohere in a multilocular pericarpium.

The 2nd sub-class, *Endogens*, has but two great divisions—The *Glumaceæ*, those provided with glumes, as the grasses; and the *Petaloideæ*, having flowers with petals.

CELLULAR PLANTS.

The 2nd class of cellular or flowerless plants has three sub-divisions. *Filicoideæ*, (ferns) those having a distinct axis, and vascular system—*Muscoideæ*, (mosses) having a distinct axis, but no vascular system; and—*Aphylleæ*, (mushrooms, lichens, &c.) having neither axis nor vascular system.

The whole of the preceding divisions may be compared to the volumes of a great work. Each volume contains sections and chapters, in which the individual subjects are treated of.

The natural *orders* of plants are those in which besides some of the above described points of general resemblance, many additional points of identity are found. Botanists have formed about 272 such groupes or orders, of which 228 are found in the Exogenous sub-class, 31 in the Endogenous—the remainder in the Cellulares, or flowerless division.

The distinctions of the natural orders are founded on a multitude of characters; take for example the 1st tribe of Exogens, the Angiospermæ, we find the following characters chiefly dwelt on—1st. *Apocarpæ*—the flowers unisexual—flowers hermaprodite—*fruits* in a fleshy disk, or not—*anthers* bursting by valves curling backwards—or by longitudinal slits—stipulæ present, and the leaves with or without transparent dots. Stipulæ absent, and the albumen soft or solid—seeds with an arillus or not, and ovarium solitary or manifold. Leaves sheathing at the base, or with a taper leafstalk—albumen none, and leaves with or without pellucid dots. Stigmas capitate, or terminal, or linear—petals being sepaloid.

Proceeding to the *Syncarpæ*, we find—ovarium multilocular with ovula attached to the base of the partitions, or the ovarium celled with the ovula attached to the walls of the ovary. Placentæ linear, contracted, stamens two, corolla regular or irregular. Sepals four, stamens tetradynamous—disk glandular or not, ovarium sessile. Stamen indefinite, disk continuous, enlarged, ovarium stalked, &c. &c.

Continuing the analysis, we find characters drawn from the hilum, and the relative position of the ovum—from the nature of the vernation—the dehiscence of the capsule—the œstivation of the calyx—the structure of the anther—the surface of the seed—the symmetry or irregularity of the flower, the position, and peculiarity of the embryo—the nature of the fruit—the junction or separation of styles, stigma, or anther—the leaves being alternate, opposite, or deciduous, stipulate, &c.

Such are the chief distinguishing signs by which the natural orders are formed. It is apparent from this sketch, that it is chiefly, if not exclusively, from the organs of reproduction the characters are derived.

The organs of nutrition, namely, the root, stem, leaves, &c. mark the differences between species and individuals, as will be subsequently seen.

It would be profitless to enter here into more detail. We prefix to each natural order a general account thereof, and to each individual a detailed description. The whole is closed by a synoptical view of all those in the classes in which medicinal articles exist, as an aid to the memory of the student, and as a guide to his future researches.*

* Lindley's admirable synopsis of the natural system, and his tabular classification of fruits, are given in the Appendix.

PART IV.

PHYSIOLOGICAL AND CURATIVE ACTION OF MEDICINES.

The agents which we name medicines, and employ in the treatment of disease, are those which independently of any mechanical operation are capable of producing changes in the structure or function of the animal fabric, and thereby of correcting or nullifying diseased action.

Of these substances several can exercise such powerful agency on the structure and functions of the higher animals, as to destroy the former, and fatally disturb the latter. These are termed poisons;—the difference of action between the medicine and the poison, thus frequently depends merely on the difference of quantity of the agent which acts on the living body.

The action of a *medicine*, as we have above described it, presumes the existence of *disease*. Although the majority of our medicines are capable, it is true, of inducing manifest effects in the healthy body, nevertheless there are some, and those of great value, which arrest or cure diseases, although they do not in the same quantities induce in the healthy body any powerful or even perceptible action.

To give examples of the preceding statements; foxglove, tartar emetic, nux vomica, opium, &c. in small doses, are *medicines*—in large quantities, *poisons;* small doses of quinine or anarcotine arrest or cure intermittent fevers, although in the healthy body they usually produce no perceptible alteration of structure or function.

The basis of the following classification of medicinal agents is afforded by the tables published by the late Dr. Duncan, Professor of Materia Medica in Edinburgh, and which appear to us to combine all the advantages of a therapeutical and physiological system. We have given many additional details as to the mode of action of each class, rejected several of the agents, and added others peculiar to this country.

Classification of Materia Medica.

External agents act on the body,

I. As *Aliments*, or articles of diet.	
a, By being digested or absorbed and adding to the quantity of its watery constituents.	Diluents. Drinks.
b, By being digested, and either during or after that process, allaying pain and soothing irritable surfaces...	Demulcents. Foods.
II. *By Evacuation.*	
a, By the skin, ...	Diaphoretics.
b, By the mucous membrane of the nostrils, ...	Errhines.
— of the glottis, trachea, and lungs,	Expectorants,
— of the stomach, ...	Emetics.
— of the intestines, ...	Purgatives.
— of the uterus, ...	Emmenagogues.
c, By the glandular organs.	
α, the kidneys, ...	Diuretics.
β, the salivary glands, ...	Sialogogues.
III. External agents act	
By *stimulating* the vital powers.	Stimulants.
This stimulation may be——	
a, LOCAL and external.	
Causing redness, ...	Rubefacients.
— blackness, ...	Nigrefacients.
— serous secretion, ...	Vesicants.
— purulent secretion, ...	Suppurants.
b, LOCAL and internal, ...	Carminatives.
Or STIMULANTS may act generally.	
If temporary, ...	Diffusible stimulants.
If durably, ...	Tonics.
If by constricting fibres and coagulating fluids, ...	Astringents.
If by checking spasmodic action,	Antispasmodics.
If by exciting spasmodic contraction.	Convulsives.
IV. External agents act	
By depressing the vital powers.	
a, By diminishing the generation of heat,...	Refrigerants.
b, By influencing the brain, or spinal chord,...	Narcotics & narcotic antispasmodics.

V. External agents,
Act chemically.

a, as	Acids.
b, as	Alkalies.
c, By destroying structure, ...	Caustics or corrosives.
d, as Solvents of urinary concretions,	Lithontriptics.

FIRST DIVISION.

§ 1.—*On Diluents, Emollients, and Demulcents.*

Water and aqueous beverages, such as solutions of gum, gelatine and sugar, and mixtures of oily and glutinous, albuminous or gelatinous matter suspended in water, constitute the chief diluents and emollients of the physician. Starchy solids, jellies, &c. are termed Demulcents.

In the healthy body these agents internally taken are digested, absorbed, and assimilated; in disease they are sometimes absorbed, and are administered for that view, as in cholera, in which the blood has lost much of its natural water; sometimes again no absorption takes place, or is desired, and diluents are given to lubricate and sheathe inflamed or irritable structures. Occasionally diluents are used as auxiliaries to promote the action of more powerful remedies, such as emetics, diaphoretics, and cathartics.

In inflamed or irritable states of the urinary organs diluents are used to dilute and render less acrid the urinary secretion.

Externally, various emollients and demulcents are used to relax the tissue to which they are applied. Inflammation is thus often checked, or suppuration promoted, or pain much relieved. Poultices or cataplasms are usually formed of emolient or demulcent substances, sometimes alone, sometimes combined with other medicinal agents.

Ointments and cerates in their simple state come under the same head, and will be described in the Pharmacopœia.

We give in the Appendix a copious table of articles of this class, to which belong fully four-fifths of the remedies used by the native practitioners, and to which numerous imaginary virtues are attributed—The individuals marked with an asterisk are however really of value, and are described minutely in the Pharmacopœia.

SECOND DIVISION—MEDICINES ACTING BY EVACUATION.

§ 1.—*Sudorifics or Diaphoretics.*

Sudorifics are agents capable of causing increased perspiration, sensible or insensible, from the skin and the mucous membrane of the lungs.

The natural quantity of total transpiration from a healthy man daily, has been experimentally ascertained by Dalton to amount to 37½ ounces, of which about two-thirds are water, the remainder carbonic acid.

The quantity of transpiration from the skin is influenced by several causes. It is much augmented by the contact of moist air, the warm bath, increased clothing, friction, by currents of dry warm air, by diminished atmospheric pressure, by external heat, by the process of digestion, by exercise, and all other causes which direct the circulation towards the skin.

Many diseased conditions diminish or suppress the cutaneous secretion. Thus in ardent fevers we find the skin hot and dry; in dysenteric inflammation of the lining membrane of the intestines, and in diabetes, or morbid discharge of urine, the same symptom is witnessed; the kidneys and gastric intestinal mucous membrane thus alternating with the skin as secreting organs.

Several causes, on the other hand, which depress the vital powers, simultaneously occasion increased cutaneous secretion. In cholera, for example, in fainting, and in the last stages of pthisis, and many other fatal diseases, the skin is bathed in cold sweat. In cholera the urine is at the same time suppressed, and the sweat contains its peculiar principle, urea.

There are again many substances, which when taken into the stomach occasion even in healthy persons an unusual diaphoresis.

Thus if the skin be kept warm, and the body be covered, copious draughts of diluents cause profuse sweating.

Several substances, such as spirituous liquors, sulphur, guaicum, camphor, acetate of ammonia, &c. enter the circulation, reach the skin, stimulate its minute vessels, and the same effects are observed.

In disease sweating is produced by many measures, of very opposite character, according to the cause by which the dryness of the skin is occasioned.

Thus in the exanthematous or eruptive diseases, the exposure of the skin to moderately cool air is frequently followed by diaphoresis, as the result of diminished inflammatory action on the surface.

In ardent fevers, the affusion or application of cold water is often followed by the like result. Again, in internal inflammations the remedies for that state, such as bleeding and tartar emetic, when successful, often act as diaphoretics also; and the appearance of moisture on the skin evinces to the physician the success of his remedial measures.

The medicines which contain antimony, and ipecachuana, given in small doses, are remarkable for their sudorific action; they are much used in the treatment of dysenteries and fevers, when increased cutaneous secretion is not only a favorable symptom, but may be made a powerful auxiliary in the treatment of the disease. The action of the remedies in such diseases we believe to partake of the nature of both cause and effect. The state of the skin must be modified before the transpiration commences, but this secretion when established and encouraged, acts most powerfully and favorably on the original source of the diseased condition.

Diaphoretics are chiefly used in the treatment of fevers; acute inflammations, especially dysentery; in affections of the lungs; in diabetes, or morbidly increased secretion of urine; in dropsies; in gout, rheumatism, and syphilis, and in numerous diseases of the skin.

In the descriptions of the several articles the rules will be given for their use, and form of administration.

---

§ 2.—*Errhines.*

Under this head all modern writers on Materia Medica arrange those substances capable of exciting a discharge from the nostrils, by direct application to these organs—and also of producing sneezing. They are all local irritants, generally of an acrid nature; many produce extremely violent and dangerous effects, such as gangrene of the parts, apoplexy, &c. As in our entire experience in the practice of medicine we have never deemed it expedient to prescribe a remedy of this class, and as their use is likely to lead to the worst results, we have decided on omitting the list which Dr. Duncan has given. All the substances he enumerates possess additional properties, for which they will receive due notice under a different head.

---

§ 3.—*Expectorants,*

Or medicines causing evacuation from the mucous membrane of the glottis, trachea, and air-cells of the lungs.

The existence of this class is still disputed, and in several works of high merit it is altogether omitted.

The mucous membrane of the lungs in its healthy state continually exhales a mixture of gases and watery vapour, and is moistened with thin mucus. In this state there is no demand for any further evacuation. But in disease two opposite conditions may occur. The air-cells may be overloaded with mucus, or pus, or other fluids, preventing the aeration of the blood, and thus occasioning difficulty of breathing. Or, again, the natural secretion of vapor and mucus may be deficient, and the membrane dry, occasioning a painful sense of constriction, rendering the breathing laborious, and causing frequent, harsh, and violent coughing.

Either of these states may affect the whole of the lungs, or only a part thereof. Different causes too may be concerned in the production of the same condition. Thus chronic inflammation of the mucous membrane may cause the cells to be overcharged with mucus—or great debility, as in old persons, may lead to the same results. Pthisis causes accumulations of pus; and empyema, terminating in ulceration, may pour large quantities of the same fluid into air-cells previously healthy.

We find again that the secretion may be deficient in consequence of inflammation, or, on the contrary, of deficient vascularity. It must be obvious that expectorants must in all these various conditions act in a different manner.

Mechanical compression, such as that occasioned by sneezing, or coughing, or vomiting, very frequently causes the expulsion of mucus or pus from the air-cells, and thus acts as a decided expectorant. Again, there are medicines, for example the antimonial preparations, which by their tendency to subdue inflammation relieve that cause either of undue dryness or of increased secretion. Some substances also are known, such as benzoic acid, myrrh, ammoniacum, garlic, &c. which in their course through the circulation enter, and stimulate the minute pulmonary vessels, which may have become torpid through general debility or old age.

Sometimes when the cause of the symptoms is understood, we are enabled to apply our remedies directly to the seat of the malady. Thus the vapors of water, spirit, weak ammonia, of volatile oil, chlorine, iodine, carbonic acid, carburetted hydrogen, of tobacco, hemp, stramonium, and other narcotic vegetables, have been employed for this purpose, and often with great advantage.

Various vessels are used in the inhalation of these gases, and vapors, all of which act on the principle of the hookah.

The precautions to be adopted with each remedy will be pointed out under its particular head.

We should not omit to mention an indirect method of producing expectoration, sometimes advantageously resorted to. The irritation of the lungs and their mucous membrane often spreads to the orifices of the air passages. By swallowing diluent drinks, or by allowing saccharine or gelatinous matters to melt in the mouth, the demulcent effect produced on the parts with which these substances actually come into contact, is extended by sympathy to the distant organs, and free expectoration is frequently produced.

---

§ 4.—*Emetics*,

Or medicines used for exciting Vomiting.

Vomiting is an inverted action of the stomach, accompanied by spasmodic contraction of the respiratory and abdominal muscles, by means of which the stomach is emptied of its contents. Vomiting is often preceded by a sensation of extreme sickness (nausea), and is usually followed by faintness, weakness of the pulse, and copious diaphoresis.

During the act of vomiting the circulation being much impeded, the veins of the head and neck become tense and swollen, and the countenance red and turgid. Instances are on record in which these blood-vessels have burst under this distension, and death been the consequence. Vomiting may be produced in many ways.

1. By nervous sympathy. By tickling the fauces with a feather, or touching them with the finger.

2. By the contact of acrid and irritating matters with the mucous membrane of the stomach; for instance, by mustard, sulphate of copper, sulphate of zinc, &c.

3. By peculiar excitement of the nerves of the stomach, as by ipechacuana, tartar-emetic, the kanoor, (Crinum asiaticum), &c.

These substances will produce vomiting if injected into the blood, or the rectum, or applied to a wound.

4. By mental impression. In many individuals it is easy by mere description to excite disgust to such an extent as to occasion vomiting.

5. By distension of the stomach by large quantities of food or drink, or pressure on this organ by adjacent enlargements of the spleen or liver.

6. Lastly, by several mechanical injuries, as great operations, blows on the head, &c. &c. Sea sickness, violent

rotatory motion, &c. may be enumerated as common causes of vomiting.

Emetics are very much used by practitioners, especially in the treatment of diseases of children, and of persons labouring under the effects of the narcotic poisons.

The operation of emetics is in most cases much promoted by draughts of tepid water. In narcotic poisoning the stomach, and the system generally, are frequently so torpid that stimulants are simultaneously used; of these one of the best is a mustard cataplasm applied to the epigastrium.

Where all attempts at evacuating the stomach by emetics prove unsuccessful, the stomach pump is resorted to, and often with perfect success.

The Stomach Pump.

The stomach pump consists of a brass syringe with two valves, as shewn in the drawing; and two elastic pipes made of caoutchouc.—By means of this instrument fluids can be injected into the stomach and pumped from it at pleasure.

Directions for use. The patient being placed in the sitting posture, a piece of perforated wood (see *fig.* 107) is placed across the mouth, to prevent the tube being injured by the teeth. The long tube, previously oiled, is then carefully introduced by pressing it horizontally to the very back of the throat and then depressing its point by raising the right hand, so as to make a gentle curve. The tube thus enters the gullet, and passes freely into the stomach. By neglecting to bring it fairly in contact with the back of the throat the point of the tube may enter the larynx (top of the windpipe), and cause immediate suffocation, or irreparable injury. The long tube is then connected with the orifice of the syringe *a*, while the short tube is dipped in a basin containing the liquid to be injected.

The operator must hold the syringe vertically. In the drawing, fluid is shewn as being thrown into the stomach from a basin; to pump from the stomach it is only necessary to transfer the end of the tube in the stomach to the lowest aperture of the syringe. This may be readily done without removing the tube from the stomach. These directions apply to Reid's instrument.*

* In another instrument (Weiss') by a rather complex valvular arrangement fluid can be thrown into, or extracted from, the stomach without changing the tubes. The student should consult for the use of this instrument the maker's directions which accompany each case.

§ 5.—*Purgatives.*

Purgatives are those medicines which excite a transitory irritation of the internal surface of the alimentary canal, causing the contents of the intestines to be evacuated by the rectum, in quantities greater than the natural excretion, or when the natural excretion is prevented.

Purgatives may produce this effect in various ways.

1. By stimulating the mucous membrane of the alimentary canal to secrete an unusual quantity of watery fluid, and subsequently by causing increased action of the intestinal muscles. Of such purgatives we find the best examples in sulphate of soda and of magnesia, jalap root, kaladana, and scammony; these are called hydragogue cathartics.

2. By diluting the solid contents of the intestines, lubricating the passages, and stimulating the muscles. Ex.—Castor oil, the pulp of Cassia fistula, &c.

3. By increasing the flow of bile and pancreatic juice into the alimentary canal. Ex.—Mercurial pill, and calomel, colocynth, rhubarb.

4. By acting on the muscular contractility—chiefly colocynth, aloes, scammony, and jalap.

Several of these if in solution, and injected into a vein, applied to a wound, or even to the undivided skin, will produce their specific effects on the intestines.

Purgatives differ in the interval between their administration and action. This chiefly depends on their solubility, and on the particular tract of the intestine they affect. Thus croton oil may act in half an hour; the neutral salts in one or two hours; senna, kaladana, and jalap in two to four hours; aloes, on the contrary, takes several hours before its operation commences, and then seems only to affect the large intestines.

Purgatives are also named Cathartics, and are termed *laxative* if mild, and *drastic* if severe in their operation.

All purgatives may be administered by injection into the rectum, in the form called an enema, clyster, or "lavement." For the preparation, use, and administration of these remedies directions are given under the head *Enema.*

Purgatives are chiefly employed in the treatment of fevers, inflammations, spasmodic or other intestinal obstructions, apoplexy, and dropsy.

They are to be avoided as much as possible during the prevalence of epidemic cholera. The more drastic kinds are unsuitable for menstruating or pregnant females in consequence of the irritation they occasion extending to the womb, and in the latter often inducing premature labour.

§ 6.—*Diuretics.*

We have already described the physical and chemical properties of urine.

The average quantity of urine secreted by healthy European adults may, from Dalton's experiments, be estimated at 48 ounces daily.

This quantity may be diminished by various unusual states of the secreting organs, or of the general system; for example—by inflammation of the kidneys, by paralysis of their nerves, by too copious perspiration, by excessive purging, by general febrile action in the system, &c.

The measures directed to the relief of these causes become indirect diuretics by their secondary effects.

In the healthy state, again, there are many substances which much increase the quantity, and even alter the quality of the secretion. Most of these are absorbed in the digestive tubes, taken into the circulation, come directly into contact with the kidneys, and pass off by the urine, in which they may be often detected.

Lastly, where morbid accumulations of fluids have taken place, as in dropsies of various kinds, we may employ medicines in the first place to stimulate the absorbent system to take up the fluid; and this entering the circulation may be eliminated by the kidneys without any more direct use of diuretics; or while we act on the absorbents, the kidneys may be simultaneously urged by such remedies into unusual action.

All diluent fluids may be considered diuretics, especially if the surface of the body be kept cool.

---

§ 7.—*Emmenagogues.*

These are remedies supposed to possess the power of restoring or bringing on the menstrual discharge.

The menstrual fluid (catamenia), is a red secretion discharged monthly from the internal surface of the uterus in human females, from the age of puberty to between 40 and 50 in the European, and 30 and 40 in the native of Bengal. The secretion contains water, albumen, red coloring matter, and the saline constituents of the blood, but no fibrine;—it does not coagulate. It has been seen in the monkey, and traces of it occur in some other mammalia.

The secretion may be suppressed by many causes, such as organic disease of the uterus, inflammatory condition of that organ or its appendages, by local debility, by general diseased action, such as fever, by pregnancy, &c.;—the secretion may take place and find no avenue for its escape, as in cases of imperforate hymen or vagina.

It is very doubtful whether any remedy, with perhaps one exception, possesses any direct influence over the uterus. Still Amenorrhea, or defective menstrual secretion, may be obviated by many measures, directed according to the indications above mentioned. We thus frequently observe that in young females of full constitution and sanguine temperament, the secretion is impeded at a time when the pulse is full and strong, and there is every appearance of increased action in the system. Bleeding, leeches, saline purgatives, and cupping over the loins constitute the proper remedies in such cases.

On the other hand, where the amenorrhea co-exists with a pallid countenance, general torpidity, a weak pulse, depraved digestion, and confined bowels, we find the use of certain stimulant remedies and tonics most beneficial; of these the ergot of rye, the oils of sabine and of rue, and the tincture of the muriate of iron, may be mentioned as the most beneficial, and under the heads of these articles will be found proper directions for their use.

Where the general health is good, and the defective secretion is caused by local debility, shocks from the Leyden jar, or the use of the electro-magnetic machine—the current being directed from the pubes to the sacrum—together with blisters, aloetic pill, and turpentine enemata give the best promise of success.

In applying leeches in such cases it is always expedient to do so as nearly as possible at the period when the discharge would naturally be expected; most females know the time exactly; indeed the older physicians believed that all females menstruated about the same day in the month, but this opinion is no longer entertained.

In adopting measures in amenorrhea, it is necessary to ascertain carefully that the patient is not pregnant, otherwise abortion may be produced by the remedies had recourse to. A black circle or areola round the nipple, of the size of a rupee, with whitish lines radiating from it over the breast, milk in the nipples, morning sickness, and occasional vomiting, will in the earlier months of pregnancy identify the case. In the later months the size of the abdomen, and the evidence afforded by the stethoscope will remove all doubt. The stethoscope is simply a cylinder of light wood, about a foot long and an inch and a half in diameter.—Sound passes with great readiness through this instrument, and by its use we are enabled to study various natural and morbid states of the heart, the lungs, and other organs within which sounds are generated, and which we could not otherwise investigate.

To use the stethoscope in such cases, apply one end of the instrument midway between the umbilicus and pubes, the other end to the ear, and listen attentively. The contractions of the fœtal heart will be distinctly audible. They are much more rapid than those of the mother's heart, which may be counted at the same time by the pulse at the wrist.

---

§ 8.—*Parturifacients.*

These substances bring on premature* or increased contraction of the muscular coat of the pregnant womb, by which the fœtus is expelled. There is but one known agent unequivocally endowed with this power—the ergot of rye, and the nature of its operation is still a mystery. For further details, see "Ergot of Rye."

Sabine and Rue are popularly considered to act powerfully on the uterus. The ripe pine-apple in some parts of India is believed to possess the same property. Facts are wanting to enable us to decide fully on these opinions.

---

§ 9.—*Sialogogues,*

are substances capable of inducing increased secretion from the salivary organs, viz. the mucous membrane and follicles of the mouth, the parotid, sublingual, and submaxillary glands.

Sialogogues are either direct or indirect. Among the former we place all irritating and acrid substances, such as pepper, anthemis pyrethrum (akurkura), the acrid spices, and tobacco. The indirect sialogogues are chiefly mercury, iodine, and prussic acid.

Direct sialogogues are chiefly used in local paralytic affections, unnatural dryness of the mouth or fauces, for the relief of hoarseness, temporary loss of voice, tooth-ache, earache, and some forms of head-ache. They have been employed too with success in the cure of salivation resulting from other causes.

Indirect sialogogues are usually employed in the treatment of general diseases, such as syphilis, scrofula, and rheumatism, but their effects and mode of administration must be noticed under the separate heads of Iodine, Hydrocyanic

* Many practitioners are of opinion that it is only at the full period of gestation that this influence is exerted.

acid, and Mercury. It is necessary to add, that it is mercury only which induces increased salivation as an invariable effect. Under the same heads will also be found descriptions of the best methods for relieving those who suffer from excessive salivation.

THIRD DIVISION.

External agents, acting as stimulants of the vital powers.

(*a*) LOCAL AND EXTERNAL.

Causing *redness* of the skin, *rubefacients*—*blackness, nigrefacients.*

Causing serous secretion beneath the epidermis—*blisters.*

Causing the formation of pustules—*suppuratives.*

---

§ 1.—*Rubefacients or Nigrefacients—Blisters.*

There are many substances which when applied to the skin cause inflammatory action in its minute vessels. If the skin be white, redness is produced, and there is great and irritating pain of the parts. If the skin be dark, increased blackness ensues.

Mustard, the plumbago, or lal-chitra, ammonia, acetic acid, turpentine, hot water, and alcohol, are the chief and most valuable agents of this kind.

If applied longer than necessary to produce the reddening or blackening effect, vesication or blistering ensues, and watery fluid is secreted in such quantities that it lifts the epidermis up so as to form a bulla or vesicle.

The Melöe cichorei, or native fly, the *Cantharis vesicatoria*, or Spanish fly, and the Lal-chitra, *Plumbago rosea*, are the only remedies of this kind had recourse to. The fly is used either in ointment or as a tincture. The Lal-chitra in pulp or paste made with water.

---

§ 2.—*Suppuratives.*

Suppuratives are those which cause an eruption of pustules resembling those of the small pox. Tartar emetic, the citrate of antimony, croton oil, and hydriodate of potash, are the best agents of this kind.

The anacardium, or ballataka, and the juice of the Burmese varnish tree produce a peculiar inflammatory action of the skin very difficult to cure, and consequently these substances are not employed in medicine.

Uses of Blisters, Rubefacients, &c.

All these remedies are used—1st as derivatives; 2d. as counter-irritants; 3rd. as general or local stimulants.

Derivatives act by the inflammation which is occasioned, and the consequent secretion diverting a like action from some important part or organ.

Thus, in fevers when effusion on the brain is threatened; in abdominal inflammation where ulceration is proceeding on the mucous membrane of the intestine; in acute inflammations of important viscera or joints; in pericarditis, gout, in visceral congestions, rheumatism, &c., blisters often attract, as it were, the inflammation to some part of less importance, and thereby prevent a fatal termination.

In many painful diseases, such as neuralgia, tic doloroux, and the like, the irritation occasioned by a blister, or any other of these remedies, causing intense pain in the part to which it is applied, the distant part often experiences corresponding relief.

Lastly, as mere stimulants, we daily observe the beneficial effects of these applications in the treatment of amaurosis, of several local paralyses, in cholera, asphyxia, apoplexy, in cases of narcotic poisoning, in debility or atrophy of the limbs or joints or viscera, and in a multitude of similar affections.

THIRD DIVISION—*(b.)* LOCAL AND INTERNAL STIMULANTS.

§ 1.—*Carminatives.*

This term is applied to aromatics and condiments which stimulate the stomach and intestinal tract, and lead to the expulsion of flatulence.

---

§ 2.—*Temporary, or Diffusible Stimulants.*

§ 3.—*Permanent, or Tonics.*

§ 4.—*Astringents.*

The two first of these sections agree in the general nature of the effects they produce on the system, and vary chiefly in the time required to produce the effect, and in the degree of permanency with which this influences the body.

Diffusible stimulants very soon after being taken into the stomach, or inspired, or thrown into the rectum, cause a sensation of fulness and warmth in the part, thence extending over the body to the skin;—we also observe increased fulness and frequency of the pulse, augmented vascularity of the skin, and unusual exhilaration of ideas. This state constitutes what is termed excitement, and is usually succeeded, after a variable time, by a proportionate ebb or sinking of the actions described below the healthy conditions. This state is termed collapse. All diffusible stimuli however differ in this respect from each other. In some instances the collapse is scarcely perceptible (for example from the nitrous oxide gas, and the gunja); in others, it may proceed to a fatal degree, as in cases of excessive inebriation from ardent spirits, and in the effects of opium.

Of the diffusible stimuli, those most generally employed are alcoholic liquors, ammonia, sulphuric ether, nitrous ether, acetic acid, opium, gunja, musk, camphor, nitrous oxide, and the essential aromatic oils.

The chief cases in which these are employed are, in fainting, narcotic poisoning, asphyxia from drowning, the collapse of cholera, in hæmorrhages, especially those occurring during labour, in the convalescence from fevers, or similar severe maladies, in delirium tremens, or the 'horrors,'—the singular nervous state induced by long continued intoxication, and the sudden disuse of spirituous stimulants.

Permanent tonics,

are so called from the tone or elastic tension they gradually impart to the muscular and fibrous system. Less immediate than the previous class in their effects, their action indeed is often imperceptible. By degrees we find however that under their use various debilitated organs regain their natural health, the appetite increases, digestion is regularly performed, the secretions become natural, the spirits revive, and fitness for muscular exercise is accompanied by the wish for its enjoyment.

The remedies of most importance in this class, may be divided under two heads,—those of direct and indirect action; of the latter class it suffices to say that where general debility proceeds from a local cause, such as increased secretion or discharge, hæmorrhage, suppuration, &c—arresting the local discharge will prove tonic in its general operation.

The direct, or general tonics, chiefly recommended, are Peruvian bark, sulphate of quinine, anarcotine, the vegetable bitter remedies, such as gentian, cherayita, quassia, the *creat* or Justicia paniculata, the preparations of iron and arsenic. Of these, some possess, besides their tonic property, a marked power of interrupting periodical returns of disease, as in ague, and other intermittent disorders; quinine, anarcotine, nux-vomica, and arsenic, are the most remarkable examples of this class.

Others, again, appear to act as *tonics*, by improving the condition of some natural secretion; small doses of mercury are often known to produce this effect by slow and almost imperceptible influence. Sarsaparilla and the Hemidesmus Indicus are reputed to possess similar powers in syphilis; iodine in scrofula; mudar in elephantiasis—all these are termed *alteratives*. Their mode of action is very obscure, but their effects generally unquestionable. The preparations of iron and iodine exercise a like influence over many forms of spleen disease, removing enlargements of that organ, and at the same time promoting the restoration of the general health.

Antispasmodic Tonics.

In certain debilitated states, of the nervous system especially, spasmodic contractions of the voluntary muscles occur, and assume the various forms of convulsive diseases, exemplified by hysteria, chorea, and epilepsy. Tonics, especially the preparations of iron, arsenic, and quinine, aided by moderately diffusible stimuli and aperient remedies, frequently prove of essential service in these affections. In all cases however an attentive diagnosis is absolutely requisite. These diseases may proceed from very opposite causes,—from inflammation, irritation, or congestion, in the digestive organs, in the brain or spinal chord; from organic changes of structure in these parts; from the presence of worms in the intestinal canal, and many other causes, all of which would be aggravated by a stimulant or tonic treatment.

The tonic and stimulant remedies used for this purpose are called *Antispasmodics*. Assafœtida, galbanum, ammoniacum, myrrh, valerian, and musk, are those generally employed.

Convulsive Tonics.

On the other hand, again, there is a tribe of tonics which act as such only when used in small doses, and when taken too freely themselves cause convulsive movements, resembling those witnessed in tetanus, and which may even prove fatal. The nux-vomica bark, seeds, and leaves, strychnine, brucine, the viscum monoicum, (kuchela-mulung), all these prove powerfully tonic, stimulating the nervous system to increased and permanent activity, and thereby remarkably influencing the muscular apparatus. It is not uncommon to find such remedies inducing slight spasmodic twitchings of the limbs, even when given in the most cautious doses. When this happens their use must be forthwith given up, or at least intermitted.

It is especially in paralysis that this tribe of tonics proves most useful, and many remarkable cases are on record of the successful treatment of such diseases by the remedies now described.

Astringent Tonics.

Astringent tonics are those which have the special power of causing the contraction of the parts to which they are applied, either by the permanent shortening of the muscular fibre, or the coagulation of albuminous fluid.

All vegetable substances containing *tannic* and *gallic* acid are remarkable for producing this effect, and are therefore capable, under many circumstances, of arresting profuse secretions and discharges, by mechanically contracting the orifices from which the discharge proceeds—or by producing chemical changes on surfaces in a raw ulcerated state.

Gall-nuts, Peruvian bark, babul bark, the cœsalpinia, and rohun, may be cited as astringent remedies owing all their virtue to the presence of tannic and gallic acid.

Some inorganic substances, especially alumn, the salts of lead, iron, and copper, and corrosive sublimate, have this property to an extraordinary degree. The salts of lead even seem to exercise it generally (that is on parts to which they are not immediately applied) as for instance, when administered by the stomach they check bleeding from the lungs or uterus.

It rarely happens, however, that we are enabled to employ astringents uncombined with other remedies. The parts which demand their use are often inflamed, or very irritable, and in either case narcotics or sedatives may be required to deaden the sensibility of the part, and enable the astringent to act upon it with efficacy. Thus in cholera, dysentery, diarrhœa, and many similar states, we use opium or hyoscyamus with acetate of lead or sulphate of copper.

FOURTH DIVISION.

Agents acting by depressing the vital powers.

a. By diminishing the generation of heat. *Refrigerants.*

b. By diminishing the action of the brain and spinal chord. *Narcotics.*

§ 1.—*Refrigerants.*

The temperature of the human body in health averages 96° of Fahrenheit's thermometer. This heat is under ordinary circumstances constant, that is to say, it does not rise or fall with that of surrounding bodies, as is the case with inanimate matter, and with several of the lower animals. Thus in experiments instituted by Sir Charles Blagden and others, they exposed themselves to a heat of nearly 300° without the temperature of the body rising higher than 99½°. On the other hand, in the Arctic voyages of discovery while the external air was so cold as the point at which mercury freezes (—39°), the temperature of the body remained constant, provided the apparel worn was of the proper non-conducting quality.

In some diseased conditions, especially in inflammation, tropical fevers, and scarlatina, we find the heat of the skin to increase several degrees. In scarlatina it has been noticed as high as 108°. In other morbid states, for example in the malignant cholera, the heat of the body falls even below that of surrounding objects. In May, at Calcutta, while the thermometer is at 98° or 100° in the shade, it is not uncommon to see cases of cholera in which the thermometer applied to the skin indicates 64°.

The physiological cause of animal heat is not clearly understood. The arterial blood in circulating through the body gradually changes in color from that of vermillion to a deep purple. It loses oxygen and becomes impregnated with carbonic acid and water. These facts shew that in the minute arterial terminations, and during the functions of secretion and absorption, carbon and hydrogen combine with oxygen. As a necessary consequence of this union, according to the existing state of chemical knowledge, heat must be evolved. By interrupting the circulation of a part we diminish or destroy its natural warmth. On the other hand, increased circulation is almost always attended by a proportionate increase of temperature.

But the subject is still fraught with very great difficulty.

The division of the chief nerve leading to an organ destroys its heat as effectually as the interruption of the arterial circulation. What the precise relation between the circulating and nervous systems may be, how far one is dependent on the other, or whether in the circle of actions constituting the phenomena of life, one system can ever play an independent part, the state of physiological knowledge does not yet enable us to determine.

But difficult or impossible although it be to reach the causes of the phenomena of heat, we still possess many powerful agents by which its degree may be either increased or diminished.

Under the head of "stimulants" will be found a general description of the agents by whose operation the heat of the body is increased. The student will observe that none of these act in accordance with any chemical or physical views.—We do not administer highly oxygenated salts or acids as theory might indicate, but we rely on agents acting chiefly on the nervous system—either quickly and transitorily as the diffusible stimulants—or more slowly, but permanently, as the tonics and astringents.

Refrigerants, or cooling agents, are of two kinds—external and internal.

External Refrigerants.

Of these there are several kinds—

1. Those which act by the direct abstraction of heat, such as cold air, ice, or iced or cold water—cooling mixtures of ice, or solutions of neutral salts *(See Table, page 46)*, especially the *muriate of ammonia.* While these salts undergo solution, heat is rendered latent, the temperature falls several degrees, and applied in this state to the skin, the solution abstracts its free caloric till equilibrium of sensible heat takes place.

Other external refrigerants act by rendering heat latent by evaporation—thus spirit, sulphuric ether, or acetic acid, undergoing evaporation on the skin, this organ parts with its heat very rapidly as the fluid evaporates.

The effects produced by the sudden abstraction of heat from the skin, are proportionate to the extent of the tissue affected, to the degree of cold applied, and the mean temperature of the air in which the individual is accustomed to reside. To the inhabitants of the tropics the sudden fall of 10 to 15 degrees of external warmth causes tightness and shrinking of the skin, diminished capillary circulation, shivering, and internal congestion, and may lead to the occurrence of fevers and inflammatory states of the liver, lungs, intestinal mucous membrane, &c. A still lower temperature or prolonged exposure, may cause the loss of life by the remote action on the nervous or vital powers, but still without influencing the texture of the skin itself.

Cold, moreover, especially when applied locally and in great excess, may lead to two sets of injuries. The circulation totally failing, frost-bite and gangrene of the part may occur, and this is constantly exemplified in cold countries in the loss of the ears, the nose, fingers, &c. the parts most exposed to the contact of an intensely chilling atmosphere. Or if the cold be concentrated and intense, as when frozen mercury is applied to the skin, speedy destruction of the part may ensue, its tissue having nearly the same appearances as those occasioned by fire.

External refrigerants are chiefly used in the treatment of ardent fever, of apoplexy, of inflammations of the limbs, in wounds, and strangulated hernia. The cold affusion, or subjecting the patient to the action of a dash of cold water; sponging the body with cold water; the application to the head of ice, or of a solution of muriate of ammonia, or of cloths dipped in sulphuric ether, are remedies continually had recourse to in the treatment of the fevers of this country.

Internal Refrigerants.

Chemical science has hitherto pointed out no remedy acting in exact conformity with physical theories, and by the internal use of which the heat of the body can be reduced.

The nitrate of potash was long considered a powerful refrigerant, and much used in the treatment of fevers. Dr. Murray attempted to explain its action in conformity with Crawford's hypothesis, that animal heat was occasioned by the combination in the lungs of the carbon of the venous blood with the oxygen of the air; that the heat thus caused was rendered latent in the arterial blood, and again set free in the course of the circulation; lastly, that nitrate of potash being highly oxygenated, and thus providing the blood with the element it required from the air, the changes above described did not occur in the lungs. The theory of Dr. Crawford, as well as its adaptation by Dr. Murray, are justly rejected by modern physiologists, as being either at variance with facts, or unsupported by experimental evidence. Nitrate of potash in small doses doubtless does produce some refrigerating effect, but when it does so it always proves at the same time powerfully diuretic. The determination of blood towards the kidneys, which must precede this increased secretion, diminishes the circulation in the minute vessels of the skin, and thus it appears most likely it is that the cooling effect is occasioned.

Many neutral salts, indeed, as well as other promoters of secretion, whether local or general, on this obvious principle diminish morbid excess of heat. Thus purgatives—sudorifics, especially antimonials, and ipecachuanha—diuretics, and chiefly digitalis, produce this effect in a remarkable degree, and accordingly are highly valued in the treatment of ardent fevers.

There are however certain agents which seem to direct their action primarily on the nervous system, the powers of which they directly lower; this sedative effect extending to the circulating system, general cooling of the body follows. Foxglove (digitalis) may be cited as an excellent example of this kind. The cautious use of small doses of this remedy in the fevers of Bengal is frequently followed by extraordinary benefit. It is especially useful where fever coincides with an irritable or inflamed state of the alimentary canal, a condition which antimonials seldom fail to aggravate.

The only other refrigerant we deem it necessary to notice prominently, is the hydrocyanic acid. In doses of one or two drops, given with half an ounce of water, this energetic remedy rapidly depresses the vital powers, and produces retardation of the pulse, and lowering of the temperature. Its use, however, as well as that of digitalis, demands great care and close observation, and is scarcely to be entrusted to any inexperienced practitioner.

FOURTH DIVISION,—*(Continued.)*

b. External agents acting on the brain, or spinal chord, or on both.

§ 1.—*Narcotics.*

This highly important class of remedies, demands more special consideration than we have bestowed on the preceding sections.

Narcotics, properly mean those remedies which have the power of occasioning stupor (narke, ναρκη). They are also called hypnotics, from their generally inducing sleep, (hypnos υπνόσ), also anodynes, from their alleviating pain, (odune οδυνη), and sedatives, from the calming influence they exercise. Narcotics may act first locally, that is on the part to which they are directly applied—secondly, by entering into the circulation, and coming into direct contact with the nervous centres—or lastly, by the sympathetic influence which distant organs and their states may exercise on each other.

The brain, spinal chord, and nervous system, are primarily affected by these agents, and various organs experience remotely, or indirectly, special effects from different narcotics.

Most narcotics when given in small doses prove stimulant, as alcohol, opium, and gunjah; and even in large doses these exercise a stimulant effect before the sinking of the vital powers is witnessed. Some narcotics, on the contrary, produce no perceptible excitement; of these hydrocyanic acid and digitalis are the best examples.

Sleep is not an invariable sequel of the effects of narcotics when given in remedial doses. Although digitalis and tobacco can produce sleep, it is morbidly deep, amounting almost to apoplexy, or the state termed coma.

Opium, while it first excites, generally terminates by causing an invincible tendency to sleep; in excessive doses, profound coma, &c. supervenes, with stertorous breathing; and as a sequel to this state, in cases of recovery, constipation is a general effect. The pulse throughout may be full and soft; sometimes convulsions occur; the pupil is generally contracted; the temperature continues undiminished, the skin commonly moist. Should the dose be greater than life can support, the body on examination presents few appearances worthy of remark. Congestion of the vessels of the brain, effusion of serum into the ventricles, in rare cases extravasation of blood—such are the only leading phenomena, and these are evidently not peculiar to this narcotic.

It is but rare that in the excitement stage of the effects of opium, any mental delusion prevails, or any violent intoxication is observed. Reverie and calm enjoyment, or at most cheerfulness, are witnessed.

Hyoscyamus, or henbane, the action of which approaches that of opium, causes, in large doses, loss of voice, dilatation of the pupil, coma, and delirium, often of a furious kind.

Belladonna, or the deadly nightshade, and its near ally the mandrake, are remarkable for the great degree of dilatation of the pupil they occasion, even when externally applied, or taken internally in very small doses. In larger quantities extravagant delirium first occurs, and afterwards coma: convulsions are very rare.

Stramonium, or the Datura, is chiefly marked by its occasioning deep comatose sleep, with dilatation of the pupil, and in some cases, insensibility to light. Furious delirium, and paralysis of the lower extremities have also been noticed.

Gunjah, or the Indian Hemp, in small doses, proves powerfully excitant, occasioning singular laughing, or extatic delirium, followed by cataleptic rigidity, and deep sleep; in large doses there is less excitement, the cataleptic state less pronounced, and the coma more profound.

Tobacco when swallowed or otherwise taken by persons not habituated to its use, causes great paleness, sinking, tremors, violent nausea and vomiting, purging, coldness of the skin, smallness and acceleration of the pulse, dilatation of the pupil, and in extreme cases, convulsions, coma, and death.

The effects of hydrocyanic acid and digitalis have been already adverted to.

Such is an epitome of the effects occasioned by the principal narcotics employed in medicine. The study of these effects naturally points to the morbid conditions in which their use is of greatest benefit.

To produce the stimulating effects of narcotics, in excessive fatigue, exhaustion, cholera, &c. *small* doses of opium, gunjah, or hyoscyamus are successfully resorted to.

To alleviate pain, as in cases of neuralgia, sciatica, tic doloroux, &c. opium or gunjah in *full* doses, alone or united with ipecachuanha, or antimonials, will often prove successful.

In sleeplessness and anxiety, as in the disease termed delirum tremens, (occasioned by the excessive use of spirituous liquors), opium or gunjah when freely given will be found in a large proportion of cases to effect a cure, the diminution of tremor, or the return of sleep, being the first evidence of the disease yielding.

In several spasmodic diseases, such as hydrophobia and tetanus, opium in excessively large doses has been tried, but without the benefit anticipated. The gunjah in such cases seems to promise better results. In cases of cholera, where cramps are frequent and severe, in convulsive paroxysms occasioned by the strychnos poisons, and in several other spasmodic or convulsive maladies, such as asthma and hooping cough, these narcotics have been tried with advantage.

The narcotics which so remarkably influence the pupil, belladonna, hyoscyamus, and stramonium, especially the first, are used accordingly in many diseased conditions of the eye, in which it may be deemed essential to prevent the edges of the iris from being agglutinated together.

In many febrile and inflammatory diseases, hydrocyanic acid or opium, either alone or combined with other remedies, especially calomel, have been used with the utmost advantage. Thus in peritonitis, full doses of opium at the same time alleviate the agony of the patient, and seem to check the progress of the disease.

Lastly, lacerated wounds and burns may be specified as cases in which opium frequently produces the most valuable results.

It is necessary to remind the student that habit often exercises a powerful influence on the quantities of narcotics which may be administered in practice, or taken for the purposes of intoxication. Enormous quantities of opium have been consumed daily by many individuals. Violent disease also, such as tetanus and hydrophobia, renders the system so insensible to these narcotics, that excessive doses are borne with impunity. It does not seem however that hydrocyanic acid is thus affected. Digitalis is distinguished by its often *accumulating* in the system, without producing any particular result from each dose, until at length overwhelming collapse sets in, the whole quantity exercising its powers at one time. Several fatal cases have thus occurred, which point out the necessity of extreme caution in the use of this energetic and somewhat capricious remedy, especially in the treatment of remittent fevers.

FIFTH DIVISION—CHEMICAL AGENTS.

a. Destroying tissue—*escharotics, caustics.*
b. Solvents of urinary stones or gravel—*lithontriptics.*

§ 1.—*The Actual Cautery—Moxa.*

There are several substances which are capable of totally destroying the tissue of any organic matter with which they come in contact; of these the most remarkable are—ignited bodies; the mineral acids; the alkalies; some of the salts of mercury, silver, copper, and zinc.

Ignited bodies, or the actual cautery, afford a formidable agent, which at once subverts the composition of the part to which it is applied. It was much used by the old surgeons, and is still by veterinary practitioners, and among savage nations. It is chiefly resorted to for the destruction of carious or sloughy parts, as a counter-irritant in rheumatism, sciatica, and other neuralgic diseases, and for the purpose of restraining hæmorrhages by scorching and shrivelling up the mouths of the divided vessels. Amputated stumps were thus treated by the older European surgeons, and are still so in Nipal, and in many parts of the East.

When actual heat is employed as a counter-irritant, the *moxa* is generally had recourse to. The *moxa* is the cottony down which envelopes the leaves of some species of artemisia. It is formed into a cone, generally an inch in diameter at the base, and 1⅛ inch high; this is secured on the skin by a brass ring with a wooden handle; the tip of the cone is then touched with a match, and the ignition urged by a bellows or by the breath. Before the flame reaches the skin the heated air generally occasions a blister, producing at the same time excessive pain. When the flame is within a line of the skin, the ring should be lifted off. A slough usually follows after a variable interval, and leaves an open, healthy sore.

Raw cotton dipped in a weak solution of saltpetre, then dried and compressed, is an excellent substitute for the true moxa.

Dentists are sometimes accustomed to apply the actual cautery to nervous filaments lying exposed in the hollow of a carious tooth. The best mode of accomplishing this object is by the ignition of a small platinum wire placed in the circuit of a galvanic battery of 12 plates. Two twisted copper wires, 10 feet long, and each covered with silk, terminate in a platinum loop at one end, and two diverging naked wires at the other. The loop is first introduced cold into the tooth, and then by bringing the wires into contact with the battery poles the platinum ignites, and the nerve is instantaneously destroyed.

The actual cautery, in its various forms, is sometimes resorted to in the collapse of cholera, and in asphyxia from drowning. A cup filled with boiling water, covered with a thick towel, and then swiftly inverted on the part, offers a quick, safe, and effectual method of employing heat in these desperate cases. Gunpowder flashed on the skin, or spirits kindled on its surface, are sometimes resorted to on similar emergencies.

Caustics and Escharotics.

The mineral acids, alkalies, and some of the salts of silver, mercury, copper and zinc, afford the best examples of these agents.

Acid, Alkaline, and Silver Caustics.

The skin is composed ultimately of carbon, nitrogen, oxygen, and hydrogen. These elements under the operation of chemical caustics undergo changes of arrangement on which the peculiar physical effects of the caustic depend.

Sulphuric acid having a very powerful affinity for water, causes the oxygen and hydrogen of the skin to combine to form that fluid; carbon is set free, forming a black stain, and various gaseous compounds are disengaged, causing a brisk effervescence.

Nitric acid, if very strong, produces similar changes, but it forms carbazotic acid with the carbon, and produces a bright yellow stain on the part.

Nitrate of silver (lunar caustic), acts on the proximate principles of the skin; the albumen unites with the oxide of silver, and the acid further produces the effects above described; a white stain is first occasioned, which rapidly blackens on exposure to the light. The new combination being solid does not spread, so that we can limit the action of the caustic to such parts as we desire to affect.

The *Caustic alkalies*, potash, soda, and ammonia, combine with the oily and gelatinous tissues, and convert these into a soap. Attracting water from the atmosphere the two former deliquesce, and spread, so that it is necessary to defend the parts in the vicinity from being injured. This is usually managed by the application of adhesive plaster, perforated where we desire to effect the cauterization.

To moderate the effects of potash, and soda, these caustics are frequently made into a paste with lime.

Mercurial Caustics.

These are chiefly corrosive sublimate, bin-ioduret of mercury, and the acid protonitrate and pernitrate of that metal.

The *corrosive sublimate* (bi-chloride of mercury) is reduced to the state of protochloride by the contact of animal tissue, the disintegration of which it very speedily causes. It is never used as a remedial caustic.

The *bin-ioduret of mercury* acting in the same way, but also remotely producing the specific effects of mercury and iodine, occasionally proves a very useful caustic, especially in the treatment of scrofulous and syphilitic ulcers.

The *acid nitrates of mercury* have been highly recommended by Dupuytren, and some other French surgeons, as caustics in sloughing venereal sores, and in hospital gangrene.

Copper Caustics.

Sulphate of copper produces effects much resembling those of lunar caustic. It is a cheap, manageable, and very useful article, much used in repressing excessive granulations, and in promoting cicatrization.

The nitrate and acetate of copper enter into the composition of ointments occasionally used as cauteries or stimulants.

Zinc Caustics—Arsenic.

The chloride of zinc has recently been discovered to possess considerable caustic energy, attacking morbid, while it seems to spare healthy, tissue—producing merely inflammation in the latter, while the former is corroded or dissolved. For the uses of the chloride of zinc in cancer, see "*zinc preparations.*"

Arsenic is in some works erroneously described as a caustic. It always acts by producing inflammation.

---

§ 2.—*Lithontriptics.*

These are agents supposed to possess the property of effecting the solution of stony or sandy deposits in the bladder.

By reference to the account of the urine, it will be seen to contain, in the natural state, several earthy and solid ingredients, especially phosphates of lime and magnesia and uric acid. In the healthy state the two former exist in solution in the free acid of the urine; the latter is in minute quantity, and probably combined with soda, which enables it to remain in solution.

Should any circumstance tend to render the urine alkaline, the necessary consequence will be the precipitation of phosphate of lime or of magnesia, or of both these bases. The circumstances under which uric acid is precipitated are not so clearly understood. The condition which favors an alkaline state of the urine encourages the solution of uric acid, and perhaps its formation in larger than usual quantities. If under this state an acid condition should alternate, the uric acid will then be deposited.

Paralysis of the bladder is one of the causes which leads to the alkaline state of the urine. Preternatural acidity is usually the result of a more remote morbid state, affecting the secretion itself as formed in the kidneys.

Accordingly we find stones or sand to be generally either phosphate of lime, phosphate of lime and magnesia, uric acid, alternations of these substances, carbonate of lime, the mulberry calculus or oxalate of lime. Rarer varieties, such as the cystic and xanthic oxide, and fibrinous calculus, are described, but require no notice here.

These calculi we may divide thus,

Soluble in acids.	*Soluble in alkalies.*
Phosphate of lime.	Uric acid.
——— of magnesia.	Lithate or urate of ammonia.
Ammoniaco-magnesian phosphate.	
Oxalate of lime.	

The object of lithontriptics is to produce in the urine the most favorable state for inducing the solution of the particular stone. An acid state is occasioned by the cautious use of the nitric or muriatic acids,—the alkaline state, by means of soda, potash, cream of tartar, the citrates of potash and soda, &c. A reference to the Table of Diuretics, in the appendix, will give further particulars on this subject.

Some surgeons have proposed to inject the solvent directly into the bladder. This attempt however has proved always intolerable, through the excessive irritation occasioned to the patient.

Dumas some years since proposed to attack the calculus by introducing the poles of the galvanic battery, one into the rectum, the other into the bladder. The form of battery then in use occasioned severe shocks, and was moreover of little decomposing power. We are now in possession of far superior instruments, effecting powerful decomposition without occasioning pain to the most sensitive organ. Still the proposal seems unpromising, from the very great difficulty with which *solid* substances undergo decomposition. In numerous experiments made by the editor of this work, calculi were exposed to a powerful and constant current for several days without any practical diminution of their weight. The apparatus used was a glass cylinder closed at one end by a membrane, and placed in a vessel containing urine, which was frequently renewed. A plate of platinum was inserted in each vessel, and connected with a 12 plate battery. The urine in contact with the calculus could thus be rendered acid or alkaline at pleasure, still without the desired effect being obtained.

PART V.

THE VEGETABLE MATERIA MEDICA ARRANGED ACCORDING TO THE NATURAL SYSTEM.

Division I.

VASCULARES OR COTYLEDONEÆ

Classes.

1st.	2nd.
Dicotyledoneæ,	*Monocotyledoneæ,*
or	or
Exogenæ.	*Endogenæ.*
Increasing by external layers. Leaves with branching veins, wood and bark distinct.	Increasing by internal layers, no distinction of bark and wood, veins simple.

Class I.

Dicotyledoneæ, or Exogenæ.

Sub-classes IV.

1. *Thalamifloræ.*—Petals many, distinct, and with the stamens inserted into the receptacle.
2. *Calycifloræ.*—Petals many, distinct, or united at base, with the stamens inserted into the calyx.
3. *Corollifloræ.*—Petals united into one, bearing the stamens, and inserted into the receptacle.
4. *Monochlamydeæ.*—Corolla wanting, or united with calyx—staminiferous.

Sub-class 1—Thalamifloræ.

Section 1.—Ovaries numerous, aggregate, each having a style; rarely solitary, from abortion or coalition. Stamens indefinite, or if definite opposite the petals, and either 5 or a multiple of 5.

NAT. ORDER I.—RANUNCULACEÆ.

This important natural family consists of herbaceous, shrubby, or rarely climbing plants, with fascicular, fibrous, or tuberous roots, and alternate, sometimes opposite, rarely amplexicaul leaves. The calyx is distinguished by the sepals being from 3 to 15 in number, distinct, deciduous; æstivation usually imbricated, sometimes valvular; corolla occasionally deficient (as in Thalictrum); petals from 5 to 15; stamens numerous; anthers adnate, opening externally, inserted with petals below the pistils; pistils seated on a torus, united in each of the flowers; ovaries one-celled, with one ovule—or many-seeded, capsular, baccate—or follicular as in Aconite; seeds albuminous; embryo minute; albumen horny; style lateral, sometimes long and feathery.

The Ranunculaceæ are chiefly natives of temperate climates, a few only being found in India within 25° north latitude; of these, all but eight or nine are, according to Dr. Wight, natives of the hilly districts. Nearly 100 species have been discovered in the Himalayas.

The majority of the Ranunculaceæ contain an acrid principle, volatile at the temperature of boiling water, and capable of producing inflammation and vesication if brought in contact with the skin. The taste is stimulating and acrid; if swallowed either in substance or solution, many of these plants occasion violent purging and vomiting, sinking of the pulse, cramps, collapse, and death. Some contain a powerful narcotic alkali named *Aconitina*, of much value in the treatment of rheumatism, and neuralgic diseases. Others are bitter tonics, devoid of poisonous properties, or slightly aperient. Lastly, the seeds of one species (Nigella) contain a somewhat aromatic essential oil, are valued as a spice, and much used as a popular stimulating medicine.

Dr. Wight remarks, that of the species found in lower India, none have been noticed by Rheede or Ainslie, while the few which Roxburgh knew, he merely gives a botanical account of; neither have these been assigned any medicinal virtues by native writers.

The order is subdivided into five tribes—the Clematideæ, Anemoneæ, Ranunculeæ, Helleboreæ, and Pæoniaceæ.

Tribe 1—Clematideæ.

Involucre 0, or resembling a calyx below the flower. Sepals 4—8, coloured, valvate—Petals 0, or shorter than the sepals. Achenia numerous, terminated by a long feathery, hardened, tail like style—Seed pendulous—Perennials, usually with permanent half shrubby stems—Leaves exactly opposite. (*Lindley's Flora Medica, p.* 61.)

This tribe is acrid and poisonous; the leaves and fresh stems if bruised and applied to the skin cause vesication. Royle describes 10 Himalayan species. There is one, the *Clematis gouriana,* abundant among the ruins of Gour, and which doubtless participates in the properties of the others. In France the *C. vitalba* is used by mendicants to cause artificial sores for the furtherance of their impostures. In Cochin China, according to Louriero, the *C. sinensis* is used as a diuretic and diaphoretic. At the Mauritius the *C. mauritiana* is employed to blister the cheek for the relief of tooth ache.

No species of Clematis is admitted in the British pharmacopeiæ—still from the experiments of Storck, Wendt, and Mueller with several species, in the treatment of syphilis, scrofula, and rheumatism, there seems much reason to hope for beneficial effects from the cautious trial of the Indian kinds. Storck used an infusion of 2 scruples of the dried leaf in a pint of boiling water, the dose 4 ounces thrice daily.

Tribe 2—Anemoneæ.

Calyx and corolla imbricate in the bud, petals absent or flat, carpels one seeded, indehiscent, usually ending in a tail or point. Seed pendulous, leaves allineate or radical. Herbs; rarely even shrubs.

This subdivision contains only herbs. The leaves of all are acrid and irritating, and cause blistering if applied while fresh to the skin. The roots are generally purgative, and so uncertain in their action that few have been much employed in medicine. The *Anemone pulsatilla,* and *nemorosa* are described by Fee, Lindley, and others, as exceedingly acrid and corrosive. The *A. cernua,* however, according to Siebold is in high repute among the Chinese as a tonic bitter, under the name of Hak-too-woo.

Genus I.—Thalictrum.

Involucre none, calyx of 4 or 5 deciduous, petal-like sepals; petals none; carpels 4 to 15, pointed, stalked, or sessile. Roots perennial, stems annual, flowers corymbose, panicled, somewhat racemose, green, white, and yellow.

Of this important genus Royle notices 9 species, natives of Mussooree, Kunawur, and Cashmere. The following is the most remarkable—

Species 1. *Thalictrum foliolosum*, Wall. (*Vern.* Pelijuree; Shuprak.) Off. The *root*.

This plant is found at Mussooree, and generally on the Himalayas. For specimens of the roots we are indebted to Dr. Falconer of Seharunpore.

The roots are fibrous, fasciculate, about the thickness of a crow quill, dark brown externally, internally yellow, rather difficult to pulverize, bitter to the taste. They yield to water 25 per cent. of a yellow bitter extract, to alcohol 15 per cent. The watery solutions do not blacken the salts of iron, and give no precipitate with infusion of gelatine, but yield a slight precipitate when treated by ammonia. A sufficient quantity was not at our disposal to enable us to ascertain if this precipitate contains any peculiar or alkaline principle.

The bruised root having been given to large dogs in the quantity of 10 grs. to ʒij. no particular effects were observed.

It has been used in the Hospital of the Medical College in several cases of ague, and as a tonic in the convalescence from acute diseases.

5 grs. of the powder, or 2 grs. of the watery extract given thrice daily, have in some cases prevented, and in several moderated, the accession of fever, and at the same time acted gently on the bowels. The only sensation experienced was warmth at the epigastrium, and a general comfortable feeling.

Another species of Thalictrum (flavum) is common in France, where it is termed "the poor man's rhubarb", as a substitute for which medicine it is generally employed. The Indian species is easily procurable from the hills, though not known in the bazars of the lower provinces.

It deserves extensive trial, and promises to succeed well as a febrifuge of some power, and a tonic aperient of peculiar value.

Dose of the powder—5 to 10 grs. as a tonic and aperient, in the interval of intermittent fevers, and in convalescence from acute diseases.

Officinal preparations. Powder, tincture, and extract, for which see the Pharmacopœia.

Under the sub-division *Anemoneæ*, Fée further notices the *Knowltonia vesicatoria*, used commonly as a blister at the Cape of Good Hope, and the *Hydrastis canadensis*, or Canadian yellow root, a valuable bitter tonic, and useful yellow dye-stuff.

Tribe 3—Ranunculeæ.

Calyx and corolla imbricate in the bud—Petals sometimes wanting—sometimes irregular, bilabiate, nectariferous—Calyx petal-like—Corolla capsular, dehiscent, many-seeded, leaves radical or alternate—Herbs.

(*Don's Gen. Syst. p.* 3.)

This sub-division contains several plants of great poisonous energy. They are extremely acrid and corrosive, and so unmanageable as to be excluded from medical use by all modern practitioners. The *R. sceleratus* (*R. indicus* of Roxburgh, *R. carnosus*, Wall.) and *ficaria* are described by Fée. The former is common in northern India, and used as a blister by the natives. These with the *R. acris* and *bulbosus* all agree in their vesicating, and acrid properties.

Draughts of tepid water constitute the best remedy in cases of poisoning by these plants, by diluting the acrid juices on which their effects chiefly depend.

Tribe 4—Helleboreæ.

Calyx and corolla imbricated in the bud, petals sometimes wanting, sometimes irregular, bilabiate, nectariferous; calyx of 5 petal-like sepals, carpels capsular, many seeded, opening on the inside.

Gen. 1.—Coptis.

Calyx of 5 or 6 coloured petal-like, deciduous sepals—petals small, cucullate; stamens 20 to 25; capsules 6 to 10 on long stalks, somewhat membranous, 4-6 seeded, pointed, with the style stellately disposed. Small, smooth, and stiffish perennial herbs, with divided leaves, and small white flowers.

(*Don. Syst. p.* 46.)

Sp. 1. *Coptis Teeta*, Wall.

(*Vern.* Mishmee Teeta, *Assamese.* Honglane, *Chinese.* Golden-thread root of Assam.) Off. The *root.*

Leaves trisected, segments being petiolate, lobed and pinnatifid, lobes deeply divided. Scape with few flowers, internally of a dark golden colour. Leaves erect, glabrous, with long petioles of firm texture. Petiole slender, dilated at the base. Scape round, erect, thin, slightly striated, bearing flowers (seldom more than three) on its apex, the flowers being small, alternate, and pedunculate; sepals oblong, lanceolate, pale, with parallel veins. Petals lanceolate or strap-like, obtuse, thrice shorter than the sepals; stamens and pistils numerous; anthers plano-rotund, pale; unripe carpella membranous, terminating in an obtuse net; style cylindrical. Bracteæ under each peduncle.

The Coptis Teeta is a native of the mountainous regions bordering on upper Assam, and is in high repute among the Mishmee, Lamas, and Assamese. Dr. Wallich, in a paper in the VIIth volume of the Transactions of the Medical and Physical Society of Calcutta, informs us that quantities are sent down to Assam in neat little baskets with open meshes, made of narrow strips of rattan, and measuring 3 to 4 inches in length by 2½ in breadth, and 1½ in width; each basket contains about an ounce of small pieces of the root from 1 to 3 inches long. The roots are nearly cylindrical, and uneven, scabrous, more or less curved, of a greyish brown colour externally, internally bright yellow, varying in thickness from the size of a crow quill, to double that diameter. The root is perfectly dry and brittle, occasionally a few fibrillæ issuing from one end. The taste is intensely and purely bitter, very lasting, with only a slight aroma. On mastication the root tinges the saliva yellow.

In North America the Coptis trifolia is much employed as a bitter tonic, and has been accurately described by Bigelow. The chemical properties of the American correspond exactly with those of the Assamese root, which contains neither tannic nor gallic acid, but abounds in a yellow bitter principle, soluble in alcohol and water.

The Coptis Teeta has found its way through the drug shops of Bengal, and is even occasionally exposed for sale in the upper provinces; it brings a very high price, and is deemed a tonic remedy of the greatest value. It has been used extensively in the General Hospital by the late Mr. Twining, who reported that its influence in restoring appetite, and increasing the digestive powers, were very remarkable, and that it might be said to possess all the properties of our best bitter tonics.

Further trials in the College Hospital were equally satisfactory. It did not seem to exercise any febrifuge virtue, but under its influence several patients recovering from acute diseases, manifestly, and very rapidly, improved in strength. The dose was 5 to 10 grs. of the powder, or an ounce of the infusion thrice daily.

Officinal preparations. Powder, tincture, infusion, and extract.

Gen. 2.—Nigella.

Calyx of five deciduous, petal-like sepals.—Petals five to ten; carpels five, connected. Styles very long.

(*Don's Gen. Sys. p.* 3.)

Sp. 1. *Nigella sativa.* Small Fennel flower.

(*Syn.* Siah daneh, *Pers.* Hab. Sinde, *Egypt.* Mugrela, *Bengal.* Kala-jira, *Hind.* Μελανθιον of Dioscorides.) Off. The *seeds.*

This plant is a native of the south of Europe, Egypt, Barbary, and the Caucasus, and is extensively cultivated in India.

The stem is erect, 1-2 feet high, many flowered, downy. Leaves capillary, cut into numerous fine segments. Petioles downy; flowers naked, dirty white; anthers, ovate, obtuse; capsules muricated, united up to the point into an oval fruit, terminated by 5 erect styles.

The *seeds*, resembling coarse gunpowder, are triangular, slightly compressed, obtuse above with oblique bases, rugose, black externally, internally of a greenish white hue. The capsules are polyspermous, oblong, and pointed at the side.

The seeds are of strong aromatic odour, and flavour resembling sassafras or cubebs. These properties are due to an essential oil, of which the seeds yield from 5 to 10 per cent.

The nigella seeds have been long used in medicine, and are praised by Hippocrates as a tonic condiment. At present they are chiefly employed by the native Hakims and Baidas as aromatic adjuncts to purgative or bitter remedies. In Bengal they are given to nurses, in the belief that they increase the secretion of milk, and facts have been laid before us which tend to corroborate that opinion. In eruptions of the skin Dr. Ainslie informs us, the seeds reduced to powder and mixed with sesamum oil, are much used as an external application.

The seed will seldom be prescribed in substance. The tincture is a useful, warm stimulant, and may be added conveniently to numerous draughts and mixtures intended for other purposes. The popular mode of giving the nigella to nurses is by mixing the powdered seed with curry, to which however it communicates a very heavy and disagreeable flavour.

The price of the seed in the bazars is from one to two annas the seer,—2lbs. avoirdupois.

Officinal preparations. Powder and tincture.

Gen. 3.—Aconitum.

Calyx of 5 petal-like, irregular, deciduous or marcescent sepals; upper sepal helmet-shaped; petals or nectaries two within the helmet, on long stalks, tubulate above, spurlike below; spur straight, hooked, or twisted. Herbaceous, perennial, with tuberous, fibrous, or napiform roots; leaves palmate, partitions toothed, and racemes terminal, with one flowered pedicels rising from the axillæ of the bracteæs; flowers large, irregular, blue, yellow, cream-colored, or white. All species are poisonous except *A. atees.*

Sp. 1.—***Aconitum ferox.***

(*Vern.* Bish. Bikh. Meetha Teelia. Metha zuher. Ati Singeea Bish. Bishnak.)

Off. The *root.*

A native of the Himalayan mountains, Sirmoor, Kemaon, and Nipal, and one of the most celebrated articles in Indian medicine and toxicology. The plant was first identified and described by Dr. Wallich in his Plantæ Asiaticæ Rariores.

The tubers are 2 or 3, fasciculate, fusiform, 2-4 inches long, blackish externally, pale inside. Stems erect, 2 to 3 feet high, smooth at base, slightly downy upwards, branches villous; leaves roundish, heart-shaped, deeply 5 parted, lobes incised, pinnatifid, wedge-shaped at base, generally hairy along the veins on the lower side. Racemes terminal, long, downy; flowers large, deep blue, hairy; helmet gibbous, semicircular, about an inch long, with a short beak in front; hooded petals cylindrical, narrow, slightly incurved.

The roots (which enter into several formulæ constantly employed by the native practitioners, and which are also doubtless too often used as convenient instruments of poisoning) are sold in every bazar in India, and may be purchased in large quantities for about 10 annas the seer.

The root is brittle, breaks with a resinous fracture, and is readily reduced to a coarse powder; in this state it is destitute of smell, slightly bitter to the taste, the tongue being subsequently benumbed wherever touched on. 1000 parts yield to water 280; to alcohol, 360. The watery solution is copiously precipitated by ammonia. The precipitate re-dissolves in water acidulated with sulphuric acid. If again thrown down by ammonia, and re-dissolved by boiling alcohol, on cooling, and spontaneous evaporation, the solution deposits crystals of an alkali named *Aconitina.* (See Pharmacopœia.)

Aconitina is soluble in 150 times its weight of cold, 50 of boiling water; crystallizes from the saturated alcoholic solution, is soluble also in ether, and decidedly alkaline. The salts it forms with acids are not crystalline, and are very bitter.

Aconitina is too formidable a poison to be used internally; externally it is employed, with much advantage, in neuralgia and tic doloroux, in the form of ointment, composed of one grain of aconitina to ʒi of lard.

Aconitina was first discovered by Pallas in 1835, in the root of the Aconitum napellus, or monk's hood, a species included in the European Pharmacopeiæ, and long known as a most energetic acrid narcotic. It is associated with a peculiar vegetable acid which has lately been examined by Braconnot, and described in the *Journal de Pharmacie* for 1838. It is to the aconitina alone, however, that the bikh root owes its medicinal and poisonous properties.

In the recent state, all the species of aconite, especially our article and the Acon. Napellus, exercise the most powerful influence on the animal economy. If swallowed in large doses, vomiting and purging, burning in the throat, gripings, distension of the abdomen, convulsions, intoxication, delirium, or stupor, are the effects which in a period varying according to the dose, terminate in death. All these symptoms are attributable to inflammation of the alimentary canal, and to a remote action on the brain and spinal chord. If taken in small doses aconite exerts, on the contrary, a more simply narcotic influence, benumbing the parts with which it comes into actual contact, and often exercising a remote action on other organs, producing diuresis or perspiration, and very frequently alleviating the pain in neuralgic and rheumatic affections.

All the effects of the aconite are witnessed in a concentrated state when the extract is introduced into a wound. Mr. Pereira, in some experiments made some years ago, found that one grain of the spirituous extract introduced into the peritoneal sac of a rabbit killed it in 9½ minutes.

A preparation of the root is much used in all the hilly districts in India to poison arrows for the destruction of wild beasts. We seldom however obtain the root sufficiently fresh in the plains to produce such effects as would explain its alleged utility for this purpose. It has been used on several occasions to poison wells and tanks, and doubtless might be made a formidable means of defence against the invasion of the territories in which it abounds.

In medicine the Bish is chiefly employed by the natives in the treatment of leprosy, fever, cholera, and rheumatism. In Europe the wolf's bane, or monk's hood (A. Napellus) has long been deemed efficient in many painful and spasmodic affections. The extract has been generally employed, commencing with half of a grain repeated thrice daily, and gradually increased until a tingling sensation of the affected part is produced. From three to five grains daily have thus been taken not only with impunity, but with the effect of checking or even removing many forms of nervous disease.

We have employed the Indian species in the form of tincture, internally, in the treatment of a great number of cases of chronic rheumatism. We commenced with 10 drop doses thrice daily, and proceeded gradually to two drachms in twelve hours. The effects observed, were numbness of the mouth and fauces, diuresis, increased appetite, in a few cases slight giddiness, and in about three-fourths of the cases alleviation of the rheumatic pains. The tingling described by Dr. Duncan occurred in several instances, and was the certain precursor of the suspension or cure of the disease. We did not notice any effect on the bowels; in those who had no diuresis, gentle perspiration usually occurred; no tendency to sleep followed in any of our cases.

Externally we have used the extract made into an ointment, as directed in the Pharmacopœia, in a few cases of severe facial neuralgia, and painful nodes. From one to two drachms of the ointment were rubbed on the affected part, which was then covered with a plantain leaf; numbness generally followed in half an hour, then a sensation of warm tingling, and usually a distinct remission of the pain for several hours. These frictions may be repeated thrice daily with perfect safety.

Our experiments were instituted in imitation of those made by Dr. Turnbull in England with the alkali aconitina. Our results fairly bear out his statements, and shew the method he introduced to be one of great practical value. In England aconitina costs 1*s.* 6*d.* a grain, which high price is an almost insuperable obstacle to its extensive use. The extract however may be used in a large proportion of cases with equal benefit.

Off. prep. Tinct. Extract, the alkali aconitina, and the ointment of the Extract.

Sp. 2. *Aconitum heterophyllum*, Wall. (*Vern.* Atees.)
Off. The *root.*

The root of this plant has long been celebrated in Indian Materia Medica as a tonic and aphrodisiac medicine. The plant was first described and identified by Dr. Wallich (see Plant: Asiat: Rariores), and has received additional notice from Prof. Royle.

It occurs in abundance on the lofty mountains of Choor Shalma and Kedarnath, and varies greatly in the size and form of its leaves, from which circumstance it derives its specific name.

The root is composed of two oblong tubera, of light ash colour externally, white internally, and of pure bitter taste. Under the name of *atees*, however, and very like the true root, there is commonly sold in the bazars of Bengal an insipid and totally inert substance, which we have reason to believe to be the dried tubera of the Soota mooli, or *Asparagus sarmentosus.*

The true bitter atees is devoid of any astringency, yields to water 18 per cent, to alcohol 32.

The watery solution is not precipitated by ammonia, and does not contain aconitina. The atees may be given in substance to large dogs to the extent of 60 grains, without producing any serious effect.

In any trial of this medicine prescriptions should invariably give the vernacular name, to prevent confusion with the formidable aconite of the preceding article.

The two preceding plants are noticed by Mr. G. Don in his General System, under the name of Nirbisia or Nirbisi. The Aconitum ferox of Wallich, is apparently Don's Nirbisia bisma. The A. heterophyllum, Wall. seems to be Don's Nirbisia Hamiltonii. Don was evidently unaware that *nirbisi* means an *antidote*, or he would not have applied this term to one of the most powerful of vegetable poisons.

Nirbisi is a tuberous root, without poisonous properties. The name is applied in Sirmoor to the Delphinium pauciflorum. The best article however comes from Lahore.

Mr. Colebrooke applied this term to the roots of Curcuma Zedoaria, on account of the Persian and Arabic synonyms being Judwar and Zudwar. Clusius gives a plate of this Zedoary, the roots of which strikingly resemble those of A. atees. The Persians describe five kinds of Zedoary—Chinese, Nipalese, Tibetan, Dukunee, and Spanish. There can be little doubt but the Nirbisi is the true Zedoary of ancient writers, but its source is as yet unknown.

Gen. 4.—Helleboreæ.

Calyx permanent, rather coriaceous, of 5 sepals—Petals 8 to 10—Capsules coriaceous, sessile.

Sp. 1.—*Helleborus niger*, or black hellebore.

(*Syn. Melampodium. Vern*: Katuroum, *Sanscrit.* Kalikootkie, *Duk.* Khertick, *Arab.* Kherbeck seea, *Pers.*)

Off. The *roots.*

Under these native names two kinds of Hellebore root are brought from Nipal and from the Red Sea, and are commonly sold in the bazars; they are much used by farriers, and occasionally by the native practitioners as a powerful cathartic in maniacal and dropsical cases.

The roots of one kind, sold under this native name, occur in pieces four to six inches long, are black all through their substance, externally of a greyish colour, with numerous joints. The second variety is in similar pieces, but of a whitish colour internally.

The Hellebores though formerly much extolled, especially in the treatment of insanity, are now seldom or never prescribed.

The *Helleborus fœtidus*, or stinking hellebore, is common in England, and used as a popular purgative. It is a dangerous and uncertain substance, and justly neglected by scientific practitioners.

Gen. 5.—Delphinium.

Sp. 1. *Delphinium Staphisagria*, Stavesacre or Louse-wort.

This is a biennial plant, a native of the Levant, Teneriffe, and Asia Minor. The seeds are irregularly triangular, blackish on the outside, yellowish within, of a very nauseous, bitter, and acrid taste, and heavy smell. Reduced to powder and taken internally in small doses, they act as a violent cathartic and emetic, and so uncertainly, that they are now never administered. Their energy is due to the presence of an alkali named *Delphinia*, obtained by acting on the bruised seeds with water acidulated with sulphuric acid, and adding carbonate of potass as long as a precipitate falls. This is to be collected, dried, and acted on by boiling alcohol, which deposits the alkali on cooling in white flakes.

Reduced to powder and made into an ointment in the usual way, this seed is still used as an external application, especially for destroying vermin in the hair. The seeds are also used in the Levant for intoxicating fish.

Several species of Delphinium occur in the Himalayas, and have been described by Prof. Royle in his work on the Botany of these regions. The *D. Ajacis* (*Hind.* Na-furman) is cultivated in gardens in India during the cold season (Royle). The properties of the seeds doubtless agree with those of the stavesacre kind.

Tribe 5—Pæoniaceæ.

Anthers bursting inwards, leaves radical, alternate. Herbs, rarely shrubs.

Gen. 1.—Pæonia.

Sp. 1. *Pæonia officinalis*. Peony.

A native of the south of Europe; seeds emetic and cathartic; root believed to be antispasmodic.

The *P. Emodi*, Wall. occurs on the Shalma mountain, Kemaon.

GEN. 2.—ACTEA.

Sp. 1. *Actea spicata*, Baneberry. A native of the Caucasus and Siberia. Roots astringent; the whole plant acrid and poisonous.

The *A. Acuminata*, Wall. is found on the Choor and Acharanda mountains.

GEN. 3.—XANTHORIZA.

Sp. 1. *Xanthoriza apiifolia*, a native of the United States. Root intensely bitter, and a valuable tonic medicine.

No Indian species of Xanthoriza has yet been discovered.

NAT. ORDER II.—PODOPHYLLEÆ.

Sepals 3. Petals 6—9. Stamens 12—18. Fruit fleshy, celled, many-seeded, crenated, sessile stigma.

Of this order, but two species deserve attention.

The *Podophyllum peltatum*, (may-apple) is a native of the United States, where the root is considered to be a valuable, and powerful cathartic. The *P. Emodi*, Wall. occurs in Nipal and Kemaon, and on the Choor mountain in the Himalayas, at an elevation of 10,000 feet. A specimen of the root was forwarded to the Committee by Dr. Falconer, of Seharunpore, but the quantity obtained was too small for the requisite experiments being instituted upon its virtues. The *P. hexandrum* was found by Dr. Royle on the Kedarkanta mountain, at an elevation of 12,000 feet.

NAT. ORDER III.—PAPAVERACEÆ.

This is a small order, but one of great importance to the medical practitioner. It is composed of annual or perennial plants, with fibrous roots; leaves alternate, simple, penninerved, toothed, or with pennate lobes. The flowers are white, red, or yellow, never blue.

They contain a proper juice, of white, yellow, or blood-like colour, and in which the medicinal properties of these plants reside. In the genus Papaver the juice is milky, and contains several alkalies; for example, the narcotic principles morphine and codeine, with anarcotine. In the concrete state this juice constitutes the opium of commerce. The juice of the Argemone mexicana is yellow, and also contains an alkali, *argemonine*, destitute, however, of any remarkable medicinal virtues. The Sanguinaria Canadensis is emetic and purgative in large doses, and has a blood red juice, containing an alkali, called *Sanguinaria*. The seeds of the Papavers, (poppies)—of the Argemone mexicana, (shialkantu)—and of the Sanguinaria Canadensis, (puccoon) agree in containing a bland, nutritious, colourless fixed oil.

Gen. 1.—Papaver.

Sepals 2, convex, deciduous; petals 4; stigmas 4—20; sessile upon the crown of the ovary; capsule celled, spheroidal, opening by pores beneath the lobes of the stigma; placentæ opposite the stigmatic lobes; many seeded.

Sp. 1. *Papaver Rhoeas,* (corn poppy). This unimportant species is found in gardens in upper India. The capsule is obovate, smooth, sepals hairy, stem many flowered, rough, with spreading setæ, leaves pinnatifid with elongated, toothed, acute lobes.

The petals are of a beautiful red colour, and are used to colour a syrup, the Syrupus rhoæados of the English pharmacopœia; no active or narcotic principle has been found in this species.

Sp. 2. *Papaver somniferum,* (Opium poppy): var. *a* with black, var. *b* with white seed.

(*Vern.* Post, *Hind.* Khuskush, *Arab.* and *Duk.* Kooknar, *Pers.* Chosa, *Sans.* Μήκων of the Greeks.)

This most important plant is a native of the south of Europe and Asia Minor, and is now naturalized by cultivation in India.

The stem is erect, smooth, rather glaucous, from three to four feet high; leaves amplexicaul, with rather blunt teeth; petals large, dull white, often with a purple spot at the base; capsules obovate or globular, smooth, rather hard, with numerous small oily seeds.

The *capsules* are employed in medicine for the preparation of a sedative decoction and syrup, much used for children. They are devoid of odour; of slightly bitter taste. If collected before the concrete juice is removed in the manner subsequently described, the capsules contain a minute portion of all the active principles of opium; for medicinal purposes those should be rejected which are marked with longitudinal and parallel cuts resulting from the extraction of opium. An infusion of poppy heads in cold water should strike a red colour with permuriate of iron.

Off. prep. Decoction, syrup.

Poppy Oil. The seeds of the poppy yield by expression 56 per 100 of a bland and very valuable oil, of a pale golden colour, fluid to within 10 degrees of the freezing point of water, Sp. Gr. 939; it dries easily, is inodorous, of agreeable flavour, is partially soluble (8 in 1000) in alcohol, dissolves the oxides of lead. The mass from which the seed is expressed is found to be extremely nutritious to cattle. This oil is for all pharmaceutical purposes equal to that of the olive employed in European pharmacy, and we have accordingly recommended it in our formulæ for Hospital use.

CONCRETE JUICE.—OPIUM.

(*Vern.* Afeem, *Duk.* Ufyoon, *Arab.* Sheer i khushkush, *Pers.* Apaynum, *Sans.* Μήκωνιον or Οπος of the Greeks.)

This invaluable remedy, and important article of commerce, requires to be treated of in considerable detail, we shall therefore notice the extraction of the concrete juice, the chemical properties of the opium, and the mode in which the juice is prepared for medicinal and commercial purposes in the great factories of Behar and Benares; we shall then describe the leading varieties of the drug used in European medicine. The manufacture of morphia and anarcotine which should follow here, will be treated of in the Pharmacopæia; lastly, we will give an outline of the most important uses of opium in the treatment of disease.*

Preparation of Opium.

Towards the end of March when the plant is nearly ripe the bleeding of the capsules takes place. This operation is performed in the evening, and consists of tracing four parallel lines with a sharp knife or shell, penetrating the epicarp and sarcocarp of the capsule; a milky juice immediately exudes and its flow is promoted by the deposition of dew during the night; each set of incisions yields on an average one grain of opium. This is removed the ensuing morning, and the incisions repeated as long as any milk flows. The whole of the opium collected daily, and which is necessarily mingled with variable proportions of dew, is mixed together in earthen or wooden vessels. Should the quan-

* Some information regarding the cultivation of the poppy, the quantity grown in Bengal, and the adulterations of the drug, is given in the Appendix.

tity of dew have been excessive, a partial solution of the opium occurs, and an exudation of drops of a black, shining liquid (Pasewa) occurs on the surface of the opium. This pasewa contains many of the active principles of the drug, and should be mixed with it again to secure the uniform power of the mass. The proportion of pasewa is often much increased by the fraudulent admixture of water by the growers, in hope of having their opium purchased by the gross weight.

When brought to the factories the opium is usually of the consistence of 64 to 68, that is, containing that proportion of solid matter per 100. It is then placed in large tanks of brick work, or in wooden vats, with the upper surface exposed to the air. From these reservoirs portions are daily removed and exposed on wooden trays three inches deep by four feet long and two broad; evaporation takes place under such circumstances with tolerable rapidity, and the opium eventually reaches the consistence of 70—the standard of the factory for the Chinese investment.

The degree of inspissation is estimated on the purchase of the drug, as well as during its subsequent evaporation, by drying average portions of 100 grains each, on a metallic table heated to 208° by steam.

A sufficient quantity of opium, of average quality, is permitted to attain the consistence of 80°, and in that state is issued under the name of "Abkaree" to the licensed dealers of the bazars. Lastly, the finest opium which can be procured is set apart for medical purposes, and allowed to lose by evaporation nearly the entire of its water.

The *Chinese investment opium* is of a rich chesnut colour, translucent at the edges of thin masses, tears into portions with ragged margins; its structure is granular, its taste hot and bitter, its smell rich, peculiar, and agreeable; if a small portion be rubbed between the finger and thumb for a few seconds it draws out into long colourless threads, and from the number, fineness, and tenacity of these threads the Chinese form their first estimate of the value of the drug.

The *abkaree*, or Bengal bazar opium is more solid than the Chinese investment drug, of a darker colour, and often of a heavy ascescent smell.

For the Chinese investment the opium is made into cakes, each containing 4 lbs, and enveloped in a case made of the petals of the poppy, and agglutinated with a paste made of opium and water, (Lewa). The abkaree opium is also vended in balls weighing 2 lbs. covered by strips of a coarse kind of silk cemented by a mucilage of gum. The medicinal opium is solid, brittle in the cold season, of a brown colour, and fine smell. The medicinal drug is packed with great care in 4lb. and 2lb. squares, covered with layers of talc, and further defended by a case of brown wax ½ an inch in thickness.

Besides the above, several kinds of opium are to be met with even in Indian commerce—that from Malwah demands most attention.

Of the *Malwah* opium there are many varieties, some of which the Committee have had opportunities of examining through the kindness of Dr. Morehead of Bombay. The specimens were (average) 1½lb. in weight, hard, brittle, containing from five to ten per cent. of moisture, mixed with fragments of leaves and seeds, and impregnated with oil, apparently used in the collection; the colour was almost a rusty brown, the odour very powerful, and taste intensely bitter and lasting.

Besides the opiums above mentioned, it is necessary to notice the chief varieties alluded to in works on European Materia Medica. *M. Berthemot*, in a paper published in the "Journal de Pharmacie," for September 1838, describes three principal kinds, viz.—1st. the opium of Alexandria; 2d. of Constantinople; 3rd. of Smyrna.

The *Alexandrian* opium is in small, very dry, pieces, enveloped in fragments of leaves, of a very deep brown colour, clean and shining fracture, of faintly virose smell.

The *Constantinople* variety is in two forms, usually in flattened morsels contained in large leaves, sometimes rather soft, occasionally dry and brittle, softening between the fingers, and translucent when pressed into thin layers. The smell is stronger than that of the former kind, and is deemed a sufficient distinguishing sign between both.

The *Smyrna* opium, lastly, is either in flat pieces, or roundish balls; one kind is very dry, wrapped up in large leaves, of shining fracture, reddish brown colour internally, of bitter, acrid, and enduring taste. The second kind is rolled in seeds of the Rumex, is soft, and easily torn, of fawn colour internally, but darkens rapidly on exposure to the air, transparent when drawn out, and often mixed with the seeds which constitute its outer covering.

The Smyrna opium is the most valuable of the varieties now described, containing the largest proportion of the narcotic alkali morphia, and in a state which permits this principle to be purified with greatest ease.

Chemical composition of Opium.

All the varieties of opium, above mentioned, are partly soluble in water, partly in alcohol, and contain ingredients insoluble in either of these fluids. The preparation used by the Chinese is a watery extract, which they term *chundoo*, and which is subsequently described (*see* EXTRACTS). The watery solution varies in colour from that of pale sherry, to a deep brown tint. The amount of extract differs too according to the variety of the drug; and in tint of colour, the extract ranges from a pale brown to deep blackish red. In the 6th vol. of the Transactions of the Medical and Physical Society of Calcutta, Dr. Smyttan, lately Opium Inspector at Bombay, has published a tabular view of the different proportions of extract in a great number of specimens he subjected to examination. In the editor's Manual of Chemistry the results of several similar experiments are recorded. From all it appears that Patna and Benares opium yields about 40, Malwah and Levant opium from 75 to 80 per 100 of watery extract.

Very little was known of the chemical nature of opium till 1803, when M. Derosne discovered the alkaline principle, which he termed narcotine, on the supposition that it was the narcotic principle or essence of the drug. As this supposition has since been remarkably falsified, we have in our Pharmacopœia adopted for the same principle, which is a most important febrifuge remedy, the modified term of *Anarcotina*, simply prefixing the Greek negative particle *a* to the old denomination.

In 1817, M. Sertuerner found, however, the true narcotic principle, a crystalline alkali, which he called *morphine*. He also discovered at the same time a peculiar acid, which he termed the *meconic*, from *μήκων*, a poppy. In 1830, M. Couerbe found a third alkali, which he called *meconin*. In 1832, M. Pelletier discovered and described *narceine*, and in the same year M. Robiquet detected the alkali *codeine*. Lastly, a substance named *thebaine* has been found by M. Theboumery, and ascertained to possess very distinct chemical properties.

Besides these peculiar principles, opium contains several others, common to many concrete juices, such as resin, gum, colouring matter, caoutchouc, and woody fibre.

Of all these, three only are of value to the practitioner, namely morphia, anarcotina, and meconic acid.

Morphia

is a white alkali, which crystallizes in four-sided prisms, insoluble in water; soluble in 40 parts of cold and 30 times its weight of hot alcohol; also soluble in fixed and volatile oils, and in solutions of caustic potash and soda. On ultimate analysis it yields

34 atoms Carbon, ...	204
18 ditto Hydrogen, ...	18
1 ditto Azote, ...	14
6 ditto Oxygen, ...	48
Atomic equivalent, ...	284

The quantity of pure morphia present in opium varies according to the kind:

Bengal investment Opium contains,...	2½ per 100.*
Medicinal opium, ...	4
Malwah ditto,...	6
Garden opium, Patna, ...	10½
Turkey opium, ...	9
Smyrna opium, ...	10½

Morphia forms salts with the acids, which are all soluble in water and alcohol, and are precipitated by the alkalies, especially ammonia. They are reddened and destroyed by nitric acid; and with permuriate of iron strike a deep blue colour.

Nitric acid, however, produces a similar effect with strychnine, brucine, emetine, infusion of cloves, corydaline, and many other substances.

The mode of preparing morphia is described in the Pharmacopœia.

Taken into the stomach in substance, it produces little narcotic effect, owing to its extreme insolubility, but if previously combined with an acid it acts as a powerful narcotic in very small doses, (see Morphia and its Salts—Pharmacopœia.)

Anarcotina.

A white alkali, in needle-shaped crystals of pearly lustre, and often procured as large as ½ an inch in length, by one

* The official returns by the Opium Examiner of Calcutta for the last four years, shew the following per centage of *morphia* in a "tolerably pure" state.

1836	1837	1838	1839
3.7	3.8	4.0	3.9
4.1	4.1	3.9	4.0
3.6	4.1	4.0	3.7

line in breadth. It neutralizes acids, and the resulting salts are of most intensely bitter taste. They are devoid of any narcotic properties, and are capable of arresting the paroxysms of intermittent and remittent fevers. (*See Anarcotina*, Pharmacopœia.)

On analysis, Anarcotina yields

Carbon, ...	40 atoms,	=	240
Hydrogen,.. ...	20 „	=	20
Nitrogen,... ...	1 „	=	14
Oxygen, ...	12 „	=	96
Atomic equivalent			370

The proportion of Anarcotina present in various opiums is very variable;

Bengal investment contains, ...in	100	parts,	3.
Malwah, ...	100	=	3.
Abkaree of Bengal, ...	100	=	$4\frac{1}{2}$.
Turkey, ...	100	=	1.

Codeia.

A white crystalline solid, soluble in boiling water and in ether. It is distinguished from morphia by not becoming blue on being tested by the permuriate of iron, not being reddened by nitric acid, and not being precipitated by ammonia from its solution in muriatic acid; its salts crystallize readily. In its physiological effects it resembles morphia, but it is apt to occasion vomiting when taken even in small doses.

Narceine.

Narceine is white, crystalline, slightly bitter, soluble in 230 parts of boiling water, and fusible at 198°. The sulphuric, nitric, and muriatic acids much diluted with water dissolve it freely, and the solution is of a light blue colour. It does not produce a blue compound with permuriate of iron, but assumes that colour when heated with iodine. Its physiological effects are not yet thoroughly understood. Two grains have produced very little effect when injected into the jugular vein of a dog.

Meconine.

This is a white crystalline solid, fuses at 194, may be distilled unchanged at a higher temperature; soluble in 18 parts of boiling water. It contains no nitrogen, is soluble in the acids, and the solution in dilute sulphuric acid when concentrated becomes green and then purple; with chlorine it forms a blood red compound, and is changed into mechloic acid. It appears to possess no action on the animal economy.

Meconic Acid.

This acid, with the sulphuric and acetic, exists in all varieties of opium, and holds the alkaline principles in combination.

When pure it is white, crystalline, scaly, soluble in water and alcohol, of a sour taste, reddens the vegetable blues, unites with bases to form salts; if boiled in water it is partially decomposed, carbonic acid is set free, and a new acid called the meta-meconic remains. It contains no nitrogen.

If the meconic acid or any of its salts be added to a solution of permuriate of iron a deep red colour is immediately produced; this character has been much relied on as a test for detecting opium in cases of poisoning, but it is very liable to fallacy. The saliva produces the same effect in consequence of its containing sulphocyanic acid; infusion of mustard, and several other vegetable products also occasion a red colour in solutions of the persalts of iron; several methods have been proposed for distinguishing between these colored solutions, but none appear to us deserving of confidence.

Meconic acid has been given in large doses to men and other animals without producing any remarkable effect.

Besides the preceding ingredients, opium, like most other vegetable juices, contains resin, gum, caoutchouc, and ligneous fibre.

Effects of Opium on Animals and Vegetables.

Opium in excessive doses acts as a narcotic poison on all the higher animals; in man producing stupor, apoplexy, convulsions, or paralysis; in other mammalia the symptoms of irritation are more prominent, convulsions being more frequent than stupor or coma; on the lowest classes of animals, and the contractile vegetables, opium acts as a relaxing or paralysing agent.

In small doses as far as one grain, opium taken by healthy men generally acts as a stimulant, the pulse being slightly increased in strength and frequency, and the mind excited to a train of happy imaginations. This condition is succeeded by drowsiness, thirst, and loss of appetite, and is ultimately followed by some degree of constipation. All these effects diminish remarkably by the habitual use of the drug, so that there are very numerous examples of persons having acquired the power of consuming several drachms of solid opium daily; nor does it appear to be ascertained that this habit has a direct tendency to shorten life; on the contrary, the longevity of opium-eaters is in many parts of the East of proverbial notoriety.

In somewhat larger doses, say two to four grains, after a brief period of excitement, followed by giddiness, profound sleep soon ensues, the pupils are slightly contracted, the pulse slow and full, the breathing slow, the temperature of the body somewhat increased.

Beyond four grains to healthy persons not accustomed to opium it may be considered to act as a poison. Dr. Christison says,* "the symptoms of poisoning with opium, when it is administered at once in a dangerous dose, begin with giddiness and stupor, or generally without any previous stimulus; the stupor generally rapidly increasing, the person becomes motionless and insensible to external impressions, he breathes very slowly, generally lies quite still with the eyes shut and pupils contracted, and the whole expression of the countenance is that of deep and perfect repose. As the poisoning advances the features become ghastly, the pulse feeble, and imperceptible, the muscles exceedingly relaxed, and unless assistance is speedily procured, death ensues; if the person recovers, the torpor is succeeded by prolonged sleep, which commonly ends in 24 or 36 hours, and is followed by nausea, vomiting, giddiness, and loathing of food."

In the effects thus described, opium seems to act by the impression produced on the parts with which it comes directly into contact; and, secondly, by being absorbed into the circulation, and conveyed to distant organs. It has been detected in the blood, urine, and serous fluids of persons who had taken it even in medicinal doses.

Mr. Pereira in his excellent lectures on Materia Medica, published in the Medical Gazette for 1836-37, gives a most useful analysis of the effects of opium on the several organs of the human frame. We subjoin an adequate summary of this author's observations.

The action of opium on the *cerebro-spinal* system is indicated, first, by the excited, secondly, by the depressed state of the functions of these organs. An accumulation of blood in the cerebral vessels is indicated by the swollen state of the veins, the lividity of the countenance, and is further proved by the facts observed on dissection in such cases. Sometimes, however, delirium and convulsions are observed without torpor; or convulsions with low unconscious muttering, and utter insensibility to all external objects.

The effects on the digestive organs in exciting thirst, allaying hunger, diminishing secretion, and lessening the contractile power of the muscular fibres, we have already noticed. The urinary organs are similarly influenced, the secretion from the kidneys being diminished, and the contractile power of the bladder weakened.

The *heart and arteries* are also affected in their functions. Sometimes the heart's action is increased, at other times, however, its contractions are lower than natural, and its force diminished. These conditions are, however, the secondary consequences of the first impression on the cerebro-spinal system. The *respiratory functions* are also modified in like manner, the general paralysis of the muscles affecting those essential to the respiratory process, which thus becomes mechanically impeded, and death by suffocation is the frequent consequence.

The sensibility of the skin is often materially altered; in some individuals great itchiness is experienced, even after small doses of opium; in others, on the contrary, the surface of the body becomes nearly insensible. Perspiration is generally much increased.

The functions of the generative system in either sex, and in the healthy state, appear to be but little affected by this agent.

On the dissection of persons who have died of the effects of opium, few morbid appearances of any importance are observable. Death may have been thus occasioned without any structural change, or altered state being observable. Congestion of the cerebral vessels, effusion of serum on the surface, in the ventricles, or at the base of the brain, very rarely the extravasation of blood—such are the appearances generally seen, but all these may be produced by other and common diseases.

Effects of Opium-smoking.

The vice of opium-smoking is now so prevalent in Calcutta, not only among the Chinese, but the degraded, and depraved of every sect and nation, that we have had many opportunities of witnessing the results to which it leads.

Stupor, reverie, and voluptuous listlessness are the immediate effects produced. In this state the individual can be at once and easily aroused to exertion or business. No sickness, constipation, or any other functional disturbance supervenes on each indulgence; gradually, however, the appetite diminishes, the bowels become irregular, emaciation takes place, sexual tendencies are destroyed, and premature old age speedily comes on. This we admit is an extreme case; when the habit is but moderately followed it appears to occasion no greater evil than the proportionate indulgence in wine or other spirituous liquors.

Medicinal uses of Opium.

From the preceding facts we may derive many useful conclusions as to the states of disease in which opium is likely to prove beneficial or injurious.

The chief diseases in which opium has been beneficially used are—fever, delirium tremens, inflammations and mortification, rheumatism, hæmorrhage, spasmodic and painful diseases, cholera, in irritant poisoning, in syphilis and diabetes.

In *fever*, when no symptoms of cerebral congestion are present, such as headache, lividity of the features, oppressed respiration or stupor, opium is often beneficial by obviating wakefulness, allaying pain and restlessness, checking diarrhœa, and inducing perspiration; its use however requires the utmost caution, for if given during congestion of the cerebral blood vessels, we may expect an aggravation of all the symptoms. A hot dry skin and parched furred tongue, and an unnatural state of the pupils, should warn the practitioner against this medicine; delirium however does not always forbid its use, especially that low muttering form, accompanied by twitchings of the tendons and a cool skin and weak pulse; in this state, and in advanced stages of the disease, full doses of opium and wine are often of the most remarkable utility.

In intermittent fevers (ague) opium has been used with the twofold object of alleviating the current paroxysm, and in the interval of preventing a return of the disease. A full dose, say sixty drops of the tincture of opium, given on the first accession of the cold stage, has very frequently been known either to stop the paroxysm or materially diminish its violence; the antiperiodical virtues of the drug are however scarcely procurable from any safe doses, and depend on the anarcotina it contains. For the use of this substance in the treatment of agues, see Anarcotina, (Pharmacopœia.)

In *Delirium tremens*, the "horrors" of the European drunkard (a singular disease, usually brought on by long continued excess in spirituous liquors, and characterized by obstinate wakefulness, the strangest visions, and tremblings of the limbs) no medicine but the Hemp, at all approaches opium in efficacy. It requires to be given in full doses, two to four grains, repeated every second or third hour until sleep is produced. When this takes place the disease generally yields without further difficulty.

Inflammation in many of its forms is much under the controul of this agent, especially the inflammation of the great serous membranes of the body, the peritoneum, and the pleura. Full doses of opium though perhaps inadequate to effect a cure without bleeding and leeching, still are invaluable auxiliaries, allaying the excruciating pain of the disease, arresting cough and spasm, and inducing sleep. In inflammation of the mucous membrane of the stomach, gall ducts, bladder, and kidneys, in chronic catarrh, in diarrhœa, and in mild cholera dependent on irritation or inflammation of the mucous membrane of the alimentary canal, opium is of signal utility. Combined with blue pill or acetate of lead, it is given with the utmost benefit in *dysentery*, both acute and chronic. On the same principle we use opium freely to allay the pain, irritation, and inflammation occasioned by many acrid poisons, such as cantharides and arsenic; in all these cases however the poison must first be removed from the stomach and alimentary canal, otherwise the use of opium would but mask the symptoms, while the poison is still doing irreparable mischief.

When inflammation has terminated in *mortification*, and when this state is accompanied (as it frequently is) with excessive pain, opium gives great relief, and often enables us to arrest the progress of the disease.

It must be borne in mind, however, that experience has shewn the impropriety of using this medicine in congestion or inflammation of the parenchymatous substance of the brain, lungs, and liver.

In acute *Rheumatism*, opium combined with calomel given so as to induce gentle salivation affords us one of our best modes of treatment; in the chronic form of the disease, combined with ipecachuana or mudar, in the form of Dover's powder, it acts as a powerful diaphoretic, allays pain, brings on sleep, and often gives permanent relief.

In *Diabetes*, or excessive discharge of urine, no remedy produces such decided benefit as this, although it can scarcely be said to have ever effected a positive cure.

Hæmorrhages, or discharges of blood, when induced by

irritation or inflammation, are often arrested by opium in various forms and combinations.

Off. Preparations. Anarcotina, muriate of anarcotina, morphia, muriate of morphia, extract, Chinese extract, tincture, compound powder, &c. &c.*

GEN. 2.—CHELIDONIUM.

Sp. 1. *Chelidonium majus,* (great celandine,) a native of shady places all over Europe, not found in India; biennial, two feet high, flowers bright yellow, juice of hot bitter taste—a violent *acrid* poison acting as a drastic purgative and emetic; a popular remedy for warts and opacities of the cornea.

In England the juice of the Chelidonium glaucum is used in veterinary practice, and Dr. Grainger states that two drs. of the seed in a pint of water make a good emetic.

GEN. 3.—ARGEMONE.

Sp. 1. *Argemone mexicana,* (*Shial kanta* of Bengal.)

This plant is abundant all over Hindustan, and is easily recognized by its prickly, thistle-like leaves, and bright yellow flowers. It is a native of South America, now naturalized, and exceedingly common about Calcutta; the seeds are used in Jamaica as an emetic, a thimbleful being bruised with water. Barton again describes them as being more powerfully narcotic than opium.

The Editor has subjected the seeds to numerous experiments, and has never found them to shew any emetic or narcotic influence; they contain a bland oil resembling that of the poppy, and which can be used in ounce doses without producing any purgative effect.

The juice, which exudes on wounding or bruising this plant, is of a bright yellow colour, and is used by the natives as an application to indolent ulcers, and to remove specks on the cornea. It has by some writers been described as possessing the activity of gamboge. If this expressed juice of the plant be rendered alkaline by ammonia a precipitate falls which is partially soluble in hot alcohol, giving a rich golden tincture; on cooling and spontaneous evaporation, silky crystals of an alkaline principle are deposited, which we propose to term *argemonine.*

* In the sequel of this work will be found directions for counteracting the effects of over-doses of opium. See article "poisons;" section, "opium."

We have given this argemonine in considerable quantities to dogs, and did not find it induce any acrid or narcotic effects. It has not been as yet tried in hospital practice.

Gen. 4.—Sanguinaria.

Sp. 1. *Sanguinaria canadensis.*

Puccoon, blood root, red root. This plant is a native of the United States and Canada, but is not found in India. The root yields a very red juice, which acts as a powerful emetic and purgative. It contains an alkali named *sanguinaria.*

Gen. 5.—Meconopsis.

Sp. 1. *Meconopsis aculeata.*

A native of Nepal, Choor, Kedarkanta, Peer Punjal.

The roots are reputed to be exceedingly narcotic. A fine drawing of this plant is published in Royle's Illustrations of the Botany of the Himalayas.

An alcoholic extract of one drachm of the root given to a small dog produced no perceptible effect.

NAT. ORDER IV.—FUMARIÆ.

The plants of this order have watery juice, are common in the Himalayas from Nipal to Cashmere, and contain a bitter principle. One species, the Fumaria officinalis, or Fumitory, is used as a bitter tonic, and diaphoretic in Europe. The Fumaria parviflora, (Pitpapra), is considered to be identical with the χαπνοσ of the Greeks; it is much used in the Upper Provinces, mixed with black pepper, in the treatment of intermittent fevers.

Ainslie under the head F. officinalis, gives the following synonymes—*Shatra*, Pers. and Duk.—*Pit-papra*, Hind. *Buck—lutulmelic*, Arab. He states he found the dried plant in a druggist's shop in Trichinopoly, and that the Hakeems consider it diuretic. Among European practitioners it was long regarded as a valuable tonic and alterative.

Several trials of this plant were made by the Editor on specimens obtained from the Botanic Garden of Calcutta, but none led to any encouraging results.

GEN.—CORYDALIS.

Sp. 1. *Corydalis cashmeriana.*

Sp. 2. *C. govaniana.* Wall. (*Vern.* Bhootkes) common in the Choor mountains, above 8000 feet of elevation, where it is regarded as a charm against evil spirits. For specimens of the roots we are indebted to Dr. Falconer. They are long, fibrous, tough, and exceedingly bitter; dark brown externally, yellow within. The tincture rendered alkaline by ammonia, and allowed to evaporate spontaneously deposits abundant crystals of the alkali, termed *Corydalia.*

Corydalia occurs in pearly crystals, is soluble in acids, with which it forms salts, which do not crystallize; and which are intensely bitter to the taste. Nitric acid communicates a deep red, permuriate of iron a rich blue color to the alkali, and its salts. Twenty grs. have been given in solution to dogs without inconvenience.

The *Corydalis tuberosa,* and *fabacea* in Europe have a bitter acrid root, usually sold as *aristolochia* root, and used chiefly as an external application to indolent tumors.

The small quantity in our possession alone prevented the Corydalia and its salts from being extensively tried in the treatment of ague. The chemical properties of the salts are closely analogous to those of morphia and anarcotine; an interesting fact, as it strengthens the resemblance already detected by botanists between the Papaveraceæ and Fumariæ. More extensive trials will, we hope, be made with this very promising article.

NAT. ORDER V.—CRUCIFERÆ.

The cruciferous plants receive their name from the cruciform disposition of the four petals of which the corolla is composed; they are herbaceous or shrubby, constitute one of the most natural families, and include over 1000 species, of which not more than twenty are found in tropical regions; many additional species however occur in the Himalayan mountains; all are pungent, bitterish, agree remarkably in composition, containing fixed and volatile oil, starch, sugar, azote, and sulphur; one species, the Isatis (woad), yields a blue coloring principle like indigo; many are alimentary; for instance the Brassica rapa, turnip, (shulgum), Brassica oleracea, cabbage, (kobee), Brassica erucoides, (suffed shurri), cultivated for its oil. Some are used in medicine, and none certainly known to possess poisonous properties.

In the mustards a compound principle named sinapisin has been discovered, which will be subsequently described.

Botanical characters. Sepals four cruciate; petals four cruciate, alternate with the sepals; stamens six, tetradynamous, that is, two short and four longer, in pairs opposite the anterior and posterior sepals. Disk with various green glands between the petals and stamens and ovarium; ovarium superior, unilocular, with the placentæ usually meeting in the middle, and forming a spurious dissepiment. Stigmata two, opposite placentæ; fruit a siliqua or silicula, one-celled or spuriously two-celled, dehiscing by two valves, separating from the replum, or indehiscent. Seeds attached in a single row by a funiculus to each side of the placentæ, generally pendulous; albumen none; embryo with the radicle folded upon the cotyledons; leaves alternate, flowers usually yellow or white, seldom purple. (*Lindley's Intr. to Nat. Syst. p.* 14.)

The cruciferæ have been arranged by Don in 21 tribes and 110 genera. It would be inconsistent with the objects of this work to observe his minute and complicated divisions. We shall therefore follow the arrangement by Decandolle as modified by Fée, as the best and clearest with reference to the medicinal and economical uses of these plants.

Tribe 1—Arabideæ.

Gen. 1.—Nasturtium.

Sp. 1. *Nasturtium officinale.* Water-cress. (*Syn.* Sisymbrium nasturtium. *Vern.* Loot putiah, *Duk.* The seeds are called *Huruf* in the bazars.)

The leaves of the water-cress are gently stimulant and diuretic. As a salad, they are wholesome and palatable, and eminently serviceable to persons affected by scorbutic diseases.

Gen. 2.—Cheiranthus.

Sp. 1. *Cheiranthus Cheiri.* Wall-flower. *Vern. Khueree.* The dried petals are much used in upper India as an aromatic stimulant. It has been long discarded by European practitioners.

Tribe 2.—Alyssmeæ.

Gen.—Cochlearia.

Sp. 1. *Cochlearia Armoracia.* Horse-Radish. Europe.

Root white, thick, taper, long, acrid, stems erect, two feet high, branched, and those which flower smooth and angular, radical; leaves stalked, very large, oblong, line leaves smaller and sessile, flowers white; calyx, spreading; silicles elliptical, usually abortive. *(Lindley's Flora Medica, p.* 91.)

The root of this plant is stimulant, diaphoretic, and emetic, and externally rubefacient; a compound infusion is much used in medical practice in Europe as an adjunct to other remedies.

The root of the Hyperanthera Moringa (M. pterygosperma *Gaertn. Vern.* Suhunjuna) common all over India, has precisely the same properties as this plant, and is accordingly substituted for it in our formulæ.

The *Cochlearia officinalis*, or scurvy grass, was long in repute for its supposed anti-scorbutic virtues, and doubtless is very beneficial owing to the stimulant and nutritious principles in which it abounds.

Tribe 3—Thlaspideæ.

Four species of the genus Thlaspi are mentioned in the French codex (Fée). They are altogether inert.

Tribe 4—Anastaticeæ, and 5—Cakalineæ.

They also contain no useful article.

Tribe 6—Sisymbrieæ.

Several species of the genus Sisymbrium are officinal in various countries on account of their possessing properties resembling those of the Scurvy grass. The *Erysimum perfoliatum* is cultivated in Japan for its oil seeds.

Tribe 7—Lepidineæ.

Gen.—Lepidium.

Sp. 1. *Lepidium sativum.*
Garden cress. Haleem, *Duk. Bengal.*
Aliverie of the bazars.

The aliverie seeds of the bazar, which were referred by Rottler and Ainslie to the Arabis chinensis, have been ascertained by Dr. Wight to belong to the garden cress, which Roxburgh informs us is cultivated universally in Asia during the cool season. The seed is of reddish colour, agreeable warm taste, and is used by the native physicians as a gentle stimulant. Bruized and mixed with lime juice it is deemed useful for checking local inflammation. *Ainslie*, vol. ii. p. 12.

Taken whole in half drachm doses, we find also that it answers as a gentle and warm aperient.

Tribe 8—Isatideæ.

This tribe is chiefly remarkable from one of its species, the Isatis tinctoria (Woad, *Eng.* Pastel, *French*) containing a blue dye, much used as a substitute for indigo. The colouring principle is manufactured by a process nearly the same as that by which indigo is prepared.

The *Camellina sativa* (Myagrum) Μυαγρον of Dioscorides, is cultivated in Europe for the extraction of an oil used only by the soap-makers, and for lamps.

Tribe 9—Brassicaceæ.

This tribe contains several very important alimentary species, viz. the *Brassica oleracea,* cabbage, and the red-leaved variety of that species; also the *B. campestris* and *rapa* (rape), *B. napus,* turnip, and the variety *oleifera,* cultivated for its oil, which is consumed to an immense amount in France for illuminations. The oil is purified by being mixed with dilute sulphuric acid (water 100 parts, sulphuric acid 2 parts). The mixture is allowed to rest for a week, and then the dilute acid removed. The acid acts by coagulating and removing an albuminous substance with which the oil is naturally combined, and which interferes with its combustion.

Gen.—Sinapis.

Calyx equal, spreading, petals obovate, stamens distinct, entire, oblique, tapering, two-celled, two-valved, cells many-seeded, valves concave or keeled with a central nerve, style either short and acute or rostrate, subulate, conical or ensiform, seedless or one-seeded, seeds one rowed, globose. (*Lindley, op. cit.* p. 92.)

Sp. 1. *Sinapis nigra.* Black mustard. Off. The *seeds.* (*Vern.* Surson. Rai. *Duk.* and *Hind.* Khurdal, *Arab.* Sirshuf, *Pers.* Rajika, Sarshapa, *Sans.*)

The mustard flour imported from England is the ground seed of this plant, which is extensively cultivated in Europe. The seeds are small, round, of a blackish brown colour, and beautifully veined externally, internally yellow. They are devoid of odour, but are acrid, bitter, and oily to the taste.

The most remarkable constituents of mustard are fixed oil, volatile oil, and sinapisin, or sulpho-sinapisin.

Fixed and Volatile Oil.

100 lbs. of English mustard yield about 20 lbs. of fixed oil, of a brown yellow colour, faint smell, and mild taste. It is possessed of mild aperient properties. The cake left after the oil is expressed, when reduced to powder affords the "mustard" used by Europeans with their food, and employed as a rubefacient poultice under the name of *sinapism.*

Volatile oil. This is prepared by distilling the powdered seed with water. The oil is formed in consequence of the addition of water, for alcohol and ether in which the oil is freely soluble, remove none from the bruized seed unless water be first employed; the oil is yellow, of intensely pungent taste and smell, heavier than water, and soluble in alcohol. According to Pelouze it is composed of,

Carbon,...	49.84
Hydrogen, ...	5.09
Nitrogen, ...	14.41
Sulphur, ...	20.48
Oxygen,...	10.11

This oil is a powerful vesicatory when applied to the skin, mixed with water it is an energetic stimulant; on its presence depends the uses of the mustard poultices so often prescribed. Acids, excess of fixed oil, or carbonate of potash prevent its formation from the mustard seed paste, and should consequently never be mixed with sinapisms.

Sinapisin, or *Sulpho-sinapisin.*

This is composed of,

Carbon, ...	57.920
Hydrogen, ...	7.795
Nitrogen, ...	4.940
Sulphur, ...	9.657
Oxygen, ...	19.688
	100.00

This substance exists in the infusion and tincture of mustard seed, and as it powerfully reddens the persalts of iron is by many chemists deemed a compound of sulpho-cyanic acid. Mustard previously freed of its oil by sulphuric ether gives to alcohol a deep red tincture, which on evaporation to the consistence of a syrup yields crystals of sinapisin.

Medical uses. Internally in small doses mustard flour is a valuable condiment, promoting digestion and occasioning gentle perspiration. In the dose of two drachms carefully diffused through water it operates as a quick and most effectual emetic, which has been much employed in the treatment of malignant cholera. It is the best of all emetics in narcotic poisoning.

The whole seeds of this variety, and of the *Sinapis alba* have been much used in England in the dose of half a drachm to one drachm in dyspepsia. The action is described to be diuretic and purgative. The practice has however fallen into disuse.

Sp. 2. *S. alba.* White mustard.

This species differs only in the colour of the seeds, which are spherical, yellowish, and much larger than the black kind. The properties of the white seed are less energetic than those of the black. In other respects they agree altogether.

Sp. 3. *Sinapis ramosa,* (Beng. Raee.) See Roxburgh, vol. iii. pp. 119, 120.

In India we have several species of Sinapis, of which Royle enumerates Sinapis ramosa (raee), S. glauca (toria), S. dichotorna (kalie surson), S. juncea, (bunga surson), the three last of which are extensively cultivated for their oil. Roxburgh mentions several others, of which the following claim a place in this work.

It being generally believed that the indigenous mustard would not yield a flour fit for sinapisms, we instituted several experiments on the subject, and found that by first carefully expressing the fixed oil the powder of the oil cake mixed with water afforded as powerful a sinapism as an equal weight of the best English mustard.

Officinal preparations. Powder, volatile oil, and poultice.

Sinapisms are compounds of mustard flour and water, crumb of bread is sometimes added. We recommend the paste being made of mustard flour and water alone.

Magendie informs us that the volatile oil diluted with its own weight of alcohol is an excellent rubefacient, its action being almost instantaneous; if the friction be continued for a few minutes the surface rises into blisters.

Tribe 10.—Raphanus.

This tribe contains the Radish, *Raphanus Sativus*, and some other alimentary and anti-scorbutic species, but none of any medicinal importance.

NAT. ORD. VI. AND VII.

MAGNOLIACEÆ AND WINTERACEÆ.

The Magnoliaceæ are frutescent or arborescent plants, with alternate, generally entire leaves, terminal or axillary flowers. The most remarkable principle they contain is an essential oil often united with a bitter substance, sometimes with tannic acid.

None of this order are known to be poisonous, and many are cultivated for the fragrance, and beauty of their flowers. There is no European species. India and America have several.

The *Winteraceæ* were long included in the order now described, but have lately been separated. They afford two medicinal substances of some value, the *star anise-seed, and Winter's bark.*

GEN. 1.—ILLICIUM.

Sp. 1. *Illicium anisatum.*

Star anise, Badian Khutai, or Chinese anise—a native of the countries extending from $23\frac{1}{2}°$ to $35°$ of N. latitude, or from Canton to Japan. The capsules constitute a rather important article of commerce, and are sold in all the bazars.

The fruits are shortly pedunculate, formed of from five to twelve capsules arranged like a star, each segment being oval, compressed, wrinkled, hard, brittle, of an iron brown colour, four to five lines long, shining within; seeds smooth, oval, compressed, obtuse at both ends, convex at one side, rather hard, brittle, and of rust-brown colour.

Both capsules and seeds evolve a powerful odour of anise; the taste is similar, very mild, sweet, and somewhat acidulous. The kernel of the seed is oily.

The capsules and seeds abound in an essential oil easily procured by distillation with water; this oil is rather brown, lighter than water, more difficultly congealed than the true aniseed oil, but in other respects exactly of the same properties.

Large quantities of the capsules are used in Europe in the preparation of liqueurs.

The powdered capsules are used by the Mahomedan practitioners as stimulant carminatives. For the colics of children the essential oil is given with advantage, in the mode subsequently described.

Off. Prep. Essential oil.

Gen. 2.—Wintera.

Sp. 1. *Wintera aromatica.*

Syn. Drymis Winteri. Hab. Straits of Magellan, Chili, Peru, &c. Off. *The bark.*

A very aromatic tree, sometimes reaching forty feet in height.

The bark is found in the shops of the European druggists in rolled, hard, compact pieces, from one to fifteen inches long and one to nine lines thick, nine to twenty-five lines in diameter; colour externally ashy or yellowish gray, or pale red, internally pale buff; fracture compact; odour penetrating, resembling a mixture of cloves and cascarilla; taste acrid, burning and persistent.

Tannic acid, volatile oil, and resin, are the chief ingredients of this bark; in European practice it is still much used as a stimulant tonic, and diaphoretic, but it is not likely ever to become an object of importance in Indian medicine.

Gen. 3.—Magnolia.

Sp. 1. *Magnolia glauca.*

Swamp sassafras. Hab. middle and southern states of America. Bark bitter and aromatic, an excellent substitute for guaiacum, and said to be especially useful in chronic rheumatism.

Several species of Magnoliæ exist in Nipal, and in the hills beyond Sylhet.

GEN. 4.—LIRIODENDRON.

Sp. 1. *Liriodendron tulipifera.*

Tulip tree. Forests in the United States.

Bark very bitter, and strongly fragrant; stimulant, tonic, and aromatic; used in fevers, agues, and rheumatism with the best results.

Dr. Emmet, of the Virginia University has found in this bark a principle intermediate between camphor and the resins, and which he terms *liriodendrine.*

GEN. 5.—MICHELIA.

Sp. 1. *Michelia Champaca. Champa.*

The bark of this well known tree is bitter, and aromatic, and on several trials appeared to us to possess the properties attributed to the Magnolia glauca.

It may be given in powder in intermittent fevers in doses of from 10 to 30 grains. Its aromatic properties are dissipated by boiling either in water or spirit, and on evaporation a bitter extract remains, which contains tannic and gallic acid.

NAT. ORDER VIII.—ANONACEÆ.

This order is made up of trees and shrubs—is tropical in its habits, inhabiting thick forests, and reckoning in India about 100 species, according to Dr. Wight's estimate.

The custard apple, Anona squamosa, (Gunda gutra, *Sans.* Shurifa, *Pers.)*, and the bullock's heart, A. reticulata, are the best known species in India. The roots of the Uvaria narum are employed in the Mauritius in decoction as tonics and stimulants, and are externally applied for destroying vermin. The powdered seeds of the custard apple are used in Bengal for the same purpose. The fruits of some African and American genera are highly aromatic, the Habzelia for example, and afford an article known in commerce as Æthiopian pepper. The Xylopiæ of the West Indies have intensely bitter wood, bark, and berries. The bitter is accompanied by an agreeable aroma; the wood is much used as a tonic remedy.

The Guatteria longifolia, or Debdaroo of the Hindus, deserves examination,—indeed the properties of the Indian species are very little known.

NAT. ORDER IX.—MENISPERMACEÆ.

This is an important order to the physician, containing several very valuable remedies, and more than one formidable poison.

The Menispermaceæ inhabit only warm climates; the stalk is sarmentaceous, the leaves alternate, petiolar, simple or compound, the flowers axillary.

The pervading principle is a bitter substance, associated with mucilage or starch, and a yellow colouring matter of great intensity. The fruits of several contain a bitter poisonous acid, the *picrotoxic* acid, and are used for the purpose of stupifying fish, and for fraudulently increasing the intoxicating power of malt liquors.

GEN. 1.—ANAMIRTA.

Sp. 1. *Anamirta paniculata, Colebrooke. A. Cocculus, Wight and Arnot.*

Syn. Menispermum Cocculus, L.—M. heteroclitum, Roxb.

Vern. Kakmari, *Sans.*—The seeds are called Kakmari ke beenje, in the bazars.

A strong climbing shrub, with the bark corky, ash-coloured, and deeply cracked into fissures; leaves roundish, acute, very slightly cordate, sometimes truncate at the base, hard, leathery, shining, smooth, with five digitate ribs, six inches long and as many broad; stalks shorter than the leaves, tumid at both ends; flowers in lateral compound racemes. Drupes two to three, globose, cotyledons distinct, linear, oblong, very membranous.—(*Lindley's Flora Medica*, p. 41).

A native of Malabar and the eastern Islands, and cultivated in the Botanical Garden.

The seeds of this species are well known in commerce under the name of Cocculus indicus, or "*Coques du Levant*;" they are roundish, kidney-shaped, enclosed in a blackish brown, dry, and wrinkled perisperm, within which the fruit is white, bivalvic and unilocular; the kernel is oily. They are devoid of smell, of extremely bitter taste, and poisonous in moderate doses. These properties are due to the presence of a peculiar principle named *Picrotoxic acid.*

This acid is prepared by making a watery extract of the berries, and precipitating a watery solution of this extract by acetate of lead; filter, evaporate to dryness in a water bath, dissolve in spirit, filter a second time, and continue evaporating and redissolving until the extract is perfectly soluble in alcohol and water. It now consists of picrotoxic acid and colouring matter. The latter may be separated by the careful addition of a small portion of water; the colouring matter is removed, and the picrotoxic acid remains.

This acid crystallizes in silky needles, in transparent plates, or in granular masses; it is soluble in twenty-five times its weight of boiling, 150 of cold water. The taste is intensely bitter; its acid properties are feeble, but distinct; sulphuric acid gives it a saffron yellow colour; by nitric acid it is converted into the oxalic acid. It is composed ultimately of carbon 12, hydrogen 7, and oxygen 5 atoms.

Besides the picrotoxic acid, these seeds contain resin, gum, fatty matter, malic acid, mucus, starch, and lignine, with salts of lime, potash, and iron. Recent experiments have detected in the pericarp two alkaline principles, named Menispermine and Paramenispermine, which seem however to possess no very remarkable properties.

The seeds are poisonous to all animals, and even to vegetables. The general effects produced on the former are nausea, vomiting, tetanic convulsions, and insensibility; ten or twelve grains of the picrotoxic acid are sufficient to destroy a dog. The chief use of Cocculus indicus is for stupifying fish; mixed with crumbs of bread and thrown into ponds the fish which eat the crumbs become intoxicated, float on the surface, and are easily taken. It is well known that fish thus caught are exceedingly dangerous. The seeds are often added to beer, which they render more intoxicating, but proportionately injurious to the health.

The only use of the Cocculus indicus in medicine is as an external application, as a powder or ointment, to destroy vermin in the hair, and in the treatment of some cutaneous diseases.

Gen. 2.—Cocculus.

Sp. 1. *Cocculus palmatus.*

Syn. Menispermum palmatum. Cocculus colombo.

Off. The root, Colombo kejur *Hind.* Colombo root *Eng.*

Root perennial, composed of fasciculated, fusiform, branched, fleshy, curved, and descending tubers, from 1 to 2 inches thick, epidermis thin and brown, marked with transverse warts; flesh of deep yellow colour, excessively bitter, inodorous. Stems annual, herbaceous, 1 or 2 from one root, about ½ an inch thick, twining, simple in male plant, branched in the female, rounded, green, hairy in the grown plant; leaves alternate, the younger thin, pellucid, bright green, 3 lobed, the older remote, about 8 inches in breadth, nearly round, deeply cordate, 5 to 7 lobed, dark green above, pale beneath, hairy on both sides. Petiole as long as the leaf, thick below. Racemes axillary, or two together; fruit a drupe or berry, very hairy, tipped with a black long gland.

(*Lindley op. cit. p.* 369.)

A native of the shores of Oizo and Mozambique, introduced into Madras, and now successfully cultivated in the Calcutta garden. The root is common in the bazars, being brought from Ceylon, whither it comes from Africa. Colombo having been long the intermediate stage in the traffic, has given its name to the root.

In commerce Colombo root is met in slices of one to two inches diameter, half an inch thick, often perforated in centre, much wrinkled, greyish externally, bright yellow within; the taste is excessively bitter, smell heavy, powder of a greenish grey colour, and very apt to attract moisture from the air. The commercial parcels are often adulterated with the roots of the *Costus indicus, C. speciosus, and C. arabicus,* (Kust, Kushmut, Putchuk, Kemooka, *Vern.*) with *bryony* dyed with turmeric, and with the root of another species of *Cocculus* which we will subsequently describe.

The dry roots contain one-third their weight of starch, a large quantity of yellow colouring matter, a crystalline principle named *Colombia,* traces of volatile oil, woody fibre, and the usual salts; they are free from the astringent acids, and consequently give no precipitate with the salts of iron, or with solutions of gelatine.

Colombia is prepared by acting on the powdered root with sulphuric ether till it ceases to be discoloured; by spontaneous evaporation crystals are obtained, but in the very small proportion of one part in sixty-four. It may also be prepared by acting on the root with alcohol, Sp. Gr. 835, distilling off ¾ of the tincture, and allowing the residual liquid to stand for some days; impure crystals are obtained, which on washing with cold water and solution in alcohol may be rendered nearly pure. The liquor from which the crystals are deposited may be evaporated to dryness, mixed with powdered glass, and digested in sulphuric ether, which dissolves wax, colombia, and the fatty matter; distil off the ether, and boil the residue with acetic acid; on evaporation crystals are separated.

Colombia crystallizes in prisms, is very bitter, is neither acid nor alkaline; sulphuric acid gives it first a yellow, then a red colour. It contains no nitrogen, being shewn by Liebig to consist of carbon 12, hydrogen 7, oxygen 4 atoms.

Colombo root is one of the most valuable tonics we possess; it seldom occasions any unpleasant sensation in the stomach or alimentary canal; it improves the appetite and digestive powers, does not constipate, and though destitute of absolute febrifuge qualities, is one of the best remedies for persons convalescent from fevers. The dose of the powdered root is xv grs. to ʒi. The tincture is the best form, as the spirit dissolves all the active, and removes none of the inert ingredients; the dose of the tincture is from one to three drachms. The watery infusion is very apt to spoil, on account of its containing a large proportion of starch.

(*False Colombo.*)

A root called American colombo is very commonly met with. It is the root of the *Frasera Carolinensis*, or *Walteri*, a native of North America, of the natural order Gentianeæ. It may be at once distinguished by the absence of starch, in consequence of which it does not give a blue colour with tincture of iodine. It also contains tannic acid, which may be detected by the deep black colour struck with the permuriate of iron. The true colombo contains no astringent principle.

Another spurious colombo arrives in Europe from Algiers, and may also be distinguished by the tests above-mentioned. The Costus speciosus and Arabicus are at once known by their very different appearance, and violet smell. The adulteration by *bryony* is rare. This root is white, and cold water will remove the turmeric employed to dye it yellow. But even to the eye of an inexperienced person the characters of true colombo once carefully examined, are so decided that no mistake can be apprehended.

It is not improbable that the roots of other species of Cocculus may resemble the colombo sufficiently to be substituted for the latter, not only in trade, but in medicine. Experiments with this family are however peculiarly dangerous, on account of the presence in some of the bitter and very poisonous picrotoxic acid.

Off. prep. Infusion. Tincture and compound tincture.

Sp. 2, *Cocculus cordifolius.*

Syn. Menispermum cordifolium, see *Fl. Ind.* iii. p. 811.

Vern. Guluncha, Gudancha, &c.

Off. Root and stems.

This is one of the most common and valuable plants in India. The stem is twining, perennial, succulent, running over the highest trees. Bark thick, corky, with many elevated scabrous specks; from the branches there drop filiform fibres, which continue lengthening till they enter the ground, and form additional stems and roots, some of which Dr. Roxburgh states measure thirty feet in length, not being thicker than twine; leaves alternate, petioled, broad, cordate, five-nerved, entire, curved, smooth, about four inches each; petioles round, smooth, swelled at the base; racemes axillary or terminal, or from the insertion of former leaves, with frequently a few flowers in separate axils. Flowers numerous, small, yellow. MALE-flowers, calyx six-leaved, leaflets oval, petals six, wedge-formed, half the length of the calyx, margins inflected, and embracing the filaments; filaments six, clubbed, spreading rather longer than the petals, anthers immersed in the fleshy extremity of the filaments. FEMALE-flowers calyx and corolla as in the male, filaments six, fleshy, sterile; germs three, superior, resting on a tumid receptacle, style single, very short; stigmas torn; berries one, two, or three, generally one; two rarely, all three come to maturity, of the size of a small cherry, smooth, red, succulent, with very glutinous pulp, each resting on a tumid receptacle; seed single, kidney-formed, on the inside there is a deep pit which receives its receptacle. *Roxb.*

The root is large, soft, and spongy, and when fresh is used extensively by the natives of Bengal, being mixed with sour rice gruel, and sugar, for the cure of heat of urine in gonorrhœa. On the mode of preparing the goluncha in its various forms, and its uses in disease, some very curious information is given by the Dewan Ramcomul Sen, in a paper published in the Trans. Medical and Physical Society of Calcutta, 1827, vol. iii. p. 294. An extract called *Palo* is procured from the stem, and is used dissolved in water for the same purpose. The stems, roots, and leaves are bitter, and afford a decoction called *Pachana*, much used as a bitter tonic, in convalescence from fevers and acute diseases generally.

The *Palo* is prepared by cutting the stem into small pieces, which are cleaned and bruised in a mortar, then soaked in water for 24 to 48 hours. The mass is then squeezed between the palms of the hands, and the woody particles separated from the fluid, which is strained through a cloth. The solution is evaporated to dryness before the sun, and when dry the residue resembles sugar; the dose is half a rupee to one rupee weight, taken with sugar, milk, and rice gruel.

The decoction *Pachana* is made from 2 to 5 rupees weight of the stem cut into small pieces, bruised in a mortar, and boiled with a pound (½ a seer) of water down to two ounces; this is then strained and drank with honey. An infusion in cold water is also prepared, and is much employed in the treatment of cutaneous diseases.

In the IVth vol. of the Transactions of the Medical and Physical Society of Calcutta, p. 431, 1829, is a paper by Mr. Piddington, detailing some experiments on guluncha. The species employed by Mr. Piddington, he names the *Menispermum verrucosum* and *glabrum*, neither of which properly refer to our article. The *M. verrucosum*, though cultivated in the Botanic Garden is not indigenous, it is a native of Java and Amboyna, and is now known to be the *Funis felleus* of Rumphius. It is a much more powerful bitter than the gulancha. Mr. Piddington's experiments indicated the presence of starch, mucilage, and extract, and of a crystalline principle, apparently possessed of alkaline properties, but of which too minute a quantity was at his command to allow a satisfactory examination of its nature. The alcoholic extract Mr Piddington described as likely to prove of great value in the treatment of intermittent fever. The highly satisfactory effects of *M. verrucosum* in Java and Manilla promised indeed similar advantages from the use of gulancha here. Dr. Hardie of Oudepore and Dr. Stewart of Calcutta used the extract in several cases of intermittent fever in 1829, and reported on it very favourably.

Our article, in common with all the order, should be collected during the hot season, when the bitter principle is most abundant and concentrated.

In several trials made at the College Hospital, the gulancha was found to be a very useful tonic, but we could scarcely attribute to it any very decided febrifuge effect. The decoction, or cold infusion used in the same manner as sarsaparilla was of very great utility in the treatment of several cases of chronic rheumatism, and of secondary venereal affections. Its action is decidedly diuretic and tonic in a very high degree.

Off. prep. Extract, tincture, infusion, and decoction.

Gen. 3.—Cissampelos.

Sp. 1. *Pareira brava*, or wild vine.

Gries wurzel German, or gravel root.

Off. The root.

A climbing shrub, a native of South America.

The root occurs in flattened, angular, or in cylindrical pieces, some two inches thick, and over a foot long, with a dark brown rind, furrowed longitudinally, and wrinkled transversely; transverse section of yellowish grey colour, marked by numerous concentric circles; fracture fibrous, taste sweetish, aromatic, and subsequently bitter. The stem is often fraudulently mixed with or substituted for the root.

Fenueille states that the root contains resin, a yellow bitter principle, a brown colouring matter, starch, an azotized substance, and various salts of ammonia and lime. Its effects on the system are those of a tonic diuretic, and in large doses slightly aperient. Over chronic inflammation of the bladder Mr. Brodie says it has a great influence, lessening very materially the secretion of the ropy mucus, which is itself a very great evil. The same distinguished surgeon considers that it also diminishes the inflammation and irritability of the bladder.

The Pareira brava may be given in powder in doses of ½ a drachm to 1ʒ—or one to two ounces of the infusion of ʒvi of the root in 20℥ boiling water. Sir B. Brodie's formula constitutes the compound decoction of this Pharmacopœia.

Off. prep. Powder, extract, tincture, infusion, compound decoction.

Dr. Roxburgh, Fl. Indica, vol. iii. p. 848, describes six species of cissampelos, viz.

C. Glabra, (*vern.* Peergrug,) a native of Sylhet, root acrid and used in medicine by the natives. C. hexandra, (*vern.* Neemooka,) a native of Bengal. C. convolvulacea, a native of Coromandel and Malabar. C. Caapeba, from the

Moluccas. C. hernandifolia, a native of Chittagong; and C. tetrandra, brought from Amboyna.

The C. glabra, hexandra, hernandifolia, and convolvulacea, natives of the Peninsula, are all referred by Wight and Arnot to the same species, which differs from C. Pareira chiefly in the form of the sepals, and the length of the staminal columns.

We have used the Neemooka of Bengal with decided advantage under the same circumstances as the *Pareira brava* would be employed in. With this and the Menispermum cordifolium we are but little dependent on other countries for the valuable remedy so justly lauded by Brodie and others.

To enable the reader to identify the Neemooka, we subjoin the description from Wight and Arnot's Prodromus, p. 15.

Cissampelos, generic characters of—

Dioicious.—Male, sepals four, in a double series; petals four, united into a cup-shaped corolla, with usually an entire margin; stamens united into a slender column dilated at the apex, bearing two-celled anthers, opening horizontally; cells placed end to end, and forming a four-lobed, four celled ring round the top of the column.

Female, calyx of one lateral sepal; corolla of one petal in front of sepal; ovary solitary; stigmata three; drupe obliquely uniform, not compressed, wrinkled round its margin; seed solitary, uncinate. Embryo long, terete, inclosed in a fleshy albumen. Twining shrubs, leaves peltate or cordate, mucronulate at apex. Racemes axillary; of the males usually trichotomously branched, and somewhat corymbose, with subulate small bracteas, or with none at all; of the females simple, elongated, bearing broad alternate foliaceous bracteas, with several one-flowered pedicels in the axils.

Sp. C. convolvulacea.

Stem pubescent, leaves cordate, usually obtuse or acute, sometimes accuminated, rarely emarginate; sinus narrow or wide. Upper side glabrous or slightly pubescent; under side more or less pubescent, sometimes tomentose; petioles inserted at the margin, or sometimes slightly extra marginal. Male racemes three to four, shorter than the petiole; sepals orbicular, unguiculate; columns of stamens longer than the entire, externally hairy, cup-shaped corolla; female racemes usually in pairs, sometimes solitary and forked, in flower scarcely as long as the petiole, in fruit often much longer than the leaf; drupes hairy.

In the genera above described there are several species

much used in other countries, and some of popular notoriety in India, though of little actual utility. Of these the following notice will suffice :—

Cocculus bakis, Senegal Root, diuretic and very bitter, used in intermittents and gonorrhœa.

C. fibraurea, Cochin-China, and China; used by the Malays in agues and liver diseases.

C. cinerascens, Rio Janeiro. Root, used in intermittent and liver diseases.

C. platyphyllus, Brazil, do.

C. crispus. Syn. *Menispermum verrucosum*, (see page 200.) Java, Amboyna. The whole is extremely bitter, and is used with complete success by the Malays as a febrifuge remedy.

C. acuminatus, Coromandel and Bengal. Syn. M. polycarpon, (Rox. vol. iii. p. 816.) Tiliacora racemosa, (Colebrooke, Trans. Lin. Society, xiii. 67).

Used as an antidote to snake bites, being rubbed between stones and mixed with water. It is the Naga-mushadee of the Hindoos, Tileakora of the Bengalees. It is the third sort of mushadee of the Telingas, the first being the nux-vomica tree, the second the naga-mushadee, or snake-wood tree, subsequently described.

Pereira medica, Lindley, Syn. Menisp. fenestratum. Wood and root.

The Wonivol of Ceylon—considered in Ceylon an excellent stomachic.

Clypea burmanni. Syn. Menispermum peltatum, Malabar, Coromandel, Ceylon; very bitter; used in fevers, dysentery, and piles.

Abuta rufescens, white Pareira brava, Cayenne and Guyana. Root used for the same purpose as the Cissampelos Pareira.

NAT. ORDER X.—BERBERACEÆ.

This order, which is nearly allied to Menispermeæ and Podophylleæ, is composed of small trees or shrubs, with dry or succulent fruits, the latter of which contain large quantities of malic acid. The bark and wood are very bitter. A yellow colouring matter and an azotized bitter principle called *Berberite* exist in all the species. These are chiefly confined, as Mr. Royle observes, to the temperate zone of the northern hemisphere. In India, species occur in the uncultivated state only in the hilly regions.

Bot. Char. Calyx inferior, free, of 3, 4, 6 early deciduous sepals, which are often coloured or petaloid, surrounded by several bracteoles, ranged in a double series, with the margins overlapping each other previous to the opening of the flower. Petals equalling the number of sepals, and placed opposite to them; filaments short, occasionally so irritable that on being slightly touched on the inner surface near the base they spring forward with elastic force and strike the anther against the stigma. Anther two-celled, cells bursting with elasticity by recurved valves from the base to the apex, and not according to the more usual form by pores or a longitudinal slit. Ovary superior, one-celled, with several ovules usually springing from the base, erect; style short, stigma thick, orbiculate; fruit a fleshy berry, or indehiscent capsule, with few exarillate, erect, albuminous seeds; albumen fleshy or horny, with the straight embryo in the axis. *(Wight's Illustrations, p. 22.)*

Gen. 1.—Berberis.

Sp. 1. *Berberis Lycium.*
— 2. *Berberis Aristata.*

Vern. Chitra, Kushmul. Wood—darhuld and darchob. Extract, hoosiz, rusot, the Λυχιον of the Greeks. Common in the Himalayas.

—*B. Lycium*—(Royle's Illustr. p. 64.) Off. *Root and bark.*

Spines three-parted, conical, leaves 5—8 in a cluster, pale, leathery, veiny, oblong, lanceolate or obovate, tapering to the base, mucronate, margins spiny, toothed, or entire. Racemes twenty-flowered, erect, spreading, becoming pendulous in fruit. Pedicels long, simple, flowers small. External scales lanceolate; ovaries smooth, four-seeded. Fruit ovate, obtuse at each end.

A watery extract called *Rusot* is prepared in the hilly districts of India from the sliced root, stem, and branches of this plant. This extract is to be found in all the bazars, and is much employed by the native practitioners. Dr. Royle has very ably traced the history of this substance, and identified it perfectly with the celebrated λυχιον ινδιχον of Dioscorides, the *Hoosiz hindee* of the Arabs. Alone, or rubbed with equal parts of opium and alum, and diffused through water, it is chiefly used as an external application in incipient or chronic ophthalmia, being applied around the eye. Mr. Playfair, Dr. Royle, and other high authorities speak in very favourable terms of the success of this practice.

Rusot of best quality is a pale yellow, uniform, pasty extract, soluble in water and alcohol, to which it communicates a brilliant yellow colour; exceedingly bitter to the taste, of rich heavy smell, blackened by salts of iron, precipitated by solution of gelatine, and consequently containing tannic and gallic acid.

The bitterness of this extract is due to the presence of a principle called *Berberite*, discovered in the bark of the root of a European barberry by Buchner in 1835, and which we have found ourselves in the rusot of the bazar.

Berberite is obtained from rusot by the process described in the 3rd part. It is a light powder, formed of minute silky yellow needles, devoid of smell, excessively bitter, little soluble in cold water, but hot water dissolves it freely; soluble also in alcohol, insoluble in ether. It has no alkaline or acid properties, is rendered green by sulphuric, red by tannic acid, and is precipitated by gallic acid. In alkaline solutions the yellow colour is indistinct, but returns on saturation with acids. Berberite is precipitated from its solutions by corrosive sublimate, nitrate of silver, tartar emetic, and several other metallic salts, but not by acetate or sub-acetate of lead. It is very easily destroyed by a temperature not much exceeding that of boiling water.

On analysis *Berberite* is found to contain azote 1, carbon 33, hydrogen 18, oxygen 12 atoms.

The trials instituted on the medicinal virtues of rusot have led us to some satisfactory results.

We were induced to use it internally as a tonic, in consequence of the popular reputation in Europe of the bark of the common barberry, as a remedy for agues. We were also aware that M. Buchner had used *Berberite* as a tonic as far as ten grain doses, with considerable benefit. Lastly, the intense bitterness of this principle, and its yielding azote on ultimate analysis, led us to anticipate its utility in the treatment of periodical fevers.

In our experiments we employed a specimen of extremely fine *rusot*, supplied by Dr. Campbell of Nipal, and also an extract prepared at the Medical College from the bark and stems of the Berberis Asiatica, obtained from Dr. Wallich from the Botanic Garden.

Rusot is best given as a febrifuge in half drachm doses diffused through water, and repeated thrice, or still more frequently, daily. It occasions a feeling of agreeable warmth at the epigastrium, increases appetite, promotes digestion, and acts as a very gentle, but certain aperient. The skin is invariably moist during its operation.

In over thirty cases of tertian ague, (several complicated with spleen), we have succeeded in checking the fever on an average within three days after commencing the rusot. In eight cases of quartan six were cured. The cases of common quotidian thus successfully treated were so numerous that they were not recorded. In no instance was head-ache or constipation produced, but we have seen rusot exasperate the symptoms of chronic dysentery and hepatitis when complicated with ague.

On the whole, we deem the rusot a most important accession to our Materia Medica, and worthy of being substituted in a multitude of cases for cinchona bark. Its aperient action renders it especially valuable.

The rusot is manufactured in Nipal and the Dhoon, at about eight annas the seer. What is found in the Bengal bazars is usually of a very inferior description, old, mouldy, black, and mixed with half its weight of impurities.

Berberite may be given in five-grain doses. We have not employed it much, as it is a preparation very troublesome to make in a pure state, and as the administration of the extract proved so satisfactory.

Off. prep. Extract and Tincture.

Of other species it is only necessary to notice—

Berberis Aristata, Nipal. *Vern.* Chitra. Fruit (sun-dried) used as raisins; bark and root used for making rusot.

B. ‡*Kunawurensis*, found in Kunawur, and similarly employed.

B. Asiatica, or tinctoria, Neelgherries, used for dyeing yellow.

B. Vulgaris, the common European Barberry; bark used in periodical fevers, and the root as a purgative.

NAT. ORDER XI.—CAPPARIDEÆ.

This order is of very trivial importance to the medical reader. It is chiefly tropical in distribution, and consists of shrubs or thorny trees.

The calyx is four-parted, petals 4, torus small, stipes of the ovary slender, stamens numerous, fruit siliquose, somewhat baccate, stipitate. In chemical produce this order is allied to the Cruciferæ. Many species contain an acrid volatile principle.

The *Capparis spinosa*, or caper plant, is well known through its young flower buds, which constitute the capers of the shops. The buds of the *C. sinaica*, or caper of mount Sinai are the *filfil-jibbel*, or mountain pepper of the east. The fruit of the *C. aphylla* of India, (*vern.* Kureel,) is also used as a pickle.

Of the genus CRATÆVA we may notice the *C. gynandra*, a native of the West Indies. The bark of the root is said to blister like cantharides. The *C. tapia* (*Vern.* Birmi ke chawl. Tapia and Varana *Sans.*, garlic pear *English*,) is a native of Ceylon, also common in Malabar. The juice of the astringent bark is used as a tonic, and febrifuge. The *C. religiosa* is common in India. The leaves are called Bel-ka-pat, are slightly bitter and aromatic, and much used by native practitioners. The *C. marmelos* (Bilva or Mahura) formerly considered a species of this genus, is now referred to the order Aurantiaceæ, and called *Ægle marmelos*.

The genera CLEOME and POLANISIA, embrace several species of supposed medicinal virtues. Ainslie describes five species. The *Cleome felina* (cat's cleome, *Eng.* Swarnakshira, *Sans.*) is used as an astringent in northern India and Ceylon. The *C. pentaphylla*, (*Vern.* Hurhuriya, *Beng.* Caraila, *Hind.* Hoolhool, *Duk.* Caravela and Varsar, *Sans.*) affords small, black, rather aromatic seeds, used by the natives in decoction as a stimulant drink in low fevers, and in some forms of convulsion. The expressed juice too is considered stimulant, and sudorific. The *C. viscosa*, or viscid Cleome (*Vern.* Hoorhoorya, *Hind.* Svana barbara *Sans.*) is also celebrated for its seeds, the *Chorie-ajooain*, of the bazars. These are believed to be vermifuge and stimulant, and are given to the extent of a tea spoonful twice daily (Ainslie.) The *C. dodecandria* and *icosandria* of Ainslie are identical with this plant, and are described by Lindley as *Polanisia icosandra*. In Cochin China the whole plant bruised is used like sinapisms for counter-irritation, and blistering. This fact deserves attentive experimental investigation.

NAT. ORDER XII.—FLACOURTIACEÆ.

This group is of very little interest, containing but two species requiring particular notice.

GEN. CHAULMOOGRA.

Sp. 1. *Chaulmoogra odorata.*
Vern. Chaolmoogra, Petarcura.
Off. Seeds.

A native of Sylhet, and the seed employed extensively in the treatment of cutaneous diseases.

The seeds are various in shape, nearly oval, smooth, grey, hard. Embryo white.

The seeds yield by expression about 10 per cent. of a thick fixed oil, of unpleasant flavour, and rather offensive smell; ʒi given to a dog caused violent vomiting in 15 minutes. They are much used by the natives in the treatment of cutaneous disorders, being beaten up with ghee into a soft mass, and applied three times daily.

The *Hydrocarpus venenata* of Ceylon, allied to this order, has poisonous fruit, and induces intoxication.

The *Flacourtia cataphracta* (*Vern.* Talisputrie, *Duk.* Panayala, *Beng.* Talisha, *Sans.*) affords a popular medicine in Behar. The small leaves and shoots resemble rhubarb in flavour, and are used as gentle astringents in the dose of half a drachm in powder. An infusion of the bark in cold water is also employed as a remedy in hoarseness.

NAT. ORDER XIII.—BIXINEÆ.

This order only contains one species requiring notice, viz. the *Bixa Orellana*, or Annotto plant; a native of Cayenne, also indigenous in India; cultivated in the Calcutta Botanical Garden. Capsule two valved; seeds 8—10 attached to each placenta, with a red pulp. This red pulp separated from the seeds and sun-dried gives the annotto of commerce. It is chiefly employed for tinging cheese and butter, to which it imparts various shades of colour from yellow to red. It is also mixed with chocolate as a colouring ingredient.

NAT. ORDER XIV.—VIOLACEÆ.

This interesting family is very extensively distributed, and at least seventeen Indian species have been pointed out. It is divided into three tribes, of which the first, the Violeæ, alone concerns the medical inquirer. Many species possess a delicate and peculiar fragrance, for which they are highly prized; several contain the emetic principle *Emetine* in small quantities, and an analogous substance called *violine;* the family is composed of herbs and small plants having usually blue flowers.

Gen. 1.—Viola.

Sepals 5 unequal, prolonged into appendages at the base; Corolla unequal, 2 lipped, of 5 petals, the lower calcarate; stamens 5, hypogynous, syngenesious, unequal, the 2 anterior having anthers that are often calcarate; capsule many seeded, 3 valved.

(*Lindley Flor. Med. p.* 97.)

Sp. 1. *Viola odorata.*
Vern. Banopsha.
Off. Whole plant.

The plant in the dry state is sold in all the bazars, and is prescribed in infusion by the Hakims as a diaphoretic in the treatment of fever. It nauseates slightly, owing to its containing a very minute quantity of the principle termed *violina*, closely resembling the emetine, on which depend the virtues of the ipechachuana of Brazil.

The Viola odorata, as sold in the bazar, has dry, thready, fibrous roots of a pale yellow colour, knotty, some as thick as a quill. The leaves are heart-shaped; flowers blue. The entire plant retains slightly the delightfully sweet smell characteristic of this tribe. Under the name of Beg-banopsha, or violet root, and having precisely the smell of the fresh flower of our article, is sold in the bazar the well known " orris root" or Iris florentina. Excellent issue peas are made from this root.

To obtain violina the alcoholic extract of the plant is treated with ether to dissolve some fatty and green colouring matter. The residue is boiled in water, acidulated with sulphuric acid, and the solution is precipitated by hydrated oxide of lead. The precipitate contains *violina* and oxide of lead. The mixture boiled with alcohol, and the solution evaporated, yields the violina as a pale yellow matter, which may be rendered white by washing with cold strong alcohol.

We have separated Violina from the bazar " Banopsha," but in the very small proportion of about 1 from 200 parts.

Violina is alkaline, somewhat soluble in water, insoluble in ether and the oils. It acts as an emetic in doses of two to three grains.

The root of this violet separated from the plant and reduced to powder, proves emetic in doses of from two to four drachms made into a decoction by boiling water. The emetic operation is preceded by much nausea, and is often followed by purging. Our experience on the whole leads us to prefer as an emetic the *Crinum toxicarium*, subsequently described. The infusion of one drachm of the root in half a pint of water, is a very good nauseant and diaphoretic. We did not succeed in our attempt to substitute the violet root for ipecacuanha in the preparation of Dover's powder, or of Twining's antidysenteric pills.

Several species of violet possess similar properties. Royle has figured three Himalayan species, V. serpens, V. reniformis, and V. kunawurensis, the first of which is found in Mussooree, the second on the Choor mountain, the last in Kunawur.

Gen. 2.—Ionidium.

Sp. 1. *Ionidium ipecacuanha.* A native of Brazil, the roots emetic, substituted for, and used for adulterating ipecacuanha. The root contains 5 per 100 of emetine.

Sp. 2. *I. microphyllum,* C. uinchunchulla of the Andes. This plant is stated to be a specific in elephantiasis, and enjoys a great reputation in South America.

Sp. 3. *I. suffruticosum.*
Syn. Viola suffruticosa, (L.)
Vern. Ruttun puruss, *Duk.* Charati, *Sans.*

A rugged and somewhat prickly reclining herb, having a small crimson flower. It is common over the peninsula of India, and is used as a demulcent. We have examined carefully specimens obtained from the Calcutta Garden, but did not detect the least trace of the active principles emetine or violine.

NAT. ORDER XV.—POLYGALEÆ.

This order is made up of trees, shrubs, or herbs, with scattered leaves; many species are found in India, some of which are reported to possess medicinal properties. The Polygala Senega, and Krameria triandra, are included in most European Pharmacopeiæ, and are asserted to be very useful as expectorant and tonic remedies. An Indian species of Polygala is employed in the treatment of snake bites.

Gen. 1.—Polygala.

Sp. 1. *Polygala Senega.* Snake root.
Off. The roots.

A native of North America. The roots are formed of large fleshy fibres, twisted, knotty, ash-coloured, wrinkled transversely. Epidermis grey, thick, and resinous-like substance white, hard, and brittle. Smell peculiar, taste at first weak and mucilaginous, and subsequently acrid and nauseous. Powder of a grey colour.

The active principle of the Polygala Senega is a bitter acid, which has been recently described by M. Quevenne, (*Journ. de Pharmacie*, xxii. 449, 1837.)

The polygalic acid is obtained by boiling the powdered root in water, precipitating by acetate of lead, filtering, treating the filtered liquid with sulphuretted hydrogen to separate excess of lead, filtering, evaporating to dryness, treating the dry matter with alcohol at 837, and evaporating to dryness again.

The alcoholic extract is then washed with ether, redissolved in water, and subjected again to precipitation by subacetate of lead, to sulphuretted hydrogen, and purification by solution in boiling spirit.

Polygalic acid is a white inodorous powder, tasteless at first, subsequently acrid, pungent, and causing a sensation of contraction of the jaws; soluble in hot water and in absolute alcohol, insoluble in sulphuric ether and the fixed and volatile oils. The polygalic acid is turned yellow by nitric acid; sulphuric acid gives it first a yellow, then a rose red colour, which subsequently becomes intense violet, and after 24 hours disappears altogether. The salts of the polygalic acid, though quite neutral, are not crystallizable.

Two grains given to a dog occasioned vomiting, and four grains caused death after an interval of three hours.

Senega root was introduced into medical practice as a remedy in snake bites, but its efficacy in the treatment of these accidents is very questionable. In scruple doses the powdered root proves cathartic, often diuretic, occasioning much griping and distress. In smaller doses it seems to stimulate the kidneys or skin, according to the temperature at which the body is kept. Its expectorating effects are strongly marked in many cases of catarrh, dependent on debility, and seem to shew a decided action on the bronchial mucous membrane. The nature of this action it is however difficult to comprehend. Though comparatively little used, senega root is still employed by some experienced practitioners in the treatment of typhoid fevers, of chronic rheumatism, and as an indirect uterine stimulant in amennorrhea.

Dose of the powder from ten to twenty grains—of the decoction, one to three ounces.

Off. prep. Tincture, decoction.

Several species of Polygala are similarly employed in Germany, South America, and Java. In Nipal and the Himalayas, the P. crotalarioides is used as a snake antidote. Of this species the stem is branched from the base, suffruticose, decumbent, downy; leaves obovate, wedge-shaped at the base, stalked; racemes 8—10 flowered, wings roundish, obovate, as long as the orbicular, ciliated capsule.

In the Moluccas the *Soulamea amara* (Rex amaroris) is stated to be employed with great advantage in cholera, and in ague. All parts, especially the roots and fruit, are excessively bitter.

Gen. 2.—Krameria.

Sp. 1. *Krameria triandra.*

This plant is a native of Peru, and yields the Rhatany root of the Pharmacopœia; a powerful astringent, but destitute of any other virtues. Under the head of *Diospyros* will be found a most efficient indigenous substitute for this article.

NAT. ORDER XVI.—PITTOSPOREÆ.

Several species have a liquid resin round the seeds, which deserves examination.

NAT. ORDER XVII.—DROSERACEÆ.

This order consists of small herbaceous plants, of bitter, acrid, severe caustic flavour. Applied to the skin they cause pain and inflammation. None have been used in medicine.

NAT. ORDER XVIII.—ELATINEÆ.

This contains no medicinal article.

NAT. ORDER XIX.—CARYOPHYLLEÆ.

All these plants are herbaceous, with opposite leaves and terminal flowers. Of several hundred species scarcely any possess the least activity. The *Dianthus caryophyllus*, or clove flower, is fragrant and aromatic; and the petals being of a lovely pink tint are used in some parts of Europe for preparing a syrup and conserve. The Dianthus chinensis is of analogous qualities, and is cultivated in Indian gardens under the name of *Kurunphul.*

The genus SAPONARIA includes an article well known in India, the *Saponaria vaccaria*. The properties of this plant are identical in every respect with those of the *S. officinalis*, or soap wort, the Στρουθιον of Dioscorides. The taste of the entire plant is bitter, the roots are cylindrical, two to three feet long, the thickness of a swan quill, branching above, epidermis ruddy, thick, and easily separable ; parenchyma white and solid. The taste of the root is bitter and mucilaginous ; the infusion is blackened by salts of iron, and the decoction froths like a solution of soap. According to Bucholz' analysis these properties are due to the presence of a mucilaginous extractive called *saponine*, regarding which an additional notice will be found under the head of *Sapindus emarginatus*.

NAT. ORDER XX.—LINEÆ.

This order occurs chiefly in Europe and the north of Africa; in India one species, the *Linum usitatissimum*, is cultivated all over the plains in the cold season. The seeds of all the species are mucilaginous and oily. The leaves of the *L. catharticum* are purgative and emetic.

GEN.—LINUM.

Sp. 1. *Linum usitatissimum*. (*Vern.* Atees, Tisi, Mushina, *Hind.* and *Beng.*)

Off. The seed.

Root slender, herb, very smooth, stem 18 inches to 2 feet high, round, straight, leafy, corymbose, leaves alternate, sessile, acute, 3 ribbed, rather glaucous, the lowermost short and blunt; flowers several, erect, in a corymbose panicle; calyx with three prominent ribs, with a membranous irregular margin; petals thin, delicate, roundish, wedge-shaped, readily dropping off, blue, glossy, and with numerous veins.

The seeds are oblong-oval, flattened, with sharp edges, thinned towards the summit, smooth, brilliant, about a line in length, brownish internally, white and oily, contained in a fruit formed of ten capsules, apparently forming one. They dehisce longitudinally on ripening, and each capsule contains a single seed.

The seeds yield an abundance of oil and mucilage, the former being contained in the substance, the latter in the envelope of the seed.

Linseed mucilage. This mucilage resembles a thick solution of gum arabic, and is precipitated in white flakes by alcohol and by acetate of lead. Being tasteless and inodorous it is justly considered one of the most valuable emollients or demulcents which can be used in medical practice. Besides gum it contains an azotised principle, free acetic acid, acetate of potash and lime, &c.

The seed when bruised or powdered gives out its mucilage to water with great facility, and hence it forms an excellent external application. The formula for the linseed poultice will be found in the Pharmacopœia.

Linseed oil. This oil is obtained by expression from the seeds, which are first slightly roasted in order to destroy the mucilage. The oil is clear, yellowish brown, fluid, not congealed even by the most intense frost, smoking very much when burned, readily becoming rancid, dries speedily on exposure to the air. By age it becomes of a deep colour, very acrid, and nearly opaque. The odour is peculiar and disagreeable, the taste disgusting.

Linseed oil is one of the chief ingredients in oil varnishes and in printer's ink; by boiling with litharge its drying properties are much improved. It does not seem improbable that the spurious white "atees" roots of the bazar are occasionally obtained from this article, or from the *Goola shoopré*, or Linum trigynium, indigenous in the Lower Provinces.

The leaves of the *Linum catharticum* while fresh are strongly purgative, but are uncertain in their action.

NAT. ORDER XXI.—MALVACEÆ.

This important order includes herbs, shrubs, and trees, and numbers over 800 species, the majority of which are natives of South America; several are found in the plains of India, and a few on the Himalayas at moderate elevations.

The Malvaceæ are all mucilaginous, of faint flavour, but some very acid. The majority are inodorous, three or four species however exhale a strong smell of musk. In the genus Gossypium the seed is surrounded by the well known cotton. The perisperm of the seeds yields a very mild fixed oil. No remedy of any energy, and no poisonous substance is found in this order.

Gen. 1.—Malva.

Sp. 1. *Malva sylvestris.* Marsh-mallow.
(*Arab.* Khabazee and Anjil. Khitmie, *Pers.* the seed, *towdrie.*)

Off. The root.

This is a plant common in all parts of Europe, and much used for preparing the emollient drinks and ptisans in which the French practitioners repose so much confidence. All its virtues are attributable to the mucilage in which it abounds. It is indigenous in Cashmere, and cultivated in Indian gardens.

The *Malva mauritiana,* L. *Kungee ke pat,* the seeds of which are brought from Hydrabad, is cultivated in most parts of this country, and may be used instead of the article in the text. *M. rotundifolia,* L. is likewise cultivated in India. V. Roxb. vol. iii. p. 181.

Gen. 2.—Althæa.

Sp. Althæa officinalis. Hollyhock.
Vern. Gool Khirree.

Off. The root.

A native of Europe and of Cashmere, and used precisely as the preceding species. Besides gum, the root contains a large proportion of a crystalline acid, called the *aspartic,* combined with ammonia—the asparagin of Robiquet. This principle is prepared by slicing the roots and macerating the slices in cold water, filtering and evaporating the liquor. The aspartic acid is separated by boiling the aspartate of ammonia with baryta water. The aspartate of baryta is soluble in hot water, and in that state is decomposed by sulphuric acid. By filtering, the sulphate of baryta is separated, and as the solution cools the aspartic acid is deposited in small crystals.

The Althæa, under the name of *Guimauve,* may be considered almost the staple of French pharmacy. The leaves are used as emollients for cataplasms and fomentations; the flowers are ingredients in the pectoral or cough mixtures; the roots are used in simple and compound syrups, in pastilles, pastes, oils, powders, pills, &c. Notwithstanding the great esteem in which it is held, it is difficult to specify the reason, for it certainly acts as a mere demulcent, and not more effectually than mucilage in any other form.

In India the Althea rosea is widely cultivated in gardens, and may be substituted for this article.

Gen. 3.—Sida.

Sp. Sida acuta, Burm.
Syn. Sida lanceolata, Retz.
Vern. Pata, Sanscrit.
Off. The root.

A native of the peninsula, and found also in the hilly districts. Plant shrubby, branches without tubercles under the leaves; leaves narrow, lanceolate, accuminated, glabrous, or slightly sprinkled above and on the nerves beneath with bristly hairs, coarsely simply serrated, the serratures open. Stipules linear, accuminate, stiffish, striated, with several longitudinal nerves, ciliated, often longer than the petiole; pedicels axillary, solitary, not shorter than the petiole, not longer than the stipules, jointed above the middle, sometimes arranged in a short axillary almost leafless branch; carpels 5—9.

The root resembles common liquorice, is very bitter, strikes a blue colour with salts of iron, does not precipitate gelatine, yields to boiling water 23 parts—to alcohol 19 parts per 100. Crystals of aspartate of ammonia are deposited on spontaneous evaporation of the watery solution. The extract dissolved in water is precipitated by ammonia.

Dr. Ainslie informs us that an infusion of this root combined with ginger is given in intermittents and in chronic diarrhœa. The leaves bruised with oil are applied externally as a poultice to accelerate suppuration.

We have used an infusion of the root with some advantage in the cases alluded to by Ainslie, but we could not satisfy ourselves as to its febrifuge action. It promotes perspiration, increases the appetite, and is in many respects a useful substitute for more costly bitters.

An electuary is prepared from the expressed juice of the *Sida* in Bengal, and used in the treatment of worms in the intestinal canal. We have learned from some experienced native practitioners that no reliance can be placed on its efficacy.

Care must be taken not to confound the classical name of this plant with the *Sidhee* of the bazar, which is a mixture of the dried leaves and young capsules of the Indian hemp, a powerful narcotic.

Gen. 4.—Abelmoschus.

Sp. 1. *Abelmoschus longifolius*, Wall. (Hibiscus, Roxb.)

Abelmoschus esculentus, Wight and Arnott, (H. esculentus, L.) according to Roxburgh, is a distinct species from the above, and a native of tropical America. It is possible they may be one and the same plant, as they are considered by Wight and Arnott.

Vern. Okra. Dharoos, *Beng.* Bendee, *Tel.* Ramturai, *Hind.*

Dr. Roxburgh says that he never found this plant wild, and that it is much cultivated throughout India. The other sort (A. esculentus) is a native of the West Indies. We subjoin Dr. Roxburgh's admirable description of this plant.

"*Root* ramous, annual. *Stem* erect, ramous, from three to six feet high, round, towards the base somewhat ligneous, and in a good soil as thick as a man's wrist, tender parts covered with sharp bristles, and often spotted with purplish specks. *Leaves* alternate, petioles the inferior ones only angular, about the middle of the plant palmate, while the superior ones are sub-digitate, with the divisions lanceolate-oblong, all are serrate, and somewhat bristly; the general size of the whole leaf is from eight to twelve inches each way. *Petioles* round, bristly, as long as the leaves, generally more coloured than the stem, or branches. *Stipules* often paired. *Flowers* axillary, solitary, short-peduncled, very large, pale yellow, with a dark crimson bottom. *Calyx;* the *exterior* one from six to twelve leaved; *leaflets* linear, bristly, caducous; the *interior* one spathiform, bursting on one side, of a remarkably soft texture. *Coral stamens,* and *germ* as in the genus. *Stigmas* as many as the cells in the capsule. *Capsule* from six to twelve inches long and about one in diameter, somewhat bristly, particularly the ridges, their number corresponding with that of the cell and valves, viz. from five to eight, with a single row of round, smooth seeds in each cell.

"This is one of the best, if not the best, of the esculent herbs of India; the plant is easily raised from seed, and produces abundance of fruit, the only part which is eaten. The whole plant, particularly the capsules, is replete with much mild mucilage, which I consider as highly nourishing as well as mucilaginous, and might no doubt be employed to advantage in all diseases requiring emollients and demulcents. Some tender branches placed in water for examination soon rendered it gelatinous, almost as much so as if the branches of *Pedalium murex* had been standing in it. Dr. Cullen observes that coughing is often caused by acrid vapour rising from the lungs, irritating the glottis and its neighbourhood; that by besmearing these parts with demulcent matter, we often lessen the irritation and frequency of coughing. A mild, palatable, culinary preparation of the very young capsules of this plant, would, I think, stand as fair a chance to answer this intention as any thing I know, and at the same time prove a nourishing part of the diet.

"The stigmas are replete with a very beautiful deep purple juice, which they communicate to paper, and which is tolerably durable.

"*H. esculentus*, the West India *Okra*, possesses virtues nearly similar, though I believe inferior; this I have also cultivated for many years in the Botanic Garden, and it differs from this very conspicuously, both in the shape of the leaves and capsules." *Roxb. Fl. Ind.* iii. p. 210.

Without exactly admitting the correctness of Dr. Cullen's views as to the cause of the irritation of the glottis, experience amply shews the value of the practice recommended by that able physician; in the third part will be found a formula for the preparation of a *demulcent lozenge*, which we have devised in the hope of meeting the object Roxburgh points out. We can recommend this lozenge strongly as a very pleasant nutritive and soothing preparation.

Sp. 2. *Abelmoschus moschatus.* (Musk Hibiscus).
Syn. Hibiscus Abelmoschus.
Vern. Hubb-el-musk.
Off. Seeds.
A native of the East Indies and South America.

Stem herbaceous, hisped, with wide spreading hairs, not prickly, leaves and long petioles hisped with rigid hairs, but otherwise glabrous, unequally and coarsely toothed, 5·7 lobed, lobes all spreading, oblong or lanceolate, acuminated, pedicels harshly pubescent, axillary about as long as the petioles, involucral leaves 6—10, linear hairy, somewhat persistent, capsule oblong, acuminated, hairy.

The seeds are found in all the bazars, and are much esteemed for their cordial, stomachic, and antispasmodic virtues. Reduced to powder the Arabs use them as an adjunct to coffee.

The seeds are brown, kidney-shaped, the size of hemp seed, slightly compressed, striated, with parallel streaks, and covered with points slightly hollowed. In smell and taste these seeds resemble a mixture of musk and amber, and on burning a similar odour is evolved.

In the *Journal de Pharmacie*, vol. xx. p. 381, M. Bonastre has given an account of the chemical composition of these celebrated seeds. M. Bonastre obtained the following substances:—

Parenchyme and moisture, ...	52
Gum, ...	36
Albumen, ...	5·6
Fixed oil, solid crystalline matter, odorous principle and resin, ...	6·4

The fixed oil is greenish yellow, fluid at 32, solidifies gradually by exposure to the air. The solid crystalline matter is deposited from the hot alcoholic solution of the seeds. It is white, pearly, of pleasant taste, soluble in ether, from which it crystallizes in rays, fusible at 95° Fahr.

The odorous matter is a light green fluid, which has a strong smell of musk. It is not volatile, and indeed it is remarkable that these seeds did not yield an essential oil, at least in M. Bonastre's experiments.

Dancer states the seeds to be emetic. We have not found this to be the case in our experiments.

Gen. 5.—Hibiscus.

Sp. 1. ***Hibiscus Sabdariffa***, Rozelle. West India Sorrel. The fleshy acid calyx of this plant is well known to yield excellent jelly, and very palatable tarts.

Sp. 2. ***Hibiscus Rosa sinensis***, Shoe-flower plant.
Vern. Jasoon, ***Duk.*** Jaba, ***Sans.***

This plant is common in India; the leaves are used as emollients, anodyne and gentle aperients; the flowers, for giving a red tinge to spirituous liquors. The flowers are deep scarlet, and yield a juice which turns rapidly to a dark purple, and is very mucilaginous. Applied to soft, unsized white paper, this colour is nearly as sensitive a test for acid as the celebrated litmus.

Gen. 6.—Thespesia.

Sp. — ***Thespesia populnea***, *(Soland).* Portia tree.
Syn. Hibiscus populneus, L.
Vern. Paris-ka-pul.
Sooparshavaka, Sans. ***Poursunghai***, Tamul.

Arboreous leaves broad—cordate entire, smooth; exterior calyx scarcely any, interior one almost entire, capsules ovate, spheroidal, and bristly, seeds downy. *Roxb.* The same writer describes at greater length an H. populneoides, which Wight and Arnott deem identical with the *populnea.* The trunk is straight, from 15 to 25 feet to the branches, thicker than a man's body, branches numerous, young shoots covered with bronze-coloured scales, *leaves* about the extremities of the branches alternate, petioled, cordate, waved, leathery, entire, from 5 to 7 nerved, long pointed as in Ficus religiosa; the corolla large, yellowish-white; fruit yellow and shrivelled, 5 celled, many seeded, with much yellow juice.

Ainslie informs us that the bright yellow juice is employed as an external application in various cutaneous diseases, especially the Malabar itch, and that a decoction of the bark is given internally.

Besides the preceding species, several others are common over India, which may be used as effectual substitutes for any of the preceding articles. We may mention the Abutilon asiaticum, G. Don. *Noogoo banda*, (Tamul), (Sida asiatica, L.) &c. well known in gardens in Bengal, Sida rhomboidea, R. (Lal Barela of Hindostan,) and also Pavonia zeylanica, the flowers of which are of a pale rose tint in the morning and deepen to a red colour in the evening, and the Pavonia odorata, (Bala बला Sans.) of which the sweet smelling roots are given in infusion; the root of this species is light coloured, about the thickness of a quill.

NAT. ORDER XXII.—DIPTEROCARPEÆ.

This highly important order requires to be noticed with more than ordinary minuteness, from the great value of the products it affords, and the abundance of its species throughout India.

From the writings of Roxburgh, Wight, and Royle, we observe that the distribution of this order is almost exclusively Indian, species being found only as far as 31° N. L. Two species only are of foreign origin, (Wight.)

It is principally composed of large, handsome, fine flowering trees, abounding in resinous juice; the leaves are alternate, marked with strong parallel veins, occurring from the midrib to the margin, furnished with deciduous convolute stipules, terminating the branches in a point; the racemes of flowers are either terminal and panicled, or axillary, solitary, or several from the same leaves, and from the axils the flowers often secund. Calyx persistent, somewhat tubular at the base, five lobed, lobes at first slightly unequal, afterwards enlarged, usually two of them much more so than the rest, becoming wing-like; æstivation imbricated, petals hypogynous, free, or slightly combined at the base; æstivation twisted; stamens indefinite, distinct, when numerous attached to a broad somewhat elevated torus, occasionally irregularly polyadelphous; when few, adherent to the base of the petals; filaments dilated at the base; anthers frequently terminating in a bristle, or tipped with a gland-like point, two celled, opening by terminal fissures; ovary three-celled, with two pendulous ovules in each, style and stigma simple. Fruit coriaceous, one-celled by abortion, three-valved or indehiscent, surrounded by the calyx. Seed solitary without albumen, cotyledons twisted, or crumpled, or unequal, and obliquely incumbent, radicle superior. (*Wight's Illustrations*, p. 86.)

Gen. 1.—Dryabalanops, Gaertn.

Sp. 1. *Dryabalanops Camphora*, Colebr.

Syn. Shorea camphorifera, *Roxb.* (see Colebrooke, As. Researches, vol. xii. p. 535.)

A very large tree, a native of Borneo and Sumatra, where it is sometimes found six to seven feet in diameter.

In the cavities of the trunk there occur collections of solid camphor, and of a light fluid called camphor oil. The solid camphor is often deposited in long pieces, weighing over ten pounds. This camphor is highly prized by the Chinese and Japanese, and so rarely finds its way to Europe that it is seldom found even in the richest collections of Materia Medica. Mr. Pereira informs us that he has only met with it twice. Dr. Duncan had specimens, of which he published a detailed and interesting account. It occurred in tabular plates, readily reduced to powder, compact, ringing when shaken in a bottle; it sinks in water, and does not sublime spontaneously. In these characters it differs from common camphor, (See Laurus Camphora). The fluid camphor is transparent, pale yellow, bitter, slightly viscid, Sp. Gr. 887. On distillation, it yields a volatile oil, and a camphor-like white substance remains in the retort.

For specimens of camphor oil we are indebted to Mr. Evans, late of Calcutta. The characters correspond well with those Dr. Duncan describes, and which we recollect from having assisted at his experiments. The oil we may add is a good solvent of caoutchouc, copal, and resins in general.

For additional details relative to the properties of camphor and camphor oil, see the article Camphora Officinarum, in the sequel of this work.

GEN. 2.—SHOREA, Roxb.

Sp. — *Shorea robusta*, Roxb. Saul.
Vern. Uswukunida, *Sans.*
Sal of the bazars.
Off. The resin, *dammar.*

This is a tree of great size, a native of Morung, the Paulghat mountains, &c. Sepals 5, afterwards changing into 5 long wings, petals 5, stamens 15, filaments capillary below the anthers, anther cells short, obtuse, connectivum filiform, produced beyond the cells into a more or less elongated, coloured, deciduous bristle, ovarium 3 celled, with two pendulous ovules in each cell. Seed solitary, cotyledons stalked, not crumpled, radicle superior, leaves coriaceous, oblong, obtuse, often emarginate at the base, panicles numerous from the axils of the fallen leaves, branches and pedicels glabrous.

The Shorea robusta, and indeed some other species, yield abundance of the resin called dammar, (also *dhoona* and *ral*,) the superior kinds of which are efficient substitutes for the pine resin of the European Pharmacopœiæ.

From Captain Jenkins of Assam, we have received specimens of this resin, perfectly transparent and colourless; in the bazars the colour ranges from pale amber to dark brown. It is devoid of taste or smell. Spec. gravity 1·097 to 1,123, easily fusible, partially soluble in alcohol, (83·1 per 1000) almost entirely in ether, perfectly in oil of turpentine and the fixed oils; sulphuric acid dissolves, and gives it a red colour. By dissolving this resin in oil of turpentine and boiling it with a solution of potash till all the turpentine is expelled, we obtained a compound of resin and potash entirely soluble in water.

Dammar unites with the oxide of lead and forms plasters. For its numerous applications in Pharmacy, see 3d part, article *Plasters*.

Two parts of colourless dammar and 2½ of oil of turpentine make the best varnish for lithographic drawings.

GEN. 3.—VATERIA.

Sp. — *Vateria indica.*
Vern. *Piney marum*, Pandum.
Product. East Ind. Copal.

This is a very large and stately tree, a native of Malabar, and lately found also in Mysore.

The young shoots, and all tender parts except the leaves are covered with fine stellate pubescence, leaves alternate, petioled, oblong, entire, from emarginate to obtuse, pointed, smooth, coriaceous, from four to eight inches long and two to four broad, petioles round, about an inch long; stipules oblong, panicles terminal, ramifications rather remote; flowers rather remote, pedicelled, pretty large; bractes oblong, one-flowered; calyx 5, cleft to the base, divisions oblong, obtuse, villous on the outside, corolla five-petalled, petals oval, emarginate, broader but very little longer than divisions of the calyx, filaments from 40 to 50, short, broad, inserted between the petals and the base of the germ, anthers linear, with a single filiform beak; germ superior, conic, downy, three celled, cells containing three ovules each, attached to the top of the axis, style longer than the stamens, stigma acute, pericarpium a coriaceous, fleshy, oblong, obtuse, one-celled, three-valved capsule, general size about $2\frac{1}{2}$ inches long and $1\frac{1}{2}$ in diameter, seed solitary, of same shape as the capsule. *Roxb. Fl. Ind.* p. 601.

The substance called East Indian Copal, and sold in England as gum anime, exudes abundantly from this tree.

It occurs of all shades of colour between pale green and deep yellow. The finest pieces are called *kahroba,* and sold as *amber* in the bazars of Bengal.

The resin before it hardens is the "piney" varnish of Malabar. This soon hardens by exposure to the air. We are indebted to Dr. Wight for the publication of a formula by which the hard resin can be dissolved in drying oil, and thus used as an excellent varnish. *(See appendix.)*

Besides the uses already alluded to, candles are made of this resin in Malabar, which Dr. Wight informs us diffuse in burning an agreeable fragrance, give a fine clear light, with little smoke, and consume the wick without snuffing.

Gen. 4.—Dipterocarpus.

Calyx of one piece, five cleft, two of the segments when in fruit expanded into long ligulate, scarious wings; petals five; stamens numerous; anthers long, linear, tapering; ovarium three-celled; with two pendulous ovules in each cell; seed solitary; cotyledons crumpled; radicle superior. Flowers in racemes white tinged with red.

Sp. 1. *Dipterocarpus laevis, Hamilt.*

Syn. D. turbinatus, Roxb.

Vern. Tilea gurjun, Bengalee.

A native of Chittagong, Pegu, Assam, Tippera, &c. The trunk grows to an immense size, bark deeply cracked, young branches compressed, 2 edged, leaves ovate-oblong, or ovate, retuse at the base, acute, shining on both sides, with numerous prominent veins, petioles glabrous, tube of the enlarged calyx slightly ventricose, but scarcely contracted below the limb, even; capsule ovate, even *(Hamilt.* in Werner. Soc. Trans. vol. vi. p. 299.)

This tree yields in abundance the thin balsam well known in all the Indian bazars, and called the gurjun or wood oil. To procure the balsam, Dr. Roxburgh informs us a large notch is cut in the trunk of the tree near the earth, where a fire is kept up till the wound is charred, soon after which the liquid begins to ooze out; a small gutter is cut in the wood to conduct the liquid to a receiver. The average produce is said to be 40 gallons in each season, during which it is necessary to cut off the charred surface from time to time, and burn it afresh. The process is performed during the cold season.

The gurjun balsam varies in consistence from that of thick honey to a light oily liquid. The colour of a fine specimen of thick gurjun obtained from Captain Jenkins of Assam, was a pale grey; specimens sent from Rangoon by Mr. Speir were a light brown. As found in the bazar this substance generally occurs as a brown, oily looking, semi-transparent liquid, in odour strongly resembling a mixture of balsam of copaiba with a small portion of naptha. The Sp. Gr. is 0.962. It is totally insoluble in water, freely in warm alcohol at 835°, and difficultly in ether. Submitted to heat about 5 per 100 of water first passes over; a yellowish white matter then sublimes and covers the upper part of the retort; this substance is solid, crystallizable, soluble in essential oils, and possesses many of the properties of benzoic acid. Its proportion is not more than 1 per 100. Continuing the distillation, from 35 to 40 parts per 100 of essential oil are obtained, and a thick resin remains in the retort.

The essential oil when freed from water by prolonged contact with dry chloride of calcium, and distilled a second time, is transparent and nearly colourless, of specific gravity 934, boils at 240°; it is soluble in alcohol, ether, naptha, and the essential and fixed oils. It dissolves caoutchouc, copal, vateria resin, and solid gluten. Potassium and sodium retain their lustre in it, and undergo no change; the taste is acrid, sweetish, and heavy, its odour closely resembles that of the essential oil of copaiba.

The residual resin is light brown, easily fusible, of copaibic smell, and faintly acrid taste; absolute alcohol divides it into two parts, *a* and *b*, of which the insoluble part *b* dissolves in spirit at ·835. Both possess acid properties, and are closely analogous to the copaiba acid resins. Like one of these the gurgun resin *a* forms a saline compound with magnesia, which dissolves in a mixture of the resin *b* and essential oil.

The close resemblance in the physical and chemical properties of this gurgun and copaiba balsam led to the institution of an extensive set of experiments by the Editor on the medicinal effects of the former in the treatment of gonorrhœa. The results, which have been laid before the profession, and which have been confirmed by trials made by other practitioners, seem perfectly conclusive that in the treatment of gonorrhœa, gleet, and similar affections of the urinary organs the essential oil of gurgun is nearly equal in efficacy to the South American drug.

The essential oil may be given in 10 to 30 drop doses in mucilage, milk, rice water, or thin gruel, and repeated thrice, or still more frequently daily. It generally causes a sensation of warmth at the epigastrium, eructations, and sometimes slight purging. It communicates a strong smell of turpentine to the urine, which it increases remarkably in quantity. Some obstinate cases of chronic gonorrhœa and gleet, which had long resisted copaiba and cubebs, have been cured by this remedy in the course of the experiments alluded to.

For additional suggestions relative to the mode of administering this remedy, see Copaiba. In the Pharmacopœia we have given a formula for a solution of the essential oils of gurgun and cubebs in sulphuric ether, which affords a cheap, but perfectly efficacious substitute for the celebrated "Frank's Specific."

Besides the above species, the D. angusifolius of Wight and Arn. (D. costatus of Roxb. but not of Gaertn.), D. costatus, Gaertn. (D. incanus, Roxb.) and D. alatus, Roxb. of Pegu, afford this fluid in great abundance. Its price in the bazar ranges from 3 to 5 rupees the maund. Besides its uses in medicine, it is likely to be found a perfect substitute in the arts for the expensive balsam of copaiba, now much used in the preparation of colourless varnishes and drying paints. In the coarser kinds of house and ship painting, gurjun balsam is used as an excellent substitute for linseed oil.

Dr. Wight and other writers speak confidently of the good effect of the gurjun oil mixed with dammar in preserving wood from the ravages of the white ant.

NAT. ORDER XXIII.—TERNSTRÖMIACEÆ.

This order, so important in a commercial and social light, as yielding the varieties of tea, affords but one plant, the *Cochlospermum gossypium*, which claims a place in this work.

Gen.—Cochlospermum, (Kunth.)

Sp. 1. *Cochlospermum Gossypium.* Yellow-flowered cotton tree.

Syn. Bombax Gossypium, L.

Off. product. Kutira gum of the bazars.

Dr. Roxburgh describes this tree as common on the Arracan mountains.

It occurs also in Bundlecund, on the hills round and near Adjigurh and Kalingur, as well as on those near Hurdwar, and the Kheree pass.

The calyx is of five, oblong, oval, unequal sepals, at length reflexed, the two exterior smaller; bracteoles none, petals five, emarginate, unequal sided; æstivation twisted, stamens numerous. Anthers linear, acuminate, attached by the base, opening by a pore at the apex. Ovary seated on an elevated disk, styles united up to the apex into one, long, and filiform; capsules shortly obovate, 3-5 celled, 3-5 valved, valves bearing incomplete dissepiments in the middle; seeds numerous, somewhat kidney-shaped, covered with cotton; albumen fleshy, embryo slender; leaves five to six inches long, five-lobed, hoary beneath, on cylindrical downy stalks; panicles terminal; flowers large, bright yellow.

The trunk of this tree yields the gum called *Kutira* in the Upper Provinces. This gum is useless in the arts; in medicine it is simply a demulcent and emollient, and may be used for making lozenges.

NAT. ORDER XXIV.—STERCULIACEÆ, OR BYTTNERIACEÆ.

Gen. 1.—Sterculia.

Sp. 1. *Sterculia urens,* Roxb.

Vern. Bulee.

Off. The *gum.*

A native of the mountainous parts of Coromandel and Hindostan.

The trunk is erect, very straight, top large and shady, bark light ash-coloured, very smooth, outer coat thin, transparent, covered with a farinaceous substance, inwardly fibrous and netted; leaves about the extremities of the branches, alternate, petioled, 5-lobed, 5-nerved, lobes acute, very downy, from 9 to 12 inches each way. Petioles nearly as long as the leaves, round, downy. Panicles terminal, pretty large, covered with a glutinous farinaceous yellow down; bractes lanceolate; flowers small, numerous, yellow; male and hermaphrodite mixed; calyx campanulate, 5-toothed, leathery, divisions acute, with an obcordate hairy gland on the inside of each division next the base; corolla none; filaments ten, alternately longer, united below into a thin sheath; anthers 2-lobed, alternately larger; ovary 5-lobed; style single, short, thick; stigma 5-lobed; follicles covered with yellow down, and many stiff stinging hairs; seeds 36.

The gum, which exudes spontaneously during the hot season, occurs in large light brown transparent tough masses. Immersed in water they swell like a jelly, but do not dissolve but by protracted boiling. The solution is not adhesive, and is destitute of the thickness of solutions of ordinary gum.

The uses of this gum are very limited; the want of adhesiveness renders it unsuitable for the arts, while its difficult solubility renders it inferior to most other gums for medicinal purposes.

A similar gum called Kutira is afforded by the Cochlospermum gossypium of Coromandel, Travancore, and Ceylon, a large tree, with bright yellow flowers. See p. 225.

For an account of the properties and uses of the true tragacanth gum, which the Kutira much resembles, see *Astragalus*, natural order "Leguminosæ."

The roasted seeds, which contain starch and fixed oil, have much the flavour of chesnuts, and are eaten by the natives of this country.

The *Sterculia fœtida*, distinguished by the abominable fæculent smell of its flowers, is common on the continent of India and Java, where the fruit is used in the treatment of gonorrhœa. The leaves are deemed aperient, and a decoction of the fruit mucilaginous and astringent. The seeds are oleaginous, but are deemed unwholesome.

The *Sterculia Tragacantha*, now called *Southwellia Trag.* is a native of Sierra Leone, and on being wounded yields a gum resembling Tragacanth.

Gen. 2.—Guazuma.

Sp. 1. *Guazuma tomentosa*, K. (Bubroma Guazuma, Willd). A native of South America and of the West Indies, and now common in gardens in India, where the wood is called the bastard cedar; the old bark is used in the West Indies as a sudorific; the young bark is very mucilaginous, and employed for clearing sugar.

The bark of the *Kydia calycina* (*Choupultea*, Hind.) a native of Coromandel, Nepal, and the Nilgherries, is used for the same purpose in this country.

GEN. 3.—THEOBROMA.

Sp. Theobroma Cacao, Chocolate tree.

This remarkable tree is a native of the West Indies, but thrives well in the Calcutta Garden. The fruit is yellow or red, oval, about three inches long, with a fleshy rind nearly half an inch thick. The seeds are about twenty-five in each fruit, and when toasted, and beaten into a paste with annotto, vanilla, &c. constitute the chocolate of commerce. The nutritive properties of chocolate depend on a concrete oil or butter, of most agreeable flavour, of which 1000 parts of the seed yield 386.

GEN. 4.—ERIODENDRON.

Sp. Eriodendron anfractuosum, (DeCand.), Cotton tree.
Syn. Bombax pentandrum, L.
Vern. Suffed simul.

An elegant tree, common on the Coromandel coast; the leaves fall during the cold season, and the blossoms appear in February before the leaves. The trunk is perfectly straight, the seeds numerous, smooth, black, and enveloped in very fine soft silky wool.

The gum is termed *Huttian ke goond*, and is given in solution with spices in bowel complaints.

GEN. 5.—BOMBAX, L.

Another tree, the *B. malabaricum*, D.C. (*Bombax heptapyllum*, L.) is the *Ruckta-simul* of Bengal; it yields a gum resin called *Moocherus*, and its roots constitute the *sufed mooslie* of the bazars.

The Moocherus occurs in knotty, opaque, dark brown pieces, often with internal cavities; 100 parts yield 56 to water, consisting of gum, tannic and gallic acids. The remainder is a mixture of a tasteless resinous substance and caoutchouc.

Few remedies are more extensively employed by the natives than their white and black *mooslie*. Blume says that the bark of the root is emetic, and the statement is confirmed by Rumphius, but is contrary to our own repeated trials.

The white *mooslie* is a small brittle root, which in the dry state contains sixty per hundred of gum, fifteen of starch, with traces of resin, the remainder being woody fibre. The powdered root forms a thick mucilage with cold water, and answers admirably as a nutritious demulcent for convalescent persons.

Gen. 6.—Helicteres.

Sp. Helicteres Isora.
Vern. Merowrie, *Hind.* Avurtunnie, *Sans.*
The capsule consists of five fibres twisted together like a screw, and varies in length from 1 to 2¼ inches; reduced to powder and mixed with castor oil it is employed as an application to sores behind the ears.
The powder of the fruit has also been used in griping pains of the bowels, but solely because the twisted fibres of the capsule were considered to stamp it as a remedy, according to the ancient doctrine of signatures.

Gen. 7.—Adansonia.

Sp. 1. *Adansonia digitata.*
Syn. Baobab.
Now cultivated in India, and remarkable for being the largest of most trees with single trunks. The trunk is sometimes thirty feet in diameter. It is throughout emollient and mucilaginous. The leaves dried and reduced to powder are called *lalo* by the Africans, and are used to diminish excessive perspiration, (Royle); the fruit is slightly acid, and the expressed juice mixed with sugar is used as a cooling drink in fevers; a thick mucilaginous juice is obtained by tapping from all parts of the tree.
The reddish spongy pulp of the fruit mixed with tamarinds is much used by the natives of Senegal in the treatment of dysentery. In Merat and de Lens Dictionaire de Matiere Medicale, Dr. Louis Frank gives an account of the mode of using this remedy. The patient at first is confined to a very spare diet, and drinks only a weak decoction of tamarinds. If this does not succeed he takes the Baobab pulp with small doses of rhubarb; should this also fail the powdered bark of the fruit is employed, made into a paste with water, and the size of a chesnut being given repeatedly daily. Dr. Frank speaks highly of the success of this practice, which however we deem applicable to none but the very mildest cases of this disease.

NAT. ORDER XXV.—TILIACEÆ.

This order agrees in many respects with the last, especially in the mucilaginous and demulcent properties of some of its constituents. Only one species demands our notice.

GEN.—CORCHORUS.

Sp. Corchorus olitorius.
Vern. Bhunghee, *Bengalee.*

An annual plant common in Bengal. There are two varieties, the green (Pat, *Beng.*), the reddish, (Bun-pat, *Beng.*) both are used for their fibres, which are called *jute* and *pat*. A coarse kind of cloth (*tat*) is woven from the jute, and affords the materials of the well known gunny bags. The leaves are ovate, acuminated; peduncles 1—2 flowered, capsules nearly cylindrical, 10 ribbed, 6—8 times longer than broad, glabrous, rostrate, with sometimes 5 terminal points, 5-celled, 5-valved; seeds numerous, with nearly perfect transverse septa.

An infusion of the leaf is much employed as a fever drink among the natives of the Lower Provinces, and Mr. Twining mentions the practice with approbation in the 2d. vol. of his admirable work on the diseases of Bengal.

NAT. ORDER XXVI.—AURANTIACEÆ.

A numerous order, which derives its characters from the lime and orange tribe, and which seems almost exclusively peculiar to tropical or juxta-tropical regions; all are characterized by pellucid dots on the leaves and bark, denoting the presence of glands which contain much volatile oil; several exude gum, and some afford a bitter tonic principle. The fruit of one variety moreover abounds in a valuable acid to which it gives its name—the citric acid.

Gen. characters. Trees or shrubs, with simple, alternate, petiolate leaves; calyx pitcher-shaped, three to five cleft; corolla five to eight petals, stamina numerous, 20—60; filaments combined into several bundles; anthers oblong; style round, stigma hemispherical; fruit baccate with 7—12 many seeded pulpy cells, filled with little vesicles containing an acid or sweet juice, and readily separable from each other.

Gen. 1.—Citrus.

Sp. 1. *Citrus medica*, Citron.

(Μηλεα μεδικη of Dioscorides.)

Petioles naked, leaves oblong, acute, finely-toothed, stamina 40; fruit oblong, wrinkled, with thick rind, and juice slightly acid.

Sp. 2. *Citrus Limonum*, Lemon tree.

Vern. Jambira, *Sans.* Nimbooka, Neboo, Lemboo, *Beng. Hind.*

Petioles somewhat winged, leaves oblong, acute, dentated, stamina 35, often without a pistil; Flowers purple externally; rind thin; juice very acid.

The fruits are ovoid oblong, nippled at top, external skin thin, smooth, highly odoriferous, pale yellow, marked all over by small cells filled with essential oil; beneath this epidermis occurs an inner white spongy skin of variable thickness in different varieties, covering an acid sarcocarp of from 7 to 11 compartments, separated by prolongations of the endocarp; each compartment has two seeds containing a very white and bitter kernel.

Essential Oil of lemons.

This oil is yellow, light, very volatile. It is prepared by rasping the lemons until the oil-vescicles are removed. These are then pressed between glass plates, and the expressed juice allowed to stand till the impurities subside. This oil is composed of 10 atoms carbon, 8 atoms hydrogen, (citrene). If a current of muriatic acid gas be passed through it at a low temperature, it concretes into a solid mass of neutral crystals, containing 1 atom of muriatic acid, and forming a salt called muriate of citrene.

This oil is used chiefly to give flavour to various medicinal mixtures, and is seldom or never employed by itself.

Lemon peel.

This is of pale yellow colour, rough, dotted, odorous, and bitter; it is used principally, like the oil, for imparting its aromatic taste to medicines, and as a gentle stomachic stimulant.

Lemon juice.

Lemon juice contains nearly 2 per 100 of citric acid, water 97½, the remainder being gum, malic acid, and extractive matter.

It is a most grateful and useful material for the preparation of cooling drinks. Mr. Pereira gives a good formula for these beverages, which are particularly useful in fever cases; —two lemons sliced, two ounces of sugar, two pints of boiling water, mixed and allowed to settle and cool.

In scurvy, lemon juice has long been esteemed as a certain specific. As it is difficult to preserve the juice on long voyages, citric acid and the essential oil have been in most cases substituted for the juice itself.

For the preparation and properties of citric acid, see section *Acids*, Pharmacopœia.

Sp. 3. *Citrus Limetta*, Bergamot lime, or Sweet lime.

This species is chiefly remarkable for the abundance of essential oil afforded by the rind, and which constitutes an important article in commerce, under the name of oil of Bergamot—much used by perfumers.

Sp. 4. *Citrus Aurantium*, Sweet orange.

Vern. Narungee, *Sans.* Kumla, *Beng.*

Petioles nearly naked, leaves ovato-oblong and acute, stamina 20, fruit globose, cortex thin, pulp sweet.

The leaves are rather bitter, and contain essential oil. A still more fragrant oil, called oil of *neroli* by the perfumers, is afforded by the flowers. The berries while unripe are gathered, dried, and turned in the lathe to the size of peas, and are used in issues on account of their fragrant odour.

The bitter matter of the unripe orange is a substance named *Hesperidin*, discovered by Lebreton in 1838. The white part is freed from the green part and also from the inside of the fruit; it is then steeped in water from 75 to 86, the liquid filtered and evaporated to one-fourth. Some albumen separates, and is to be removed. The entire must now be saturated with lime and evaporated to the consistence of syrup; this being heated with alcohol at 817, leaves gum, albumen, malate of lime, &c. and the hesperidin is dissolved; filter again, and evaporate. A granular extract is obtained, which is to be mixed with distilled vinegar; the clear liquor being allowed to evaporate spontaneously deposits the hesperidin in soft silky crystals, which are tasteless at first, but subsequently leave a bitter flavour.

The properties of hesperidin deserve investigation; its bitterness leads us to suppose that it may possess considerable febrifuge powers. It does not however seem to possess a decided alkaline or acid reaction.

The rind or peel of the orange is bitter and aromatic, and affords a very useful stomachic tincture and syrup. The juice of the ripe fruit contains sugar, malic and citric acids, citrate of lime, mucilage, albumen, and gum. Like the lemon juice it makes an excellent cooling drink, and is an invaluable specific in the treatment of scorbutic diseases. The seeds of the orange yield oil by expression.

Sp. 5. *Citrus vulgaris*, Bitter Seville orange.

Syn. C. Bigarradia, (Duhamel.)

The leaves differ from those of the sweet orange by the petiole only. The flowers are alike in both species.

The rind of the fruit is bitter, acrid, and hot to the taste, the pulp acid and bitter, the seeds excessively bitter. The bark of the tree participates in these qualities. The rind of the fruit is used in making the celebrated liqueur *curacoa.*

The bitter orange deserves attentive examination, and is likely to yield on due analysis a bitter principle of considerable value in medicine as a tonic and febrifuge remedy.

Sp. 6. *Citrus Decumana*, Pumplenose, Shaddock.

Vern. Batavi neemboo.

The fruits are as large as a child's head. They are of no importance in medicine.

It would be inconsistent with the object of this work to enter into details regarding the numerous varieties of the species above noticed, which can merely interest the horticulturist, and are unimportant to the medical student.

Gen. 2.—Bergera.

Sp. Bergera Königii.

Vern. Bursunga, *Beng.* Karivepa, *Tel.* Karivepilli, *Tam.* Kristna neemboo, *Sans.*

A small tree, a native of the mountainous parts of the coast, cultivated also generally in gardens for its leaves, which are used in curries. It flowers in the hot season; the leaves retain their flavour when dry.

Leaves stalked unequally, pennate, leaflets alternate, short stalked, ovato-lanceolate, rhomboidal, oblique, smooth or downy, somewhat serrated; corymbs terminal, compound, shorter than the leaves; spreading bractes pressed close to pedicels, small, solitary, lanceolate, deciduous.

The bark and root are used as stimulants, and are applied externally to parts bitten by venomous animals. The green leaves are given raw in dysentery, and also applied externally to cure eruptions. *Roxb.* An infusion of the toasted leaves Ainslie states to be used by the Hindoos to stop vomiting.

GEN. 3.—FERONIA.

Sp. 1. *Feronia Elephantum.* Wood-apple.
Capitha, As. Res. vol. iv. p. 230.
Vern. Kathbel, *Beng.* Yelanga, *Tel.* Vellanga, *Tam.*

A large tree found in most parts of India. Flowers often polygamous, calyx flat, 5 toothed, petals, 4, 5 or 6, spreading, stamens 10, filaments dilated and united at the base, anthers linear, oblong, tetragonal, ovary seated on the elevated disk, 5-6 celled. Ovules numerous, style scarcely any, stigma oblong, fruit baccate with a hard rind, 5 celled, many seeded, seeds immersed in a fleshy pulp, leaves pinnate, leaflets 5-7, nearly or quite sessile, obovate, very slightly crenulated, pellucid, dotted along margin, common petiole slightly winged, racemes lax, few flowered, terminal and axillary.

Branches armed with simple spines, leaflets small, obovate, smooth, teeth of calyx pink, petals paler, anthers crimson.

Fruit fleshy, extremely acid before maturity, when ripe filled with a brown sub-acid agreeable pulp, containing 5 parcels of roundish oblong flat woolly seeds, adhering to placentæ by long stalks. Both leaves and flowers have a strong odour of anise. The young leaves are used by native practitioners as a gentle stomachic stimulant in the bowel complaints of children.

A large quantity of gum (*kavit ka goond*) is procured from this tree. It very much resembles gum Arabic in its chemical and sensible properties. The babul tree also furnishes much of the gum found in the Bazars. The nim, mango, cassia auriculata, cotton tree, and several others, yield this principle, and the products of all are mixed for sale by the native druggists.

For the properties and uses of the best gum, see *Leguminosæ*, art. *Acacia*.

GEN. 4.—ÆGLE.

Sp. 1., *Ægle Marmelos.* Cratæva Marmelos, L.

Vern. Covalum, *Hortus mal.* Tanghula, *Malay.* Maredoo, *Tel.* Bilanus, *Rumph.* Bivalva, *Sans.* Bilva and Mahura, *As. Researches.* A large tree, a native of all parts of the East Indies.

Trunk pretty erect, bark ash-coloured, branches few and irregular, thorns axillary, single, or none, very sharp and strong, leaves ternate, leaflets oblong, or oblong-lanceolate, thinning away to a bent point, crenulate, of various sizes, the exterior being always the largest; panicles small, terminal, and axillary, flowers large and white, hermaphrodite, calyx 4-5 toothed; petals 4-5, filaments about forty, short, anthers linear, erect; ovules numerous in each cell, style very short, and thick, stigma capitate; berry large, spheroidal, smooth, with a hard shell, and 10-15 cells, which contain besides the seeds a large quantity of a tenacious, transparent juice, which can be drawn into very long threads. These on drying become very hard, but continue transparent. Seeds from six to ten in each cell, oblong, a little compressed, woolly, attached to the inner angles of their cells.

This tree flowers during the hot season, and the fruit ripens after the rains.

The statements we find in works on oriental Materia Medica are very various as to the qualities of this tree and its products. Rheede says a decoction of the bark of the root is considered in Malabar to be very useful in hypochondriasis, melancholy, and palpitation of the heart; and that the leaves are used in decoction in asthmatic complaints. The same author adds that the unripe fruit is of use in diarrhœa. Among the Javanese the fruit is deemed very astringent. Roxburgh correctly states the fruit to be delicious to the taste, and very fragrant. (*Ainslie, vol.* ii. *p.* 189.)

In the Asiatic Researches, vol. ii. p. 349, we find it stated that the fruit is nutritious, warm, cathartic, its taste delicious, its fragrance exquisite; its aperient and detersive qualities, and its efficacy in removing habitual costiveness, have been proved by constant experience. The mucus of the seeds is for some purposes a very good cement.

NAT. ORDER XXVII.—HYPERICINEÆ.

This order in most of its botanical properties resembles the Guttiferæ, and like these, some of its species yield a yellow very cathartic juice. That of the Vismia guianensis is called *American Gamboge*, and resembles this drug in all its qualities.

NAT. ORDER XXVIII.—GUTTIFERÆ.

A tropical order of very great interest, in consequence of several of its members yielding the gamboge of the druggists. The Guttiferæ chiefly occur in Siam, Ceylon, and Malabar, and some species extend all over the Peninsula.

We shall first notice the leading species supposed to yield gamboge, and then describe the properties of this valuable remedy.

Gen. 1.—Hebradendron.

Sp. 1. *Hebradendron gambogioides.* (Graham.)
Syn. Cambogia Gutta, L. Mangostana Morella, (Desroup.)
Vern. Gokatu, or Kana goraka, *Cing.*
Off. The concrete juice, gamboge.

A moderately large tree, indigenous or cultivated in Ceylon; from the tender twigs, and from fissures in the bark there exudes a bright yellow juice, which concretes into a hard resinous substance, identical with the best gamboge of commerce, which however is brought from Siam.

Sp. 2. *Hebradendron pictorium,* (Graham).
Syn. Garcinia pictoria, Roxb. Fl. Ind. ii. p. 27.

A tall very branchy tree, a native of Wynaad. Bark thick, of deep rust colour, with yellow specks, and containing in its substance masses of gamboge; leaves opposite, short, petioled, oblong, bellied, rather acute, entire, smooth on both sides, 3 to 4 inches long, 1½-2 broad. Hermaphrodite flowers axillary, solitary, sessile, of middling size, and yellow colour, calyx of two integral pairs of concave obtuse leaflets, permanent. Petals four, oval, longer than the calyx, filaments united into four bodies, again joined at the base into a narrow ring round the bottom of the young ovary, divided above into 2 to 6 single, unequal, short filaments; anthers 10—15, oblong, two lobed, ovary superior, round, four celled, one ovule in each, attached to the axis. No style; stigma four lobed, permanent. Berry size of a large cherry, oval smooth, slightly four lobed, crowned with the sessile, four lobed, warty, permanent stigma; rind leathery, pretty thick, rather spongy, one-celled; seeds four, oblong, kidney-shaped. Male flowers, calyx, and corolla, as in the female; filaments numerous, inserted on the crown of a square fleshy receptacle in the centre of the flower, obovate, angular; anthers peltate. *(Roxb.)*

This tree flowers in February, and the fruit ripens in May and June.

The gamboge exuded by this tree was pronounced by Dr. Roxburgh superior in colour, while recent, to the Siam article; no trials have been made of its medicinal qualities.

Closely allied to these species are *Garcinia pedunculata* (Tikul, or Tikoor of Rungpore) a tree 60 feet high; trees when 7 years old are 20 feet high, 25 inches in circumference. Flowers from January to March. Fruit ripens in hot season. Fleshy part of fruit and arillus large, firm, very sharp, and acid, used in curries and for acidulating water; cut and sliced it retains its qualities, and is recommended as a succedaneum for limes and lemons during long voyages.

Garcinia mangostana. The celebrated mangosteen of the Eastern Islands; from the rind of the fruit we have obtained small quantities of fine gamboge.

Garcinia cornea. Of this species there were two trees in Col. Kyd's garden, said to have come from Malacca, and to exude yellow juice.

Gen. 2.—Stalagmites.

Sp. 1. *Stalagmites ovalifolia*, Brown and Graham.

Syn. Xanthochymus ovalifolius. (Roxb. ii. p. 632.)

A native of the Southern provinces of India and of Ceylon. The seeds were sent from Ceylon by General Hay MacDowal, to the Calcutta Garden, under the Cingalese name *Ambul Ghorka;* in 7 to 10 years the trees began to blossom during the whole of the hot season, and in July 1812, when ten years old, they produced perfectly ripe fruit. Dr. Wight is of opinion that this tree yields one kind of gamboge in Ceylon. It is desirable to ascertain what may be the produce of the trees in the Calcutta Garden.

Sp. 2. *Stalagmites pictoria.*

Syn. Xanthochymus pictorius. (Roxb. ii. p. 633).

Vern. Dampel, *Beng.* and *Hind.* Kata Ghorka, *Cing.*

A native of the mountainous districts of India; leaves opposite, linear, lanceolate; flowers in lateral fascicles, berry ovate, pointed. Fruit ripens in November and December, and the tree yields a large quantity of inferior gamboge.

Gamboge.

Vern. Mukki, *Tamul*, and Ossara rewund, *Arab.*

Besides the trees above described, there are supposed to exist others from which the bulk of the gamboge of commerce is obtained. The article is prepared almost exclusively in Siam, none being obtained from India or Ceylon.

In Siam, according to Koënig, the juice is collected by breaking off the leaves or young branches. From the fracture the gamboge exudes in drops, and was therefore called *gum gutta.* It is received on leaves, cocoanut shells, earthen pots, or in bamboos; it gradually hardens by age, and is then wrapped up in leaves prior to sale.

There are three varieties of Siam gamboge—1st. rolls, or solid cylinders; 2d. pipes or hollow cylinders; 3d. lumps or cakes.

Fine gamboge is brittle, fracture shelly, surface opaque, and brownish yellow with lustre. It forms a yellow emulsion when rubbed with water; powder bright yellow, inodorous, nearly tasteless, but leaving a faintly acrid flavour.

Analysis. Dr. Christison has recently published a very elaborate analysis of the three varieties of this drug, and which exhibits the subjoined results:—

	Cylinder, or Pipe.		Cake, or Lump.		Coarse.	
Resin, ...	74·2	71·6	64·3	65·0	61·4	35·0
Soluble gum, Arabin,	21·8	24·0	20·7	19·7	17·2	14·2
Woody fibre, ...	trace.	trace.	4·4	6·2	7·8	19·0
Fecula, ...	——	——	6·2	5·0	7·8	22·0
Moisture, ...	4·8	4·8	4·0	4·2	7·2	10·6
	100·8	100·4	99.6	100·1	101·4	100·8

The *resin* is obtained separately by heating powdered gamboge with sulphuric ether, and evaporating the solution. It is brittle, of deep orange colour, powder light yellow, insoluble in water, soluble in alcohol and ether. It also dissolves in solutions of caustic potash, and is separated by acids in its original state. Undervorben has shewn that this resin possesses acid properties. It forms yellow compounds with oxide of lead and with lime, brown with protoxide of iron, green with the oxide of copper. When precipitated by acid from its alkaline solutions, and redissolved in caustic potash, the liquor assumes a blood red colour. In doses of five grains this resin occasions copious watery evacuations without pain or uneasiness.

The gum of gamboge is nearly identical with gum Arabic. The starch occurs only in the inferior varieties, and is considered an adulteration. It is a curious fact, well worth recording, that under the name of *Ossara rewund* Dr. Falconer, of Seharunpore, obtained from the Himalayas a fine extract of the Rhubarb of that territory.

Medical properties. In small doses gamboge acts as a hydragogue cathartic, and diuretic. In larger quantities, nausea and vomiting, griping, and profuse watery evacuations are occasioned. When taken in poisonous doses it produces all the symptoms of violent inflammation of the alimentary canal.

It is much given in dropsies, the object being to occasion watery stools, and also that it should act as a diuretic. As a purgative it is usually joined with jalap or cream of tartar; its diuretic operation is said to be much facilitated and increased by dissolving it in a solution of carbonate of potash; half an ounce of gamboge, 1 oz. of carbonate of potash, and 12 oz. of brandy digested together for a week, give a tincture of which the dose is 40 to 60 drops, and which is stated on good authority to be a powerful diuretic.

In *tape worm*, a compound of gamboge, scammony, and calomel gained great celebrity as Madame Bouffer's specific, but the Indian pomegranate seems a much more certain remedy. A similar formula is much used in America in the treatment of obstinate constipation; there are few remedies superior to these compounds in their action on the bowels, especially in the treatment of apoplexy and dropsies.

The full dose of gamboge powder is 5 to 15 grains. It is however usually given in 3 grain doses, repeated until the desired effect is produced, but it is not in ordinary cases to be carried beyond the total quantity of 20 grains.

Off. prep. Powder, tincture, compound tincture, pill, &c.

Gen. 3.—Calophyllum.

Sp. 1. *Calophyllum inophyllum.*

Vern. Poonamarum, Poona, *Tel.* Sultana champa, *H.*

The seeds yield oil *(surpun ka tel)*, the roots a resin, the latter deemed the same as the Bourbon *Tacamahaca;* the fixed oil is fragrant, and used as an external application in rheumatism.

The seeds are bitterish.

The balsam seems analogous to myrrh, and is useful in indolent ulcers.

It occurs in all parts of India, and is in flower and fruit most part of the year. In Java the tree is said to be diuretic.

Sp. 2. *Calophyllum calaba.*

A native of Travancore, produces true East India tacamahaca resin. This resin is rarely met with it, it is yellow, translucent, adhesive, of acrid taste, and pleasant aromatic smell.

Gen. 4.—Mesua.

Sp. Mesua ferrea.

Vern. Nagsara or Nagkesur, (As. Researches, iv. 295.)

Found chiefly in gardens in Bengal, where it flowers in the beginning of the warm season. The dried anthers are fragrant; the flowers and leaves are used in Bengal as antidotes to snake poison.

NAT. ORDER XXIX.—CANELLEÆ.

Gen. 1.—Canella.

Sp. 1. *Canella alba,* (wild cinnamon.)

Off. The bark.

A native of the Caribbean Islands and South America, cultivated in the Botanic Garden, Calcutta.

A tree from 40 to 50 feet high, inner bark thick, smooth, of pale orange colour, with a sharp aromatic taste; leaves scattered, shining, yellowish green, obovate, wedge-shaped at base, dotted when young, opaque when old; flowers small clustered, purple, petals concave, erect, thick, deciduous; berry the size of a pea, fleshy, smooth, blue or black, hot and biting while green, seeds generally two.

The bark occurs in dry, buff pieces, often in thin cylinders or long canes, sometimes in large and thick fragments, both lined with a white membrane. The former are to be preferred for medicinal uses. The taste is bitter and hot, smell pepperish, powder white. The bark contains resin, volatile oil, extractive and colouring matter, gum, starch, albumen, acetates of potash and lime, muriates of potash and magnesia, and oxalate of lime. It contains neither tannic nor gallic acid, nor oxide of iron, by the absence of which substances it is easily distinguished from the bark of the *Drymis wintera,* with which it is often adulterated. Petroz and Robinet describe a substance as existing in the bark, of a saccharine nature, resembling *mannite.*

The leaves are excessively pungent, yield a volatile oil on distillation with water, but still retain their pungency when stove-dried; dried and reduced to powder and treated by boiling alcohol a green tincture is obtained, which on spontaneous evaporation affords very large transparent crystals. These crystals are neutral, and much resemble piperine; we propose to term them *canelline,* pending a complete investigation of their properties. They may probably be found identical with the saccharine matter of Petroz and Robinet.

Medical uses. Canella bark is employed with much advantage as an aromatic tonic in diseases of debility, such as the latter stages of typhoid fevers, in chronic rheumatism, and in some forms of secondary syphilis. In cold infusion it is a valuable vehicle for preparations of iron, of quinine, or anarcotine.

The powdered leaves yield their active principles and colouring matter to melted lard or concrete vegetable oils, and give a good substitute for savine ointment for exciting a discharge from blistered surfaces.

Off. prep. Tincture, compound powder, ointment of leaves.

[In the five following orders, viz.,
Hippocrataceæ, Erythroxyleæ, Malpighiacæ, Acerineæ, and Hippocastaneæ, there is nothing which requires attention].

NAT. ORDER XXX.—SAPINDACEÆ.

This is a remarkable order, from the saponaceous properties of one of its genera; it is almost exclusively tropical in its distribution, and abounds especially in Sylhet.

Some of the species, viz. the Paullinea australis, Magonia pubescens, and Senaria triternata are acrid and narcotic, and used for stupifying fish. Of the genus Sapindus most of the species are remarkable for being used as substitutes for soap, a property dependent on a principle named Saponin or Æsculic acid, described below; the root and bark of several species are saponaceous, as well as the fruit. Edible fruits also abound in the order, of which we may mention the *lichi* as one of the best of those produced in India.

The Sapindaceæ are either trees, shrubs, or even herbaceous plants; the leaves are alternate, and often compound.

GEN. 1.—SAPINDUS.

Calyx 4, 5 partite, petals as many as sepals (rarely one abortive), naked or hairy, or with a scale above the claw; torus a disk occupying the bottom of the calyx, entire or crenulated; stamens 8—10 inserted between the margin of the disk and ovary, ovary 3, rarely 2 celled, ovule erect at base of each cell, style crowned with a 3, rarely with 2 lobed stigma; fruit externally fleshy, 1, 2 lobed from abortion, rarely 3 lobed, lobes globular, indehiscent, 1 seeded, seeds without arillus. Embryo curved or straight; the trees have leaves without stipules, usually abruptly pinnate, sometimes unequally pinnate, or from abortion having only one leaflet; flowers racemose; berries saponaceous.

Sp. 1. *Sapindus emarginatus*, Vahl.

Vern. Ritah, *D.* Rishta, *D.* Bindake, *Hindee.* Arishta, Phemla, *Sans.* Rarak, *Malay.*

Petiole simple, terete, pubescent, leaves abruptly pinnate, leaflets 2, 3 pairs, oblong, retuse or emarginate, quite entire, upper side glabrous, under very downy. Racemes in terminal panicles; calyx, segments five oblong; petals five, equidistant, oval, outside densely hairy, margin very woolly with a small woolly appendage on each side about the middle, inside nearly glabrous, or with a few scattered hairs about the middle; stamens eight, woolly; ovary densely hairy; fruits 1, 4, but usually three lobed, lobes very hairy on the inside on the insertion of the seeds. (W. and A.)

The dry fruit is about ¾ inch in diameter, globose, corrugated, with three very obtuse angular projections; brownish yellow. The *pericarp* is about 1-10 inch in thickness, the *endocarp* soft, dark brown, of peculiar sweetish bitter taste, and nauseous cheesy smell. Dr. Ainslie states that the Hindoo physicians deem it a useful expectorant. In the Bazars the nut is usually extracted, and the pericarp alone sold.

When this substance is mixed with water it froths like soap, and is used instead of that substance for many important purposes. Dr. Sherwood has mentioned that the seeds pounded with water often put an end to the epileptic paroxysm, a small quantity being introduced into the patient's mouth.

Another species, the *S. Saponaria*, has been used in medicine in the treatment of chlorosis, in the form of the tincture or extract of the soapy matter of the capsule.

The nuts themselves are exceedingly hard and tough, and as they take a fine polish are employed for necklaces and beads.

The kernels of the small black nuts of the S. Saponaria are eaten in the West Indies, and deemed as palatable as the hazel nut or almond. The roots as well as the capsules are used in washing, but it is stated that the fabric washed is rapidly corroded; this however requires confirmation. (Feé, vol. ii. p. 48.)

Sir Stamford Raffles, in his work on Java, states that the Soap berries of that island have been examined, and the constituent principles of the best soap obtained. M. Feé also speaks of the sarcocarp being oily, and containing potash. These statements are however disproved by the analyses of several chemists, which have shewn that the soap-like substance is chiefly formed of a principle termed *saponine* by Bussy, and *æsculic* acid by M. Fremy, who obtained it also from the fruits of Æsculus hippocastanum, (Horse chesnut).

Saponine, or Æsculic Acid.

Saponine is prepared by boiling the root or fruit for a few minutes with alcohol, Sp. gr. 837. The solution being filtered and left to cool deposits the saponine, which is pressed between blotting paper and dried. It is a white pulverescent mass, of very acrid taste, and occasioning violent sneezing when applied to the nostrils. It is very soluble in water, and the solution froths like soap lather. Insoluble in ether, soluble in absolute alcohol. Solutions of saponine are partially coagulated by nitric acid. The alkalies do not saponify this principle—with subacetate of lead a copious precipitate is occasioned, composed of saponine 72.8, oxide of lead 27.2.

With potash, soda, and ammonia, saponine forms gelatinous compounds, supposed by Fremy to be æsculates of these bases; they dissolve in and crystallize from alcohol, Sp. gr. 928.

Among other genera we find *Paullinia pinnata*, of Brazil, acrid and narcotic, used to poison fish, and *Magonia pubescens*, also of Brazil, the ashes of which are extremely alkaline, and the bark used for the irritation on the skins of horses occasioned by stings of insects.

Schmidelia serrata.

Syn. Ornitrophe serrata. Roxb. Fl. Ind. ii. p. 266. Bengal, Coromandel.

Vern. Rakhal phul, *H.* Tualika, *Tel.*

Ripe berries eaten. Root astringent, employed to check diarrhœa.

Schleichera trijuga.

Vern. Roatangha, *Tel.* Roxb. Fl. Ind. ii. p. 277.

Various parts of India.

The bark is astringent, rubbed up with oil the natives use it to cure the itch. The wood is very hard. The pulpy subacid oil is edible and palatable. (*Lindley.*)

NAT. ORDER XXXI.—ÆSCULACEÆ. (Lindley.)

Æsculus Hippocastanum. Europe. Part of India ? Persia.

A magnificent tree, one of the chief ornaments of European landscapes. The *bark* is very astringent, and is used to check diarrhœa, also as a febrifuge. The seeds contain *æsculic* acid, a substance supposed to be identical with saponine. This tree holds a place in the British pharmacopœia, but its products are never used in medical practice.

NAT. ORDER XXXII.—MELIACEÆ.

This order is closely allied to the Sapindaceæ. It is found chiefly within the tropics, but the Melia azaderachta, an important species, has been completely naturalized in the south of France ; another is found near Pekin, and a third in New Zealand.

Some botanists divide the order into two tribes—Meliæ and Trichiliæ; and the latter again into Cedreleæ and Swieteniæ. Some species of all these are found in India.

GEN. 1.—MELIA.

Calyx five partite; petals five, patent, stamen-tube 10-cleft at apex, with ten anthers in the throat, segments 2, 3, partite, anthers opposite to segments, and a little shorter, oblong, slightly apiculate; ovary seated on a short disk, five-celled, cells each with two superposed ovules, style columnar, breaking off from the top of the ovary; stigma five lobed; fruit a drupe with one 5-celled bony nut ; cells, one seeded. Trees. Leaves alternate, bipinnate, leaflets in pairs, with an odd one, toothed. Peduncles axillary, simple below, above panicled, branched, and many flowered. W. and A.

Sp. 1. *Melia Azedarach*, Persian Lilac, (Hill margosa, *Dek.*)

In the present species the leaves are deciduous, leaflets about five, obliquely ovate, lanceolate, serrated finely, acuminated, glabrous, petals nearly glabrous. The number of parts of the flower are occasionally increased by a fifth.

This species flowers in the Botanical Garden of Calcutta during the hot season ; it thrives luxuriously, and becomes a large useful timber tree, of very great beauty. Its flowers are like those of the lilac, and sweetly fragrant. (Roxb. ii. p. 395.)

Sp. 2. *Melia sempervirens*, or Bukayun.

Bukayun, Bukain, *Pers.* Bān, *Arab.* Maha nimba, *Beng.*

A smaller tree than the M. Azedarach—the flowers blueish.

Gen. 2.—Azadirachta.

Sp. Azadirachta Indica, Juss.

Syn. Melia Azadirachta, Roxb. Fl. Ind. ii. p. 394. *Nim*, or *Margosa*. Royle, p. 140.

Vern. Nimba, *Sans.* Vepa, *Tel.* Neem, *Beng.* Vepam, *Tam.*

Calyx five partite, petals five, patent, stamen tube bearing 10 anthers in the throat, short, ten-lobed, lobes reflexed, anthers opposite to the lobes, and about equal to them, oblong. Ovary seated on a short disk, three-celled, ovules two in each cell, collateral, pendulous. Style columnar, stigma three partite, the lobes conical, fruit drupaceous by abortion, one-celled and one-seeded, leaves simply pinnated, leaflets unequal sided, glabrous, serrated, panicles axillary, number of parts of flower occasionally decreased by a fifth.

A middling sized, very common, beautiful, and very useful tree; flowering time the hot season; it differs from all the other species in having a one-celled, one-seeded nut, though the germ has uniformly five cells with one or two ovula in each. Roxb. ii. p. 394.

There is much confusion in the names of the different plants above quoted. We have deemed it expedient to submit their botanical characters under the received nomenclature; we shall however, to avoid further confusion, notice their chemical and medicinal relations under the native appellations.

The author of the "Mukhsun-ul-udwieh" describes four kinds of Neem, or Melia—1st. Nim; 2nd. Bukayun; 3rd. Dek; 4th. an unknown species, which Royle supposes to be the Melia composita of the Peninsula.

1st—*Nim*, (Melia Azadirachta. Azadirachta Indica. Margosa tree).

Every part of this tree, especially the bark, is bitter; the bark is also astringent, the leaves are bitter and very nauseous; from the ripe pericarp of the fruit a very bitter fixed oil is expressed; the trunk of the tree yields gum, and the young trees when tapped yield a saccharine sap or toddy, capable of undergoing the vinous fermentation.

The leaves are employed all over India as poultices to tumours and open sores; the seeds (*nibuolee*) are blanched, powdered, and mixed with water, and used for cleaning the hair. The bark is considered by native practitioners as amongst their most valuable tonics, and is given with aromatics in fever and rheumatism; in Java the bark is considered vermifuge, the dose being half a teacup full of a decoction twice daily.

The oil is also thought anthelmintic, and is applied externally to foul ulcers, and used as a liniment in rheumatic and spasmodic affections, and in headaches from exposure to the sun. The wine or toddy is believed to be stomachic, the dose being one ounce and a half every morning.

Dr. White of Bombay used the bark of this tree as a substitute for Cinchona, and found its success nearly equal as a febrifuge remedy. Mr. Skipton has related a case of hysteria (Trans. Med. Phy. Soc. Calcutta, vol. i. p. 123) in which a decoction of the leaves was used with the best effect.

In the Trans. Med. and Phy. Soc. Calcutta, vol. iii. p. 430, Mr. Piddington described a crystallized sulphate of the bitter principle of the Nim, which he termed sulphate of Azedirine, but he did not communicate the process for its preparation, nor any account of its properties. The late Mr. Twining, who had seen the small specimen sent by Mr. Piddington to the Society, described it as being whitish, in the form of grains or minute crystals, of slightly bitter taste, but possessing no other sensible properties. No trial was made of its medicinal properties.

2.—*Bukayun*, (Bān, Azad-i-durukt, Melia Bukain, or Sempervirens—Maha nimba).

The seeds are called Hub-ool-Bān, and are considered emetic, laxative, and anthelmintic, the bark bitter and anthelmintic.

3.—*Dek.* (Melia azidarach. Persian lilac, Hill margosa).

In general and medicinal properties this species corresponds with the first.

Gen. 3.—Trichilia.

Sp. Trichilia emetica, Elcaja, Forskäl.

Fruit pale yellow when ripe, pulp bitter, and reputed to be poisonous; properties as yet but little examined.

Common on the mountains of Yemen and in Senegal.

The fruit is used by the Arabs under the name of *Djous el kai,* and in powder mixed with oil is employed against the itch.

GEN. 4.—GUAREA.

Sp. Guarea trichilioides.

Bark a violent emetic and purgative.

GEN. 5.—XYLOCARPUS.

Sp. Xylocarpus Granatum.

Syn. Carapa moluccensis. (Lamark).

Roxb. Flora Ind. ii. 240. *Beng.* Pussoor—a native of the Sunderbuns. Fruit ripens in June and July.

In the vii. vol. Journ. de Pharmacie p. 411, there is a very interesting paper by M. Virey on the "Carapa tree," and other neighbouring species.

The Carapa of Guiana was first described by Aublet. It yields fruits, the almonds of which are white, solid, oily, and bitter. The oil he described as being used by the Galebi savages to anoint their skins and hair, in order to keep off insects.

Rumphius described a similar but smaller tree in the Moluccas, under the name of "Madahul," "or *Granatum litoreum.*" This Wildenow described as Xylocarpus granatum. The Xylocarpus is mentioned as a tree with elegantly veined wood, used in India in cabinet work, and its bitter root being employed in bilious fevers. A starchy substance, used as an article of food, is also found beneath the bark of the capsule.

In the same periodical, vol. v. p. 49, we find a description of the Guiana Carapa, and its products, by M. Cadet. M. Cadet describes the process for extracting the oil, and narrates several unsuccessful attempts at separating the oil from the bitter principle with which it is associated. In 1821, M. Boullay published further experiments, by which it appeared he had separated from the oil a minute quantity of a distinctly alkaline principle; M. Petroz and Robinet in the same year communicated to the Academie Royale de Medicine their analysis of specimens of the Carapa bark, received from Cayenne, where it had been used with great success as a febrifuge by M. Mille. These writers give a minute description of the bark, and the action of reagents on its solutions. As the result of their analysis, they described an alkaline substance, an acid (kinic?), red and green coloring matter, and a salt of lime. They did not name the alkaline principle, nor indeed had they a sufficient quantity to examine it thoroughly. Its clinical effects remain altogether open to investigation.

Gen. 6.—Walsura.

Sp. Walsura piscidia.

Vern. Wallursi, *Teling.* Walsura, *Tamul.*

A native of the Circar mountains; flowers during cold season. Roxburgh informs us that the bark thrown into ponds intoxicates the fish, which are consequently very easily taken. The fish are not deemed unwholesome.

Another species of Walsura, (Robusta) exists in Sylhet, but the bark is not employed as a fish poison.

NAT. ORDER XXXIII.—CEDRELACEÆ.

This order comprises several genera of considerable value in medicine, and the arts.

Gen. 1.—Swietenia.

Sp. Swietenia Mahogani. Mahogany tree.

Indigenous in South America, and naturalized in some parts of the Peninsula of India. A large tree, with very rough tuberculated bark, leaves equally pennated, leaflets opposite, very smooth, ovate, lanceolate; flowers in axillary panicles, small, whitish; fruit the size of a hen's egg,(Lindley.)

The bark is used in the West Indies as a substitute for cinchona. It is very astringent, but contains no alkaline principle, and is not used by European practitioners.

Gen. 2.—Soymida.

Sp. Soymida febrifuga.

Syn. Swietenia febrifuga.

Vern. Rohun Rohitaka, *Hind.* Wond Marum, *Tam.* A large forest tree, a native of several of the mountainous districts of India, in the Rajamundry Circars, the district of Cuddapa, the Chunar hills, and the jungles to the south of Hazarebâg. Royle indeed states that it occurs in all the central and southern parts of India.

Bot. Char. of the genus Soymida. Sepals 5, spreading, unguiculate; stamen tube cup-shaped, 10 lobed, each lobe with 2 teeth at the apex, and an anther between the teeth below them; ovarium seated on the disk, which is broader than itself, and covers the bottom of the tube, five celled, ovules 12 in each cell, style short, equal, five angled, stigma thick, peltate, five angled; capsule oblong, obovate, five celled, five valved, dehiscing from the apex, septifragal, the thin woody sarcocarp in each valve becoming detached from the endocarp, and both from the large persistent five angled axis; seeds pendulous, winged all round, especially upwards and downwards; leaves abruptly pinnate, leaflets opposite, 3-6 pair, oval, oblong, obtuse; panicles large, terminal, or in the axils of the uppermost leaves. In the Soymida febrifuga the leaves are alternate, abruptly pinnated, in 3-4 pairs, about a foot long, leaflets opposite, oval, obtuse, or emarginate, unequal at the base, smooth, shining, 3-4 inches long by 2-3 broad. Panicle terminal, large, diffuse, smooth, sepals five, ovate, deciduous; petals ovate, obtuse, concave, spreading, stamen tube urceolate, 10 toothed, each tooth bifid, anthers 10, oval arising from within the tube below its crenatures. *Lindley*, *Fl. Med.* p. 155.

The bark of this tree has enjoyed much celebrity as a substitute for cinchona. Its use was introduced by Dr. Roxburgh. Dr. Duncan made it the subject of his inaugural dissertation in 1794, and Mr. Breton published an Essay on its properties in the Med. Chur. Transactions of London, vol. xi. p. 324. The same writer also published in Calcutta, a lithographed pamphlet on the uses of this bark.

The bark is of a dull red colour, epidermis rough and gray, fracture fibrous and woody. The bark found in the Bazars varies from the thickness of a quill to flat or rolled pieces 1-2 inches in breadth or diameter.

In vol. iv. Trans. Med. Phys. Soc. of Calcutta there is a paper by Mr. Piddington on the Rohuna bark, and the sulphate of its bitter principle. Mr. Piddington stated that he had applied to the bark the process described by Paris, (Pharmacologia, Vol. ii.) for preparing sulphate of quinine, and with perfect success. He presented to the Society a small specimen of the alleged sulphate of Rohuna, and described in full detail the process for its preparation. In 1836, however, it was ascertained by the Editor of this work that the salt prepared by Mr. Piddington was sulphate of *Brucine*, and that the bark he operated on was that of the nux-vomica tree. On inquiry in the bazars it was found that in several shops the nux-vomica bark was sold for the Rohun.

The nux-vomica bark *(Kuchila)* is thin, black internally,

very brittle, is grey externally, and stained with bright rust-coloured spots; nitric acid gives a blood-red stain to the inner side of the bark, and changes the red exuberance to green. In powder, rohun bark is red, nux-vomica bark dark grey. The infusion of the former is deep red, of the latter nearly colourless.

The Editor has made several ineffectual attempts to obtain an alkaloid principle from the true rohun. The bark is much less bitter than is generally described, but is very rich in gallic and tannic acid, and contains a great quantity of red colouring matter. It is necessary to add, that when subjected to the usual processes for preparing sulphate of quinine it yields an abundant crop of spicular crystals, which are merely sulphate of lime, but which may readily deceive an inexperienced observer. The sulphate of lime is known by its not being decomposed at a red heat.

Mr. Breton and others have spoken very highly of the efficacy of this bark in the treatment of periodical fevers. It seems to us to be exactly similar to the mahogany bark, useful where astringent tonics are applicable, but of very questionable efficacy as a true antiperiodic. Although we cannot advise its use in the treatment of obstinate or dangerous cases, still for mild ague, in which doubtless like all other astringent tonics it will often succeed, we recommend it to be given in the form of the *extract* described in our officinal preparations.

Off. prep. Extract.

GEN. 3.—CEDRELA.

Sp. Cedrela Toona. (Toon).

Vern. Tunna, *Beng.* Loodh, *Sans.*

This noble timber tree is common in Bengal; it flowers in February, and the seeds ripen in May and June. The trunk grows to a great height, and is quite erect.

Bark smooth and grey. Branches numerous, forming a large beautiful shady head. Leaves alternate, abruptly pinnate, drooping, from 12—18 inches long, leaflets 6—12, pairs, opposite or nearly so, short, petiolated, obliquely lanceolate, the upper half broadest, and extending further down the petioles than the lower; margins waved, smooth on both sides, tapering to a long acute point, from two to six inches long; petioles and petiolets round and smooth, stipules none; panicles terminal, nearly as long as the leaves, pendulous, composed of numerous diverging compound ramifications, smooth in every part; bractes minute, deciduous. Flowers very numerous, small, white, and possessing a fragrance like fresh honey, calyx five-parted, petals five, oblong, margins ciliate, the apices incurved over the stamens, and keeled on the inside near the base; nectary consisting of five large, hairy, orange-coloured glands, sitting round the lower half of the germ; filaments erect, inserted into the centre of the five nectarial glands, rather shorter than the petals; anthers bent in towards the stigma; germ superior, oblong, internal structure, and contents as in the capsule; style length of the corolla, stigma large, flat, composed of five lobes; capsules oblong, rather larger than a field-bean, smooth, five-celled, five-valved, valvelets opening from the apex, and falling off with the seeds. Seeds numerous, imbricated, both the ends of the exterior membrane winged, affixed to the upper end of the sharp ridges of the receptacle, perisperm in very small quantity, and more like a fleshy interior integument. Embryo inverse, cotyledons oval, three-nerved, radicle obliquely superior.

The wood of this tree closely resembles the inferior kinds of mahogany, and is much used in India. The bark is powerfully astringent, but not bitter. The native physicians use it in conjunction with the powdered nut of the Cæsalpinia bonducella, an intense bitter.

For these details, we are indebted to Roxb. Fl. Ind. vol. i. p. 635.

M. Nees Von Essenbeck has published an account of some experiments on the bark, which indicated the existence of a resinous astringent matter, a brown astringent gum, and a gummy brown extractive matter, resembling *ulmine*.

The bark was used in Java by Blume in epidemic fevers, diarrhœa, and other complaints. Horsfield gave it in dysentery, but only in the last stage, when inflammatory symptoms had disappeared.

Gen. 4.—Chickrassia.

Sp. Chickrassia tabularis.

(*Swietenia Chickrassa*, Roxb. Fl. Ind. ii. 399). This tree occurs in the mountainous countries to the East of Bengal. The timber is very beautiful, and much admired for furniture; the bark is powerfully astringent.

Gen. 5.—Khaya.

Sp. Khaya Senegalensis.

A forest tree found on the banks of the Gambia; the bark is very bitter, and called Cailcedra. It is much used by the negroes in infusion and decoction, in the treatment of the violent fevers of that country.

NAT. ORDER XXXIV.—VITACEÆ, OR AMPELIDEÆ.

This order is remarkable chiefly on account of its including the grape-vine. Several genera are common through the Indian peninsula. A temperate climate, however, is that which is most favourable to the development of the saccharine and aromatic principles on which the value of the grape depends.

Vines are climbing sarmentaceous shrubs, all the parts of which are acid. The fruits of the cultivated species are sweet when ripe, but the wild kinds remain always acid. Some species of Cissus are excessively acrid.

GEN.—VITIS.

Sp. Vitis vinifera, the Wine grape.

Αμπελος οινοφορος. Dioscorides.

Booangoor, *Malay*. Ungoor, *Persian* and *Duk*. Draksha, *Sans*. Dakh, *Hind*. Inub, *Arab*.

A native of the south of Asia Minor, now universally cultivated.

The stalks are long, sometimes climbing to the loftiest trees, knotty, provided with branching spiral tendrils for attachment to surrounding objects; the leaves are alternate, petiolate, heart-shaped at the base, and divided into 3—5 toothed lobes; the flowers are greenish, and in lateral clusters.

The fruit is disposed in a thyrsus which gives its name to this form of inflorescence. The grape itself is rounded and one-celled, with from 1 to 5 bony small seeds. The colour, size, consistence, &c. of the grape vary infinitely according to innumerable circumstances connected with its cultivation. The leaves and fruit are inodorous, the flowers agreeably fragrant.

M. Feé, from whose admirable work we derive the arrangement of this action, divides the products of the grape vine into the *natural* and *artificial*.

Natural products. M. Feé observes that the fresh grape is simply an article of food, but also is slightly laxative and soothing, and has often induced favourable changes in the condition of patients who were altogether despaired of. M. Feé here alludes to the "grape treatment" of consumption on the banks of the Rhine, of which a full account is given by Dr. Granville in his journey to St. Petersburgh.

Several varieties of dried grape fruit (raisins) are described by M. Feé, but their slight importance in medicine obliges us to pass them over. Raisins are employed to impart sweetness to some officinal preparations, and for such the "Kishmish" of India may be employed.

Artificial products.

Must is the expressed juice of the ripe grape. It readily undergoes fermentation. A syrup is prepared from it in France, for which Parmentier has given the following formula. Take white ripe grapes, express the juice, add 1 per 100 of sulphuric acid to destroy the leaven or fermenting principle, and subsequently neutralize the acid by chalk. Tartrate, malate, citrate, and sulphate of lime are simultaneously precipitated. Decant, filter, and evaporate very quickly to the consistence of a thin syrup. Good Must gives 25 per cent. of syrup, which will yield 18½ parts of brown muscovado, or raw sugar. From 500 parts of this 175 of solid white sugar may be procured.

Fermented Must gives two products, *wine*, and *vinegar*.

Wine. Wine is a white, rosy, or red liquid, according to the kind of grape used, and the process followed. It is fluid, limpid, and more or less alcoholic, &c. Sugar is present in some kinds. The smell and taste vary indefinitely.

The wines chiefly employed in Hospital practice are two—port (Oporto) and sherry, (Xeres).

Port is deep red, approaching to crimson, slightly astringent. The extract consists of tannic and gallic acid, sugar and colouring matter. By distillation port wine of best quality yields of alcohol 23 per 100.

Port is very much employed in diseases of debility, scurvy, typhus fevers, cholera, the last stages of dysentery, consumption, &c.

Sherry (Vin de Xeres) is light amber coloured, sweetish, 100 parts contain 18 of alcohol. There is no astringent matter, but traces exist of citric and malic acid.

Sherry is employed as a stimulant, but is apt to produce an aperient and even cathartic effect.

Various fraudulent substitutions are daily used in the preparation of wines, to detect which M. Feé gives the following rules, which we have found to be correct.

The alcoholic solution of caustic potash changes pure wine, ... *Green.*
If coloured with mulberries, ... *Violet.*
——— with logwood, ... *Violet red.*
——— with Brazil wood or beet root, ... *Red.*
Acetate of lead precipitates
Pure wine, ... *Green.*

Wine adulterated with elder berries, logwood, or myrtle berries, ...	*Deep blue.*
—— with red sandal wood, beet root, or Brazil wood, ...	*Red.*
Alum precipitates,	
Wine coloured with litmus,...	*Clear violet.*
———— logwood, ...	*Deep violet.*
———— Brazil wood, ...	*Red.*

Lead sometimes exists in wine, and is detected by adding carbonate of soda; carbonate of lead is thrown down, which will be turned black by sulphuretted hydrogen gas. Alum, which is often present, is detected by the wine affording a precipitate with ammonia, carbonate of potash, and acetate of baryta.

The manufacture of wine is carried on, on a very simple plan. The ripe grapes are trodden by men or cattle in a vat, and the juice which is thus forced out is called the *Must*. The *Marc* or solid parts being mixed with the Must again in wooden tanks, fermentation soon takes place, much heat is developed, and carbonic acid gas is copiously disengaged; the Marc now rises to the surface of the tank, and when the effervescence ceases the subjacent wine is drawn off from below, and the Marc subjected to strong pressure.

If the wine be bottled before the fermentation has terminated, it has the property of foaming in the glass in consequence of the sudden liberation of carbonic acid; champagne is thus manufactured. In the preparation of white wines the Marc is removed before fermentation.

According to Humboldt, the conditions of climate essential for the manufacture of good wine are, a range of temperature from 62° to 50° or even 47°, provided the winter heat is not lower than 38°, nor that of summer below 66° or rather 68°. At a higher mean temperature the juice passes too rapidly into the acid fermentation. The manufacture of wine thus becomes impracticable in the plains of India; moreover the rains set in so soon after the ripening of the grape, that the manufacture of raisins by sun-drying is equally impossible.

Mr. Royle informs us of the existence of luxuriant vineyards in Kunawur, between N. lat 31° and 32° (or nearly that of Madeira) at an elevation of 9000 to 10,000 feet, the grape being of delicious flavour, and the climate exactly suited for both the wine and raisin manufacture. Grapes are also abundant in Cashmere, at Cabul, and Bokhara, and afford both raisins and wine.

The most celebrated of eastern wines however is the *Shiraz*, prepared in the district of Khol-lar, near the village of Bend Emir. There are two varieties, red and white, the former containing 15½, the latter nearly 20 per 100 of alcohol.

The different kinds of raisins called *Monuka*, *Kishmish*, and *Bedana*, are, Mr. Royle states, brought chiefly from Istaulik.

ALCOHOL, *see* Pharmacopœia.

ACETIC ACID, or *wine vinegar*, see as above.

Sp. 2. *Vitis carnosa*, Wall.

Syn. Cissus carnosa, R.

Vern. Kusar, *Hind.* Kanapa tiga, *Tel.*

Remarkably arid, roots used in native medicine; it is common in hedges and forests in Bengal, and it flowers in the rainy season.

The Cissus setosa is in all its parts excessively acrid, and Roxburgh states that the leaves toasted and oiled are applied to indolent tumors to bring them to suppuration. The young tender and succulent stems of Vitis (Cissus) quadrangularis are very generally eaten in India. When old this plant is deemed acrid, and a useful medicine; in Arabia it is used as an external application in rheumatic pains of the back and loins.

The Cissus arborea of Forskahl is the Salvadora persica of modern writers, and possesses some remarkable and valuable properties—see art. *Salvadoreæ.*

NAT. ORDER XXXV.—GERANIACEÆ.

The Geraniums and Pelargonums are common in most temperate climates, and abound especially at the Cape and St. Helena. They are great favourites as flowering plants, from the richness and variety of odour they generally exhale; none have been used in medicine, with the exception of one or two species, which are extremely astringent; remedies of this kind are so abundant in India, that it is unnecessary to introduce any from this order.

NAT. ORDER XXXVI.—BALSAMIFLUÆ.

This order contains several trees which yield a resinous product of some celebrity in medicine, and called *liquid storax.*

Gen.—Liquidambar.

Sp. 1. ***Liquidambar Altingia.***
Vern. Rasamala, *Malay.*
This is a superb forest tree, a native of the Java mountains. The bark is bitter, hot, and aromatic, and when wounded, affords the balsam called liquid storax.

Sp. 2. ***Liquidambar orientale.***
A small tree, indigenous in Cyprus and the Levantine islands. Yields a balsamic fluid resembling turpentine.

The solid *storax* of the druggists is obtained from the *Styrax officinale* of the Levant. See art. *Styraceæ*, for the properties of this drug.

NAT. ORDER XXXVII.—OXALIDEÆ.

Small shrubs or herbs with alternate, rarely opposite or sub-verticilled leaves, simple, or differently composed. All are acid, containing the oxalic acid combined with potash. Their flavour is very agreeable, and readily imparted to water. The expressed juice clarified yields crystals of the oxalate of potash, which is a dangerous poison. The leaves and fruits of several species are eaten as salad.

Gen. 1.—Oxalis.

Sp. 1. ***Oxalis acetosella.*** (Wood sorrel.)
This plant is common in groves and shady places in Europe. It is a small perennial with a subterranean woody stock, with numerous scaly joints; leaves ternate, inversely heart-shaped, hairy; peduncles radical, single-flowered, sepals five, distinct or united at base, petals five, stamens ten. Filaments slightly monadelphous, the five exterior alternately shorter; stigmas pencilled or capitate; capsule five-cornered, oblong or cylindrical.

The binoxalate of potash is extracted in large quantities from the leaves of this plant, and sold under the absurd name of the Essential Salt of *Lemons.* 20lbs. yield 6lbs. of juice, and from this 2¼ ounces of the pure salt are obtainable by crystallization (Neumann). The salt is used for dissolving stains of the peroxide of iron (iron-mould) from clothes. It is also added to whey, in quantities sufficient to give an agreeable flavour, in drinks for fever patients.

OXALIC ACID.

This acid though never used in medicine, is important as a powerful poison, and demands a brief notice in this work.

It crystallizes in long, white, and transparent prisms, and is powerfully acid; while dissolving in water its crystals give a very distinct snapping sound. It is also very soluble in strong spirit.

Oxalic acid is composed of carbon, oxygen, and water, in the proportions of carbon 2, oxygen 3, water 3 equivalents. When suddenly heated to 450° it emits water, and is decomposed, yielding formic acid, and carbonic oxide and acid; acted upon by an excess of strong sulphuric acid, it yields carbonic acid and oxide in equal volumes.

Besides the Oxalideæ, this acid in combination with potash or lime exists in several other vegetables, especially the rumex and rhubarb; the roots of the latter often contain 20 per 100 of this salt.

Oxalic acid is a formidable poison; in large doses it produces symptoms of the most violent irritation of the alimentary canal, and moreover acts with such fearful rapidity on the nervous system, that it has been known to prove fatal in ten minutes; sometimes life is prolonged for several hours, under the most distressing agonies; torturing pain referred to the stomach, violent vomiting, sometimes of bloody matter, failure of the pulse, a cold clammy skin, and extreme anxiety of the countenance are the most prominent symptoms. Few poisons are more certainly fatal, instances being known of vomiting having instantaneously occurred, and death nevertheless taken place so soon as in twenty minutes after the dose was swallowed.

On dissection signs of violent inflammation are observed; extensive destruction of the coats of the stomach has been noticed; the mucous membrane of the throat and gullet seems as if scalded by boiling water, and there is a general pulpy appearance of the soft parts dependent on the solution in the oxalic acid of the gelatine these contain.

Antidote. As oxalic acid forms a perfectly insoluble compound with lime and magnesia, chalk (the powdered plaster of walls answers perfectly) should be given instantly in large quantities, and followed by draughts of milk, and strong emetics, such as the sulphate of zinc or of copper; several persons have recovered who have been treated without loss of time in the manner now described. After the poison has been removed or rendered insoluble, leeches may be applied to the region of the stomach, a mild oily purgative administered, and the patient restricted to low diet until all symptoms of inflammation have been subdued.

(For the detection of oxalic acid, see Apendix, article Detection of Poisons.)

Sp. 2. *Oxalis corniculata* (Three-leaved sorrel.)

Vern. Umbuti, *Duk.* Pullachinta, *Tel.* Amrool, *Hind.* Chukrika, Ambashta, Amlika, *Sans.* Chooka-tiputtee, *Beng.*

This species is common all over India, possesses exactly the same properties, and yields the same products as the European sorrel.

The small leaves, tender shoots, and flowers, are given in electuaries by the Hindoos as a cooling medicine in fevers, to the extent of two tea-spoonsful daily.

Gen 2.—Averrhoa.

Sp. 1. *Averrhoa Carambola.*

Vern. Kamarunga, *Hind.* and *Beng.*

The Kamarunga tree is common in Bengal. The five-cornered, green, and juicy fruit contains a large quantity of quadroxalate of potash. It is used as a pickle, in curries, and as an ingredient in several native electuaries. The dyers also employ it very extensively.

Sp. 2. *Averrhoa Bilimbi.*

Also common in Bengal; the fruit resembles a small cucumber, and contains an abundant acid juice of similar properties to those of the preceding species. A syrup is prepared with the juice, and a conserve with the flowers, by the native physicians, who use it in the treatment of fevers.

NAT. ORDER XXXVIII.—CONNARACEÆ.

This order contains nothing of importance in medicine.

NAT. ORDER XXXIX.—ZYGOPHYLLEÆ.

The only medicinal species of much interest in this order is the *Guaiacum officinale.*

Gen.—Guaiacum.

Sp. Guaiacum officinale.
Syn. Lignum vitæ.
Off. Bark, wood, and resin.

A lofty tree, a native of Jamaica and Hispaniola. The *bark* is hard, woody, stiff, thick, in flat pieces, externally pale, within slightly streaked lengthwise, brittle, fracture slightly lamellar, shewing little crystalline points, odour feebly resinous, taste analogous to the smell, and rather bitter, powder of greenish white colour.

The *wood* is very solid, heavy, and hard, abounding in resin; it is found in commerce in large blocks, still covered with bark; the shavings of the wood are used in medicine; while cold it has but little odour, its taste is acrid, bitter, and sharp; the powder is yellow, turning to green by the action of light, a change owing to the presence of the resin.

Both the bark and wood are used as sudorifics in the treatment of gout, rheumatism, and chronic or secondary syphilis. It is asserted that a native of St. Domingo first made known to Europeans the sudorific virtues of this tree. The wood from its extreme hardness is much used for screws, presses, blocks, and pullies.

The trunk of the guaiac tree is from 60 feet upward; in temperate climates the growth is exceedingly slow, not more than one line annually; even in its native country the growth is very slow, and there is every reason to think that the supply will be soon exhausted. For medical purposes however an allied species, the *Guaiacum sanctum*, is deemed equally effectual.

Guaiac Resin.

This resin is obtained either by spontaneous exudation, or by taking a billet of wood with a hole bored through its centre, lengthwise, and setting fire to the upper end—the melted resin flows along the tube to a receiver placed beneath it.

The resin is met with in the wholesale druggists' shops in shapeless, hard masses, attached to fragments of bark; brittle, opaque, though transparent in thin flakes, generally green externally, and in any casual fissures; softening in the mouth. Sp. gr. 1228. The smell resembles slightly that of benzoin, and is increased by heat and friction; the taste is sweet, then bitter, lastly very acrid, and fixing in the throat; powder greenish white, becoming of deeper colour by exposure to the air, very irritating to the throat, and occasioning cough when inhaled.

This resin is by some writers called Guaiacine, it is often adulterated with Colophony (turpentine resin), but this may be easily detected by the smell of turpentine developed by flinging the suspected resin on hot charcoal; moreover oil of turpentine will dissolve colophony, but leave the guaiac resin.

Water takes up 9 per 100 of extractive matter; ether and alcohol dissolve the resin freely. The tincture is greenish brown, turning to milk-white by the copious affusion of water; sulphuric acid dissolves and destroys it; nitric acid affords with it no astringent matter, but abundance of oxalic acid.

Guaiac resin is changed green by nitric acid, and its vapour; and gives a blue colour to solutions of gluten, milk, gum arabic, and starch.

Medicinal uses. Internally taken, either wood or resin excites a sensation of warmth in the stomach, and dryness of the mouth and throat, (Duncan). It increases the heat of the skin, accelerates the pulse, and proves diaphoretic if the patient be kept warm, or diuretic if the surface of the body is exposed to the air. In large doses Dr. Duncan says it acts as a purgative.

Besides the diseases before mentioned, guaiac is given in cases of foul ulcers, hospital gangrene, thickened ligaments, mercurial ulcerations, and in various forms of scrofula.

The wood is used in decoction, the resin in pills, emulsion, or tincture; 10 to 30 grs. may be given daily. Dr. Duncan states that half an ounce of the tincture with three ounces of water is a sudorific dose for an adult, if he attend to keep himself warm.

Off. prep. Decoction of wood; compd. decoction; compd. decoction of sarsaparilla; ditto of ununtamul. Tincture; compound tincture. Compd. calomel pill. Guaiac mixture, &c.

Among other genera we may notice the following articles.

Tribulus terrestris, used in Cochin China as an astringent, in the South of Europe as an aperient and diuretic.

Zygophyllum. This genus is bitter, and astringent; the *Z. Fabago* is employed as a vermifuge and astringent.

Porlieria hygrometrica, a native of Peru and Chili, has the same properties as the Guaiac, but in a weaker degree; the leaves shut close in wet weather.

Melianthus. This genus contains some fœtid plants, the smell of which resembles that of stramonium. From a nectary-like gland, placed between the petals, there exudes a great quantity of honey-like juice, from which these plants derive their name.

Balanites ægyptiaca, is common about Dehli, and in the Doab as far as Allahabad, and especially on the banks of the Jumna. (Royle, p. 154.) Dr. Roxburgh describes the pulp as exceedingly bitter, and having an offensive greasy smell; the nut is used in native fire-works, the kernel being scooped out the shell is filled with gunpowder, and explodes with a very loud report.

NAT. ORDER XL.—RUTACEÆ.

The true Rutaceæ constitute an order, the species of which are extensively distributed. They contain a bitter principle combined with an essential oil, and have long been deemed valuable remedies in some maladies of the uterine system, in worm diseases, and several affections to which children are liable. The following species are admitted into the British Pharmacopœiæ.

Gen. 1.—Ruta.

Sp. Ruta graveolens. (Rue.)

Off. The herb.

A small shrubby plant, a native of the South of Europe. The smell is strong, and taste bitter; leaves while fresh excessively acrid, the leaves yield on analysis three per 100 of volatile oil, with green wax, extractive, albumen, malic acid, gum, starch, and fibre.

Med. use. The expressed juice of the herb in the dose of a tea-spoonful for children of three years and upwards, is frequently deemed useful in worm affections. The volatile oil is given in menstrual obstructions to the extent of two to three drops daily, diffused through water by sugar.

Ruta albiflora, (white-flowered rue) is common on the Himalayas, at an elevation of 5000 to 8000 feet.

Ruta augustifolia, (narrow-leaved rue,) (Sudab) is met with in gardens in India, and used medicinally.

Peganum Harmala, a closely allied species, occurs in many parts of India, and is found in the Taj garden at Agra. The seeds are used in native medicine, and called Lahoree Hoormul. In the "Mukzun-ul-Udwieh," the seed is called *Moolie;* the same as the μολη of Discorides. Royle, p. 155.

The three preceding species appear identical in properties and effects with the article of the British Pharmacopœiæ.

Gen. 2.—Galipea.

Sp. *Galipea Cusparia.*

Syn. Cusparia febrifuga. Bonplandia trifoliata. (*Angustura bark* of Humboldt.)

Galipea officinalis, Hancock in Med. Bot. Transactions, 1829, t. ii. p. 25.

Off. The bark.

A native of the Highlands of Carony, and southern and back Missions of the Orinoko.

Dr. Hancock, a zealous naturalist and able physician, who spent many years in South America, has published a very interesting account of this once celebrated bark, in the work above quoted. He says, "I am fully convinced, from ample experience, of the virtues of this bark, that it is one of the most valuable febrifuges we possess, being adapted to the worst and most malignant bilious fevers, while the fevers in which cinchona is chiefly administered are simple intermittents, for the most part unattended with danger; the natives also use the bruised bark as a means of intoxicating fishes, which affords a very singular coincidence with what is mentioned by Dr. Saunders, of the same use being made of cinchona bark by the American Indians."

The genuine bark found in the shops retains its epidermis, is rolled, sometimes flattened, thin at the edges, 3 to 15 inches long, very brittle; steeped in water it softens, and may be readily cut with scissors. The epidermis is thin, wrinkled, and fissured, and is sometimes covered with a corky, soft, yellowish gray exuberance. Internally the bark is of a fawn colour, its fracture compact and resinous; its thickness varies from half a line to the tenth of an inch; the odour is strong, resembling some animal secretions; the taste very bitter, nauseous, and persistent; powder of a pale yellow colour.

In Mr. Brande's experiments 3840 parts of the powdered bark yielded to alcohol 144 parts of resin, and 300 of an acrid unctuous matter, with 1500 of dry gummy extract. By distillation the same quantity yielded 26 of essential oil. Solutions of the bark have the peculiar property of striking a deep red colour with the persulphate of iron.

Spurious angustura. Several cases of poisoning having occurred in Hamburgh some years since, in persons who had taken supposed angustura, the specimens were found to differ altogether from the genuine bark. The true nature of the adulteration was not ascertained, however, till the occurrence of a similar effect from a supposed rohun bark in Calcutta in 1835, led the Editor to discover that the false angustura was the bark of the Strychnos nux vomica. For a description of that bark, see *Strychnos*.

Med. use. The experience of European physicians corroborates to a great extent Dr. Hancock's statements of the effects of this bark in South America. It acts as a powerful aromatic bitter, is also tonic and stimulant, and seems of great utility in the latter stages of continued fever. There is however no evidence to shew that it has any antiperiodic virtues even in the treatment of simple agues.

Dose. *Powder,* 5—20 grs. alone, or with rhubarb, lime, or carbonate of magnesia: of *Infusion,* one drachm in four ounces of water twice or thrice daily: of *Tincture,* one or two drs. in dyspepsia. Dr. Duncan quotes the statement of Humboldt that the Catalonian Capuchins in South America prepare an extract of the bark for use in their convents, but he doubts its efficacy. A fermented infusion is also made, and much esteemed in the treatment of rheumatism and fevers.

These facts are worth the attention of the student. Although the Galipea is not indigenous, it is more than probable that similar virtues may be found in the bark of some of the Indian species of this order.

A bark called *Malambo* is found in Colombia, and is possessed of strong bitter and aromatic properties; it is supposed by Bonpland to belong to a Galipea, or some allied plant.

Two species of *Ticorea*, natives of South America, are quoted also by Lindley as being possessed of similar properties in a very high degree.

The *Evodia febrifuga* (Essenbeckia feb :) is also a native of Brazil, and much valued in the treatment of fevers.

Gen. 3.—Barosma.

Sp. Barosma crenulata, (Buchn.)

Syn. Diosma crenulata.

Off. The leaves.

A small shrub, a native of the Cape of Good Hope.

Leaves elliptical, lanceolate, margin finely serrated and glandular, upper surface smooth, and of a clear shining green, inferior surface paler and beset with scattered glandular points, translucent when held between the eye and the light, (Duncan); odour and taste mint-like and very strong, but neither bitter nor astringent.

According to the experiments of M. Cadet de Gassicourt, the leaves contain in 100 parts,

Essential oil, ...	0.665
Gum, ...	21.17
Aqueous and alcoholic extract, ...	5.170
Chlorophylle, ...	1.100
Resin, ...	2.151

The rest being woody fibre.

Med. use. A powerful diuretic, and an admirable remedy in many diseases of the urinary organs, especially the irritable state of the bladder which frequently follows gonorrhœa. An infusion of half an ounce of the dried leaves to a pint of water may be taken daily.

Several other species of Barosma are found at the Cape, but none have yet been discovered in any part of India.

NAT. ORDER XLI.—XANTHOXYLACEÆ.

This family, which contains some very important articles, is chiefly indigenous in tropical Asia and America, but several are found in India, especially in the lower hilly regions. They resemble the orange tribe in many of their parts, especially the leaves and fruit, being provided with vesicles of essential oil, to which many of them owe their great pungency. In one of the order, a bitter principle called Xanthopicrite has been detected.

Gen. 1.—Xanthoxylon.

Generic characters—Diæcious, calyx short, 3, 4, 5, partite petals, as many and longer than the sepals, very rarely wanting. *Male*,—stamens as many as the petals, equal to or longer than them, inserted round the base of the gynophore; pistillum rudimentary, simple, or compound. *Female*,—stamens usually wanting, sometimes very short, and either with or without abortive anthers; ovaries (1—5) as many as the petals, or fewer, seated on a globose or cylindrical gynophore, ovules two in each, all suspended, collateral; styles 1, from the apex of each ovary, either distinct or united at the apex, sometimes very short, or scarcely any; capsules 1—5, sessile or stalked on the gynophore (receptacle), 2 valved, 1, 2 seeded, seeds when solitary globose, when in pairs hemispherical, shining and black, embryo straight or slightly curved.

Trees or shrubs, with prickles usually on the branches, petioles, and nerves of the leaves; leaves usually pellucid, dotted, alternate, or opposite, simple, ternate, or pinnated, either with or without an odd one, flowers small, inflorescence axillary or terminal, various. W. and A.

Sp. 1. *Xanthoxylum alatum.* (Roxb. Fl. Ind. iii. 768.)
Vern. Durmur, *Hind.* (As. Res. vi. 378.)

A native of Nipal, and the hilly countries north of Bengal, Rohilcund, and Oude; flowering in Calcutta in the hot and rainy seasons.

Roxburgh states that every part of the plant possesses a peculiar aromatic pungency, and that the seeds are used medicinally by the natives.

Xanthoxylum Avicennæ, (Fagura A.) a native of China, is a powerful stimulant, and used as an antidote against poisons. X. *fraxineum*, or prickly ash, a native of the United States, is much employed in North America in chronic rheumatism and as a local stimulant to secreting surfaces and ulcerating parts. X. *Clavis-Herculis*, (Hercules' club) is common in the West Indies, where its bark is much used in malignant ulcers, both internally and externally, and the tincture is reported by Dr. Gillespie to be a good stimulant and febrifuge. X. *piperitum* is a powerful aromatic, used by the Chinese in the room of ginger and pepper. The active principle resides chiefly in the fresh leaves, the dry bark, and the pericarp. The physicians of the country apply a poultice made of the bruised leaves and rice flour in sore throats.

For the preceding details we are indebted to Lindley's Flora Medica, p. 215. Royle further informs us, p. 157, that in India X. *Budrunga*, *Rhetsa*, *alatum*, and *hostile*, are used wherever indigenous for the warm, spicy, pepper-like pungency of their capsules, a property which is participated in by their bark and other parts. The capsules and seeds of X. hostile, called *tejbul* by the natives, are employed in Northern India for intoxicating fish, and chewed as a remedy in tooth ache. They are also described as the Fagureh of Avicenna.

We are indebted to MM. Chevallier and Pelletan for a description and analysis of the bark of the X. Clavis-Herculis of the Caribbean islands.

The bark is of variable size, with thick, wrinkled, and cracked epidermis, giving rise to pyramidal, short, sharp prickles with large bases. Colour rather yellow, cortical layers very yellow and greenish, readily split into flakes, and of irregular fracture. The bark evolves an odour resembling that of liquorice, its taste is strongly bitter and styptic, its powder yellow, and very difficult to prepare.

On analysis this bark yielded essential oil, acetate of ammonia, extractive matter, red and yellow colouring matter, and a crystalline principle *Xanthopicrite*.

Xanthopicrite is prepared by digesting the bark in alcohol, evaporating the tincture to the consistence of an extract, acting on the extract with water and ether in succession; the residue dissolved in boiling alcohol gives crystallized Xanthopicrite on cooling and evaporation. It is of a greenish yellow colour, very bitter taste, devoid of acid or alkaline properties, little soluble in water, insoluble in ether, but freely in alcohol, especially when heated. Nitric acid gives it a red colour.

Gen. 2.—Ptelea.

Sp. Ptelea trifoliata.

A native of the United States, has bitter and aromatic fruit and leaves; the fruit is used as a substitute for hops, the young shoots as an anthelmintic medicine.

Gen. 3.—Toddalia.

Sp. Toddalia aculeata.

Syn. Scopolia aculeata, Roxb. vol. i. 616.

Vern. Kaka toddali, *Rheede.* Conda cashinda, *Tel.*

This is one of the most common bushes on the coast of Coromandel.

The stem is irregular, bark corky, branches exceedingly numerous, climbing. Prickles innumerable, scattered over every part of the younger branches; tender shoots, petioles, and nerves of the leaflets recurved, very acute; leaves alternate, ternate, armed, leaflets oblong, or broad lanceolate, notched, emarginate, smooth, about an inch and a half long, and half or three-fourths broad; petioles channelled, armed like the branchlets, racemes axillary, generally compound, the length of the leaves; flowers small, white, calyx inferior, small, glandular, five-toothed, petals five, oblong, spreading. Filaments five, nearly as long as the petals, spreading, anthers oblong, incumbent; germ ovate, five-celled, with two ovula in each attached to the middle of the axis, style short, thick, stigma five-lobed, berry the size of a small cherry (half an inch in diameter,) compressed, five-grooved, orange coloured, five-celled; seed one in each cell. *(Roxb.)*

Dr. Roxburgh adds to the preceding description, that every part of this shrub has a strong pungent taste—the roots when fresh cut smell particularly so. The fresh leaves are eaten raw for pains in the bowels; the ripe berries are fully as pungent as black pepper, and with nearly the same kind of pungency; from these the natives prepare an excellent pickle.

The fresh bark of the root is administered by the Telinga physicians for the cure of that sort of remittent commonly called the "hill fever." Roxburgh says, "I conceive every part of this plant to be possessed of strong stimulating powers, and have no doubt, but that under proper management it might prove a valuable medicine where stimulants are required."

In the 4th vol. of the Journal de Pharmacie, p. 298, Dr. Virey gives an interesting notice of this article. In 1818 M. Bosc received from M. Hubert, a botanist of Bourbon, the bark of a shrub employed in the East Indies, Madagascar, Bourbon, and the Mauritius as a febrifuge substitute for cinchona. The bark was described as being rolled like the cinchona, covered by brown or drab epidermis, with points or patches of a yellow farinaceous colour. The inner bark was reddish brown, intensely bitter, sharp, and pepper-like, with a sweetish flavour resembling liquorice.

The bark of the Toddalia deserves most careful trial, and will in all probability be found a very valuable medicine.

GEN. 4.—BRUCEA.

Sp. Brucea sumatrana. Roxb. Fl. Ind. i. 449.

A native of Sumatra, the Moluccas, and Cochin China, successfully grown in the Botanic Garden of Calcutta. In one year the plants were about four feet high, with a straight ligneous stem, and few branches; they then began to flower in May, and continued to blossom and ripen their seed all the year.

Leaves scattered, unequally pinnate, from 12 to 18 inches long. Leaflets from 4 to 6 pair, opposite, short petioled, obliquely ovate, lanceolate, strongly and obtusely serrate, pointed, villous underneath, from three to six inches long, very bitter, and somewhat fœtid; petioles common, round, and villous; stipules none; racemes axillary, solitary, from one to six or eight inches long, somewhat compound, dark purple, and clothed with a few white hairs. Flowers numerous, very minute, dark purple, and in all the Sumatra plants hermaphrodite; bractes subulate, hairy, very small, and caducous; calyx four-leaved, or deeply four-parted, segments small, ovate, lanceolate, deep purple, hairy on the outside, and with the corols reflexed. Petals four, longer than the calyx, lanceolate, dark purple, and hairy on the outside, nectary a dark purple, 4 lobed, fleshy cup, surrounding the insertion of the germs; filaments 4, short, purple, inserted under the margin of the nectary; anthers oval, large, and deep purple till they discharge their pollen; germs 4, superior, one-celled, with one ovulum in each, attached to the upper and inner side of the cell; styles single, short, recurved, one to each germ, stigmas simple; drupes four when all come to maturity, size of a small grain of black pepper, smooth, dark purple, one-celled; nut conform to the drupe, rugose, one-celled, inner edge thinner, and the upper half marked with a white line. *(Roxb.)*

The Wooginoos of Abyssinia (Brucea antidysenterica) is considered in that country a most valuable remedy in dysentery, and severe cases of diarrhœa. The false angustura bark was long supposed to be the produce of this Brucea, and its active principle was accordingly named *Brucine*. It is now however established that the false angustura bark is that of the strychnos, nux-vomica, (*Kuchila* tree of Bengal.)

NAT. ORDER XLII.—SIMARUBEÆ.

This order is exclusively intertropical; their leaves are alternate, pinnate, and destitute of stipulæ. All the members of the order are extremely bitter, and the bitterness pervades their entire structure.

Gen. 1.—Quassia.

Sp. 1. *Quassia amara*, Bitter quassia.

Off. The wood.

A native of Surinam, Guiana, Colombia, and Panama, and recently introduced into Bengal by Lord Auckland. It thrives tolerably well in the Calcutta Garden.

The flowers are hermaphrodite, large, scarlet, distant; pedicels bracteate at the base, pointed below the apex, calyx short, five-parted; racemes long, one-sided, simple, terminal, rarely branched; petals five, much longer, arranged in a tubular form. Stamens ten, much longer than the petals; ovaries five, placed on a receptacle broader than themselves. Styles the same number, distinct at the base, thence united into one very long one, terminating in a nearly equal five-furrowed stigma. The leaves are alternate, unequally pinnate, leaflets in two pairs, opposite, entire, smooth, elliptical, acute at each end; petiole winged, jointed, with the joints obovate. The wood is imported in large thick billets, it is light, white, solid, hard, and tough, smooth; the bark thin, pale, smooth, with black stains, brittle, and very slightly adherent. It is devoid of odour, but excessively bitter.

The bitterness is due to the presence of a principle named *quassite*, which is thus procured in the separate state. The sliced wood is boiled in water, and the filtered decoction evaporated to $\frac{1}{4}$ its bulk; on cooling this is mixed with lime water, and the mixture frequently shaken for 24 hours; pectin and some other substances are thus separated; the filtered solution is next evaporated to dryness, and the residue treated with alcohol at 831. This dissolves the quassite, and some saline and colouring matter. On evaporating this to dryness and washing it with ether, the pure quassite is obtained in small, white, prismatic crystals, of extreme bitterness. 100 parts of cold water only dissolve 0·45 of this substance: strong and hot alcohol dissolves it freely. It is but little affected by sulphuric ether. Quassite is quite neutral and anhydrous, and consists of carb. 10 at. hy. 6. ox. 3.

Med. uses. Quassia wood is a very pure and simple bitter, and has been much employed in bilious and intermittent fevers, dropsies from debility, atonic gout, and indeed in all cases in which bitter tonics are advisable. The English brewers use it freely as a substitute for hops, although it is thought to have some degree of narcotic power, a decoction of quassia being much used as a poison for flies.

Quassia is very difficultly reduced to powder, and is consequently given in the forms of extract, tincture, infusion, and decoction. (*See these preparations.*)

Sp. 2. Quassia Simaruba, Bitter, or mountain damson.

Syn. Simaruba amara, *Lindley.*

Off. The bark.

A native of Guiana, Cayenne, and Jamaica; a tree with long horizontal creeping root, and a trunk 60 feet high, and branched at the summit. The bark of the root and stem yield a milky juice. The Simaruba of the shops is the bark of the root, and is imported into England in pieces some feet long, folded lengthwise. It is light, fibrous, tough, of a pale yellow colour internally, dark coloured, rough, scaly and warty externally. The bark has but little odour, and its taste is bitter, though not unpleasant.

According to Morin's analysis this bark contains resin, volatile oil, acetate of potash, malic and gallic acids, quassine, woody fibre, and other unimportant constituents. Water and spirit extract the useful parts, and the watery infusion is found to be the best of the pharmaceutical preparations.

The medical uses of Simaruba are the same as those described in the last article. Dr. Duncan recommends a decoction of two drs. of the bark in 2 lbs. of water (boiled down to one) to be drunk in cupsful thrice daily; we would prefer an infusion prepared with one pound of hot water, allowed to cool, and then strained.

Gen. 2.—Picræna.

Sp. Picræna excelsa, Lindley's Fl. Med. p. 208.

This is the tree called Quassia excelsa and Simaruba excelsa by many pharmaceutical writers; it is a native of Jamaica, its timber is intensely bitter, and furnishes the greater part of the chips sold as quassia by European druggists.

Gen. 3.—Nima.

Sp. Nima quassioides, (Hamilton.)

Syn. Simaba quassioides, Don.

A native of the Himalayas, discovered in Nipal by Dr. Hamilton, and stated by Dr. Royle to exist in Turanda, on the banks of the Sutledge, in more than 31° of N. latitude. Dr. Royle has also met with it in valleys in Gurhwahl.

In general appearance and intense bitterness this tree is too closely allied to the Simarubeæ to permit their separation. There are still several important specific differences in structure—the stamens are five, flowers polygamous, ovaries five and single ovuled, the petals erect, and of a greenish colour.

The wood of this tree is light coloured and very bitter, and although it has not as yet been subjected to experiment, we are led from analogy to entertain the most confident opinion of its proving a perfect substitute for the West Indian article.

NAT. ORDER XLIII.—OCHNACEÆ.

Of this small family Dr. Royle observes, they possess but little sensible properties, but that little is of a bitter and rather astringent nature, so that some of the species are employed as tonics.

The only species we need notice, is *Gomphia angustifolia*, a native of Ceylon and the continent of India. The root and leaves are bitter. It is employed in Malabar in decoction, in milk, or water, as a tonic, stomachic, and antiemetic.

NAT. ORDER XLIV.—SPONDIACEÆ.

Gen.—Spondias.

Sp. Spondias mangifera.

Vern. Amarataca, As. Res. iv. 284. Amra, *Hind.* and *Beng.*

The tree when wounded, yields large quantities of a mild insipid gum. The fruit is eaten raw when ripe, and while unripe is used in tarts, pickles, and curries.

NAT. ORDER XLV.—CORIARACEÆ.

The *Coriaria nipalensis* (Vern. *Mussooree)* has, from its abundance, bestowed its name on that well known hill station in the Himalayas. It is also common in Nipal. The fruit formed by the junction of several pistils is eaten in the hills, although that of the European species is poisonous, inducing narcotism and tetanus. The leaves of Coriaria myrtifolia have been used in France for the adulteration of senna, and have occasioned some fatal accidents. All parts of these plants are very rich in the astringent acids, and are consequently much employed by dyers.

With the preceding Order terminates the First Sub-class of the Dicotyledoneæ. We now proceed to

Sub-class 2—Calycifloræ.

Petals many, distinct, or united at base, with the stamens inserted into the calyx.

NAT. ORDER XLVI.—CELASTRINEÆ.

In this order Decandolle includes the Ilicineæ of Brogniart, and the Staphylaceæ of Lindley.

Mr. Royle informs us that the properties of this Order have not been much investigated, but an acrid principle has been detected in some species, and the seeds of several yield oil fit for burning.

Gen. 1.—Elæodendron.

Sp. Elæodendron Roxburghii.

Syn. Neerija dichotoma (Roxb. Fl. Ind. i. 646.)

A native of the mountainous parts of India. The fresh bark of the root rubbed with plain water is applied by the natives to almost every kind of swelling; it is a very strong astringent, possessing scarcely any other sensible quality. (*Roxb.*)

Gen. 2.—Celastrus.

Sp. Celastrus paniculatus.

Syn. C. nutans, Roxb.

Vern. Malkungee.

A native of the Circar mountains and Mysore; from the seeds an empyreumatic black oily fluid is distilled, of the uses of which in medicine Mr. Malcolmson has given an interesting account in his excellent work on Beriberi and rheumatism.

It is administered in doses of a few drops daily in emulsions, and seems to exercise a decidedly beneficial effect.

For a specimen of this liquid we are indebted to Mr. Malcolmson. It does not differ in any sensible degree from the empyreumatic products of the distillation of the common fixed oils, containing naptha and other carburets of hydrogen. Large quantities would doubtless yield paraffine and creosote.

Gen. 3.—Maytenus.

Sp. Maytenus chilensis.

A small tree, a native of Chili. The young branches boiled with water afford a wash which is used for the swellings said to be occasioned by exposure to the vapours of a tree called Lithi. In Birmah and Cochin China analogous effects are caused by the varnish trees, and in India by the fumes of the heated "marking nut," or Ballataka.

NAT. ORDER XLVII.—AQUIFOLIACEÆ.

Gen. Ilex.

Sp. 1. *Ilex Aquifolium*, (Holly).

A lovely evergreen, common in most parts of Europe.

The leaves and bark of the holly tree have been warmly praised by Dr. Rousseau as remedies in intermittent fever; the root and bark are moreover said to be emollient and diuretic.

Ilex dipyræna is common at Mussooree and every where in the Himalayas, bearing a very close resemblance to the holly, especially in November and December, when it is covered with clusters of scarlet berries. Another lofty species, *Ilex serrata*, is also found in Mussooree, and *I. excelsa* in Nipal, (Royle, Illust. p. 167.)

Ilex vomitoria, a native of Florida and Carolina, near the sea, is used in a strong decoction, called black drink, by the Creek Indians at the opening of their councils. It acts as a mild emetic, and produces a cheerful intoxication.

Ilex paraguariensis affords the dried leaves celebrated under the name of the Paraguay tea.

Gen. 2.—Myginda.

Sp. Myginda Uragoga, Carthagena—a decoction or infusion of the root is a most powerful diuretic.

Gen. 3.—Prinos.

Sp. Prinos verticillatus, Black Alder. A native of the United States. The bark is considered a valuable tonic in great debility accompanied by fever, and especially in incipient sphacelus or gangrene. Bigelow states that the berries are emetic.

Gen. 4.—Euonymus.

Sp. Euonymus tingens. The bark is in the inside of a fine yellow colour, similar to that of Rhamnus. It is used to mark the *Tika* on the forehead of the Hindus, and is considered by the natives to be useful in diseases of the eye. *(Royle.)*

NAT. ORDER XLVIII.—RHAMNEÆ.

This order is very generally distributed, but few of its species possess any properties available in medicine.

The *Zizyphus Lotus*, a native of Africa. This is the tree celebrated in ancient poetry as the Arbor Lotophagorum, the fruits of which were said by Homer to be as sweet as honey, and when eaten to destroy the love of country. The fruits, Polybius states, constituted the staple food of the districts in which they grew, and also yielded a delicious wine.

GEN. 1.—ZIZYPHUS.

Sp. 1. *Zizyphus Œnoplia.*

Syn. Z. Napeca, Roxb. Flora Ind. i. p. 13.

Common all over India, fruit eaten by the natives, its taste being pleasantly acid. A decoction of the bark of the fresh root is said to promote the healing of recent wounds. *Roxb.*

Sp. 2. *Z. Jujuba.*

Syn. Rhamnus Jujuba.

Vern. Vadari, *Sans.* Usslie Suddir, *Arab.* Kool, *Bengalee.*

A small tree, a native of various parts of the East Indies and China, and common in gardens, where by grafting and cultivation it affords a large and very pleasant fruit called *Ber.* In Hindostan it is called *Berree* and *Jaree*, in Persia *Kinar* and *Kial*, in Arabia *Nebbek* and *Sidr.* Mr. Royle mentions that the fruit of the wild kind is dried and powdered, as was done with the lotus of the Lotophagi. This powder in Arabic is called *Suve koon nebek*, in Persian *Arud i kinar*, in Hindee *Ber choonee.* A lac insect inhabits the latter kind, and its produce is used for dyeing leather, cotton, and silk. The bark is used in the Moluccas as a remedy for diarrhœa; the root with some warm seeds in infusion in fever. The lozenges, and thickened mucilage called *jujubes* by the confectioners, are prepared from this and the Z. vulgaris, a native of Syria, Persia, and Hindostan. *Royle's Illustr.* p. 170.

A variety with long fruit, described by Dr. Wallich, is called in Bengal *Narikeli kool.*

GEN. 2.—RHAMNUS.

Sp. Rhamnus catharticus. Buckthorn.

Hedges and woods in Europe—having globular, bluish black, nauseous berries, with four cells, and as many seeds; the unripe berries are used as a yellow dye, and the expressed juice evaporated to dryness with lime water or soda forms the pigment called "sap," or "bladder green." The fruits are violently cathartic; 15 or 20 causing abundant evacuations. The operation is however usually attended with colic, dryness of the mouth and fauces, and oppressive sickness.

A syrup is officinal in the London Pharmacopœia, but neither this nor the berry are any longer used by regular practitioners.

R. frangula, or black alder, has emetic fruit.

R. infectoria, a native of the South of Europe. The unripe fruit is dried and sold under the name of "French berries," or "graines d' Avignon," and is used for dyeing leather yellow.

Gen. 3.—Berchemia.

Berchemia volubilis, or *Œnoplia volubilis*, occurs in Carolina and Virginia; the roots are prescribed in cachectic disorders, and said to be antisyphilitic.

Gen. 4.—Ceanothus.

Ceanothus americanus, United States of America. An infusion of the astringent twigs is given in gonorrhœa.

In the three following orders, Samydaceæ, Homolineæ, and Chailletiaceæ, there is no article requiring notice in this work.

NAT. ORDER XLIX.—AQUILARINEÆ.

This order is remarkable for yielding at least one kind of the celebrated Agallochum wood of the ancients.

Gen.—Aquilaria.

Sp. 1. *Aquilaria Agallocha*, aloe or eagle wood. *Roxb. Fl. Ind.* ii. 422.

Vern. Ugooro, *Sans.* Aquloogin, *Arab.* Aood-Hindee, *Pers.*

Roxburgh describes this as an immense tree, a native of the mountainous tracts E. and SE. from Sylhet, lat. 24° to 25° N. flowering in April, and ripening its seed in August. He regarded the tree as that which furnished the real Calambac or Agallochum of the ancients; in this opinion Dr. Royle coincides, and he adduces much valuable evidence in its support; at the same time that he admits that a wood of similar properties may be afforded by other trees, especially the Aloexylum agallochum of Loureiro, referred by Decandolle to the Leguminosæ. A kind of aloe wood is moreover produced by the Excæcaria agallochum, of the natural order of Euphorbiacæ. A third kind is imported from Malacca and Siam.

In Persian works, three kinds are described under the names of *Aood-i-sumudree, Aood-i-Hindee, Aood-i-kimaree,* probably the Al-cemericum of Aboo Hanifa. (*Royle.*)

Dr. Roxburgh mentions his having received plants from Malacca of the supposed eagle tree, and that they were in a flourishing condition; Dr. Hamilton met the plant near Goalpara, and Dr. Roxburgh also obtained it from Sylhet.

The chief consumption of aloe wood is in Siam and China, where it is burned in the temples. Merat and De Lens inform us it was used in Napoleon's imperial palaces as incense.

The wood is heavy, yellowish white, shaded with green, fibrous, spongy, and resinous, its taste aromatic, its odour in combustion very agreeable.

It is popularly believed that the secretion of the fragrant principle of this wood is the effect of disease. Dr. Ainslie states, on the authority of Mr. Colebrooke, that it is not until the tree has been long cut down, and allowed to decay and rot, that the wood acquires its proper fragrance, to hasten which it is for a time buried under ground; on being dug up again so much of it is selected as is dark and glossy and sinks in water; this is called *Ghark;* such as sinks partially is called *Nim ghark*, and what floats *Semeleh.*

We have met with no chemical examination of this substance. It is procurable in small quantities, and at a high price, in most of the Bazars of Bengal.

Celsus recommended this Agallochum as a tonic stimulant, and it has been used in Europe in gout and rheumatism. In Cochin China it is given in vertigo and palsies, and as a stimulant astringent in diarrhœa and vomiting. (*Ainslie*, vol. i. p. 480.)

In the articles Leguminosæ and Euphorbiaceæ some additional particulars are given relative to this celebrated substance.

NAT. ORDER L.—TEREBINTHACEÆ.

This very important and extensive family has been recently sub-divided into several groups, formed of trees, bushes, or shrubs, exuding resinous, gummy, or milky juices. The leaves are alternate, simple, ternate or pinnate, destitute of stipules, the inflorescence terminal or axillary, the pericarp frequently full of resinous or caustic juice.

This family is sub-divided into several groups, the most remarkable being the Anacardiaceæ, (marking nut tribe); the

Sumachs; the Burseraceæ; the Amyrideæ; the Pteleaceæ; and the Connaraceæ. All these groups are interesting, and differ very little in chemical constitution. The principles found in all are, fixed oil in the almond; essential oil, combined with resin in the turpentine of the pistachios; resin which flows abundantly, and either by natural or artificial processes from the trunk of nearly all the species; gum usually combined with resin as in incense, myrrh, and tacamahaca; besides these some deleterious principles have been discovered in particular species, which we shall subsequently notice in detail. (*Feé*, vol. i. p. 619.)

Tribe 1—Anacardiaceæ.

These are resiniferous or turpentine-producing trees. The resinous juice seems distributed in all their parts, but most abundantly in the bark; the fruit of some contain in the envelope an acrid, caustic, and almost corrosive juice, generally of a black colour. The almond is sweet, and contains a fixed oil like that of other oleaginous seeds. The peduncle is sometimes fleshy and eatable. The majority of these trees occur in South America, some are found in India, some in Africa, and a few in Europe.

Gen. 1.—Odina.

Sp. Odina wodier.

Vern. Ajasringha, *Sans.* Jewul, *Beng.* Cushmula, *Hind.*

A gum resin exudes from the bark, which in upper India is called *Jingun* and *Kineh-ke-goond.* Dr. Ainslie gives the latter as the synonyme of galbanum.

Gen. 2.—Pistacia.

Sp. 1. *Pistacia vera.* (Pistachio tree).

A native of the south of Europe and of Asia. According to Mr. Elphinstone it grows wild in the Hindu-kosh. The almond and pericarp are imported into India from Cabul, with a kind of gall termed *Gool-i-pista*, and a resin called *Alook-ul-imbat.* (*Royle's Illustrat.*, p. 178). The fruit (a drupe) is dry, oval, oblong, oblique, wrinkled, of ashy green colour, the nut bony, glabrous, white, with a spongy stain at the base; the almond pale green, covered with a white or brownish perisperm. The odour of the pericarp is resinous, and slightly balsamic, its taste bitter and resinous; the flavour of the almond is sweet and oily.

By expression these almonds yield a greenish, rather aromatic oil, which readily turns rancid; owing to the presence of this oil the pistachio has been much used in emulsions and cough mixtures; the chief consumption of the pistachio is however as an article of food or confectionary.

Sp. 2. ***Pistacia Terebinthus.***

Syn. Pist. vera. Terebinthus vulgaris.

Vern. Katinge Roomie, ***Arab.*** Zungbarie, ***Persian.*** Butum, ***Arab.*** Sukhur, ***Pers.*** (Royle.)

A native of Barbary, Greece, and the south of France. The trunk is lofty, leaves composed of 7—9, oblong, oval leaflets, green and shining above, the petiole enlarged, flowers small, dioiceous, in axillary panicles; stamina purple; fruits (drupes) dry, globular, and small. A resinous juice of much value is afforded by this tree and called,

Chian Turpentine.

This substance is found in commerce of thick consistence, yellowish white colour, pellucid and tenacious; its odour is strong, peculiar, and agreeable, its flavour slightly bitter; by keeping it loses its essential oil and becomes hard.

Ten parts of this turpentine afford about one of essential oil, and leave in the retort a resin similar to that obtained from other turpentines.

The Chian turpentine has been used in medicine since the days of Hippocrates, and is employed in Turkey, Persia, and the East generally as a masticatory to sweeten the breath, and preserve the teeth.

In the hot season this juice flows naturally, but in small quantities, from the tree. At first it is very fluid, but it thickens on exposure to the air. To obtain it more abundantly transverse incisions are made in the trunk and branches. To purify it, it is pressed through baskets made of willow twigs. The largest trees, it is stated, do not yield more than a troy pound of the juice; the total produce in Chio consequently scarcely exceeds one thousand pounds.

A gall forms on this tree, containing a clear and fluid turpentine, in which the larvæ of an insect exist as their natural element; the purest turpentine is indeed obtained by crushing these young galls and filtering the juice.

Sp. 3. Pistacia Lentiscus, (Mastic tree).

A native of the south of Europe, and of Asia Minor, introduced into the Calcutta Garden in 1806. The trunk is of middling size, about 15 feet high when full grown, divided into numerous twisted branches, the leaves winged, composed of 8—10 leaflets, lanceolate, hard, persistent, of deeper green on the upper than the lower surface; male flowers small, racemiform, very close, stamina with purple anthers; female flowers also racemiform, in those spikes, fruit rounded, blackish or brown when ripe.

The bark, buds, leaves, and fruit have all been used in medicine, but have been laid aside in modern times.

Mastic Resin.

Vern. Roomie mastike, *Arab.* Sakes, *Turkish.* Kinnoli, *Pers.* Koondur Roomee, or Turkish olibanum.

Manna of Lebanon. *Ulmastiga*, Spanish.

This valuable substance occurs in oval tears of variable size, smooth, diaphanous, brittle, breaking with plane brilliant, glassy, and pale yellow surfaces, and owing to its brittleness being usually covered with its own dust. Its odour is agreeable; flavour weakly balsamic; it softens in the mouth, and becomes ductile like white wax. It melts at a moderate heat, and then exhales a sweet odour.

Mastic is quite insoluble in water, it yields to alcohol 80 per 100 of soluble matter, leaving a substance resembling caoutchouc, which is slowly dissolved by ether.

This resin gives its name to the process of *mastication*, being universally chewed in the East; it is much used by dentists for filling up carious teeth; it is burned as incense; and in some parts of Greece it is added to bread in small quantities to give it an agreeable flavour. Mastic is extensively employed as a transparent varnish, dissolved in turpentine or alcohol, with other resinous bodies.

A species of mastic called *tum* is obtained in Africa from the Pistacia Atalantica. The true resin is sold in all the Bazars for about three rupees the seer.

Gen. 3.—Semecarpus.

Flowers polygamous, dioiceous, calyx five-cleft, petals five, inserted under the margin of the disk, sessile, very spreading, æstivation imbricate, stamens five, inserted under the margin of the disk, equal, distinct. Disk cup-shaped, ovary free, sessile, one-celled, styles three, stigma clavate, retuse. Fruit somewhat cordate, sessile on the enlarged receptacle, seed suspended, cotyledons thick, fleshy, plano-convex, radicle superior, minute, concealed within the apex of the cotyledons. (*Lindley.*)

Sp. 1. *Semecarpus Anacardium*, (Marking nut, Malacca bean.)

Syn. Anacardium orientale, Ανακαρδιον Ξανθοβάλανος, Galen.

Vern. Belawine, *Duk.* Belader, *Arab.* Bhela, *Duk.* Bhalataka or Arushkara, *Sans.*

A tree bearing male or hermaphrodite flowers on some, and hermaphrodite on others; a native of all the mountainous parts of India, flowers from May to August, seed ripening in January and February.

Trunk straight, covered with grey scabrous bark; bark of the younger parts smooth, light ash-coloured, its inner surface and crevices containing much insipid gum; branchlets numerous, spreading, leaves at the extremities alternate, stalked, somewhat wedge-shaped or oblong ovate, rounded at the apex, entire, firm above, pretty smooth, yet harsh and whitish beneath, from 9 to 18 inches long, and from 4 to 8 broad; petioles 1½ inches long, half round; panicles terminal, very large, composed of many simple spikes; that of the male tree much more slender, but as large and larger or branched. Bractes many, small and deciduous; flowers numerous, small, of a dull greenish yellow colour. Receptacle erect, fleshy; pear-shaped, smooth, when ripe yellow, about the size of the nut; fruit a single nut resting upon the receptacle, cordate, flattened on both sides, smooth, shining, black, the pericarp composed of two lamina, the inner one hard, the outer less so and leathery; between these are cells which contain a black, corrosive resinous juice. The juice is of a pale milk colour till perfectly ripe, when it becomes black, when dry it has all the appearance of a bitumen, being brittle, translucent, and very inflammable. Male flowers on a separate tree, smaller than on the hermaphrodite, filaments five, the length of the petals, anthers much larger than in the hermaphrodite; pistil none, or small or abortive, and in form of a semiglobular, hairy, glandular body. (*Roxb.*)

Roxburgh gives an excellent description of this tree. He says the wood is soft, and contains so much acrid juice that it is dangerous to work on. The fleshy receptacle on which the seeds rest is roasted and eaten, and tastes very like roasted apples; the kernels are rarely eaten.

The pure black acrid juice is employed by the natives externally to remove rheumatic pains, aches, and sprains; a little is rubbed over the part affected. But in tender constitutions it often produces inflammation and swelling. It is universally employed for marking cotton cloth, the colour being improved and prevented from running by its being mixed with lime water.

The juice is not soluble in water, and is not diffusible in spirits of wine, unless this solvent be previously rendered alkaline by ammonia or potash.

It unites perfectly with oils. Dr. Roxburgh further adds that the Telingee physicians use it nearly in all kinds of venereal affections, in a formula which he describes.*

The bark is mildly astringent, and gives various shades of brown dye. A brown gum exudes from the bark, but is of little value. Ainslie adds that the Hindus generally deem it a valuable medicine in scrofulous, venereal, and leprous affections. By boiling the nut an oil is prepared, which when undiluted acts as a blister. The vapours arising from the nuts during roasting have been often known to occasion erysipelatous inflammation.

A minute drop of the juice placed on the back of the hand, occasioned in the Editor of this work the eruption of an herpetic blotch, intensely itchy, and scaling from the centre towards the circumference, which did not disappear for eight months, and left a scar like that of a burn.

Gen. 4.—Anacardium.

Sp. 1. ***Anacardium occidentale.*** (Cashew tree.)

Vern. Hidgelee badam, *Hind.* and *Beng.*

A tree common in the East and West Indies. In Bengal found chiefly near the sea, and in perfectly sandy soils. Flowering time, March and April.

Trunk short, thick, and very crooked, bark considerably rough, and in old trees deeply cracked; branches numerous, very spreading, young shoots round and smooth, leaves alternate, rather short, petioled, obovate, with a rounded emarginate apex, smooth on both sides, and of a hard texture, from 4 to 8 inches long. Panicles terminal, bearing both barren and fertile hermaphrodite flowers, intimately intermixed, small and of the same size and external appearance. There may be trees which produce barren flowers only. Bractes gibbous, lanceolate, calyx inferior, 5-cleft nearly to the base, divisions oblong, conic, acute, and pretty smooth.

* *Take of the black balsam,* and expressed juice of garlic aa. ℥i.
Tamarind tree leaves, cocoanut oil, sugar .... aa. ℥ij.
Mix and boil for a few minutes. A table spoonful is given twice daily.

Petals 5 linear, lanceolate, revolute, of a pale yellow colour, with longitudinal pink stripes. Filaments generally nine, united at the base, entwining round the germ, one of them, particularly in the sterile flowers, more than double the length of the others. Anthers appear to be all fertile, that of the major filament larger, germ in the barren flowers minute, with a very short style, in the fertile flowers obliquely obcordate, one-celled, with one reniform seed attached to the side of its cell; style long, becoming convolute, as if to bring the simple stigma in contact with the large anther of the long filament. *Roxb.*

The fruit is kidney-shaped, smooth, grey, coriaceous, somewhat compressed, about an inch long; the pericarp contains between its outer and inner layer abundance of a black resinous juice of the same properties as that of the last article; the almond is white, and of agreeable flavour. The fruit is attached by its larger extremity to a fleshy, oval, succulent peduncle, the size of an ordinary pear.

The black balsam of this fruit is used for the same purposes as that of the preceding article. The peduncle, or cashew apple, is slightly acrid, but not disagreeable; by fermentation it yields alcohol.

A deep brown gum exudes from the trunk and branches, said to consist chiefly of bassorine, common gum, and gallic acid. It swells to a considerable size, but does not dissolve in water.

Under the head of Anacardiaceæ, Lindley includes the celebrated mango tree, *Mangifera indica*—the *Holigarna longifolia, Roxb. Fl. Ind.* ii. p. 80, one of the trees yielding the well known black lacquer varnish—several species of *Rhus* which we notice under the next head—the *Heudelotia africana*, or African B'dellium tree—the *Stagmaria verniciflua*, one of the black varnish trees of China—two South American species of *Schinus*—and, lastly, the *Comocladia dentata* of Cuba, remarkable for a milky corrosive juice which turns to a fixed black colour.

Tribe 2—Sumachineæ.

Trees or shrubs, with alternate leaves, often compound, oddly pinnate, with panicles more or less loose, generally axillary. A tenacious transparent gum exudes from the trunk; the bark, leaves, and fruits, contain tannic and gallic acid; several species are poisonous; the fruits of a few are however eaten in some countries; many species occur in India, chiefly in hilly districts.

GEN.—RHUS.

Sp. 1. *Rhus Coriaria*, Sumac.
Vern. Shumuk, *Pers.* Tumtum, *Arab.*

A native of Persia, Syria, Palestine, and the south of Europe, about 8 or 10 feet high, divided into numerous irregular branches; bark covered with a russet down, especially in young trees; wood soft, leaves alternate, winged, with 15 to 20 leaflets, oval, sessile, with obtuse teeth; flowers yellowish white; fruits grape-like in arrangement, and covered with russet down.

All parts of this plant are inodorous, but have a styptic taste; to the abundance of tannic acid it owes its properties and value in the arts; M. Tromsdorf has found in the berries a large quantity of bi-malate of lime.

Sp. 2. *Rhus Toxicodendron*, Poison oak.
Off. The *leaves.*

A creeping shrub with long roots and woody branches, covered with brown bark; the leaves have petiolated leaflets, with angular teeth, flowers greenish.

This plant is destitute of odour, but has an acrid and corrosive taste; from wounds in the bark, or from a broken leaf, a white milky juice exudes of excessive acridity, which by contact with the skin occasions obstinate and troublesome pustular eruptions.

The leaf of the Poison oak has been used by Dr. Hull and M. Fresnœ in the treatment of paralysis and rheumatism, and with apparent success, the first symptom of amendment being a sensation of pricking in the affected parts; half a grain to one grain was the dose employed, and repeated thrice daily. Dr. Duncan used it in larger doses, and found that in general it operated as a gentle laxative; of its antiparalytic virtues he gives a favourable opinion.

Sp. 3. *Rhus Kakrasingee.* (Royle.)

This plant has hornlike excrescences, formed probably by the deposition of the ova of some insect. It has long formed an article in the Hindoo Materia Medica. This species is found every where in the Doon, and the hills generally, at moderate elevations.

Tribe 3—Burseraceæ.

This is the most important group of the family. It is made up of trees, and resin-bearing shrubs; it furnishes turpentines and gum resins, most of which are objects of commercial value. No poisonous species has been found, and the products are so very like in all, that much confusion in their discrimination and reference has been the unavoidable result.

Gen. 1.—Boswellia.

Sp. Boswellia thurifera, Colebrooke, *As. Res.* xi. 317. xi. 158. Roxb. *Fl. Ind.* 383. Pereira, *Medical Gazette*, xx. 676.

Off. product, Male frankincense—λιβανος, Dioscorides. Olibanum.

Vern. Gunda barosa, Avul Kundoor, *Duk.* Looban, *Arab.* Koonder Zuchir, *Hind.*

A native of the mountainous tracts of Central India, and very common in the Shahabad country, from which we have obtained fine specimens of the resinous product, there called *sale gond*, or *sale lassa.* At Chandalgur it is termed *gunda biroza*, and in the dry state *sukka biroza.* Dr. Hamilton however thought the English Olibanum to be the produce of an Amyris, partly because he could not find that the sale resin was used as incense by the Hindoos.

The trunk is lofty, leaves oddly pinnate, and situated at the extremity of the branches; leaflets generally in 10 pairs, alternate, oblong, oblique, downy, toothed like a saw, flowers small, greenish, in axillary, erect spikes; fruit capsular, trivalvular and triangular; divisions of the calyx, petals, stamina, and fruit cells, variable in number.

Olibanum Resin.—Gunda Barosa.

The resin olibanum occurs in reddish or pale yellow tears, oval, oblong, and obtuse, sometimes in dense, opaque, brittle masses. The gunda barosa of the bazars is soft, ductile, opaque, greenish and white. The odour is balsamic and resinous, especially while the resin is burning; the flavour balsamic, and rather bitter. The powder, citron yellow. It is frequently adulterated by dammar, sandarach, and other cheaper resins; when chewed the hard variety softens, and dissolves partially in the saliva, which it renders white and emulsive.

M. Braconnot has published an analysis of this resin, from which it appears to contain volatile oil 8, resin 59, gum 30, and gluten 5, per 100; it is not certain however whence the specimen examined was obtained.

The *Gunda barosa* contains much more volatile oil. A very fine specimen from Shahabad, presented to the editor by Mr. J. Allan, was found to consist of 28 parts volatile oil, 37 resin, 4 gum, 11 gluten, per 100.

The essential oil has a citron-like odour; the resin is described by M. Feé as much resembling pitch.

Olibanum, or incense, has been celebrated from the earliest ages, and used in nearly all the religious ceremonies of antiquity. In burning it diffuses a thick smoke of much fragrancy. Two kinds have been long distinguished,—the Arabian and the Indian; and it seems indeed certain that a similar resin is produced by different trees of this order.

In Europe olibanum is employed only in fumigations and plasters; in the moist state it is stimulant, astringent, and diaphoretic, and is often prescribed by the natives in emulsion, with butter and water, in chronic dysenteries and gonorrhœas.

Gen. 2.—Protium.

Sp. Protium gileadense.

Syn. Balsamodendron gileadense. Amyris gileadense. (Duncan's Dispensatory.)

A middle sized tree, a native of Arabia, Ethiopia, and the East Indies, introduced into the Calcutta Garden in 1798. The leaves are alternate with short petioles, and composed of three entire glabrous leaflets. M. Feé ascribes to this tree three distinct products,—Balsam of Mecca—a wood called Xylobalsamum—and fruits termed Carpobalsamum.

Balsam of Mecca, or Gilead.

Vern. Roghen bulsan, *Pers.*

A liquid resin of syrupy consistence, limpid, yellowish. By age it thickens and solidifies. The odour is like anise, and very penetrating; flavour aromatic, bitter and hot; it is almost always adulterated with turpentine, olive oil, or wax. According to Vauquelin's analysis, this balsam is soluble in alcohol, with the exception of a very minute residue.

Prosper Alpinus and his successors, describe three varieties of Mecca balsam; one, the most valuable, obtained by incisions; the second by a short boiling of the branches and leaves; the third, by prolonged decoction.

Tradition is rich in anecdotes relative to the origin of this balsam; the Mahomedans affirm that it sprung from the blood of the slain in Mahomet's conflict with the tribe of Harb, and that the Prophet used the balsam for the resuscitation of the dead. (Feé.) It is much used in medicine by the Hakims as a stimulant, tonic, and somewhat astringent remedy, and as an external application to indolent sores. It is also employed as a perfume and cosmetic.

The Opobalsamum and Carpobalsamum require no particular notice.

Sp. 2. ***Protium Kataf.*** (Lindley, Fl. Med. p. 171.)

Syn. Balsamodendron Myrrha (Nees von Esenbeck and Kunth.)

A middling sized tree, a native of Arabia, and chiefly of Gison, on the borders of Arabia Felix. It yields the celebrated gum resin, ***Myrrh.***

MYRRH.

Vern. Balintra bolum, *Tel.* Vola, *Sans.* Heera bol, *Duk.* Murr, *Arab.* Manisan lebah, *Malay.*

A solid gum resin, in fragments or tears, reddish, half transparent, smooth or wrinkled, sometimes brittle, fracture shining. Occasionally myrrh occurs in yellow, slightly translucent and milky tears. The odour is strong, disagreeable, and aromatic, taste bitter and hot; it softens in the mouth, and is partially dissolved. It is very much adulterated in commerce.

According to Brande's analysis, myrrh contains in 100 parts, volatile oil 2, resin 22, sub-resin 5, tragacanth 9, gum and saline matters 56. It dissolves very freely in alkalies; its specific gravity is 1,360.

Myrrh exudes like gum from the bark of the tree, in a soft oily state, but soon hardens by exposure to air.

Mr. Pereira informs us that it is imported into England from the East Indies, in chests containing each from one to two cwt. He has met three varieties; the first quality, which was formerly brought from Turkey is in tears, either distinct or conglomerated, usually covered with fine powder or dust. The colour is pale reddish yellow, red, or reddish brown; the pieces are brittle, resin transparent, with a fatty kind of fracture. Some of the pieces present marks like the white spots on the nails. The odour is aromatic and balsamic; taste bitter, acrid, and aromatic.

The second quality is in distinct small tears or grains, none larger than a pea. Mr. Pereira deems this variety to be a mixture of tears of myrrh with gum arabic, and mastic or juniper resin.

The third variety is what was called formerly *East Indian*. It occurs in dark pieces, the size of a walnut.

In 1819 Braconnot published an elaborate analysis of myrrh, in 100 parts of which he found 2.60 volatile oil, resin 27.80, gum 63.70, salts and impurities 2½. The volatile oil is colourless or slightly yellow, heavier than water, soluble in alcohol, ether, and the fixed oils. It distils over with water, but not with spirit; with sulphuric, nitric, and muriatic acids it forms red solutions. The resin is of two kinds, one odorous and soft at common temperatures, and soluble in ether; the other hard, inodorous, and insoluble in ether. The gummy matter is also twofold, one soluble, the other (Bassorine) insoluble in water.

Myrrh is consequently but partially soluble either in alcohol or water separately. The alcoholic tincture is rendered milky, but not precipitated by cooling. Myrrh is freely soluble in all the alkaline solutions.

Med. effects. These are tonic and stimulant, and vary in intensity according to the dose employed. It was long supposed to have emmenaguogue properties, but this is now discredited. In dyspepsia from debility, flatulency, amennorrhæa, and chlorosis, chronic catarrh, and gonorrhœa, or cystirhæa it is still much used, and often with great advantage. We have known it employed with excellent effects in the convalescence from fever. The best form we can recommend is that known as "Griffith's myrrh mixture," for the formula of which, see the Pharmacopœia. Myrrh is also much used in the form of tincture diluted with water, as a wash for the mouth and gums —as a gargle in ulcerated sore throat, and as an application to old, foul, and indolent ulcers.

Myrrh is given in substance in the form of powder, in doses of from five to ten grains, or even twenty. It is seldom however used alone, being generally combined with aloes, iron, galbanum, or rhubarb. Numerous formulæ for these preparations are given in the sequel of this work.

Gen. 3.—Icica.

Sp. Icica Icicariba.

Syn. Amyris elemifera.

A lofty tree, a native of South America, and which produces the elemi resin of the Pharmacopœia. This resembles olibanum so closely in all its properties and uses, that we deem it needless to describe it more minutely.

The I. heptaphylla, I. Aracouchini, I. Carana, and I. Tacamahaca, produce resinous exudations of value in the districts where the trees occur, but not entitled to detailed consideration here.

GEN. 4.—COMMIPHORA.

Sp. 1. *Commiphora Madagascarensis.* (*Lindl. Fl. Med.* 173.)

Syn. Amyris Commiphora, (*Roxb. Fl. Ind.* ii. 244.) Balsamodendron? Commiphora, (*Wight* and *Arnott Prod.* i. p. 96.)

A native of Sylhet, Assam, and Madagascar; it blossoms in the Botanic Garden of Calcutta about February and March, but seldom ripens its seed. The trunk of small trees is crooked, and clothed with many spreading and drooping crooked branches down to the ground; branchlets often crooked, with thorny points; leaves alternate, petioled, oval or elliptic, serrulate. At the base or apex of the petiole at each side is generally found a small leaflet, giving the whole the appearance of a ternate leaf. Flowers short, stalked, small, red, collected in little bundles on the small protuberant buds left by the former year's leaves, disk consisting of 8 glands, alternate with the insertion of the filaments, berry drupaceous, red, smooth, but two-celled, with a single seed in each cell, calyx four-toothed, petals four. Stamens eight, with eight glands alternating with the filaments.

The trunk is covered with a light pellicle, which peels off in layers like paper.

Roxburgh states that the whole plant while growing is considerably odoriferous, particularly when any part is broken or bruised, and diffuses a grateful fragrance, like that of the finest myrrh, to a considerable distance around; on wounding much pale coloured juice exudes from the bark, and Dr. Roxburgh thus collected a minute portion of gummy matter, resembling myrrh both in smell and appearance.

A resinous substance named *Googul,* (Hind.) *Mooql* (Arab) is met with in all the Bazars. It much resembles myrrh, and is said by some good authorities to constitute the bulk of the article exported from Bengal as East Indian myrrh. Royle considers the *Googul* identical with the Bdellium of commerce, and he ingeniously traces in *Budleyoon* and *Madelkon* (the Greek synonymes of Googul) the Βδελλιον and μαδελχον of Dioscorides. A tree in the Seharunpore Garden, pointed out as the Googul tree, had scaly bark exactly conformable to Roxburgh's description of his Amyris.

Bdellium. Dr. Ainslie, vol. i. p. 29, gives an excellent summary of all the information extant when his work was published, regarding this interesting substance. He adduces as synonymes, Bdellium, Kookool, *Tam.* Googooloo, *Tel.* Googula, *Cing.* Aflatoon, *Arab.* Mukul, *Pers.* Googul, *Hind.* He describes the gum resin as semi-pellucid, yellowish, or brown, inodorous and brittle, softening between the fingers, in appearance not unlike myrrh, of bitterish taste, and rather strong smell. He states however that it is all brought from Arabia and Persia, where the tree is called *Durukht mukul.* In the Bazars, it is said that the googul "comes from the Hills." (*Royle*, p. 177.)

The medicinal properties of Bdellium are exactly like those of myrrh, and as it is much cheaper, it may be preferred for Dispensary practice.

Gen. 5.—Canarium.

Sp. Canarium Bengalense. (*Roxb. Fl. Ind.* vol. iii. p. 136.) According to Roxburgh this is an immense forest tree, a native of Sylhet and the adjacent mountainous countries, and flowering in May and June. From fissures or wounds in the bark a large quantity of very pure, clear, amber-coloured resin exudes, which soon becomes hard and brittle, and is not unlike copal; yet the natives set little or no value on it. In the Calcutta Bazar it is only valued at from 2 to 3 Rs. for seven maunds of eighty pounds each. Roxburgh does not mention the native name of this resin.

Sp. 2. Canarium commune. (*Roxb. Fl. Ind.* vol. iii. p. 137.) A native of the continent of India, the Archipelago, and Isle of France, where it is called *Bois de colophane.* It was brought from the Moluccas to the Botanic Garden, but in Roxburgh's time did not thrive, owing to the coldness of the winter months. The bark yields an abundance of limpid oil with a pungent turpentine smell, congealing into a buttery camphoraceous mass, (*Lind. Fl. Med.* p. 170.) The writer adds, that it has the same properties as balsam of copaiba; and is said to yield East Indian elemi.

NAT. ORDER LI.—MORINGEÆ.

The fruit (legume) is about a foot long, pointed, opening by three long valves, filled while fresh with a fleshy pulp, seeds covered by a solid, brittle, grey perisperm, having three very large and half transparent wings. The almond is white, and contains so much oil that it exudes on compression between the fingers.

GEN.—MORINGA.

Sp. 1. *Moringa aptera.*

A native of Sennaar, Cairo, and Palestine. The seed yields the *oil* of *ben*, much used by perfumers and by watch makers, as it neither grows rancid nor freezes readily; seeds acrid, and used as a rubefacient. They are also said to be purgative and emetic in small quantities.

Sp. 2. *Moringa pterygosperma.*

Syn. Hyperanthera Moringa.

Vern. Sohunjuna, Moongay ke-jar ke-jur, *Duk.* Sujna, *Hind.* Sigroomala and Sobhanjuna, *Sans.* Sajna, *Beng.* Moriaben, *Pers.* Seeds, Hub-ool-ban of *Arabians.*

Commonly cultivated in India for leaves, flowers, and seed vessels, which are used in curries. The roots have precisely the flavour of horse-radish, and seem identical in chemical composition. Reduced to a pulp they afford an excellent external irritant. An oil is obtained from the seeds, possessed of the same qualities as that of the first species. It is said by Royle to be aperient, and much used by the natives as an unguent in gout and rheumatism. The seeds are also used internally by the native practitioners for their pungent and stimulating virtues.

The delicate perfumes of flowers are often retained by the ben oil, by pouring it over the flowers, or strewing layers of the flower for about four hours over cotton soaked in the oil. It is thus that the jessamine, and several other very volatile odours are obtained by the perfumers. Ainslie mentions that the native doctors prescribe the green root as a stimulant in paralysis, and in intermittents, in scruple doses, and use it also in epilepsy and hysteria. In Jamaica the wood is used for dyeing a blue colour, (Ainslie i. 176).

NAT. ORD. LII.—LEGUMINOSÆ OR FABACEÆ.

The plants of this vast family are herbaceous or ligneous, the leaves generally alternate, simple, or variously decompounded. The petiole frequently dilates into a membranous wing; the flowers are in clusters or panicles.

Between 4000 and 5000 species of this family have been described, and additions are being daily made to the catalogue. Among these many are remarkable for their beauty, or the utility and importance of their products.

The form of inflorescence varies remarkably in the different species, and we also find equal diversity of chemical secretions; balsams, resins, gums, manna, sugar, fixed and volatile oils, starch, benzoin, gallic and malic acids, bitter proximate principles, &c. are found in different individuals.

Decandolle divides the Leguminosæ into ten groups; Brown's division is but threefold—Papilionaceæ, Cæsalpinia, and Mimoseæ.

Gen. 1.—Myrospermum.*

Sp. 1. *Myrospermum peruiferum*, Pereira, p. 680.

Syn. Myroxylon peruiferum.

Off. product. Balsam of Peru.

A native of Peru, New Granada, Colombia, and Mexico, and especially abundant near Carthagena. The trunk is covered with a smooth thick resinous bark. From this (as well as the bark of the *M. pubescens*) on incision, or spontaneously, there exudes the well known balsam of Peru, of which there are several kinds.

1st. ***Balsam in gourds***, opaque, in mass, of brown colour, and the consistence of honey; odour agreeably sweet, taste balsamic, but acrid, bitter, and stinging; it solidifies by time, and sometimes crystallizes, deepening also in colour, frequently adulterated by turpentines and fatty matters; affords on distillation 6 per 100 of limpid, reddish essential oil, which congeals very readily; contains 10 per 100 of benzoic acid.

2nd. *Liquid Balsam.* Opaque, in mass, colour bituminous, with a reddish tint, consistence that of turpentine, odour sweet, flavour acrid, hot, very bitter, and sharp. Adulteration very common, the essential oils and copaiba balsam being generally used for the purpose.

According to Stolze's analysis 1000 parts of this balsam contain brown resin 231, oil 690, benzoic acid 64, extractive 6; 100 parts dissolved in spirits of wine require 7.5 of carbonate of soda to saturate their benzoic acid.

A third species of Peruvian balsam, far inferior to those above described, is obtained by boiling the buds and young branches; its colour is black, but the flavour and odour are very strong and characteristic.

The effects of this balsam are highly stimulant, resembling that of the turpentines, but having little tendency to

* Lindley removes this genus with the Copaibas to Amyridaceæ.

affect the urinary organs. Its action seems more transitory than that of myrrh. Applied externally the effects resemble those of myrrh.

In chronic cough, in leucorrhea, old dysenteries, and gleets, it is occasionally used, and with some advantage. The dose is half a drachm given in pills with flour, chalk, or liquorice powder, or diffused in water by sugar, mucilage, or yolk of egg.

Sp. 2. *Myrospermum toluiferum.*
Syn. Myroxylon toluiferum.
A native of South America, yields the balsam of Tolu.

Tolu Balsam, or St. Thomas' Balsam.

This balsam is at first liquid, and resembles a thick tenacious turpentine; it soon concretes, and dries into solid, brittle, golden-yellow masses; odour balsamic and very sweet, taste sweet and agreeable; it softens in the mouth, and adheres to the teeth. Powder of amber yellow colour; sometimes it is mixed with resin, benjamin, and essential oil; distilled with water the odour and flavour are given over, and a portion of benzoic acid sublimes; dissolved in the smallest possible quantity of an alkaline solution it loses its characteristic flavour, and its taste then resembles that of cloves.

This balsam is much employed in European pharmacy. It is imported from America in earthen bottles, tin-plate boxes, or calabashes.

The effects and uses of this balsam are analogous to those of the preceding article. The flavour being much more agreeable, and the action milder, the tolu balsam is generally preferred, and it is much used in chronic catarrh and other pulmonary affections. In substance it may be given in from 10 to 30 grain doses, or an emulsion may be prepared with water, sugar, and gum; the syrup is much used, and tolu lozenges are prepared by all European confectioners.

Gen. 2.—Trigonella.

Sp. Trigonella Fœnum-græcum, (Fenugreek.)
Off. The seed.
Vern. Helbeh, *Arab.* Shemlit, *Pers.* Metha and Moothee, *Duk. Hind. Sans.* Metheeshak, *Beng.*

This plant is a native of the South of Europe, and cultivated in Asia Minor and in India.

The pod is horn-shaped, seeds oblong, cylindrical, a little compressed, truncated at both ends, covered with little hollow and yellow points, internally their colour is yellow. The odour is strong and peculiar on chewing; the seed is mucilaginous, and the taste is analogous to the smell.

Mucilage, starch, fixed oil, and colouring matter, constitute the greater part of this seed; it is used by the native practitioners in dysenteric affections, and the Arabs employ it in poultices and fomentations. (*Ainslie.*)

GEN. 3.—MELILOTUS.

Sp. Melilotus officinalis. An odoriferous and fragrant plant, occasionally used in Europe in infusion or decoction, but only as a vehicle for more active substances.

GEN. 4.—TEPHROSIA.

Sp. 1. *Tephrosia purpurea.*
Syn. Galega purpurea.
Vern. Poonkhie, *Sans.* Surpunka, *Beng.*

A native of the sandy coast of Coromandel. The root is bitter, and given by the native practitioners in dyspepsia and chronic diarrhœa. The flowers are small and purple, and disposed in a loose spike.

Sp. 2. *Tephrosia Apollinea.*
Syn. Galega apollinea.

A native of Egypt. The leaflets are obovate, oblong, emarginate, silky underneath. They yield indigo when fermented, and are often mixed with the Alexandrian senna.

The leaves of a closely allied species, *T. senna*, are indeed used instead of that drug by the people of Popaya (Lindley).

Sp. 3. *Tephrosia toxicaria.*
Syn. Galega toxicaria.

A native of Jamaica, where the young branches are used for intoxicating fish.

GEN. 5.—INDIGOFERA. (Indigo plant.)

There are several species of this important genus, all of which yield the indigo of commerce. The leaf of the *Indigofera Anil* (Vishaso Danie, *Sans.*) is used by the natives in hepatitis. Powdered indigo has been employed in Germany in the treatment of epilepsy, but with very uncertain results. When indigo is acted upon by strong nitric acid, a bitter yellow substance, carbazotic acid, is formed, which possesses some powers as a febrifuge remedy when given in small doses, but is poisonous in larger quantities.

The expressed juice of the trailing indigo *I. enneaphylla*, is given as an alterative by the native physicians in old syphilitic diseases.

GEN. 6.—GLYCYRRHIZA.

Sp. 1. *Glycyrrhiza glabra*, (liquorice.)

Vern. Jetimadh, *Hind.* Madhuka and Yastimadhuka, *Sans.* Meetha lukri, *Duk.* Usulsoos, *Arab.* Bịkh-mekeh, *Pers.*

A native of the South of Europe, Crete, and Candia, also of Cochin China. The roots are large, deep, long, partially branched, from the thickness of a goose-quill to that of a finger, with scattered radical fibres, greyish and wrinkled epidermis; internally yellow, very hard when dry; the flavour is very sweet and mucilaginous, sometimes rather acrid; powder of pale sulphur colour, when the root has been previously deprived of its epidermis. It is readily attacked by insects, on account of the sugar and starch with which it abounds.

According to Robiquet's analysis, liquorice root contains glycyrrhizine, agedoite, starch, albumen, resinous oil, phosphate of lime, malates of lime and magnesia, and woody fibre.

Glycyrrhizine is transparent, brittle, of very disagreeable sugary taste, scarcely soluble in cold water, very soluble in hot water, which on cooling becomes almost gelatinous; precipitated from its watery solution by acids, readily soluble in alcohol, insusceptible of the vinous fermentation; it yields no oxalic with the nitric acid. *Agedoite* is colourless, crystallizable in rectangular octohedra, inodorous, nearly insipid, little soluble in water, and its solution not disturbed by any reagent; it is insoluble in alcohol, evolves ammonia if heated with caustic potash. The sulphuric and nitric acid dissolve it without blackening or decomposition.

This principle is said by Boutron-Charlard, and Pelouze to be aspartate of ammonia, or *asparamide*. (*Ann. de Chim. et de Phys.* iv. 90.)

Liquorice root is most employed as an adjunct or corrective for other remedies, and it is often used in powder as an envelope for pills.

Extract of Liquorice.

This occurs in thick sticks or canes of jet black colour, above 16 inches long by 1½ in diameter, brittle, dry, with shining metallic-like fracture; the odour is strong, flavour very sweet, but rather acrid; it often contains burned particles and metallic copper, on which account it must be purified before being employed for medical purposes. To purify it, it is dissolved in warm water, the solution filtered and evaporated to dryness. The extract while soft is often moulded into very thin cylinders.

The chief use of this extract is as a demulcent in obstinate cough, irritation of the air passages, &c.

For an excellent Indian substitute for liquorice, see in this family *Abrus precatorius*, or *Gunch;* the true root however is common in the Bazars. The plant is indigenous in Malabar, and very abundant in Persia, whence it is imported into India.

Gen. 7.—Colutea.

Sp. Colutea arborescens. (Bladder senna).

A native of the south of Europe and of Asia Minor—used to adulterate the senna of Aleppo, which it much resembles in appearance and effects.

Gen. 8.—Astragalus.

Sp. 1. *Astragalus verus.*

This Astragalus, according to Olivier, furnishes the principal part of the tragacanth gum of commerce. The *A. gummifer* of Mount Lebanon, the *A. creticus* of Crete and Jonia, and the *A. aristatus* of the Peloponnesus and Cyprus also afford large quantities of this very valuable gum.

Tragacanth Gum.

Tragacanth gum is pale, yellowish, or reddish, semitransparent, smooth, horny, light, brittle, of every shape, in compressed or twisted fragments, often straight, or in vermicular tears, inodorous, tasteless, and unalterable by time; in water it swells very much, and forms a soft mucilage. If the water is in excess it does not dissolve this mucilage, which remains in a separate mass; one part of this gum renders water as viscid as 25 parts of gum arabic.

Bucholz considers tragacanth to consist of 57 parts of gum resembling gum arabic, and 43 of a principle called adragantine, or *Bassorine.*

Bassorine is a scaly mass, of dirty white appearance, readily reduced to powder, insoluble in cold water, dissolved by boiling water, unaffected by alcohol or ether, but dissolved freely by alkalies or muriatic acid.

Tragacanth gum, according to Tournefort, exudes during the hot season through the bark in slender threads, which gradually increase, harden, and form tears or worm-like pieces, such as those above described.

Several Astragali are common on the higher levels of the Himalayas, but have not yet been discovered to yield tragacanth.

This gum forms the basis of some medicinal lozenges and styptic powders. In the arts it is highly valued as an ingredient in dye stuffs, and a glaze for calico and silks.

Gen. 9.—Alhagi.

Sp. Alhagi Maurorum, Camel's thorn.

Syn. Hedysarum alhagi.

Vern. Shuturkhar, Ooshturkhar, Juwansa, *Hind.*

A native of the deserts of Egypt, Syria, Mesopotamia, Persia, and India; very common about the Jumna, especially near Delhi; used for making tattees in upper India.

An erect thorny shrub. Flowers alternate, red; legumes silky, very uncertain in size, with joints from 1 to 10 in number; corolla papilionaceous, seeds reniform; leaves simple. Although it is certain that it is to this tree that the manna of the desert is to be referred, it is known that many others produce a similar exudation.

Manna of the Desert. *Vern.* Turunjabin.

This substance occurs in small, round, unequal grains, the size of coriander seed, of yellowish white colour, caking together and forming an opaque mass, in which are found portions of the thorns and fruits of the plant; this manna is inodorous, its flavour is sweetly saccharine, followed by slight acridity.

The turunjabin is never found in the shops of Europe, but in many parts of the East it is used as a substitute for sugar. Tournefort states that it is common on the Alhagis in the environs of Tauris in Persia; at Basorah the manna is collected on a small thorny bush, also common in Khorasan, and called *el hadsje*. The turunjabin is in every respect like the manna of the sacred writings.

The Alhagi nipalensium, Nipal alhagi, (Don Pr. Fl. Nipal, p. 247,) is stated to afford this secretion.

Mr. Royle however considers this species identical with the Alhagi maurorum, and states on strong grounds that no manna is secreted by either in India, Arabia, or Egypt. Persia and Bokhara seem its proper districts, and hence the turunjabin is imported into India. In Calcutta it is difficult to procure it of good quality—when pure it sells in Bengal for 10 rupees the seer.

A good analysis of turunjabin is still a desideratum. As a medicine its effects correspond to those of the *ash manna*, subsequently described.

Gen. 10.—Agati.

Sp. Agati grandiflora.

Syn. Æschynomene grandiflora.

Vern. Buka, *Sans.* Buka angusta, *Beng.* Agati, *Tamul.* Very common in India; the bark said to be a powerful bitter tonic. The leaves are aperient.

The *Æschynomena Sesban* (Jyntee) yields an excellent charcoal, used at the gunpowder works of Ishapore.

Æ. Paludosa is the *Sola*, or light sponge wood of Bengal.

Gen. 11.—Butea.

Sp. 1. *Butea frondosa.*

Vern. Pulasa, Kinouka, *Sans.* Pulas, *Beng.* Maduga, *Tel.* Dhak, *Hind.*

A native of the mountains of India. The trunk does not surpass 15 feet in height, and is evergreen; the leaves are composed of three large, thick, round, reticular leaflets, with a terminal wedge-shaped leaflet; the flowers are bright red, and in clusters. The bark furnishes a very important exudation, the *Palass goond*, or Bengal kino.

Bengal Kino.

This substance is of brittle texture and ruby-red colour, freely soluble in the mouth, inodorous, of excessively astringent taste, soluble in water, the solution being of a deep red colour, partially soluble in alcohol, giving a pale tincture; the salts of iron blacken all the solutions.

This juice is obtained by incisions in the bark; it is at first very fluid and red, then becomes paler and hardens. Its extraction takes place during the hot season.

In the Dublin Pharmacopœia this exudation is described as a variety of Kino. We shall subsequently find that the true Kino proceeds from a different source, but in chemical properties and medicinal effects both are identical.

The Palass Kino is extremely rich in tannic and gallic acid, and contains moreover arabine and ulmine; from this composition, as might be expected, we find it to exercise the most powerful astringent effects. In two or three grain doses it is an excellent remedy in many forms of chronic diarrhœa; as an external astringent application it is quite unrivalled.

The flowers of this tree give a fine yellow dye.

Sp. 2. *Butea superba.*

Vern. Tiga maduga.

A creeper of enormous size, flowers and legumes larger than in the former species,—sensible properties the same.

GEN. 12.—ABRUS.

Sp. Abrus precatorius.

Vern. Goonch, *Hind.*

A native of India, and thence spread into Africa and America.

The roots abound in sugar, and are a perfect substitute for liquorice in every respect. The seeds are very beautiful, they are used as weights by the jewellers, also for necklaces, bracelets, and other trinkets.

No analysis has yet been made of the root.

GEN. 13.—MUCUNA.

Sp. 1. *Mucuna pruriens.* (Cowhage.)

Syn. Dolichos pruriens.

Vern. Kiwach, *Hind.* Kaunch koori, *Duk.* Atmagupta, *Sans.*

The hairs which cover the pods are mixed with sugar, and administered in the treatment of worm cases; they seem to act mechanically on the body of the worm. The round worm is the species most affected. The hairs are mixed with syrup or honey, and a tea-spoonful of the paste given as a dose. In all cases it is expedient to follow up the dose of the Mucuna by some purgative medicine. Applied to the skin these hairs occasion intolerable and almost maddening itching.

The *Carpopogon pruriens* of Roxburgh is closely allied to this species, and is now called *Mucuna prurítis*, or more properly *fabacea.*

GEN. 14.—PTEROCARPUS.

Sp. 1. *Pterocarpus Draco.*

Off. The resin. Dragon's blood. Dumul-ook-wain, *Hind.*

A native of the American Islands, and especially Guadaloupe. The bark, wood, and leaves are remarkably astringent. The dragon's blood *in mass* of commerce, according to Jacquin, is the produce of this tree. Another sort, and most likely that sold in our Bazars, is produced by the Calamus Draco of the Straits.

The supposed product of the Pterocarpi occurs in cylindrical masses or shapeless fragments, of variable size, opaque, fragile, granular, of brilliant fracture, and is enclosed in palm leaves.

For its physical and chemical properties, see *Calamus Draco.*

Jacquin is the only writer who states the dragon's blood to be the produce of this genus, and it seems probable that he was misled by some analogous red juice of the kino kind.

Sp. 2. Pterocarpus santolinus.

Red sandal (sanders) wood.

Vern. Chandana, Rukta Chundun, *Hind.*

A native of Pulicat, Ceylon, and Mysore.

The wood is compact, heavy, of a beautiful red internally, becoming brown by exposure to the air, sonorous, in squared pieces, of fibrous texture; when polished numerous cells filled with resin are exposed. The odour is weak, taste slightly astringent, it reddens the saliva, is unalterable by time; the powder is of a very beautiful red colour. According to Pelletier, water has but little action on this wood; rectified alcohol dissolves a large quantity of resin, without however removing the colour altogether; the resin is soluble in alcohol and ether, scarcely so by fixed or volatile oils, except those of lavender and rosemary.

The chief importance of this wood is as a dye stuff; the Arabs use it internally as an astringent. It is also employed as the basis of various dentifrice mixtures.

Sp. 3. Pterocarpus erinaceus, Kino tree.

A native of Senegal; a moderately lofty tree, which according to Mungo Park yields the kino originally imported into Europe.

African, or Gambia Kino.

This substance is in very small fragments of irregular form, deep ruby red colour, mixed with buds and fragments of wood; pulverulent, does not colour the saliva, crackles under the teeth, inodorous, at first insipid, then astringent; powder deep chocolate or reddish brown colour; water at 60° dissolves 7-10ths, giving a solution of brick-red colour, slightly turbid, but becoming clear on repose for some hours; alcohol dissolves two-thirds, the tincture being deep brown, and the residue colourless; ether dissolves about one-third of the matter insoluble in alcohol.

African kino is now very rare in commerce; Indian kino, the produce of Butea frondosa and Nauclea (Uncaria) Gambir, and New Holland or Botany Bay kino (that of the Eucalyptus resinifera) are the most common kinds; the Coccoloba uvifera, or sea-side grape, produces a similar substance. It has also been found in the heart of the beef-wood; we have already alluded to the Palass goond as a principle, if not identical with, at least a perfect substitute for, this article.

The *Pterocarpus Marsupium*, Peet Sal. *Beng*. a native of the Circars, exudes a red juice which hardens into a strong, simply astringent, brittle, gum-resin, of a dark red colour.

Tribe—Mimoseæ.

The Mimoseæ are a very uniform tribe, composed of trees or woody plants. Gum analogous to gum arabic exudes from the trunk; the bark contains tannic and gallic acid; the unripe fruits abound in the same principles. A few afford edible legumes. The flowers of most are inodorous, though some yield the most exquisite perfume; the leaves of many exhibit spontaneous movements, as seen so beautifully in the sensitive plants. No poisonous individual has been found in this group.

Gen. 1.—Acacia.

Sp. 1. *Acacia vera.*

Syn. A. nilotica. Mimosa nilotica. Αχανθος αιγυπτιχη.

A native of Africa from Senegal to Egypt. The trunk is lofty and thick; young branches and offsets thorny, leaves twice winged, with 6 to 8 pairs of pinnæ; leaflets linear, glands situated between the lower and terminal peduncles; flowers inodorous, yellow, small, assembled in a globe or head, and collected together at the axillæ of the leaves; the legumes are three or four inches long, flattened, glabrous, enclosing five to eight isolated seeds, contained in as many rounded pieces, separated by contractions; seeds elliptic and furrowed.

This tree affords two products, one natural, the other artificial, namely the acacia juice and gum arabic.

Acacia Juice.

(Akakia of Dioscorides and Eastern writers.)

A solid, heavy, shining, brittle, dark coloured substance, inodorous, insipid at first, flavour astringent, powder brown, soluble in water which it colours red. Solution precipitated deep blue by sulphate of iron, and copiously by gelatine, tartar emetic, and oxalate of ammonia. These results indicate the presence of large quantities of the tannic and gallic acid with lime.

Dioscorides, and before him Hippocrates, have described and highly lauded the properties of this juice. It is obtained by pounding the unripe fruit, and expressing the juice; this is thickened before the sun, and then placed in bladders in which drying gradually takes place.

The little bladders of akakia found in Europe contain about 5 or 6 ounces each; it is sold in the Bazars of Bengal in thin, very black cakes, about the size of a rupee.

Gum Arabic.

Vern. Kapitha, *Sans.* Kavit goond, *Duk.* Sumug Arabee, *Arab.*

This well known gum occurs in roundish morsels, spherical, ovoid, or formless, of variable degrees of whiteness; solid, and very hard, rarely friable, diaphanous in some varieties, opaque in others, fractures in plain, shining, glassy surfaces, Sp. gr. 1,136 to 1,431. Inodorous, and nearly tasteless; soluble in the mouth, and adherent to the teeth. Powder white in proportion to its purity, and it is remarkable that yellow gum will give a white powder unalterable by time; bleached by the sun, often adulterated by inferior gums.

Treated by nitric acid, gum arabic, like most other gums, gives saccholactic and oxalic acids; it is soluble in water, to which it gives a thick consistence; alcohol and ether do not affect it. It is decomposed by the strong acids. According to Vauquelin chlorine converts gum into citric acid. In solution, gum undergoes no fermentation or decomposition, and only develops by keeping a minute proportion of acetic acid.

Gum is consumed in immense quantities by dyers and glaziers, and enters into a great number of pharmaceutical preparations. Its nutritive qualities admit of no rational doubt, although M. Majendie denies that it can support life, chiefly because it contains no nitrogen; its composition being carbon 13, hydrogen 12, oxygen 12 equivalents.

The natives of the countries along the banks of the Niger, the Moors of the interior of Africa, the Negro gum collectors of the forests of the Gambia, as well as some tribes of Bedouins, subsist almost exclusively on this principle.

Gum exudes spontaneously, or its afflux is promoted by incisions in the bark. The *Acacia vera* is the only tree of the African desert, and its leaves yield the camel the sole forage it can meet in those arid regions.

Sp. 2. *Acacia Senegal.*

Syn. Mimosa Senegalensis.

Trunk 15 to 20 feet high; this affords the Senegal gum of commerce; it does not differ essentially from the gum of the preceding article.

Sp. 3. *Acacia arabica.*

Vern. Barbura, *Sans.* Gursoonder, *Beng.* Babula, *Hind.* and *Beng.*

The babul tree, so common all over India, affords abundance of gum *(Babula goond)* of similar properties, but inferior to, to that of the Acacia vera. The bark is a powerful astringent.

Sp. 4. *Acacia Sassa.*

Syn. A. gummifera. Mimosa gummif. οποχαλπασον, *Talleh* of the Arabs of the Desert.

A native of Africa near Mogadore, also of the Island of Bourbon; the trunk is very large and lofty, and affords the gum opocalpasum, the Abyssinian myrrh of Bruce. This substance occurs in rather large fragments of uniform texture, and brownish colour, inodorous, taste insipid and mucilaginous; in water it swells, becomes white, and acts like tragacanth. It is chiefly composed of Bassorine, but is little used except in the country wherein it is found.

Basra or *Bussorah* gum is found in irregular, white, or yellow semitransparent fragments, of variable size, but never very large. It is inodorous, insipid, and makes a peculiar noise when chewed; it swells in water, but does not mix with it completely. It is chiefly composed of the principle called—

Bassorine.

Bassorine is insoluble in water at any temperature, though it swells considerably. It dissolves in hot water acidulated with a little nitric or muriatic acid.

The solution evaporated to dryness and treated by alcohol gives a precipitate, having all the properties of gum arabic.

Sp. 5. *Acacia Catechu.*

Syn. Mimosa Catechu, αχανθη.

Vern. Khadira, *Sans.* Khuera, *Beng.* and *Hind.*

Off. product, Catechu.

A native of the East Indies.

CATECHU EXTRACT.

Vern. Kuth, Khuer.

From the root and leaves of this tree the extract called catechu (Kuth) is prepared. Mr. Kerr, and Dr. Hamilton, have described the manufacture in Behar and in Canara. Royle states that in northern India the *kuth* manufacturers move to various parts of the country in different seasons, erect temporary huts in the jungles, fell the khuer trees, and cut the inner wood into small chips. These they put in small earthen pots arranged in a double row along a mud fire-place, water is then poured in till the whole is covered. After a considerable portion has boiled away, the clear liquor is strained into one of the neighbouring pots, and a fresh supply of material is put in the first. This operation is repeated until the extract in the general receiver is thick enough to be poured into clay moulds, usually of a square form.

The catechu thus made is generally of a pale red, and is considered of the best quality, (*Royle's Illust.*, p. 182).

Ordinary catechu is dry, brown externally, reddish or pale within, fracture brilliant or dull according to the kind; in flat, round, cylindrical, or irregular pieces, inodorous, of extremely astringent taste, followed by an agreeably sweet flavour. It is often adulterated with starch and clay. According to Davy's analysis it consists of tannic acid 54, extractive 34, mucilage 6, and earthy matter 5 per 100.

Three new acids, all modifications of the tannic, and called the catechuic, japonic, and rubinic acids have been separated from catechu by Buchner; their properties are however so unimportant, that they do not demand minute notice.

Three chief varieties of catechu are described by Feé, and other eminent writers on pharmacy, viz. that of Bengal, Bombay, and the catechu in masses.

Bengal catechu is in pieces of 3 to 4 ounces each, partially rounded, of dull red colour, covered with seeds on one side, fracture dull, undulated, and often marbled; taste astringent and subsequently sweet, powder grey, tannic acid 48.5 per 100.

Bombay catechu is in pieces of 2 to 3 ounces, flattened and round, of brown colour, with seeds externally and internally, fracture shining, and rarely marbled; taste bitter, without any succeeding sweetness; powder brown grey; tannic acid 54.5 per 100.

Massive catechu is found in the Bazars in pieces of 3 or 4 ounces, fragments of larger masses, reddish or blackish brown, uniform, shining, wrapped in large nerved leaves, fracture uniform, flavour very astringent, somewhat bitter, with an after sweetness; powder orange. Proportion of tannic acid very variable.

Catechu is much used in medicine as an astringent and tonic, being usually given in combination with aromatic and earthy substances; the dose is 10 grains, repeated according to circumstances.

Off. prep. Powder, compound powder, tincture, &c.

GEN. 2.—VACHELLIA.

Sp. V. Farnesiana, (Mimosa Farnesiana, Roxburgh,) Urimeda, *Sans.* Gooya-babula, *Hind.* yields abundance of gum. Flowers very fragrant.

GEN. 3.—PROSOPIS.

A Jamaica species, by some considered to be poisonous, yields large quantities of good gum.

GEN. 4.—INGA.

Sp. Inga Sassa, Abyssinia, affords one of the false tragacanth gums. *I. fagifolia* of Barbadoes has acrid and astringent bark; the bark of *I. unguis cati* of the West Indies is said to act as a diuretic, and is employed in decoction as an astringent application.

Tribe—Cæsalpinieæ.

GEN. 1.—ANDIRA.

Sp. 1. *Andira inermis*, Cabbage tree.

Syn. Geoffrœa inermis, a native of Jamaica and Martinique.

The bark is compact, fibrous, thick, of ashy colour externally, yellow within, of resinous fracture, covered with scales and lichens, odour nauseous, taste bitter and austere. It affords an extract which smells like bitter almonds, and also much resin.

Sp. 2. *A. surinamensis.*

This species affords a bark of similar properties; both have been much praised as anthelmintic remedies.

The former bark is preferred, as being milder in its operation. The effects are powerfully cathartic, emetic, and narcotic, and fatal consequences have been known to follow.

Gen. 2.—Arachis.

Sp. Arachis hypogæa, (Earth pistachio.)
Vern. China budām.

A native of South America, Africa, and many parts of Asia; within the last fifteen years much cultivated about Calcutta.

The fruit (legume) is ovale, oblong, coriaceous, with a network of veins containing two oval, somewhat flattened seeds, covered with a brown arillus. The seeds contain abundance of fixed oil, have a faint odour, and very mild agreeable taste.

According to the analysis of MM. Payen and Henry (which the Editor has repeated with like results) these seeds contain fixed oil, resinous matter, lignin, crystallizable sugar, gum, colouring matter, sulphur, starch, and saline substances.

Arachis Oil.

This important and valuable oil is, when pure, limpid and nearly colourless, Sp. gr. 916.3, insoluble in alcohol, soluble in ether, and turpentine. It has while fresh a faint smell, and but little taste; 1950 parts of seed separated from their coverings and blanched, give 1405 of kernels, from which by cold pressure 703 parts of oil are procured. In 1840 the seeds were for sale in the Calcutta Bazar at 3 Rs. per maund of 80 lbs.; they are consumed as a cheap popular luxury, being half roasted, and then eaten with salt. The oil is calculated to serve as a perfect and very cheap substitute for olive oil for pharmaceutical purposes. It burns with little smoke, with a clear flame, and affords a very full, bright light. We have found it to answer perfectly in Argand lamps.

It is believed by the natives of Bengal to be aperient, but we have found it produce only the same effects as olive oil, given to the same patients and in the same quantities. The oil cake affords excellent food for cattle.

Gen. 3.—Dipterix.

Sp. Dipterix odorata. Tonkin Bean.

Syn. Coumarouna odorata. A native of the woods of Guiana; the fruit is fleshy, thick, yellowish, thready, with a solitary cell, sub-compressed and bivalvular.

Seeds oval, oblong, somewhat boat-shaped, 1 to 2 inches long, shining, with an oily surface, marked with a network of wrinkles; colour purple brown; odour very fragrant; taste slightly bitter, but very burning, and almost caustic.

MM. Boullay and Boutron-Charlard, state it to contain a fat saponifiable matter (coumarine) sugar, malic acid, gum, starch, fibre, and salts of lime and ammonia. *Coumarine* is crystallizable in square needles, or short prisms, very odoriferous, much resembling the volatile oils, little soluble in water, but very much so in alcohol and ether.

These seeds are only employed as a perfume for snuff.

GEN. 4.—CATHARTOCARPUS.

Sp. Cathartocarpus Fistula.

Syn. Cassia fistula.

Vern. Soovarnuka, *Sans.* Sonali, *Beng.* Amultas, *Hind.*

A native of India and Egypt, and cultivated in South America. It is a tree from 20 to 30 feet high, leaves pinnate, from 12 to 18 inches long, deciduous, leaflets from 4 to 8 pair, opposite or nearly so, the lower broad, ovate, the upper oblong and entire, generally obtuse or emarginate, polished on both sides; flowers large, bright yellow, and fragrant; legume cylindrical, indehiscent, having a large longitudinal suture, a foot or more in length, in thickness of about one inch, slightly curved, obtuse, covered with woody, brittle, and externally dark brown smooth bark; there are very numerous transverse cells, parallel to each other, with thin paper-like partitions. The cells are filled with a dark shining pulp, the seeds are solitary in each cell, and of hard consistence, odour none, taste sweetish, and slightly acid.

According to Braconnot's analysis, 20 parts of the pulp consist of sugar 12.00, gum 1.35, astringent matter, gluten, and colouring matter in small quantities, and water 3.80. The cathartic properties are held to reside in the sugar. Several pharmaceutical preparations of cassia pulp occur in the Pharmacopœiæ of Europe.

When long kept the Cassia pods become dry, and rattle when shaken; these are found by experience to be destitute of purgative properties.

The leaves of the tree are also purgative, the powdered seeds are aperient, in the dose of from four to six drachms.

The pulp is a soft, gentle, and agreeable laxative, but requires to be taken in large doses, from four drachms to an ounce being at least required. Its most valuable use is as a base for purgative electuaries, containing more active ingredients.

Off. prep. Electuary of Cassia, confection of cassia, confection of senna, compound electuary of senna, &c.

GEN. 5.—CASSIA.

This genus we take on Lindley's arrangement.

The sepals are five, combined at the base, more or less unequal, stamens 10, distinct, the three upper rarely fertile, usually with anthers of a different shape from the others, and abortive, very rarely only 4—7 and all fertile; anthers dehiscing at the apex by two pores or clefts, ovary stalked. Legume compressed, many-seeded; trees, shrubs, or herbaceous plants, leaves simply and abruptly pinnated, leaflets opposite, petioles often bearing glands.

Sp. 1. *Cassia elongata.* Senna plant.

Syn. C. lanceolata, Royle. Illustr. p. 186 and 201, t. 37. Wight and Arn. Prodr. i. 288. Wight in Madr. Journal, April 1837, p. 398. Wall. in Trans. Calc. Med. Soc. vol. viii. p. 160. Cassia Senna, Roxb. Hort. Beng. p. 31.

Off. The leaves—the *Tinnevelly senna,* or Senna mekhi, of the Bazars.

A native of the interior of India, according to some authorities; others believe it to be only naturalized.

Annual, or with care suffruticose; stem erect, smooth; leaves narrow, equally pinnate, leaflets 4—8 pairs, lanceolate, nearly sessile, slightly mucronulate, smooth above, rather downy beneath, with veins turning inwards, and forming a flexuose intramarginal line; petioles without glands, stipules softly thorny, semipartite, spreading, minute; racemes axillary and terminal, erect, stalked, rather longer than the leaves; pedicels without bractes; sepals linear, obtuse, petals bright yellow; of the stamens the five lowest sterile and small, the two next large, curved, and perfect, the three uppermost minute and gland-like. Ovary linear, downy, falcate, with a smooth recurved style; legumes pendulous, oblong, membranous, about an inch and a half long, $\frac{5}{8}$ broad, quite straight, tapering abruptly to the base, and rounded at the apex, deep brown, many seeded.

Sp. 2. *Cassia acutifolia,* (Alexandrian senna.)

Arabia Felix, Upper Egypt, Arabia, and Senaar, between the Nile and Red Sea.

This species constitutes the bulk of the senna consumed for medical purposes in Europe. It is much adulterated with the leaves of Cynanchum arguel, Tephrosia Apollinea, and Coriaria myrtifolia.*

Sp. 3. *C. lanceolata,* (of Forskäl, Suna mukee of the Arabians) and C. ethiopica, furnish other species of the same article. The greater part of the produce of C. lanceolata finds its way to India through the Red Sea, Surat, Bombay, and Calcutta. In 1838-39, the Calcutta imports were 966 maunds at 6 Rs. per maund of 82 lbs. This species has been

* For drawings of the senna leaf and of those employed to adulterate this drug, *see* fig. 107, *et seq.*

cultivated successfully by Mr. Hughes at Tinnevelly, and Dr. Royle at Seharunpore. The plants in these situations yield a drug quite equal in value to the best imported article. In the Calcutta Garden the plant does not thrive well.

Sp. 4. *Cassia obovata*. Syn. C. obtusa, Wight and Arn. p. 288. Senna obtusa, Roxb. Fl. Ind. ii. p. 344. C. Burmanni. Wall. in Trans. Calc. Med. Soc. vol. viii. p. 164. Wight in Madr. Journ. July 1837, p. 71. t. 4.

Indigenous in Mysore, Egypt, Suez, Nubia, and central Africa.

The leaves furnish the Aleppo and Italian drug. A nearly allied species, the C. obtusa, is common on the dry uncultivated lands of Mysore.

SENNA OF COMMERCE. (Suna mukhi, *Hind.* Sana pāt, *Beng.*)

All the preceding species agree in certain properties; the odour of the leaves is heavy and peculiar, taste bitter, nauseous, and glutinous, powder yellowish green.

At least eight varieties of senna leaf are known in commerce in Europe. 1. The Senna palthe; 2. Senna of Sennaar, or Alexandria; 3. of Tripoli; 4. of Aleppo; 5. of Moka; 6. of Senegambia; 7. the false or Arguel; 8. the Tinnevelly.

The Senna palthe is prepared at Boullac, and is known to contain 5 parts of the C. acutifolia, 3 of C. obovata, and 2 of the Cynanchum olœifolium. It is in this variety of the drug that the poisonous leaves of Coriaria myrtifolia have been found by M. Dublanc. The *Moka* senna is chiefly cultivated for exportation to India, where it is common in all the Bazars. The other foreign varieties do not require particular notice. The Tinnevelly drug is in species identical with the Moka.

In Egypt the senna harvest takes place twice annually, in April and September; the stalks are cut off with the leaves, dried before the sun, and then packed with date leaves.

From all parts of Upper Egypt these packages arrive at the entrepôt near Boullac, called *la Palthe*. The Palteers are tax agents of the Pasha, who has of course a monopoly of this trade; they sort, mix, and adulterate the drug, and pass it into commerce through Alexandria.

M. Lassaigne and Feneueille have given a complete analysis of the Senna acutifolia, and we have found in several experiments, that their results apply to the other varieties of the drug, especially those found in the Indian Bazars. The ingredients detected were *cathartine*, colouring matter, albumen, mucus, fixed and volatile oil, malic acid, lignin, and various unimportant saline and earthy substances.

Cathartine is incrystallizable, reddish yellow, bitter, and nauseous; soluble in alcohol and water, insoluble in ether; attracts moisture from the atmosphere.

Medical uses and effects. Cathartine in very small doses purges and excites colic, three grains having occasioned these effects in its discoverer Feneueille.

Taken in substance or infusion, senna is an extremely certain and safe cathartic, especially valuable in cases of fever and surgical injuries, in which it is desirable to produce speedy and effectual evacuations. It however often occasions vomiting, sensation of heat in the abdomen, griping, and flatulence. All authors agree in forbidding its use in cases of abdominal inflammation, and it is also very objectionable in females far advanced in pregnancy, or in persons liable to severe hemorrhoidal affections, or uterine irritation.

It is seldom or never given in substance, a compound infusion being the form preferred; in this it is usually combined with ginger and some saline aperient. An electuary is also prepared with senna leaves, which acts so mildly that it may be used with advantage, even in the cases above alluded to, in which senna is generally deemed inadmissible.

For these and several other preparations, see the Pharmacopœia.

Sp. 5. *Cassia alata.*

Syn. Senna alata. Roxb. Fl. Ind. ii. p. 349.

Vern. Daod murden, *Hind.* Dadrugna, *Sans.*

Gardens, indigenous? stem erect, as thick often as a man's leg, marked by scars of the fallen leaves, and permanent stipules like prickles; leaves scattered abruptly, pinnate, two feet long, leaflets opposite, from 8 to 14 pair, the exterior largest, linear, oblong, obtuse, or emarginate, with a point, smooth and entire veined, from three to six inches long, and from 2 to 2½ broad, petiole channelled, the channel formed by two firm yellow borders—a cross bar between each pair of leaflets, racemes terminal, and from the exterior axils, long, sometimes bifid, nearly erect, bractes large, one flowered, oval, concave, yellow, deciduous; calyx coloured like the corolla. Legume horizontal, from five to six inches long, with a broad wing on each side.

The fresh leaves bruised and mixed with lime juice are deemed a powerful specific in ring worm; we have often tried them, and with decided advantage.

The whole plant is used by the Tamuls as a remedy in venereal, in poisoned bites, and as a general tonic.

Sp. 6. *Cassia auriculata.*

Vern. Tanghedoo, *Tel.* Mayharie and Talopota, *Sans.*

A very common shrub in Coromandel; the powder of the dried seeds is introduced into the eye in extreme stages of opthalmia. The seeds are also used as tonics, in the form of electuary, the dose of which is a small tea-spoonful twice daily. *Ainslie*, ii. p. 32.

All parts of the plant have much astringency, and seem to possess no other property.

Sp. 7. *Cassia Tora.*

Vern. Kulkul, *Arab.* Prabunatha, *Sans.* Chakoonda, *Hind.*

Common all over the plains, leaves fœtid, mucilaginous, and gently aperient. They are much used for adulterating senna. The seeds ground with sour butter-milk are used with excellent effect in itchy eruptions, and the root rubbed to a pulp with lime juice has almost specific powers in the cure of ring worm.

Like all the allied species of Cassia this seems to owe its virtues to its astringency alone.

Sp. 8. *Cassia Absus.*

This shrub (described by Roxb. Fl. Ind. vol. ii.) is extremely common in the Deyra Dhoon and on the plains. It is a small biennial or triennial, covered with glutinous hairs, legumes six seeded, seeds black.

M. Delile mentions this seed as the Chychm of the Egyptians, brought by the caravans from Darfour, the powdered seeds being used as an application in cases of chronic opthalmia. Mr. Royle informs us they are used for the same purposes in India, and are known by nearly the same name, Chaksoo being the Hindostanee, Chusmuk and Chusmeeguh the Persian, Kushmeezurk and Hub-ul-Soudan, Arabic.

To this is also added *Akakalis* as a Greek name. *Royle*, p. 184—this term too we find to be well known in the Bazars.

Sp. 9. *Cassia occidentalis.*

Common in Bengal, small, very offensive, used in cutaneous maladies, and also aperient. Roxburgh gives it no native name.

Gen. 6.—Tamarindus.

Sp. Tamarindus indica.

Vern. Tinteree, *Sans.* Umli, *Hind.*

This well known tree is a native of the East and West Indies; the legume is thick, oblong, several inches in length, curved, compressed between each seed, smooth, of greyish rusty colour, externally formed of a double envelope. The pulp is contained between ligamentous plates; seeds large, four-cornered, with cartilaginous, brown shell.

The odour of the pulp is vinous, the taste acid, somewhat astringent, and saccharine. The pulp is dried by age if of good quality; if inferior it becomes mouldy and fermented. As used in Europe it is usually very much adulterated, especially with prunes and tartaric acid. Copper has accidentally become mixed with many specimens, in consequence of the dessication of the juice having taken place in copper vessels.

According to Vauquelin's analysis, tamarind pulp contains the citric, malic, and tartaric acids, supertartrate of potash, sugar, gum, vegetable jelly, fibre, and water.

The citric acid is stated to exist in the proportion of 9.40 per 1.000. This analysis requires repetition on the recent pulp. To prepare tamarind pulp for European consumption all that is necessary is to open the legumes, remove the pulp and seeds, place it in layers in barrels, and pour on a strong boiling syrup; on cooling the barrel is closed. In Guadaloupe instead of syrup, raw sugar is employed; this method gives an article of better colour, and more agreeable taste than the first.

The preserved pulp in doses of half an ounce to one ounce is a gentle purgative, which also allays thirst and feverishness. It is apt however to occasion griping, and cannot be relied on except in trivial cases of costiveness, and similar slight ailments.

Gen. 7.—Hæmatoxylon.

Sp. Hæmatoxylon campechianum, (Logwood.)

A large tree, a native of Campechy and Jamaica. It is a valuable red and astringent dye stuff, and its extract is used in medicine on account of the tannic and gallic acid it contains. A crystalline principle named *hæmatin* also exists in it, which possesses no medicinal properties.

Several species of Cæsalpinia yield similar woods; the *C. echinata* is that also known as Fernambuc, or Brazil wood.

Gen. 8.—Cæsalpinia.

Sp. 1. *Cæsalpinia Sappan.*

Vern. Patanga, *Sans.* Bukum, *Hind.*

This affords the well known *sapan* of Bengal commerce. The tree is a native of Siam and Amboyna, and constitutes an article of very important trade to Calcutta; the wood, *bukum*, is solid, heavy, hard, compact, whitish while recent, but reddening on exposure to the air. It is tasteless and inodorous, communicates a fine red colour to water, and the alkalies remove more colouring matter when water ceases to act. Alcohol forms a deep red tincture. Like logwood the sapan is considerably astringent, and contains a principle if not identical with, at least much resembling *hæmatin*. The extract may be substitued for that of logwood.

Paper dyed with the tincture is a good test for alkalies, being turned to a reddish-violet colour.

Sp. 2. *Cæsalpinia Bonduccella.*

Syn. Guilandina Bonduccella.

Vern. Kutkulega—Kutkaranga. Akulmookt of Avicenna.

A climbing plant armed with many sharp, small, recurved prickles, leaves bipinnate, pinnæ 7 pairs, leaflets 3—8 pairs, ovate oblong, more or less downy, with 1—2 small recurved prickles between them on the under side; stipules large, pinnatifid, bractes lanceolate, reflexed; racemes simple above the axils; sepals 5, nearly equal, combined at the base into a short urceolate tube; petals 5, sessile, nearly equal, stamens 10 distinct, filaments villous at the base, style short; legume oval, ventricose, compressed, prickly, 2-valved 1-seeded—seeds bony, shining, nearly globose. (*Roxb. Fl. Ind.* ii. 357. W. & Arn. 280. *Fleming, As. Res.* ii. 159.)

A native of the East and West Indies; seeds a powerful tonic, and very valuable febrifuge.

The kernels are very bitter; reduced to powder and mixed with black pepper they are used in 3 to 6 gr. doses in ague with the best results; powdered small with castor oil they are applied externally in hydrocele.

The seeds yield oil, starch, sugar, and resin. Mr. Piddington published an analysis in the Trans. Medical and Physical Society of Calcutta, in which these principles were described. Nitric acid reddens the nut, and subsequently gives it a yellow colour.

The root is deemed in Amboyna to be a good tonic.

Gen. 9.—Copaifera.

Sp. Copaifera officinalis.

Several species of Copaifera, all natives of the West Indies, Peru, and Brazil, afford by incision or natural exudation the liquid so valuable in medicine called the Copaiba, or Capavi balsam.

These plants are now referred by Lindley to *Amyridaceæ*. Lindley enumerates the Copaifera Jacquini, multijuga, Langsdorfii, and coriacea, as the chief sources of the drug. The Hardwickia binata, a nearly allied tree, thrives well in the Botanic Gardens, but has never produced any resinous juice resembling copaiba, nor afforded any other useful product.

Balsam of Copaiba.

This liquid is a compound of resin and essential oil, and varies in its properties according to the predominance of either of these ingredients. As usually met with in commerce it may be distinguished into two kinds, the Brazilian and West Indian; the former is thin, clear, and pale, of pleasant aromatic smell, and acrid bitter taste; the latter thick, golden yellow, and the smell resembles that of turpentine. It is much adulterated with castor oil. This may be detected by boiling the suspected sample with water until all the volatile oil is expelled; a brittle resin is obtained if the balsam be pure, if adulterated with fixed oil a thick unctuous and soft mass remains. Pure balsam of copaiba moreover dissolves carbonate of magnesia, forming a transparent solution. Should the common fixed oils be used as the adulteration, the fraud may be detected by alcohol, in which the balsam is freely dissolved. It must be remembered however that castor oil is also soluble in strong spirit.

The balsam of the shops generally contains in 100 parts volatile oil 38, yellow brittle resin 52, brown viscid resin 1.56, the loss being traces of extractive with water and volatile oil.

The *volatile oil* is obtained by distillation with water. When twice distilled and then allowed to remain for some time in contact with chloride of calcium all traces of water are removed; it is colourless, transparent, of acrid taste, and strong disagreeable odour; it is soluble in alcohol and ether. As it contains no oxygen it serves to keep potassium unchanged; on analysis it is found to consist of 10 atoms carbon, and 8 hydrogen.

Resin of Copaiba. This is a compound of two resins, one of which can be obtained in crystals, and has all the properties of an acid, and is soluble in rectified spirit or naptha. It is called the copaivic acid; the other resin does not possess these properties. The acid resin forms salts with bases. It is owing to the presence of this acid that the balsam has the property of dissolving the carbonate of magnesia.

Effects and uses. In small doses a stimulant diuretic. It also acts, though less manifestly, on the mucous membranes of the intestinal tube and the lungs; sometimes it occasions heartburn, nausea, and flatulence, vomiting, and diarrhœa; an eruption of red spots is not an uncommon sequel of its use. All these symptoms are much increased when larger doses are taken, and in some instances violent irritation of the urinary organs is occasioned.

Copaiba is chiefly used in the treatment of gonorrhœa, gleet, and some similar affections of the urinary organs and the mucous membranes generally.

The most distinguished English surgeons recommend copaiba to be used in gonorrhœa only after all violent symptoms have subsided, or been removed by antiphlogistic measures.

Others advise large doses at the onset of the disease, but such dangerous effects have followed the plan in several cases, that it has not been generally adopted.

In chronic inflammation of the bladder great relief is often given by this remedy, used in small and frequently repeated doses. In leucorrhea similar results are reported by many experienced practitioners. In chronic bronchitis and in old diarrhœas it often proves very beneficial.

20 to 30 drops may be taken in milk, or with gum or sugared water, or milk of almonds. With starch, gum, or calcined magnesia it may be made into pills. 2 ounces of copaiba balsam and 1 drachm of calcined magnesia mixed and set aside for eight hours form a mass which give 200 pills, (*Pereira.*) The French have introduced gelatine capsules, containing each 1-36th of an ounce of the balsam, and which are tasteless, and inodorous. Pereira justly recommends the essential oil in 10 to 20 drop doses.

"Frank's Specific" for gonorrhœa is believed to be a solution of this essential oil with that of cubebs in nitrous ether. It may be perfectly imitated thus:—Oil of copaiba 1℥, oil of cubebs ʒi, spirit of nitrous ether ℥i—20 to 30 drops for each dose.

Gen. 10.—Hymenæa.

Sp. 1. *Hymenæa Courbaril.*

A native of South America; the trunk acquires an immense height; the wood is used by cabinet makers, is very hard, and acquires a fine polish. When in a sickly state it furnishes the resin called *western Anime.*

Anime Resin

is yellowish, transparent, hard, friable, in irregular fragments, resembling copal and amber, with brilliant and smooth fracture, of balsamic agreeable odour, of weakly resinous taste, softening in the mouth, burning with a very agreeable smell; more soluble in alcohol than copal, soluble also in the fixed and volatile oils. Its chief employment is in the preparation of varnishes, and when indigenous it is used for flambeaux and tapers.

Sp. 2. Hymenæa Copal.

The first clue to the plant yielding the true copal resin was obtained by M. Bonastre's finding a flower of an Hymenæa in a polished and transparent fragment of the resin. That one variety of copal is afforded by a species of hymenæa there can be but little doubt, still the subject is far from being thoroughly elucidated.

Copal Resin.

The Hymenæa copal is solid, in large irregular fragments of very variable size, opaline, yellowish, splintery, glassy, brittle, brilliant; fracture plane or convex. The outer surface is often dull, and marked by numerous impressions of the substances with which it was in contact while soft; its hardness is very great; specific gravity 1045 to 1139; while cold inodorous, on burning odour very fragrant; it is nearly insipid, crackles when chewed, and does not soften in the mouth.

Copal is frequently adulterated, especially with anime. It is readily detected by the difference of solubility in alcohol. In this fluid too the surface of copal becomes adhesive and soft, by which it is distinguished from amber, which does not soften in the least in alcohol. Copal is difficultly soluble in alcohol, ether, and the essential oils; it dissolves in alkalies, forms tannin with nitric acid, and is insoluble in fixed oil; by means of camphor and turpentine copal is dissolved in spirit, and if softened by heat it is taken up by the oils.

The use of this resin is exclusively for the preparation of varnishes, for which it is chiefly esteemed, on account of its brilliancy, hardness, and transparency.

For additional remarks regarding copal, refer to *Vateria Indica.*

Gen. 11.—Aloexylon.

Sp. Aloexylon Agallochum.

Eagle or aloes wood, a native of Cochin China.

The wood is rather hard, in fragments of about one cubit in length, obtuse, furrowed, heavy, marbled ashy and brown, shining, brittle, very resinous; odour weak but agreeable, increased on friction, and very strong on burning the wood; flavour agreeable, balsamic and slightly bitter, and irritating to the throat.

No analysis is on record of this substance; it is only known as a curiosity in Europe, but in the East it is deemed an invaluable tonic and stimulant remedy, a delicious perfume, and becoming offering for religious ceremonies. See Aquilaria Agallocha, (Aquilarineæ); also Excœcaria Agallochum, (*Euphorbiaceæ*).

Aspalathum wood is also supposed to proceed from this or the Aquilaria in a state of decomposition, but of this nothing is known with certainty. The Rhodes wood (Convolvulaceæ) has also been called "Aspalath."

Gen. 12.—Clitoria.

Sp. Clitoria Ternatea.

Kalizer-ke-jur, *Hind.* Upurajita, *Beng.* Neela gheeria, khurne, *Sans.*

Dr. Ainslie informs us that the sweetish, somewhat warm white root of this plant (which is common all over India) is given in substance ground into powder in croup cases, that it sickens and sometimes vomits, the dose being half a pagoda weight for a child of two or three years.

We have used the root extensively in order to test its alleged emetic effects, but have never observed their occurrence; an alcoholic extract acts however as a brisk purgative in from 5 to 10 grain doses. But griping and tenesmus are often produced, and during the operation of the medicine the patient is feverish and uneasy. We cannot recommend its use.

Besides the above genera Lindley describes several others of less interest, of which the following notice is sufficient.

Gen. 13.—Anagyris.

Sp. A. fœtida, a large bush, a native of the South of Europe, the seeds acrid and narcotic.

Gen. 14.—Baptisia.

Sp. B. tinctoria, (United States) yields an inferior kind of indigo; the roots are slightly astringent, cathartic, and emetic.

Gen. 15.—Genista.

Sp. G. tinctoria, (Dyer's broom) common in Europe, the whole plant gives a good yellow dye.

Gen. 16.—Cytisus.

Sp. 1. *C. Laburnum*, the common laburnum of Europe, an ornamental and favourite garden tree. The seeds are poisonous, and contain a peculiar principle called *cytisin.*

Sp. 2. *C. scoparius*, (common broom.) The young tops in decoction are diuretic and cathartic, the seeds reputed to be emetic. The plant has been used in dropsies with advantage.

Gen. 17.—Anthyllis.

Sp. A. Hermanniæ.
Syn. Aspalathus creticus—has diuretic roots.

Gen. 18.—Psoralea.

Sp. P. corylifolia.
Vern. Hakooch—common in India, seeds considered stomachic and deobstruent. The seeds are very small, of dark brown colour.

Gen. 19.—Pueraria.

Sp. P. tuberosa, (Hedysarum tuberosum of Roxburgh), Shimeeya batrajee, *Beng.* a native of the Circar mountains, the bruised root is used as a poultice to swellings of the joints.

Gen. 20.—Sabinea.

Sp. S. florida, West Indies, flowers poisonous.
S. or *Robinia candida*, is the Balas-mundulee of Bengal.

Gen. 21.—Piscidia.

Sp. P. Erythrina, Jamaica dogwood, West Indies. The tincture of the bark is a powerful narcotic and diaphoretic; the root a common fish poison.

Gen. 22.—Coronilla.

Two species are described, having cathartic leaves and juice.

The *Coronilla picta*, is the Krishna rajam of Bengal, a plant highly esteemed for the beauty of its purple flowers, and the emollient qualities of its leaves. These are applied as a cataplasm to suppurating tumors.

GEN. 23.—ARTHROLOBIUM.

The leaves of *A. scorpioides* (Europe), blister when applied to the skin.

GEN. 24.—ORMOCARPUM.

Sp. O. sennoides, (Hedysarum sennoides of Roxburgh.) Kanana, *Sans.* Junglee moonghee, *Hind.* Root considered tonic and stimulant.

GEN. 25.—LATHYRUS.

Sp. L. Aphaca (Europe), Chuna, Burachuna, *Beng.* ripe seed narcotic. *L. Cicera* (Spain), seeds poisonous. *L. sativus*, Khesaree, Teora, *Beng.* The expressed oil of the seeds is a powerful and dangerous cathartic.

GEN. 26.—PHASEOLUS.

Sp. P. radiatus, Masha, *Sans.* Mash Kulai, *Beng.* Moong. Thikiree, *Hind.*—roots said to be narcotic by Royle.

P. trilobus, Moojanee, *Beng.* Trianguli, *Hind.*—the leaves are said to be tonic and sedative, and are used in cataplasms to weak eyes.

GEN. 27.—POINCIANA.

Sp. P. pulcherrima, Krishna choora, *Beng.* and *Hind.* Gul-i-turah, *Hind.* is said to be much used in medicine in upper India, but for what purpose, is not stated. Ainslie notices the plant under the name of *Kurish-Churrin.* A decoction of the leaves and flowers is given as a febrifuge in Tortola; the leaves are purgative, and when bruised smell like sabine: in infusion they are considered powerfully *emmenagogue.* These properties demand careful investigation.

GEN. 28.—BAUHINIA.

Sp. B. tomentosa, Usmaduga, *Sans.* a native of Ceylon, Malabar, and Coromandel; the dried buds and flowers are used in dysentery.

NAT. ORDER LIII.—ROSACEÆ.

This is a very extensive order, and contains several medicinal articles. The tannic acid is the principle which most abounds throughout the order, sugar occurs in those species having fleshy fruits, and of these many also contain the malic acid. A peculiar gum named *cerasin* is yielded by many of the trees, volatile oil is but rarely present, though fixed oil is obtained in large quantities from the kernels of many of the fruits.

That formidable poison the hydrocyanic or prussic acid, is the product of the chemical action between water and a principle contained in the leaves, bark, roots, seed, and flowers of many of the Rosaceæ; a poisonous essential oil is also obtained from several of the same species.

The flowers of the peach and rose, and the drupe of the prune are aperient; the bark of the root of the *Spirea trifolia* is emetic; the *brayera* is a drastic purgative, and has specific powers in expelling tape worm.

M. Feé adopts Decandolle's arrangement of the genera of this order.

Tribe 1—Chrysobalaneæ.

The seeds of the *Prinsepia utilis*, of Royle, common on dry rocks, near Muttiana, in N. Lat. 31½°, and at elevations of 5000 to 6000 feet, (Royle, p. 202,) yields abundance of useful fixed oil.

Tribe 2—Amygdaleæ, or Almonds.

Gen. 1.—Amygdalus.

This genus is made a separate order by Lindley; we have deemed it more convenient to adhere to Decandolle's division.

These are trees or shrubs with petiolate, entire, penni-nerved dentate leaves, with white or rose-coloured flowers; the pericarp varies much in its form; it is woody in the almond tree, and of harsh taste, dries up on the ripening of the seed, while in other genera it becomes succulent and pulpy. A bony shell covers the kernel, the oily perisperm of which is accompanied by a variable quantity of prussic acid, a bitter principle, and amygdaline; in the leaves of some the proximate elements of prussic acid are also present.

From the trunk of most of the almond trees there exudes a gum described under another head; the bark is used in tanning. The kernels, besides the principles above mentioned also yield abundance of fixed oil.

Sp. 1 *Amygdalus communis*, (common almond.)
Vern. Badamie, *Parsee.*
Var. A. sweet; B. bitter.

A native of the Himalayas, the Mauritius, Taurus, Caucasus, and Hindookosh; cultivated in Europe, abundant in Cashmere.

Nut bony, covered with a pericarp which separates on the detachment of the fruit, an inch to 1¼ inch long, yellowish, brittle, hard, marked with longitudinal chinks, back round, base angular, almond oval, compressed, sharp-pointed, covered with a brown perisperm, substance of the almond pure white, nearly inodorous. Flavour sweet, mild, and pleasant; when chewed the saliva is rendered milky; by long keeping the oil contained in the almond grows yellow and rancid, and the episperm becomes the prey of mites, which find their way into the almond to deposit their eggs in its substance.

The best analysis of the sweet almond is that by M. Boullay, published in the *Journal de Pharmacie* 1817, p. 337. He found in 100 parts,

Water, ...	3.5
Pellicles containing astringent matter, ...	5.0
Fixed oil, ...	54.0
Albumen, ...	24.0
Liquid sugar,...	6.0
Gum, ...	3.0
Fibre, ...	4.0
Loss, and acetic acid, ...	0.5

Oil of sweet almonds. Colourless, or very slightly yellow, difficultly congealed, Sp. gr. 918, taste sweet, smell light, agreeable, and resembling that of the seeds.

This oil is the basis of the greater part of the liniments, plasters, and ointments of the French and many other European Pharmacopœiæ. In all its properties and uses it is nearly identical with olive oil.

Almond milk. For the preparation of almond emulsion, or what is called almond *milk*, the almonds are blanched (deprived of their brown integument) by steeping in hot water for half an hour; half an ounce of the almonds is then rubbed in a mortar with 6½ ounces of pure water; white sugar ʒij; powdered gum arabic ʒi. The sugar and albumen are thus dissolved, and by suspending the starchy matter an excellent light vegetable milk is procured. This is much used as the basis of cough mixtures, and as a vehicle for administering camphor, gum, resins, and copaiba. It is prescribed moreover as an article of diet to children convalescent from acute diseases.

Var. B. *The bitter almond.*—(Kurwr Badam, *Beng.*

The fruit is smaller than that of the preceding variety; in every other respect the structure and appearance of the trees and fruits seem to correspond.

The taste, composition, and properties are however totally different. This leads almost irresistibly to the conclusion that there must exist specific anatomical differences between the trees. It has indeed been asserted, but on very inadequate grounds, that the sweet and bitter fruits have been gathered from the same tree. Others state that culture will change the bitter to the sweet, as it has changed the sour crab to the delicious apple, and the bitter, half poisonous wild potatoe to its present state.

On this point Lindley observes, that the sweet and bitter almond are only varieties of each other, chiefly differing in the quantity of prussic acid their seeds contain. No opinion is to be treated with more respect than that of Lindley on all botanical matters, but we must be pardoned for stating our belief that no prussic acid has yet been traced in the sweet almond.

The sweet and bitter kind are imported into the northern parts of India from Ghoorbund, and into the southern parts from the Persian gulf.

Our knowledge of the composition of the bitter almond has been much increased since the publication of M. Feé's work, chiefly through the labours of MM. Robiquet, and Boutron-Charlard.

When the bitter almond deprived of its epidermis is subjected to cold pressure it affords a large quantity of thick fixed oil, identical with that procured from the sweet almond.

When the oil cake thus obtained is reduced to powder and distilled with water, a volatile oil passes over, of golden yellow colour, of strong odour of prussic acid, extremely poisonous, and depositing crystals on exposure to the air. This oil contains a large quantity of hydrocyanic acid; the oil combines with alkalies forming soaps and a *benzoate* of the base; acted upon by nitric acid it is also oxydized, and the same acid produced. It is very soluble in alcohol and sulphuric ether.

Robiquet and Boutron-Charlard have distinctly proved that the volatile oil does not *pre-exist* in the almond, but is formed in consequence of this coming in contact with water. If almond paste deprived of fixed oil by expression be treated with anhydrous sulphuric ether, no volatile oil is separated by that solvent; but by adding water the oil is formed in abundance. On analysis it is found to consist of 14 atoms carbon, 6 hydrogen, 2 oxygen. This of course refers to the pure oil freed from hydrocyanic acid.

If we treat the pressed almond cake, first with ether, then with strong alcohol, and lastly with water, no volatile oil is formed. The alcohol removes a crystalline principle (which can only be purified by much difficulty) termed *amygdaline.*

This principle is inodorous, sweet, and then slightly bitter, decomposed by heat, unalterable by air, very soluble in boiling alcohol, insoluble in ether; caustic potash dissolves it, and ammonia is formed. According to Liebig's analysis it contains carbon=40, hydrogen=26, azote=1, oxygen=22 atoms.

The most important property of this substance however is, that when it comes in contact with a solution of the albumen of the almond in water *(emulsin)*, decomposition immediately ensues, and hydrocyanic acid and the oil of bitter almonds are formed.

Amygdalic acid. By the addition of muriatic acid to the oil of bitter almonds, and evaporation to dryness, the whole of the oil is converted into amygdalic acid and ammonia.

This acid is also easily prepared from amygdaline. If we dissolve amygdaline in cold barytes water no decomposition occurs, but by boiling the solution ammonia is disengaged. When ammonia ceases to be extricated a current of carbonic acid passed through the hot liquid throws down the uncombined barytes, and leaves in solution amygdalate of that base, from which the acid may be readily separated by diluted sulphuric acid.

This acid is deliquescent, insoluble in absolute alcohol and ether, distils slightly altered at a high temperature. On analysis it yields carbon 40, hydrogen 26, oxygen 24 eq. being 2=of oxygen more than amygdaline, which also contains 1=azote, no trace of which principle exists in the acid. It forms salts with all bases, some of which may be obtained in the crystalline state.

It is indispensably necessary to notice here some additional discoveries regarding the nature of these compounds, as they strongly illustrate the nature of many of the most interesting and important operations in the decomposition of vegetable principles.

The volatile oil of bitter almonds was long observed to have the property of absorbing oxygen from the atmosphere, and of being converted into benzoic acid. For these experiments the oil must be in the first place freed from hydrocyanic acid by being mixed with hydrate of potash, and solution of protochloride of iron—by distillation, and separation from water by quicklime. The oil thus prepared is colourless, limpid, sp. gr. 1043, boiling point above 266. In the air, whether dry or moist, and in oxygen, it is rapidly converted into benzoic acid; on analysis this oil yields carbon=14, hydrogen=6, oxygen=2. By absorbing 2 atoms of oxygen it forms,

	Hyd.	*Oxy.*	*Carbon.*
1 Water,	1	1	—
1 Benzoic acid,	5	3	14
	6	4	14

So that carbon=14, hydrogen=5, oxygen=2, must be the base of benzoic acid (benzoyle) into which it it converted by oxygen=1; the oil is therefore a hydret of benzoyle or benzoyle=1, hydrogen=1; the acid is a protoxide of benzoyle with 1 of water.

Besides several oxides there are the chloride, iodide, bromide, sulphuret, and cyanide of benzoyle, and many other compounds, for which we must refer to the works by Thomson or Liebig on organic chemistry.

Hydrocyanic Acid.

For an account of this remarkable acid, and its formidable properties, see the Pharmacopœia, art. *Acids*.

Sp. 2. *Amygdalus Persica*, (Peach tree.)

This tree was introduced into Europe from Persia, where the fruit is very fine, and called Kulloo and Kardee-aroo, and Khookh, *Arab.* It is also found of fine quality in Mysore and China, and recently cultivated with success in Bengal.

The flowers are purgative, but also narcotic. Dr. Christison relates the case of a gentleman who was poisoned by taking them in salad as an aperient. The leaves and kernels on distillation yield abundance of prussic acid. The fermented fruit gives an excellent brandy, chiefly manufactured in the United States of America.

The bark gives a large quantity of gum during the hot season.

The Armeniaca vulgaris, or Apricot. (Spanish, Albaricoque.) *Vern.* Burkook, Khoobanee, Mishmish, Bakurkhanee, is common about villages in the Himalayas, where it is also called Zurd-aloo, Chooloo, and Chinaroo). Oil of the finest kind is made by expression from the kernels, sold separately in the Bazars under the name of Badam kohee, or hill almonds. The oil is clear, of a pale yellow colour, and smells strongly of hydrocyanic acid, of which it contains usually about 4 per 100.

GEN. 2.—CERASUS.

Sp. 1. *Cerasus caproniana.* The Cherry tree. A native of Europe, the Himalayas, Caucasus, &c. In Cashmere it is called *Aloo baloo.*

The kernel of this fruit contains the elements of hydrocyanic acid, and is accordingly much used for communicating its peculiar flavour to brandy and liqueurs. The fruit of *Cerasus Pudum* is used for the same purpose in the hills. The bark is called *pudmak*, and used in medicine by the natives, as it is also in America.

The liqueur called *Maraschino*, which is chiefly manufactured in Venice, Trieste, and Zara in Dalmatia, is prepared from a variety of cherry named the *Griot marasquin;* the fruit and seed are crushed together, one part to the hundred of honey added, and the whole mass subjected to fermentation; during this process it is distilled, and the product is rectified. To the rectified spirit sugar and water are added, in proportions guided by the taste of the manufacturer, and the resulting liqueur is stored for some months before use, to free it of empyreumatic flavour.

The bark of the cherry tree is bitter and astringent; it has been used as a substitute for cinchona, but is now abandoned. It yields in certain seasons a large quantity of a gum possessed of some useful properties, but not of sufficient importance to demand minute description here. It is but imperfectly soluble in water; the insoluble part has been named *Cerasine.* It in some respects resembles gum tragacanth, but is not susceptible of such useful applications in the arts.

Sp. 2. *Cerasus Padus*, (Bird-Cherry.)
Syn. Prunus avium.

A native of the woods of Europe. It is cultivated in the Black forest, in Switzerland, and France for the manufacture of the celebrated *Kirchenwasser*, a liqueur which owes its delicious flavour to the presence of prussic acid with a peculiar bitterish substance.

Sp. 3. *Cerasus Laurocerasus.* (Cherry-laurel.)

A native of Trebizond and Affghanistan, cultivated in Europe.

The leaves are alternate, shortly petiolate, coriaceous, oval, oblong, 5 to 7 inches long, acute at top, finely toothed in the edges, smooth, shining above, with oblique, not opposite nerves. Inodorous, taste very decided, rather styptic, bitter, resembling, but stronger than, that of bitter almonds; drying destroys their powers by expelling the hydrocyanic acid and essential oil with which they are impregnated in the recent state.

The distilled water of the leaves is much used in Europe as a vehicle for opiates and other anodyne medicines. It is given in doses of from half an ounce to one ounce. Great care is essential in the observation of the exact formula given in the Pharmacopœia for this preparation, a deviation from which may render the distilled fluid a most dangerous poison.

GEN. 3.—PRUNUS.

Sp. 1. *Prunus spinosa,* (Sloe.)

The juice of this fruit is used in France as an astringent substitute for Catechu. Feé, ii. p. 109.

Sp. 2. *Prunus domestica.* (Prune). We shall only notice this as yielding the well known laxative fruit of the Pharmacopœia.

Prunes contain free malic acid, sugar, and an unknown principle in which the laxative property resides. M. Feé states that M. Bonneberg, a German chemist, obtained from 12 kilogrammes (seers) of the fruit, 1 of sugar, 3 of syrup, and 2 of spirit.

The plum of Bokhara is the fruit of Prunus Bokhariensis, (Royle,) and is called *kokamalis* (κοκυμηλεα) in Persian works on Materia Medica.

Tribe 3—Roseæ.*

GEN. 1.—SPIRÆA.

Shrubs and herbs, with few marked properties. All are astringent; the bark of Quillaia saponaria renders water frothy like soap, and is used as a detergent by wool dyers. In the *Spiræa Ulmaria* (meadow sweet) a radical principle resem-

* By itself a natural order "Rosaceæ," in Lindley's *Flora Medica.*

bling Benzoyle has been detected. It is named *Spiroil*, and gives use to a very numerous class of compounds.

Gen. 2.—Brayera.

Shrubs or herbs, whose most important constituent is the tannic acid. Some also afford essential oil; one, the *Brayera anthelmintica* is a drastic purgative, and is said by Brayer to be a perfect specific in tape-worm.

Gen. 3.—Geum.

Sp. Geum urbanum.

A native of Europe, distinguished by its smell of cloves, its styptic, and somewhat bitter taste. It is admitted into the English Pharmacopœia. It contains over 10 per cent. of tannic acid. Tromsdorff says he found 40 per 100 in some specimens.

Gen. 4.—Rubus.

Sp. Rubus Idæus. (Raspberry.)

Well known for its delicious fruit, which abounds in citric and malic acid, and sugar, and which affords the jam and vinegar of its name. *R. concolor* is the nearest species in the Himalayas.

Gen. 5.—Potentilla.

Sp. Potentilla Tormentilla.

Πενταφυλλον μελαν, *Diosc.* and *Theopr.*

A native of Europe, and officinal; the root is very rich in tannic acid.

The *Potentilla denticulosa* is common in the plains of Northern India in the cold season, and at elevations of 4000 to 5000 feet in the Himalayas; two other species are found in the Neelgherries. *Royle*, p. 202.

Gen. 6.—Agrimonia.

Sp. Agrimonia Eupatoria.

A native of all parts of Europe. It contains tannic and gallic acid, and a very small quantity of fragrant essential oil, the flavour of which resembles that of tea, for which agrimony is much used as a substitute by the poorer classes in Europe.

Agrimonia Nipalensis is very closely allied to this.

Gen. 7.—Rosa.

Bushes or small shrubby plants, with leaves usually impari-pinnate, toothed, with petiolar stipules. Flowers peculiarly fragrant in consequence of containing an essential oil. The leaves and fruits of most species are astringent, the petals laxative. The genus when Feé wrote, was known to embrace about 150 species, with an almost infinite number of varieties produced by grafting and cultivation.

Sp. 1. ***Rosa canina.*** (Dog rose, hep.) (Κυνοσβατος, Dioscorides.)

Off. Fruits.

A native of Europe; the fruit (hep) is acidulous and astringent. When reduced to pulp it gives a conserve much used in Europe in pharmacy to give due consistence to pills and electuaries of corresponding, but more active medicinal virtues.

Sp. 2. ***Rosa gallica,*** (French, or Provence red rose.)

Vern. Gul.

Off. Petals.

A native of Persia, the petals contain tannic and gallic acid, essential oil, oxide of iron, and other unimportant principles.

The petals are gathered before becoming quite ripe, they are deprived of the calyx and central attachments, and dried before the sun or in a stove. When dried they are sifted in order to separate the stamina and pistil. They are then gently compressed and kept in a dry place.

From a variety of this species, the cabbage rose, a very fragrant distilled water is prepared in England.

Sp. 3. ***Rosa centifolia.*** (Hundred-leaved rose.)

Vern. Goolab, Sudburg, Wurd. *Arab.*

A native of Syria, cultivated in Europe. The odour of this species is but partially destroyed by desiccation, and according to M. Chereau is remarkably augmented by iodine. It is less astringent than the Provence rose, and more laxative. It furnishes essential oil in small quantities, and is much employed for distillation of rose water, and in the preparation of the essential oil, or *Utr.*

The petals of this as well as the preceding species are preserved with salt by the European apothecaries for the preparation of the distilled water.

ESSENTIAL OIL, OTTO, A'THER, OR UTR OF ROSES.

This highly valuable and delightful perfume is obtained chiefly at Ghazipore in Bengal, by the process described in Dr. Jackson's excellent paper on this subject. It is also prepared in Persia, Cashmere, in Upper Egypt, and in Tunis.

The oil is nearly colourless, Sp. gr. 0,872, solid below 80, and liquefies at 84. 1000 parts of alcohol at 72 dissolve 33 of this oil. Its composition is remarkable, it being a compound of two oils, one liquid, the other solid and inodorous.

We are indebted to Dr. Jackson, late Civil Surgeon at Ghazipore, for the following interesting information on the manufacture and trade of rose water and *Utr*.

Dr. Jackson's paper was drawn up specially for this work, but in order to give it extensive publicity, without any avoidable delay, the Editor published it in the Journal of the Asiatic Society for 1839.

"CULTIVATION.

"Around the station of Ghazeepore there are about 300 beegahs, or about 150 acres, of ground laid out in small detached fields as Rose gardens, most carefully protected on all sides by high mud walls and prickly pear fences, to keep out the cattle. These lands, which belong to Zemindars, are planted with Rose trees, and are annually let out at so much per beegah for the ground, and so much additional for the Rose plants—generally five rupees per beegah, and twenty-five rupees for the Rose trees, of which there are 1000 in each beegah. The additional expense for cultivation would be about 8/8; so that for rupees 38/8 you have for the season one beegah of 1000 Rose trees.

"If the season is good this beegah of 1000 Rose trees should yield one lac of Roses. Purchases for Roses are always made at so much per lac. The price of course varies according to the year, and will average from 40 to 70 rupees. During the past season the latter was the price given for one lac of Roses towards the conclusion.

"MANUFACTURE OF ROSE-WATER.

"The Rose trees come into flower at the beginning of March and continue so through April. In the morning early the flowers are plucked by numbers of men, women, and children, and are conveyed in large bags to the several contracting parties for distillation. The cultivators themselves very rarely manufacture.

"The native apparatus for distilling the Rose-water is of the simplest construction; it consists of a large copper or iron boiler well tinned, capable of holding from eight to twelve gallons, having a large body with a rather narrow neck, and a mouth about eight inches in diamater; on the top of this is fixed the head of the still, which is nothing more than an old *dekchee*, or cooking vessel, with a hole in the centre to receive the tube or worm.

"This tube is composed of two pieces of bamboo, fastened at an acute angle, and it is covered the whole length with a strong binding of corded string, over which is a luting of earth to prevent the vapour from escaping. The small end, about two feet long, is fixed into the hole in the centre of the head, where it is well luted with flour and water. The lower arm or end of the tube is carried down into a long necked vessel or receiver, called a *bhubka*. This is placed in a handee of water, which, as it gets hot, is changed. The head of the still is luted on to the body, and the long arm of the tube in the *bhubka* is also well provided with a cushion of cloth, so as to keep in all vapour. The boiler is let into an earthen furnace, and the whole is ready for operation.

"There is such a variety of Rose-water manufactured in the bazar, and so much that bears the name, which is nothing more than a mixture of sandal oil, that it is impossible to lay down the plan which is adopted. The best Rose-water however in the bazar may be computed as bearing the proportion of one thousand Roses to a seer of water; this perhaps may be considered as the best procurable. From one thousand Roses most generally a seer and a half of Rose-water is distilled, and perhaps from this even the Attar has been removed.

"The boiler of the still will hold from eight to twelve or sixteen thousand Roses. On eight thousand Roses from ten to eleven seers of water will be placed, and eight seers of Rose-water will be distilled. This after distillation is placed in a carboy of glass, and is exposed to the sun for several days to become *pucka* (ripe), it is then stopped with cotton, and has a covering of moist clay put over it; this becoming hard effectually prevents the scent from escaping. The price of this will be from twelve to sixteen rupees. This is the best that can be procured.

"ATTAR OF ROSES.

"To procure the Attar, the Roses are put into the still, and the water passes over gradually as in the Rose-water process; after the whole has come over, the Rose-water is placed in a large metal basin, which is covered with wetted muslin tied over to prevent insects or dust getting into it; this vessel is let into the ground about two feet, which has been previously wetted with water, and it is allowed to remain quiet during the whole night. The Attar is always made at the beginning of the season, when the nights are cool; in the morning early the little film of Attar which is formed upon the surface of the Rose-water during the night is removed by means of a feather, and it is then carefully placed in a small phial; and day after day as the collection is made it is placed for a short period in the sun, and after a sufficient quantity has been procured it is poured off clear, and of the colour of amber, into small phials. Pure Attar when it has been removed only three or four days has a pale greenish hue, by keeping, it loses this, and in a few weeks' time it becomes of a pale yellow. The first few days' distillation does not produce such fine Attar as comes off afterwards, in consequence of the dust or little particles of dirt in the still and the tube being mixed with it. This is readily separated from its sinking to the bottom of the Attar, which melts at a temperature of 84o. From one lac of Roses it is generally calculated that 180 grains, or one tolah, of Attar can be procured; more than this can be obtained if the Roses are full sized, and the nights cold to allow of the congelation. The Attar purchased in the bazar is generally adulterated, mixed with sandal oil, or sweet oil; not even the richest native will give the price at which the purest Attar alone can be obtained, and the purest Attar that is made is sold only to Europeans. During the past year it has been selling from 80 to 90 rupees the tolah; the year before it might have been purchased for 50 rupees.

"GENERAL REMARKS.

"Native stills are let out at so much per day or week, and it frequently occurs that the residents prepare some Rose-water for their own use as a present to their friends, to secure their being provided with that which is the best. The natives never remove the calices of the Rose-flowers, but place the whole into the still as it comes from the gardens.

"The best plan appears to be to have these removed, as by this means the Rose-water may be preserved a longer time, and is not spoiled by the acid smell occasionally met with in the native Rose-water. It is usual to calculate 100 bottles to one lac of Roses. The Rose-water should always be twice distilled; over ten thousand Roses water may be put to allow of sixteen or twenty bottles coming out; the following day these twenty bottles are placed over eight thousand more Roses, and about eighteen bottles of Rose-water are distilled. This may be considered the best to be met with. The Attar is so much lighter than the Rose-water that previous to use it is better to expose the Rose-water to the sun for a few days, to allow of its being well mixed, and Rose-water that has been kept six months is always better than that which has recently been made.

"At the commencement of the Rose season, people from all parts come to make their purchases, and very large quantities are prepared and sold. There are about thirty-six places in the city of Ghazeepore where Rose-water is distilled. These people generally put a large quantity of sandal oil into the receiver, the oil is afterwards carefully removed and sold as Sandal Attar, and the water put into carboys and disposed of as Rose-water. At the time of sale a few drops of sandal oil are placed on the neck of the carboy to give it fresh scent and to many of the natives it appears perfectly immaterial whether the scent arises solely from the sandal oil or from the Roses; large quantities of sandal oil are every year brought up from the south and expended in this way.

"The chief use the natives appear to make of the Rose-water or the Sandal Attar as they term it, is at the period of their festivals and weddings. It is then distributed largely to the guests as they arrive, and sprinkled with profusion in the apartments. A large quantity of Rose-water is sold at Benares, and many of the native Rajahs send over to Ghazeepore for its purchase. Most of the Rose-water as soon as distilled is taken away, and after six months from the termination of the manufacture there are not more than four or five places where it is to be met with.

"I should consider that the value of the Roses sold for the manufacture of Rose-water may be estimated at 15,000 rupees a year, and from this to 20,000; and from the usual price asked for the Rose-water and for which it is sold, I should consider there is a profit of 40,000 rupees. The natives are very fond of using the Rose-water as medicine, or as a vehicle for other mixtures, and they consume a good deal of the petals for the conserve of Roses, or *Goolcond*, as they call it."*

Tribe 4—Pomaceæ.

Trees or shrubs with simple leaves, seldom stipulate, and very rarely pinnate; important for their fruits, which contain gallic, malic, or citric acid and sugar, the last is especially increased by cultivation, while the acids are diminished. A principle named *phloridzite* has been recently found in the bark of the roots of several species, and has been asserted to be of great efficacy in the treatment of intermittent fevers.

Gen. 1.—Malus.

Sp. 1. *Malus communis.* (Apple.)

A native of Asia Minor, cultivated in Europe, and recently in Tirhoot. It abounds in malic acid and sugar. The bark of the root contains—

Phloridzite.

The preparation of this substance is very simple: boil the fresh bark for two hours in water, repeat the decoction, keep the liquid of the second decoction separate; in twenty hours it deposits a considerable quantity of granular crystals

* In the Asiatic Researches, vol. i. p. 132, the reader will find another interesting account of this manufacture by Lieut. Colonel Polier.

of phloridzite, which are purified by distilled water and animal charcoal. About 3 per 100 can thus be obtained from the bark of the apple tree root. Or, digest the fresh bark in weak alcohol at 122° for eight or ten hours, distil and crystallize; 5 per 100 can thus be procured.

Phloridzite is of dull white colour, crystallizes in needles or tables, is intensely bitter, insoluble in cold, freely soluble in hot water, and in absolute alcohol. Insoluble in ether, melts at 350°, at 379° is decomposed; soluble in acids. Precipitated yellow by chlorine. No good analysis has yet been published of this substance.

Phloridzite has been used at the Military Hospital of Antwerp in several cases of ague; and the results are said to be quite equal to those from quinine.

GEN. 2.—CYDONIA.

Sp. Cydonia vulgaris. (Quince.)
Asia Minor, Cabul, Bokhara.
Off. Seeds.
Vern. Beheedana, Bedana, *Hind.*

Seeds oval, acute, plane at one side, convex at the other, often triangular, truncated at one end, of iron colour, internally white and brilliant. The coriaceous episperm contains a quantity of mucilage which is readily given out to water. The kernel is emulsive. The Beheedana constitutes an important article of commerce, being highly valued as a demulcent tonic, and restorative remedy by the Mahomedans all over the East. In 1838-39, 106½ maunds were imported into Calcutta from the Persian Gulf; into Northern India they are brought from Cabul and Cashmere.

NAT. ORDER LIV.—RHIZOPHOREÆ

includes no medicinal article. The bark of the mangrove is very astringent.

NAT. ORDER LV.—ONAGRARIÆ.

These are herbs or shrubs with simple, alternate, or opposite leaves, terminal or axillary flowers. The only plant deserving attention is the *Trapa natans*, and *T. bispinosa.* The fruit is called *singara;* these are sold in all the Bazars, and form a considerable part of the food of the inhabitants of

Cashmere, where it yields the Government 12,000*l.* of annual revenue. Mr. Moorcroft mentions that Runjeet Sing derived nearly the same share. From 96,000 to 128,000 loads of this nut are yielded annually by the lake of Ooller alone. The nut abounds in fecula, and is armed with two singular projecting spines. In China the kernel is used as an article of food, being roasted or boiled like the potatoe. (*Royle*, p. 211.)

The orders Halorageæ and Ceratophylleæ may be passed over.

NAT. ORD. LVI.—LYTHRARIÆ, OR SALICARIÆ.

This order contains but a few, and these unimportant articles. The *Lythrum Salicaria (loose strife)* was used in Europe as a mild astringent, but is now obsolete. The *Lawsonia inermis*, Mendee, *Hind.* Urkan, *Arab.* Sakachera, *Sans.* Henna, *Persian,* is an important dye stuff, and the distilled water of the flowers is used as a perfume. The extract of the flowers, leaves, and shoots is used by the Hakims in lepra, and in obstinate cutaneous diseases, half a tea-spoonful being given twice in 24 hours. The Mahomedan women in India use the shoots for dyeing the nails red, and the same practice prevails in Arabia and Barbary. In all these countries the manes and tails of the horses are stained red in the same manner.

The Grislea tomentosa, (Dhub,) yields red petals, used in dyeing, and containing much tannic acid.

GEN.—AMMANNIA.

Sp. Ammannia Vesicatoria, (Blistering Ammannia.)

Vern. Dadmaree, Bunmurich, *Beng.*

An annual found in wet land during the rains, 6 to 36 inches high, has a strong smell like muriatic acid; leaves exceedingly acrid, employed by the natives as blisters in rheumatism; and Ainslie states that the fresh leaves bruised and applied to the part intended to be blistered perform their office in half an hour, and most effectually.

We made trial of this article in eight instances; blisters were not produced in less than 12 hours in any, and in three individuals not for 24 hours. The bruised leaves had been removed from all after half an hour. The pain occasioned was absolutely agonizing until the blister rose. We should not be justified in recommending these leaves for further trial, they cause more pain than cantharides, and are far inferior to the plumbago, (lalchitra) in celerity and certainty of action.

NAT. ORDER LVII.—TAMARISCINEÆ.

This well known order occurs in many parts of the world, chiefly in hot and sandy districts adjacent to the sea or great rivers. Dr. Roxburgh describes two in India, the *Tamarix indica* (probably identical with *T. gallica*) and *dioica (jhuo)*. The *T. Furas* occurs in the drier parts of the Doab and in the neighbourhood of Dehli, where it is called *Asul* or *Atul* as in Arabia: other species are also found in the peninsula.

The Tamarices are bitter and astringent. In Denmark they are used instead of hops for making beer, and in some parts of Europe as a tonic remedy. Galls are formed on the *T. Furas,* and are called *Sumrut-ul-asul* or *Chotee mue.* On the Jhou they are named *Sumrut-ul-toorfa,* or *Burree mue.* They are imported from Moultan.

The T. gallica of Mount Sinai is at certain seasons covered with a kind of sugary exudation, said by Ehrenberg to be produced by the puncture of the Coccus maniparus. It is called Arabian manna, or Guzunjabeen; it is unknown in the Bazars of Bengal, and is not produced in India. (*Royle*, p. 213, 214.)

The Melastomaceæ and Philadelpheæ need no notice in this work.

NAT. ORDER LVIII.—MYRTACEÆ.

An important order composed of trees or shrubs, with generally opposite branches, of elegant form; leaves simple, provided with small glandular transparent points, in which exists a very odoriferous essential oil. The flowers are axillary or terminal, less perfumed than the leaves. The prevailing principle in all is volatile oil. It exists in the calices, fruits, bark, and leaves. The oil varies in its properties, in some being lighter, in others heavier than water; its odour is agreeable, its flavour hot, somewhat acid, and occasionally followed by a sense of coolness in the mouth. Tannic acid also abounds in this order. None of the species act violently on the animal economy. The juice of the Alangium is said to be purgative, but the fact is not well established, neither is the plant indisputably one of this order. The fruits of several species are eaten (ex. the guava) but as they are usually more or less aromatic, the flavour is seldom agreeable to Europeans.

The Myrtaceæ occur in Australia, New Zealand, and the Indian archipelago. In India they reach the foot of the Himalayas. They have been found moreover at the Straits of Magellan, and in the cold parts of Peru, and more than one species is cultivated in Europe with perfect success.

Gen. 1.—Myrtus.

Sp. Myrtus communis. (Common Myrtle.)
Vern. Belati mendhi, *Beng.*

A native of Asia Minor and south of Europe, common in most warm countries. It assumes the shrubby or arborescent form according to the latitude; leaves opposite, sometimes ternate, with short petioles, ovate, smooth, of a beautiful green colour, glandular and persistent, flowers axillary, 5 petalous, white, succeeded by a purple berry the size of a pea.

The plant in all its parts is most agreeably perfumed. Its flavour is aromatic, styptic, and somewhat bitter; 10 lbs. of the leaves afford about a drachm of yellow essential oil of most delightful fragrance.

The berries were employed by the Romans as a spice, but have been but little used since the discovery of black pepper. The Tuscans, however, still preserve the custom, and they also prepare from the berries a kind of wine called *Myrtidanum.* (Lindley, p. 75.) A distilled water prepared from all parts of the plant is employed as a cosmetic, and called *Eau d'ange* by the French perfumers; the bark is used for tanning and dyeing.

Sp. 2. *Myrtus Pimenta* (Pimento, allspice, Jamaica pepper.)
Syn. Eugenia Pimenta, De C.

A native of South America and the West Indian Islands, especially Jamaica, introduced successfully into the Botanic Garden of Calcutta.

The berries are about as large as a small pea, unequal, wrinkled, ash or brown coloured, marked with a prominent four-cleft umbilicus (the calyx being persistent and superior,) they are bilocular, each cell containing a black hemispherical seed; the odour aromatic, agreeable, resembling a mixture of cloves and canella; taste pleasant, styptic, not like that of pepper. These properties are dissipated by time. The essential oil is brownish red, very odoriferous, and heavy, and of pungent taste. The sole importance of these berries is in their use as a spice. They are occasionally used in medicine as a stimulating aromatic, and an adjunct to prescriptions.

Sp. 3.—*Myrtus caryophyllata*, (clove-myrtle).

Syn. Calyptranthes caryophyllata.

A native of Jamaica, Cuba, and Ceylon. The bark is compact, very hard but brittle, found in commerce in sticks composed of pieces rolled one within the other, of deep brown colour, and greyish white epidermis; the odour is strongly that of the clove, taste aromatic, hot and sharp, slightly bitter and astringent. It contains tannic acid, resin, and essential oil, and is employed chiefly as a spice.

Gen. 2.—Caryophyllus.

Sp. Caryophyllus aromaticus, (clove).

Syn. Eugenia caryophyllata.

Vern. Cramboo, *Tam.* Long, *Duk.* and *Hind.* Warrala, *Cing.* Lăvăngă, *Sans.* Chankee, *Mal.* Lawangum, *Tel.* Kerenful, *Arab.* Mykek, *Pers.*

A native of New Guinea, Amboyna, and the Moluccas.

The dried flowers and unimpregnated ovaries *(cloves)* are externally of reddish brown colour, 5 to 7 lines long, and exhibit in their centre an inferior ovary of loose texture and yellow colour; these flowers consist of an unexpanded corolla formed of 4 rounded petals attached to the internal base of the calyx, and of a quadrangular shape. Within we find the remains of the stamina, below the corolla are 4 calycinal scales, concave, stiff, pointed, and disposed like a star; the lower part of the calyx is wrinkled, elongated, and quadrangular, two of the angles being more prominent than the others; the calyx becomes thin towards its lower end, where it terminates abruptly in a little plane surface adherent to the peduncle.

Cloves should be large, heavy, brittle, brown externally, red within, and when compressed or rasped allowing a volatile oil to exude. Their odour is aromatic, very sweet, taste aromatic, strong, hot, and acrid, almost to burning, slightly bitter.

The ripe fruits dried before the sun, are also found in commerce, and are called clove berries, or *mother cloves.*

Their properties are analogous to, but much feebler than those of the article above described.

Several analyses of the clove have been published, all of which indicate the existence of volatile oil (18 per 100), Trommsdorff, caryophylline, a crystalline principle, resin, gum, extractive, and astringent matter.

The *volatile oil* is very fluid, but thickens by age, clear, transparent, at first colourless, then amber-like or brown, heavier than water, entirely soluble in alcohol, reddened deeply by nitric acid, and producing oxalic acid; odour very powerful and agreeable, taste very hot, acrid, and burning. It is much adulterated, especially with pimento oil. The oil is obtained by distilling cloves from a saturated solution of common salt in water. The salt is added in order that the liquid should acquire a higher boiling point, viz. 224.

Caryophylline is white, brilliant, satiny, soluble in boiling alcohol and in ether, and crystallizes from its solutions in beautiful starry groups.

Cloves are universally employed as spices, and enter into some pharmaceutical preparations; the volatile oil is much used by perfumers, and dentists apply it to carious teeth to cauterize the exposed nerve.

The clove plant resembles the coffee. It grows quickly, and bears while young. Its height seldom exceeds 18 feet, its trunk is straight, and sustains a large somewhat conical cyme, so tufted that it resists the efforts of the wind, and the tree is thus frequently destroyed by storms. The leaves are opposite, petioled, oval, lanceolate, very entire, glabrous, 3 to 4 inches long, 12 to 18 lines broad, shining above, and sprinkled over with small, glandular, translucent points. The flowers are white, disposed in a terminal cyme with opposite ramifications, and with smooth peduncles; these are used for the distillation of the volatile oil, which they yield in considerable quantity.

It is impossible to ascertain when cloves were first introduced into Europe.

The Chinese who visited the Molucca islands before their discovery by the English, disseminated this spice through India, whence it spread to Persia, Arabia, and Europe. After the Dutch conquest of the Moluccas they restricted the cultivation of the clove to the island of Amboyna and to Ternate. Nevertheless the plant was introduced by the French into the Mauritius and Bourbon, and by the English into Barbadoes and the Antilles, in all which localities it succeeds perfectly. *(Feé.)*

The cloves are gathered in October, or in February, either by hand or by long wands. They are exposed to smoke on earthen dishes and then dried by the sun. Each shrub gives from 2 to 4 lbs. of cloves, but in the arborescent state 20 lbs. have been produced. One clove tree is described, the trunk of which was eight feet in diameter, and which furnished annually 50 to 60 lbs. A pound of cloves contains about 5000 flowers.

The tree can scarcely be made to live in Bengal.

Gen. 3.—Eucalyptus.

Sp. Eucalyptus resinifera.

Syn. E. Kino. Metrosideros gummifera. Botany bay *kino tree*, or brown gum tree. A native of Australia, cultivated in the Calcutta Garden.

A tree with smooth, reddish, cylindrical, and angular branches, leaves alternate, slightly membranous, straight, lanceolate, glabrous, retracted at their extremities, very acute. Flowers in umbels, lateral and solitary, stamina red, placed on a resinous aromatic mass.

An astringent juice flows from this tree, named Botany Bay *kino.* Ainslie quotes *Dumul-ook-wain* as the Bazar name of this kino, but the term properly applies to the "Dragon's blood." It is infusible, occurs in fragments of variable size and form, often covered with brownish powder, brittle, thin, translucent and ruby coloured, fracture glassy and chocolate coloured, of variable depths of tint, destitute of odour. Taste austere and somewhat bitter, powder red-brown ; water dissolves about two-thirds, alcohol three-fourths, ether one-twentieth only. But there are different statements made by writers on this subject. Mr. White, who has witnessed the collection in Australia, says a single tree will yield 500 lbs. of this kino in one year by incisions practised on the bark.

The medical uses of this article correspond exactly with those of *kino*, as already described.

The bark and leaves are aromatic, but their essential oil has not been separated.

Gen. 4.—Melaleuca.

Sp. Melaleuca Cajeputi, (Cajeput tree.)

A native of Banda, Java, and Amboyna. Feé describes it as of elevated trunk, covered with a cork-like bark, branches whitish, leaves alternate, nearly sessile, entire, ovato-lanceolate, glabrous, of pale green colour, falciform, and 3 to 5 inches long, 1½ to 2 broad, 5-nerved. Flowers white, highly odorous, fruit capsular, and three-celled. The leaves yield the celebrated *Cajeput oil*, of which they smell strongly when bruised by the fingers.

Cajeput Oil (*Kyapootie ke tel*, Hind.)

This oil is very fluid, light, transparent, of a beautiful green colour; very volatile and inflammable; its odour resembles that of camphor, but is more pungent and penetrating. It is sometimes adulterated with camphor dissolved in other volatile oils, but the fraud is detected by mixing the suspected oil with sugar and water, on which the camphor immediately separates in the solid form. The green colour has been erroneously attributed to the presence of copper proceeding from bottles in which it was asserted to be sent from Banda to Europe. These statements have however been entirely controverted. Though copper may be accidentally present in some specimens, it does not exist in others of equally green colour.

Cajeput oil in doses of from 1 to 3 or 5 drops, mixed with water and sugar, has been much used as a stomachic stimulant, especially during the prevalence of cholera epidemics; it is used in spasmodic pains attributed to the stomach, and in flatulence not dependent on an inflammatory state; in malignant cholera it has been much given, but with very doubtful advantage; externally it forms a very valuable stimulating liniment and embrocation, useful in rheumatism, paralysis, neuralgic, and similar affections.

Besides the preceding, M. Feé alludes in notes to species of *Leptospermum*, natives of New Zealand and New Holland, the leaves of which are used as tea,—to *Alangium*, trees with aromatic roots, which yield a juice of violent purgative properties,—to *Psidium*, or the guava tree,—to the *Eugenia malaccensis*, and *E. Jambos* of India,—and to the *Lecythis*, the almonds of which are much esteemed, and of which two species have bitter fruit.

Gen. 5.—Barringtonia.

Sp. Barringtonia racemosa.

A native of Malabar, root slightly bitter, and considered by the Hindus to be aperient, cooling, and febrifuge. The fruit of *B. speciosa* is mentioned by Ainslie as being used in Java for intoxicating fish.

Barr. acutangula (Sumundur phul) is a native of Chittagong, and is found in a clump of trees at Saharunpore, near Mr. Grindall's house, (*Royle*, p. 216.)

NAT. ORDER LIX.—GRANATEÆ.

This order contains but one genus, *Punica;* and this but one species, the pomegranate.

GEN.—PUNICA.

Sp. Punica Granatum, (pomegranate.)

Vern. Darimba, *Sans.* Dalim, Darim, *Beng.* Anar, Gulnar, *Hind.* Buloositoon, Rooman, *Yunani.*

Off. The roots.

A native of Cabul, Bokhara, Mezenderan, and Asia Minor generally; common now in almost all warm climates; the best fruits are those of Balabagh, lying under the snowy hills, near the Cabul river. Very large quantities are annually imported into the north of India from Cabul, and Cashmere.

In the Himalayas and the plains the pomegranate also occurs, but of inferior quality; the fruit is small, and is sold in the Bazar under the name of *darmee;* the rind, *naspal*, is used in medicine and in dyeing, on account of its great astringency.

Bot. characters. Arborescent; leaves oblong, inclined to lanceolate. Flowers large, red, with a pale succulent calyx, petals much crumpled; membranous fruit, a round leathery pericarp, crowned by the prominent hardened tube of the calyx, containing several irregular cells filled with seeds, covered with a bright red, succulent, acid coat.

Calyx turbinate, 5-7 cleft; œstivation valvate, petals 5-7, stamens numerous, filaments distinct, style filiform, stigma capitate, fruit large, globose, crowned by the somewhat tubular limb of the calyx, baccate, indehiscent, covered with the tube of the calyx, divided horizontally into two parts by a very irregular confused dissepiment, the lower division 3-celled, the upper 5-9 celled, dissepiments membranaceous, placentæ in the lower division at the bottom, in the upper stretching from the side of the fruit to the middle; seeds numerous, nestling in a pellucid pulp; embryo oblong, radicle short, acute; cotyledons foliaceous, spirally convolute. Small trees or shrubs with spinescent branches, leaves deciduous, opposite, rarely verticillate or alternate, often axillary and fascicled, oblong, quite entire, not dotted, flowers 2-3, nearly sessile, on somewhat terminal branchlets, usually scarlet. (*Lind. Fl. Med.* p. 74.)

The *roots* are hard, heavy, woody, knotty, covered with a bark yellowish grey externally, internally yellow, inodorous, astringent, devoid of bitterness, very rich in tannic acid to which they owe their established vermifuge properties. The ancients used these roots for the expulsion of tape-worm, but the practice had fallen into neglect when it was revived by Buchanan and others. The bark of the root is given in a decoction of 2 ounces in 2 lbs of water, reduced by evaporation to 12 ounces. This quantity is divided into 6 doses to be taken daily, and repeated for four or five days.

Analysis. The bark of the root was analyzed by Mitouart in 1824, and found to contain tannic acid, wax, gallic acid, and a saccharine matter identical with that of manna, *(mannite)*.

The *flowers (balanistum)* are rich in tannic and gallic acid, and are used in dyeing, and in medicine as astringents; with alum they make a beautiful red ink.

The *pericarp* is hard, smooth, a line in thickness, olive brown externally, yellowish within, inodorous, extremely bitter and astringent, much used in tanning and in dyeing yellow; also as a medicinal astringent.

The juice of the fruit is acidulous and sweet, and makes a pleasant sherbet for fever patients.

Off. Prep. Infusion, decoction, &c. &c.

NAT. ORDER LX.—MEMECYLEÆ

contains no article of medicinal value.

NAT. ORDER LXI.—COMBRETACEÆ.

This order contains the celebrated Myrobalons of ancient and eastern pharmacy. Astringency is the prevalent principle, although the fruits of *Terminalia Chebula* are gently laxative also. *T. Catappa* affords edible kernels, like almonds, and also named *badam*. *T. Benzoin* in the Mauritius gives a milky juice, which becomes fragrant as it dries, and is burned as incense in churches.

Gen.—Terminalia.

Flowers often polygamous from abortion, limb of the calyx deciduous, campanulate, five-cleft, the lobes acute, petals wanting, stamens ten, in a double row, longer than the calyx, ovary 2, 3 ovuled; style filiform somewhat acute; drupe not crowned by the calyx, often dry, indehiscent, one seeded, seed almond-like, cotyledons spirally convolute;—trees or shrubs, leaves alternate or rarely opposite, sometimes crowded towards the extremity of the branches; flowers spiked, spikes racemose or panicled, bisexual in the lower part of the spike, male in the upper part. (W. and A.)

Sp. 1. *T. Chebula.* (Chebulic Myrobalon.)
Syn. Myrobalana Chebula, Gærtn. ii. t. 97.
Vern. Kadukai, *Tam.* Carakaca, *Tel.* Huldah, *Duk.* Hara, *Hind.* Araloo, *Cing.* Haritaka, *Sans.* Heleliji Kabule, *Arab.* Helileh Kelān, *Pers.* Umbed'her, *Hind.* Trivial name, *Chebula*, from *Cabul*, where it is very abundant.

Forests of Bengal—common in Mysore.

Trunk rarely straight, short, bark ash-coloured, branches numerous and spreading. Leaves opposite, or nearly so, short petioled, oblong, entire, obtuse, in young trees downy on both surfaces, spikes in a terminal panicle or axillary. Flowers numerous, small, dull white, offensive in smell, all hermaphrodite; filaments 10, twice the length of the calyx, ovary one-celled with two ovules, drupe oval, about 1½ inch long, 1 inch in diameter, smooth or greenish yellow, obscurely five-angled, one-celled, pulp hard and yellowish, nut oblong, thick, very hard, surface rough, irregularly and obscurely five-grooved, one-celled.

Fruit very astringent; in its dry state about the size of an olive. With catechu it is applied with great advantage in apthous ulcerations. The *Zengi Har* of Bengal, Singi, *Tamul.* Kurkadaga, *Sans.* (Black Myrobalon), is described by Ainslie as the unripe dried fruit, and as a brisk purge. It is deep black, oblong, pointed and slender. It is called *Ahleeluj-asood* by the Arabs, *Helileh-seeah* by the Persians, who give it as a cathartic, in doses of from 1 to 2 drachms with a little honey.

Sp. 2. *Terminalia citrina.*
Vern. Liba, *Sans.* Haria, Harra, *Hind.*

Drupe oblong, lanceolate, about two inches long, two in circumference, obscurely five-grooved, dull orange-yellow, smooth; nut oblong, deeply five-grooved, one-celled.

Fruit a gentle purgative. It is often made into a pickle.

Sp. 3. *Terminalia alata,* (T. tomentosa, Wall.)
Vern. Muddi putta, *Tel.* Urjoon, *Hind.* Arjuna, *Sans.* Maradam putta, *Tam.* Kumbuk, *Cing.*

Fruit glabrous, bark deeply cracked, astringent and febrifuge. As found in the Bazars its colour is reddish brown, taste astringent; in powder and with oil it is used in apthæ. (Roxb. Fl. Ind. ii. 440.)

Sp. 4. *T. moluccana.* (Sylhet, Moluccas.)
Drupe round, ovate, size of a large nutmeg, used as T. bellerica, for which it is substituted.

Sp. 5. *Terminalia Catappa.*
Vern. Nattoo vadom cottay, *Tam.* Budamie, *Hind.* Vodom vettello, *Tel.* Catappa, *Malay.* Ingudi, *Sans.* Budum, *Beng.*
Probably a Malayan species, cultivated in India, a valuable timber tree. Drupe three inches long, egg-shaped, grooved; kernel resembles the almond or filbert in taste and composition; yields an excellent fixed oil, and is good nourishing food.

The bark and leaves are very astringent, and yield a black paint.

Sp. 6. *Terminalia Bellerica.* (Belleric Myrobalon).
Vern. Tamkai, *Tam.* Bulla, *Duk.* Beheyra, *Hind.* Beleyluj, *Arab.* Beleyleh, *Pers.* Bahira, *Sans.*
Mountainous parts of India; common in Mysore.

Drupe oval, somewhat five-angled, size when dry of a gall-nut, and dirty brown colour; size of a nutmeg, and fleshy when fresh, with a grey silky down, very astringent; kernels eaten, and deemed intoxicating; bark abounds in gum. Ainslie reckons the fruit as astringent, tonic, and attenuant. Dose one to two direms. It is much used in the arts as an astringent, and as the basis of several colours.

Sp. 7. *Terminalia Vernix.*
A native of China.

One of the trees which affords the celebrated Chinese black lacquer.

The Emblic myrobalon (Amalaca, *Sans.* Anola, *Hind.*) is the fruit of the *Emblica officinalis,* natural order *Euphorbiaceæ.*

NAT. ORDER LXII.—CUCURBITACEÆ.

The Cucurbitaceæ, or gourds, are herbaceous, annual, very rarely perennial plants. The root of the annual species is thin, that of the perennial fleshy. The stalks, which are cylindrical or angular, are provided with claspers, by which they ascend along trees, walls, and other objects for their support. The fruit varies much in size, form, and external characters. It is generally fleshy within. Its pulp is sometimes so saturated with water that it cannot be dried. The seeds are situated in the midst of a very abundant cellular tissue; the proper tegument is thick and leathery, and encloses an almond which is at first milky, and subsequently contains oil; but few of these plants are indigenous in Europe.

The Cucurbitaceæ are mostly inodorous or fœtid, and generally the latter character indicates poisonous qualities. An acrid principle has been separated from the root of the Bryony and the fruits of the Colocynth and Elaterium; sugar has been found in many of the edible kind. The roots of several contain starch, often associated with an acrid poisonous matter, which can be separated by washing the powdered root with water, in which the acrid matter dissolves while the starch is left. The seeds of most of the order are of mild sweet taste, give good emulsions with water, and yield a fixed oil by expression.

In tropical countries this order gives the inhabitants a large portion of their food, which it often affords of the finest quality in the most arid deserts or on barren swamps and islands. In Persia, China, and Cashmere they are cultivated on the lakes on the floating collections of weeds common in these localities; in India they are everywhere abundant, either in the wild or cultivated state.

We shall first enumerate the species employed in medicine, following Lindley's excellent arrangement of this order (see *Fl. Med.* p. 83) and we will subsequently point out in a note those which are of most importance as articles of diet, or for other popular uses.

Gen. 1.—Feuillea.

Sp. 1. *Feuillea trilobata,* (Brazil.)

The bitter seeds are asserted by some, to be a powerful antidote against vegetable poisons, doubtless because they are prompt, and rather too powerful emetics and cathartics.

Sp. 2. *F. cordifolia,* West India Islands.

Properties the same as those above mentioned.

Gen. 2.—Lagenaria.

Flowers monœcious, calyx campanulate, with subulate or broadish segments shorter than the tube, corolla white, petals obovate, spreading below the edge of the calyx; ♂, stamens 5, triadelphous, the 5th distinct; ♀, stigmas three sub-sessile, thick, 2 lobed, granulated; fruit 3—5 celled; seeds obovate, compressed, tumid at the margin, 2-lobed at the apex. (*Lindley.*)

Sp. Lagenaria vulgaris. Bottle gourd. East Indies.
Syn. Cucurbita lagenaria.
Vern. Belaschora, (Rheede,) *Toombee,* (Royle,)—the Gourd of this variety is used for making the stringed musical instrument called the *sitar.*

The whole plant is of musky scent, soft, downy, stem climbing, tendrils 3-4 cleft, leaves cordate, entire, downy, somewhat glaucous, with two glands at the base; flowers stellated, very spreading; clustered anthers with their connective covered by oblong, ovate, acute papillæ. Fruit downy, smooth, tapered into a long slender stalk above the insertion of the calyx.

In the wild state the fruit is poisonous, producing symptoms like those of cholera. Dr. Lindley states that some sailors were poisoned in England by drinking beer which had been kept in a flask made of one of these gourds.

Gen. 3.—Cucumis.

Flowers monœcious, calyx tubular, campanulate, with subulate segments scarcely the length of the tube, petals scarcely adhering to each other; ♂, stamens 5, monadelphous; ♀, stigmas 3, thick, 2-parted; fruit 3-6 celled, seeds compressed, ovate, not tumid at the edge. (*Lindley.*)

Sp. 1. *C. utilissimus.*
Vern. Kankoor, kurktee, *Beng.* Kakni, *Hind.*

Higher cultivated lands of Bengal; an annual. Tendrils simple, leaves broad, cordate, more or less 5 lobed, lobes rounded, toothed slightly, the largest generally 6 inches each way. Flower leaves of the female flowers sessile and very small, male flowers axillary, peduncled, crowded, but opening in succession; female flowers axillary peduncled, solitary; both sorts yellow, about an inch or an inch and a half in diameter; fruit fleshy, generally a very perfect oval; when young, downy and clouded with lighter and darker green; when ripe perfectly smooth, variegated with deeper and lighter yellow, from 4 to 6 inches long, and 3 to 4 in diameter. (*Roxb. Fl. Ind.* iii. 721.)

The powder of the toasted seeds is described as a powerful diuretic, and serviceable in promoting the passage of sand or gravel.

Sp. 2. *C. Colocynthis.* Colocynth, or bitter apple. (Κολοχυνθις, Dioscorid.)

Vern. Indrain, *Hind.* Vishala, *Sans.* Hunzil, *Pers.* and *Arab.*

Sandy lands of Coromandel, Kaira in Guzerat, Tirhut, and the Doab, especially near Dehlee.

Stem prostrate, hispid, leaves cordate, ovate, many lobed, white, with hairs beneath, the lobes obtuse, petioles as long as the lamina, tendrils short, flowers axillary, solitary, stalked; females with the tube of the calyx globose and somewhat hispid, the limb campanulate with narrow segments. Petals small, fruit globose, smooth, six-celled, with very numerous seeds; size of an orange, yellow when ripe, with a thin solid rind and a bitter white flesh.

The seeds are oval, obtuse, compressed, smooth, of olive colour, about four lines long; they constitute (Duncan) 1¾ of the whole weight of the fruit. Pereira describes two varieties, one white, the other black or brownish; the latter very bitter, but he states both have this flavour. Duncan however, on the authority of Captain Lyon, describes the seeds as constituting an important article of food in northern Africa. The seeds of the Bengal colocynth are certainly bitter, and given in half drachm doses produce decided cathartic effects.

According to Vauquelin's analysis colocynth contains a resinous matter insoluble in ether, a peculiar bitter principle (colocynthin), fat, oil, extractive, gum, and salts.

Colocynthine is resinous, yellow, more soluble in alcohol than in water, to which however it communicates excessive bitterness. The solution in hot water is of a fine golden colour, gelatinizes on cooling, gives a white precipitate with tannic acid. According to Neuman's experiments 768 parts of the pulp give alcoholic extract 168, watery extract 216.

The pulp and seeds of the colocynth produce exceedingly powerful cathartic and emetic effects; from large doses amounting to acrid poisoning. The alcoholic or watery extract however when given in proper doses, and combined with milder purgatives, constitutes one of the most valuable of our medicinal resources. The compound extract of our Pharmacopœia contains besides the alcoholic extract of colocynth —aloes, scammony, cardamums, and soap. It is an excellent purgative, especially when given with blue pill or calomel. The dose is 5 to 10 grains. Numerous formulæ for its administration will be found in our Pharmacopœia.

We are indebted to Dr. Burn, of Kaira in Guzerat, for specimens of the colocynth of that district, and of an extract of his preparation. These articles are identical in action with the colocynth of the Doab, and both are quite equal to the best imported from Europe. These facts are of much importance, especially to the native practitioner, inasmuch as the compound extract of colocynth costs at least 1*l.* 1*s.* the pound avoirdupois. Our extract made in Calcutta costs but four rupees per lb. The colocynth of India is moreover likely to become a profitable export, either in the state of fruit or extract. We find that in 1839, 10,417 lbs. were imported into England from Mogadore or the Levant.

Sp. 3. *C. Hardwickii*, (Royle's Illustr. p. 220,) occurs at the foot of the Himalayas, and is called "puharee indrayun," or Hill colocynth.

The stems are slender, climbing, very scabrous, with white, frequently hairy glands, leaves cordate, acuminated, somewhat 5 lobed, or 5 angled, angles acute, upper surface very hairy, under less so, margins undulately crenate, minutely toothed; male flowers 1 or 2 together, female solitary, calyx of each very hairy; fruit oval, oblong, rounded at both ends, from 2—3 inches long, and about half as broad, marked with narrow white stripes, flesh very bitter.

Its qualities are described as similar to those of the colocynth.—We have not seen the article.

Sp. 4. *C. Pseudocolocynthis*, Royle.

Plains of northern India, where it is called "Indrayun," and "Bisloombhee;" stems slender, prostrate, radiating, very scabrous, leaves scabrous on both sides, with white glandlike hair-bearing tubercles, five-lobed, lobes as well as the angles rounded, the former slightly toothed, the terminal one broader, cuneate, subdivided into three smaller lobules; male flowers generally solitary, so are the females, and long peduncled. Calyx tube oblong, hispid, segments narrow, linear, and pointed; fruit oblong and smooth, marked with eight broad stripes, flesh very bitter (*Royle*).

The fruit is similar in quality to colocynth, and is substituted in northern India for the true article.

On application to Dehlee for specimens of the Bislombhee we were favoured by Dr. Macintosh, and subsequently by Dr. Ranken, with fruits which corresponded in every respect with the description and characters of the real colocynth. Dr. Burn's specimens were also identical with the true article, though called "Indrayun" and "Bislombhee." There can be no doubt then, and taking into account moreover the extreme cheapness of the dried fruit in the Bazars, that the real colocynth exists in the Doab and Guzerat, and is called by the names applied by Dr. Royle, to his *Pseudo-colocynthis.* But it is also equally evident that Dr. Royle's article is a peculiar species, perhaps more abundant than the genuine kind.

GEN. 4.—LUFFA.

Male flowers panicled, yellow. Tube of calyx hemispherical, segments longer than the tube, petals distinct, dropping off by the base, stamens 5, distinct, anthers very wavy; female flowers solitary, tube of calyx oblong clavate. Segments shorter than the tube, stamens abortive, stigmas uniform; gourd ovate, three-celled, fibrous internally, operculate. (*Lindley, Fl. Med.* p. 85.)

Sp. 1. *L. amara.*
Syn. Cucumis indicus.
Vern. Kerula, *Hind.*
Hedges, and dry uncultivated places in the East Indies.
Stems several, slender, running to a great extent, but with few branches, pretty smooth, five-sided, tendrils three-cleft, leaves slightly 5—7 lobed, rough stipules, axillary, solitary, cordate, with glandular marks on one side. Male flowers pretty large, yellow, on long erect axillary racemes, the pedicels with a glandular bract near the base, and articulated a little above it. Female flowers usually larger, axillary, solitary, peduncled; fruit oblong, three or four inches long, and one in diameter, tapering equally towards either end, ten-angled, when ripe dry, grey, and filled with dry fibres; the operculum deciduous; seed blackish grey, with elevated minute black dots. Every part extremely bitter, fruit violently cathartic and emetic, juice of roasted young fruit applied to the temples by the natives of India to cure head ache; ripe seed either in infusion or in substance used by them to purge and vomit. (*Roxb. Fl. Ind.* iii. p. 715.)

Sp. 2. *L. Bindaal.*
Diœcious, climbing, leaves five-angled, toothed; male flowers in racemes; females solitary, fruit round, citrinate, with long firm straight ciliate bristles—considered in Northern India a powerful remedy in dropsy. (*Roxb. Fl. Ind.* iii. p. 717.)

Luffa pentandra, *acutangula*, *clavata*, and *racemosa*, the two first called *Ghia* and *Kalee-tori*, are cultivated or found wild in all parts of India.

Luffa tenera receives also from Royle the name of *Kurwa-tori.*

Gen. 5.—Bryonia.

Flowers monœcious or diœcious, petals partly united at the base; *male flowers*—calyx five-toothed, stamens triadelphous, anthers flexuose; *female flowers*—style trifid, fruit ovate or globose, smooth, few seeded, seeds ovate, scarcely compressed, more or less edged. Peduncle simple, seldom forked. (*Lindley.*)

Sp. 1. ***B. rostrata,*** a native of Tranquebar.
Vern. Appakovay, *Tam.*
Stem filiform, furrowed, leaves cordate, obtuse, toothletted, scabrous, peduncles axillary and solitary, fruit ovate, angular, acuminate. The root is prescribed in India as an astringent and emollient poultice in cases of piles. (*Ainslie.*)

Sp. 2. ***B. alba,*** same as next species in properties.

Sp. 3. ***B. dioica.*** Europe.
Syn. Αμπελος λεύκη, Βρυωνια, Diosc.
Root large, white, long, fleshy. Stems annual, scabrous, climbing among bushes by their tendrils; leaves 3, 4 inches broad; berries small, scarlet, fœtid when bruised.

Root acrid and purgative, produces also violent vomiting. It was formerly a very popular remedy in Europe, but is now banished from the Pharmacopœiæ.

The active principle of this root was separated by Brande and Firnhaber. The expressed juice was mixed with water and left to rest; starch subsided, and was separated; by boiling the filtered liquid albumen was removed, and on evaporation an extract was obtained. This was digested in hot alcohol till every soluble principle was taken up. An extract was again made and treated by water to separate resin. The watery solution on being carefully evaporated afforded the Bryonite.

Bryonite is yellowish brown, intensely bitter, soluble in water, insoluble in ether, and but difficultly so in absolute alcohol; contains azote. It is quite neutral towards acids and alkalies, the latter however dissolve it freely.

Sp. 4. ***Bryonia epigæa.***
Vern. Rawkus Gudda, *Hind.*
The powder of the root is given by native practitioners as an aperient and alterative, in doses of a pagoda weight, once daily for a week, in chronic dysentery and venereal. (*Ainslie*, vol. ii. p. 158.)

The root resembles that of the colombo plant; see page 196.

Under the preceding genus, Ainslie describes—

B. scabra—Vern. Ahilaykum, *Sans.* Musmusa, *Duk.* the shoots and leaves of which are aperient, the fruit slightly bitter also.

B. callosa—Vern. Boddama Kaia, *Tel.* The bitter seeds are given in worm cases, and yield also a fixed oil used in lamps.

B. grandis—Vern. Jivaka, Vimba, Patuparni, *Sans.* Koondorie, *Duk.* Telkatcha, *Hind.* The juice of the leaves is used as an application to obstinate ulcers produced by the bites of animals. (*Ainslie, vol.* ii. p. 436.)

Gen. 6.—Momordica.

Flowers monœcious, yellow or white—male flowers, calyx five-cleft, with a very short tube, corolla five-parted, stamens triadelphous, with connate anthers; female flowers, filaments three, sterile, style trifid, ovary three-celled; fruit opening with elasticity when ripe, seeds compressed, reticulated. (*Lindley.*)

Sp. 1. *M. Elaterium.*

Syn. Ecbalium officinale, Σιχυσα γριος, Dioscor.

A native of the south of Europe; fruit oblong, obtuse at each end, hispid, disarticulating from its stalk with violence, and expelling its seeds and mucus with considerable force, in consequence of the sudden contraction of its sides.

Thomson states that for medical purposes the fruit is gathered in September, just before it is ripe. It should be sprinkled with water, each fruit cut through lengthwise, the clear juice strained through a sieve, and the cucumber also washed.

Elaterium.

These cucumbers when sliced allow a juice to subside which by standing deposits a grey sediment,—this is called *Elaterium;* it consists of resin, colouring matter, and a crystalline principle named *Elatin,* discovered by Dr. Morries of Edinburgh in 1830.

The sediment is dried before the sun, or by a stove, or on folds of calico. By boiling in alcohol the Elatin is dissolved, and is deposited in large crystals on cooling, while the resin and colouring matter remain in solution in the spirit.

Elaterium is the most powerful of all known cathartics, from $\frac{1}{8}$ to $\frac{1}{4}$ grain is sufficient to induce profuse watery evacuations. It is chiefly employed in the treatment of apoplexy, dropsies, and obstinate constipations; two varieties are found in the shops, the white and brown, they are both of equal power.

It is very liable to adulteration, chiefly with starch.

The expressed juice of this cucumber has been recommended as preferable to the deposited fecula, as being less violent in its action. It should be remembered however that the chief value of this remedy consists in its enabling us to use, under certain emergent circumstances, a substance of great activity and in small bulk.

Sp. 2. *M. mixta.*
Vern. Gol-Kakra, *Beng.*

This is erroneously named *Makal* by Ainslie, and as he also by mistake applies the same term to the colocynth plant, many errors have originated in attempts to introduce the Indian colocynth into medical practice in India. The fruit of the Gol-Kakra is large, red, and thorny, contains a yellow insipid pulp, is totally inert as a medicine, and is indeed occasionally used for food in Bengal. *Makal* is the correct name of the first species of Trichosanthes described under the next head.

Gen. 7.—Trichosanthes.

Flowers monœcious, white—male flowers, calyx somewhat clavate, five-parted, lobes setaceous, appendiculate with five exterior teeth alternating with the lobes, corolla five-parted, ciliated; stamens three, anthers combined, their cells very wavy; female flowers, calyx five-toothed, corolla five-parted, with a lacerated fringed margin; style three-fid, stigmas oblong, subulate; fruit oblong, three to nine celled.

Sp. 1. *T. palmata.*
Vern. Makal, *Beng.*

A native of all the forests of India, stems angular, very long, running over the highest trees, covered with a grey scabrous somewhat corky bark, the young green parts smooth, tendrils three cleft, leaves petioled, generally palmate, though sometimes only three to five lobed, divisions acute, slightly serrate, from three to five nerved, smooth, having frequently several round glandular hollow spots on the underside, petioles channelled, stipules single, small, axillary; male flowers racemed, large, white, most beautifully fringed with long white ramous filaments. Racemes axillary, longer than the leaves; bractes solitary, one-flowered, oval, fringed, covered on the outside with dark green glandular spots. Female flowers generally axillary, peduncled, though sometimes racemose also; fruit globular, smooth, the size of a small orange, when ripe of a deep red colour, full of a dirty looking, greenish, soft pulp, in which the seeds are placed; the seeds are reckoned poisonous. (*Roxb. Fl. Ind.* iii. p. 704.)

The taste of the rind being singularly bitter we made many experiments with the view to ascertain whether it possesses purgative, tonic, or aperient properties. In three grain doses, thrice daily, it produced no sensible effect.

Made into a paste with cocoa-nut oil, Ainslie informs us that this fruit is much used in India as an application to the sores which often form behind the ears; it is also introduced into the nostrils in cases of ozæna.

Sp. 2. *T. amara,* St. Domingo, seeds bitter and astringent, sometimes emetic.

Sp. 3. *T. villosa,* Java, fruit acts like colocynth.

Sp. 4. *T. cordata.*

Vern. Boomee koomara.

Found wild near the Megna. The root is tuberous, perennial, growing to the size of a man's head. Stem herbaceous, climbing to the length of some fathoms, 5 sided, villous, or even somewhat scabrous when old; tendrils opposite, 3 cleft, leaves alternate, petioled, cordate and cordate-lobate, finely dentate, villous on both sides, about six inches each way; petioles channelled, a little hairy, scarcely half the length of the leaves; male racemes axillary, solitary, as long as the leaves; bractes alternate, sessile, cuneate, oblong, acute, serrulate, one-flowered; flowers large, white; the fringe of the segment coarser than in the other species; female flowers axillary, solitary, short peduncled; gourd spherical, the size of an orange, and nearly the same colour, but redder; cells soft, partitions very obscure; seeds numerous, immersed in a gelatinous green pulp. (*Roxb. Fl. Ind.* iii. 703.)

The root is used in India as a substitute for Colomba.

Sp. 5. *T. cucumerina.*

Vern. Junglee chuchinga, *Beng.* Found in hedges in Bengal.

Stem 5 sided, slightly downy; tendrils 3-cleft; leaves broad cordate, angular, and sometimes lobed, toothed, downy, very various in size; male flowers racemose, small, white, and beautifully fringed; racemes axillary, erect, longer than the leaves, many flowered; female flowers, axillary, solitary, short peduncled like the males. Fruit oval, or oblong, pointed, from 1 to 4 inches long, and from 1 to 1½ inch in diameter, till ripe striated with white and green, when ripe red; seeds involved in a red pulp, lobed. (*Roxb. Fl. Ind.* iii. 702.)

The fruit is reckoned an anthelmintic. Royle says it is edible, (p. 219).

Sp. 6. *T. dioica.*
Vern. Pulwull, *Beng.*

An alcoholic extract of the unripe fruit is described as a powerful and safe cathartic in 3 to 5 grain doses, repeated every third hour till the desired effect is produced.

GEN. 8.—MURICIA.

Sp. Muricia cochinchinensis.

A native of China and Cochin China, a large shrub, berry large, reddish purple, scentless, insipid; seeds and leaves aperient, and used by the Chinese in obstructions of the liver, "tumors, malignant ulcerations, &c."—externally employed in fractures, and in dislocations. (*Lindley.*)

We subjoin a list of the chief *Dietetical species*, (Royle, p. 219.)

Cucurbita Pepo. (pumpkin,)	Meetha kuddoo.*
——— Citrullus, ...	Turbooz, ... A variety, Tentsee.
Benincasa cerifera, ...	Peetha.
Cucumis Melo (melon,)†	Kurbooza,
C. madaraspatensis, ...	Roxb. Fl. Ind. iii. p. 723.
C. patescens, ...	Wild, common near Saharunpore, becomes aromatic on ripening.
C. Momordica, ...	Phoot.
C. sativus,‡ cucumber, ...	Kheera.
C. utilissimus, ...	Kukree,
Luffa pentandra, ...	Ghia.
—— acutangula, ...	Kaleetori.
Momordica Charantia, ...	Kurella, fruit slightly bitter and tonic.
Trichosanthes anguina, ...	Chuchinga.
——— dioica, ...	Palwal.
——— cucumerina, ...	Junglee-chuchinga.

* The seeds of these yield oil by expression, and are considered "cooling medicine."
† Seeds oily, and readily become rancid.
‡ Fruits contain sugar, seed yields a mild oil.

NAT. ORDER. LXIII.—PAPAYACEÆ.

This order only contains one genus, the *Carica*, natives of South America; whence *C. Papaya*, the Papaya tree, has been introduced into India.

Gen.—Carica.

Sp. C. Papaya, Papaya.

Vern. Urun-khurbooza, *Hind.*

The fruit is formed by a large oblong pepo suspended upon the leafless part of the trunk, like the jack fruit; the surface when ripe is a pale, and rather dingy orange yellow, obscurely furrowed, and often rough, with little elevated points. The flesh is very thick, coloured, but paler than the outside, and there pass through it longitudinally five bundles of vessels; in the centre is a considerable cavity with five longitudinal ridges, thickly clothed with small roundish compressed black seeds, covered with a greyish skin or arillus, and enveloped in mucus. (*Roxb. Fl. Ind.* iii. 824.)

A milky juice exudes on incision from the rind. It is deemed a powerful vermifuge in the Mauritius, and the powder of the seeds (which taste like water-cress) is said to possess the like virtue. The milky juice very closely resembles white of egg in its chemical composition. It is alkaline, contains albumen in such quantities that it coagulates when heated to 170°, and it putrifies readily, evolving a very offensive odour.

It is stated in several works of high authority that tough meat rubbed with this juice becomes very tender and fit for the table, without any injurious property being communicated to it. The flesh of animals fed on the leaves and seeds is said also to be remarkably tender. It is even asserted that dead animals hung from the branches of the tree undergo this alteration. These ideas prevail also in Bengal, where the Mahomedan table servants frequently use the juice with the view of softening beefsteaks and old fowls. In numerous experiments which we instituted we could not trace any well marked decisive effect of this kind. Putrefaction appeared to us to be accelerated by contact with this as well as other albuminous fluids. Just before putrefaction commences muscular fibre is doubtless less rigid than at any previous time. It is thus possibly that we may best explain the effect, if any, produced by the practice in question. As to the alleged efficacy of suspending meat from the tree, we are disposed to regard it as a mere popular delusion.

The leaves are used by the negroes in washing linen, as a substitute for soap.

We cannot speak from our own experience of the anthelmintic virtue of the juice. We have given it in doses of from 20 to 60 drops, without observing any marked effects.

NAT. ORDER LXIV.—PASSIFLOREÆ.

The *Passiflora Quadrangularis*, Granadilla of W. Indies, is described as a powerful narcotic—the root is cultivated, according to Mr. Burnet, in several of the French settlements. It is said to contain an active principle, *Passiflorine;* the fruit is much eaten in Brazil. *P. Contrajerva* of Mexico, is said to be alexipharmic and carminative. *P. Fœtida* of the W. Indies is esteemed as an emmenagogue, and reckoned of utility in hysteria. (*Lind.* p. 106.)

Species of passion-flower occur in Singapore, on the Neelgherries, and in Nipal; several are cultivated in the Botanic Gardens of Calcutta and Seharunpore.

NAT. ORDER LXV.—PORTULACEÆ.

Ainslie describes fully the *Portulaca quadrifida.*

Vern. Chowly, *Duk.* Bucklut-ul-mobarik, *Arab.* Batsalikoora, *Tel.* and Oopadykee, *Sans.*

The bruised fresh leaves are prescribed as an external application in erysipelas, and an infusion given in dysuria.

The *Portulaca oleracea,* (Hind. *Loonia,*) is common in India, and eaten by the Hindoos; in Cochin China the seed is considered emollient and diuretic.

NAT. ORDER LXVI.—PARONYCHIEÆ.

Gen. 1.—Trianthema.

Sp. 1. *Trianthema obcordata,* Roxb., formerly his *T. monogynia.* Ainslie, vol. ii. p. 370.

Vern. Nasurjinghi ke jur, *Hind.* Punarnavi, *Sans.*

The root is found in Bazars; colour pale; much wrinkled, bitterish, and rather nauseous to the taste, considered cathartic, and given in powder to the extent of two tea-spoonsful twice daily with a little ginger.

Sp. 2. *Trianthema decandra.*

Vern. Beeskhupra, *Duk.* Swet punarnavi, *Sans.*

Root size of small finger, light brown on side, white within, aperient. "Four pagodas weight of bark of the root made into a decoction with 1 lb. of water and boiled down to ½ a lb. will open the bowels." (*Ainslie.*)

Gen. 2.—Achyranthes.

Sp. Achyranthes lanata. (Ainslie, vol. ii. p. 393.)
Vern. Khul ka jur, *Duk.* Astma bayda, *Sans.* Apanga, *Beng.*
Syn. Illecebrum lanatum, Roxb. ii. 504.

The root is deemed to be demulcent, and is prescribed in strangury. It is quite common in Colombo, and called *Pot kuda-pala.*

NAT. ORDER LXVII.—CRASSULACEÆ.

Ainslie describes no species. Feé mentions the *Sedum acre* as causing vomiting and purging.

The *Sempervivum tectorum,* (*house-leek*) affords an acid juice, and is used as a refrigerant internally and externally. Lindley mentions one species of Sempervivum and one of Sedum; several species are found in the temperate and cold parts of India.

NAT. ORDER LXVIII.—FICOIDEÆ.

Royle and Ainslie mention no medicinal species in this order, but allude to the genus *Mesembryanthemum,* as a ready source of soda. Feé speaks of the order as of little consequence in a medicinal view; he mentions that all the species are rich in alkaline carbonates; but this is sufficiently explained by their usually frequenting the sea shore.

NAT. ORDER LXIX.—CACTEÆ.

This order affords the species on which the varieties of the Cochineal insect feed. We must refer to the head "Cochineal" for the few details, as to these plants, with which it is necessary that the medical student should be informed.

NAT. ORDER LXX.—GROSSULARIEÆ.

This order contains the red and black currants of European gardens. Species are found in the Himalayas, but too acid to be eatable.

In the Saxifrageæ, no medicinal species are described by Royle, Feé, Lindley, or Ainslie.

NAT. ORDER LXXI.—UMBELLIFERÆ, OR APIACEÆ.

This most important family requires the careful study of the medical student. It is so strictly natural in its relations as to constitute as it were but one large genus. (*Royle.*)

The essential character is described by Lindley thus—polypetalous and dicotyledonous, stamens five, pentagynous. Carpella concrete, ovarium didymous, inferior with two styles, and solitary, pendulous ovula, leaves sheathing at the base, flowers umbellate, embryo minute in the base of a fleshy albumen. Sometimes there are three carpella. The calyx is superior, either entire or five-toothed; petals five inserted on the outside of a fleshy disk, usually inflexed at the point, æstivation imbricate, rarely valvate, stamens five, alternate, with the petals incurved in æstivation, ovarium inferior, two-celled, styles two, distinct, stigmata simple. Fruit consisting of two carpella separable by a common axis, to which they adhere by their face (commissure), each carpellum traversed by elevated ridges, of which five are primary, and four alternating with them in secondary ridges separated by channels, below which are often placed in the substance of the pericarp linear receptacles of oily matter named *Vittæ;* seed pendulous, usually adhering inseparably to the pericarpium, rarely loose. Embryo minute, radicle pointing to the Hilum.

Plants herbaceous, with fistular furrowed stems, leaves usually divided, sometimes simple, sheathing at the base, Flowers in umbels, generally surrounded by an involucrum. *Lind. Introd.* p. 4.

The Umbelliferæ abound in temperate climates; only seven wild and six cultivated species occur in the plains of India. In the hills Dr. Royle has collected not less than ninety species, the total discovered up to this time being 127 species for the Indian Flora. (*Royle's Illust.* p. 228.)

About 800 species are now known as belonging to this order.

The principle which most abounds throughout the order is essential oil. This occurs in the roots, stalks, seeds, but rarely in the flowers, which are generally devoid of odour. The oil obtained is usually colourless, lighter than water, of powerful odour, of strong and hot taste. It resides in the episperm of the seeds, and is not found in the almond, which contains fixed scentless oil. To the former (with some exceptions) the Umbelliferæ owe their medicinal virtues.

Sugar is sometimes found united with mucilage in the roots of some of the biennial species. If these do not contain an excess of the essential oil they become alimentary, (for instance, the carrot, parsnip, celery, &c.) The roots are generally devoid of much activity, even in the species which have poisonous leaves and seeds.

But should essential oil co-exist with mucilage in the roots, it usually happens that by chemical changes effected by time, the oil passes into resin, and the mucilage into gum, (as in the assafœtida, galbanum, and opoponax, &c.). These principles are secreted by the proper vessels, and are also found, but in smaller proportion, in the stems.

A powerful and very remarkable alkali, *conein*, has recently been found in a species long used in medicine,—the *Conium maculatum*, or spotted hemlock.

While M. Feé divides the Umbelliferæ into two groups, namely the "true," and the "anomalous," Lindley in his *Flora Medica* forms several sub-divisions, which we adopt in preference, as Lindley's work embraces the most recent and accurate information on this subject.

Gen. 1.—Astrantia.

Sp. A. major, Europe.

Roots acrid and purgative, sometimes mixed with those of the black hellebore, which they resemble in appearance and effects.

Gen. 2.—Eryngium.

Sp. E. campestre, (Eryngo) common in the dry plains of middle and southern Europe.

Root sweet, aromatic, and tonic, cylindrical, as large as the finger, brownish, marked with rings, white internally, brittle when dry, (Feé.) Boerhääve reckons it as the first of the aperient diuretic roots. It has been recommended in gonorrhœa, suppression of the menses, and visceral obstructions, particularly of the gall bladder and liver. It has also the reputation of being an excellent aphrodisiac; is sold candied in Europe.

Gen. 3.—Cicuta.

Sp. 1. *C. maculata*, (Snake weed, United States.)

Root a most dangerous poison, a drachm of the fresh root having killed a boy in an hour and a half. Its effects are similar to those of hemlock, but more energetic.

Sp. 2. *C. virosa* (Water cowbane.)

Ditches and banks of rivers in Europe and Siberia. A dangerous poison, effects erroneously asserted by Lindley to resemble those of prussic acid, as the cowbane causes tetanic convulsions and death usually on the third day.

Gen. 4.—Apium.

Sp. A. graveolens, (Celery.)

Vern. Kurufs, *Arab.*

A native of marshy grounds in Europe, the Caucasus, Mexico, in the Levant and Affghanistan, now cultivated in Bengal. When wild, acrid and poisonous; when cultivated, blanched, aromatic, fragrant, and nutritious. The seeds are sold in every Bazar, and used as stimulants by the native practitioners.

The roots are also employed in medicine, they are white, spindle-shaped, oval, and branched; odour increased by drying. Vogel of Munich made an analysis of celery with the subjoined results:—Volatile oil, fixed oil, sulphur, bassorine, and gelatine, extractive matter, mannite, nitrate, and muriate of potash. The essential oil dissolved in strong spirit gives an essence, a drop of which will communicate a strong and fine flavour of celery to a tureen of soup.

We have introduced a tincture of the seeds into our Pharmacopœia.

The *Apium involucratum* is the *Rhadunee* of Bengal, and *Ajmod* of Hindostan.

Gen. 5.—Petroselinum.

Sp. P. sativum, (Parsley).

Shady rocks of Europe and the Levant, much cultivated for its leaves, which have an extremely delicate bitterish aromatic taste, and are decidedly diuretic.

The seeds and roots have a place in the French Pharmacopœia, and closely resemble the preceding article in their properties. (Feé, p. 18.)

Gen. 6.—Ptychotis.

Sp. 1. *P. coptica*, (Coptic ammi) Egypt and Candia. Used as a stimulant aromatic.

Sp. 2. *P. Ajowain*, Roxb. Fl. Ind. ii. 91.

Syn. Ligusticum Ajwain, (Fleming. As. Res. xi. p. 170.) Sison Ammi, of *Ainslie*.

Vern. Ajouain, Juvanee, *Beng.* and *Hind.* Nankah, *Pers.* Amoos, *Arab.*

Cultivated in India every where. Root annual, stem erect, one to three feet high, branches alternate, smooth, slightly striated, leaves scattered, those nearest the root supradecompound, the upper less so, all with filiform divisions. Umbels terminal, erect, composed of from six to eight rays, on rather unequal peduncles, partial, of many rays on unequal pedicels, involucres both universal and partial of from five to eight linear unequal branches shorter than the umbels, petals pure white, equal, furrowed on the back and keeled within with involute points, and broad waved rather reflexed margins; fruit didymous, compressed, broad, ovate, with five scabrous ridges on each side, of aromatic smell and warm pungent taste. This is one of the most useful of the Umbelliferæ, and an excellent remedy in flatulent colic; much used in India. (*Roxb.*)

Sp. 3. *P. sylvestris*, Arub Ajwain, *Royle*, found in the Khadir lands of the Saharunpore district. Used as a stomachic aromatic and remedy in flatulence.

Sp. 4. *P. involucrata. Aneeson* of North India, *Chanoo* and *Radhooni* of Bengal, used as a substitute for parsley. (*Royle.*)

GEN. 7.—SISON.

Sp. S. Amomum. (Honey-wort,) a native of Europe.

Fruit pungent, aromatic when dry, but has a nauseous smell of bugs when fresh. Abounds in essential oil, an ingredient in the French "*Theriaque*"

GEN. 8.—CARUM.

Sp. 1. *C. Carui*, (Caraway plant.)

Meadows and pastures in central Europe; fruit narrow, bright brown, 1½ line long, with pale elevated filiform ridges and shining convex channels; similar in action to dill and anise. Flavour very agreeable, yields abundance of essential oil, which is much used in pharmacy. The oil is of yellow colour, sweet smell, and very hot taste; in Germany caraway seeds are used in bread. The essential oil is much used as an adjunct and solvent in the preparation of the resinous cathartic pills.

The roots of the caraway plant are very agreeable, and are eaten in the north of Europe.

Sp. 2. *C. nigrum.*

Vern. Zeera seeah.

Brought into India from Kunawur, and used as a carminative. (*Royle.*)

GEN. 9.—PIMPINELLA.

Sp. P. Anisum, Aniseed. (Ανισον. Dioscor.) Egypt, Scio, Levant.

Vern. Sataphuspha, *Sans.* Sonf, *Duk.* Mahoree, *Beng.*

Fruit ovate, 1½ lines long, dull brown, slightly downy, not at all shining, with the ridges equidistant, elevated, sometimes rather wavy, paler than the channels, commissure broad and flat.

Aniseed in various forms is much employed in medicine as a stomachic, especially in the diseases of children, and is also used as a condiment among all eastern nations.

The seeds are often fraudulently mixed with clay, and are liable to spoil by spontaneous fermentation in the packages. They are much richer in essential oil than the majority of the Umbelliferæ, 8 lbs. having given 3½ ounces of the oil.

Essential Oil of Aniseed.

White, yellowish, a little lighter than water, congealing at 78 Faht. into a soft mass, sp. gr. 0,985. It is liable to adulteration with spermaceti and several fixed oils, some of which may be detected by alcohol, all by leaving a greasy stain on paper when evaporated over a lamp. This oil contains nitrogen according to the analysis of Saussure. It only exists in the pericarp, the interior of the seed yielding a tasteless and inodorous fixed oil. This is often mixed with the essential oil, and is as much an adulteration as if castor or olive oil had been employed. The pure essential oil can only be obtained by distilling the seeds with water.

The oil is a good and safe stimulant, and is much used in prescriptions for children suffering from flatulence and colic. (See ***Essential oils.***)

Gen. 10.—Œnanthe.

Sp. 1. *Œ. crocata.* (Hemlock drop wort.) Europe.

Root of many fleshy knobs, full of orange-coloured fœtid juice, extremely poisonous. It has not yet been made the subject of a conclusive analysis.

Sp. 2. *Œ. **Phillandrium***, (Water drop wort.)

Also European, similar to, but less energetic than the last.

Besides these Decandolle alludes to over 20 other poisonous species.

Gen. 11.—Æthusa.

*Sp. Æ. **Cynapium***, (Fool's parsley.) Common in Europe.

Leaves poisonous, producing nausea, vomiting, headache, giddiness, drowsiness, spasmodic pain, numbness, &c. They are dark in colour, and of nauseous smell, and often prove poisonous, being mistaken for common parsley, and chervil.

Gen. 12.—Fœniculum.

Sp. 1. *F. vulgare*, (Common fennel.) Europe.
Syn. Anethum Fœniculum.

Fruit ovate, not quite 2 lines long, pale bright brown, smooth, ridges sharp, with but little space between each, lateral ones rather broadest, terminated by a permanent conical disk. An essential oil is prepared in large quantities from the seeds. The odour of the entire plant is strong and persistent, that of the roots disappears on drying.

The *essential oil of fennel* is clear yellow, easily frozen, lighter than water; sp. gr. 990.

Sp. 2. *F. dulce*, (Sweet fennel.)

Italy and Portugal, very like, but smaller, than the last in vegetation, but the fruits differ greatly, being narrow, oblong, 3 lines long, pale dull brown, smooth, ridges sharpish, with a space between each for a convex line, indicating the vittæ, lateral ones broadest; no calyx; seeds also afford a valuable essential oil, much used in medicine.

Sp. 3. *F. Panmorium.*
Syn. Anethum Panmori.
Vern. Sonf, Panmuhori, *Hind.* A native of various parts of India.

Root white, nearly fusiform, and almost simple, stem erect, branched from the base to the top, from 2 to 4 feet high, the branches erect, round, and smooth, with a uniform pale glaucous tinge, and not striated leaves, supradecompound divisions, tapering, smooth and filiform, but by no means so numerous as in the common fennel; umbels terminal, rather concave, but not regular; the convex partial umbels (of which there are generally 10 to 20), standing on peduncles of very unequal lengths. Flowers small, bright deep yellow, petals long, ovate, with their points rolled in, stamens longer than the petals, styles scarcely any; fruit exactly the same as in F. vulgare, and has the same properties. (*Roxb. Fl. Ind.* ii. p. 95.)

Used in India as an aromatic in food and in medicine.

Gen. 13.—Athamanta.

Sp. Athamantha cretensis, Cretan carrot.
Middle and South of Europe, seeds warm, aromatic.

GEN. 14.—MEUM.

Sp. M. athamanticum.

Syn. Ligusticum meum—mountainous pastures in Europe, roots fusiform, the size of the finger, aromatic and sweet. The M. mutellina has similar qualities.

GEN. 15.—ANGELICA.

Sp. A. nemorosa, Naples.

Smell of the fruit like that of the buck goat. Root acrid, and used as a remedy for the itch.

GEN. 16.—ARCHANGELICA.

Sp. A. officinalis, North of Europe in watery places.

Root large, fleshy, branched, resinous, abounds in essential oil; 500 parts yield about four on distillation with water, and 10 per cent. of resin to alcohol after the oil is removed; the roots also contain gum and inuline; pungently aromatic, stem erect, 4 or 5 feet high, 1 to 2 inches in diameter. The root is fragrant, pungent, bitterish sweet at first, leaving a glowing sensation in the mouth, and exciting salivation. A good aromatic tonic; candied with sugar it is used in Europe in chronic colds, and as a diaphoretic; insects destroy it very speedily.

GEN. 17.—OPOPONAX.

Sp. O. Chironium.

Syn. Pastinaca Opoponax. Ferula op: πανaχες ηραχλειον *Dioscor.*

Off. Prod. Opoponax, gum resin.

[OPOPONAX, *Vern.* JUWASHUR.]

Opoponax occurs in fragments of a yellowish red colour, formed of irregular tears, angular, opaque, light, and friable, pale within, thin externally, odour strong and peculiar, taste acrid, hot and bitter. According to Pelletier's analysis 100 parts contain—resin 42, gum 33, starch 4, extractive and malic acid 4, volatile oil 5, with traces of caoutchouc and wax, and 9 of woody fibre. The sp. gr. is 1622; with water it forms a milky fluid.

Opoponax is derived from ὀπος juice, παν all, and ἀχος a remedy, meaning that it is a remedy for all diseases!

In action it resembles asafœtida, but is much feebler.

3 A

The plant occurs in dry fields in the south of Europe and Asia Minor. A milky juice exudes from the root when wounded, and hardens into a fœtid gum resin, in most of its properties closely resembling asafœtida.

This resin is found in all the Bazars of Bengal, and is even exported from this country to Europe.

Gen. 18.—Ferula.

Calyx a short 5-toothed border, petals ovate, entire, acuminate, with an ascending or incurved point, fruit flattened at the back with a dilated flat border, half fruits with 3 dorsal filiform ridges, the two lateral obsolete, and lost in the dilated margin, vittæ in the dorsal channels 3 or more, 4 or more on the commissure, root fleshy, stem tall, leaves supradecompound, generally cut up into segments, involucres variable, flowers yellow. (*Lindley.*)

Sp. 1. ***Ferula Asafœtida.***

Persia, neighbourhood of Herat, mountains of Laristan and Belochistan. Hindu-kosh at 7000 feet.

Root perennial, fleshy, with a coarse hairy summit, simple or forked, leaves radical, springing up in the autumn, growing vigorously through the winter, and withering in the end of spring, 1½ foot long, shining, coriaceous, glaucous green, pinnated, with pinnatifid segments, whose lobes are oblong and obtuse, petiole terete, channelled only at the base. Stem 6—10 feet high, solid, clothed with membranous sheaths, general umbels with from 10 to 20 rays, partial one 5-6 flowered. Fruit flat, thin, reddish brown, slightly hairy or rough, obovate, six lines long, rather convex, but little thinned away at the edge; dorsal ridges slightly elevated, lateral undistinguishable, vittæ of the back 20-22 interrupted, anastomozing, and tinged with asafœtida. Vittæ of the commissure 10. (*Lindley.*)

Asafœtida.

Vern. Hing, ***Beng.*** and ***Hind.*** Ungoozeh, ***Pers.*** Hilteet, ***Arab.***

The celebrated gum resin asafœtida, is obtained by slicing the roots. A milky juice exudes, which dries rapidly into a fœtid, pasty, bitter and pungent mass.

The odour of asafœtida needs no comment. It has gained for the gum resin the epithet of the "*devil's dung;*" the taste is bitter, acrid, and very durable. Asafœtida is difficultly reduced to powder unless triturated with the carbonate of ammonia.

According to Brande's analysis, 974 parts of asafœtida

contain resin 472, gum 194, volatile oil 46, resinoid matter 16, tragacanth 64, the remainder being saline and earthy matter and water. Its sp. gr. is 1.327. It yields its active principles to alcohol and to water, and affords essential oil by distillation with this fluid. Notwithstanding its abominable smell it is used for seasoning food in the East, and even in Europe we are told it is deemed an improvement to beef-steaks to rub it on the gridiron on which they are cooked.

Asafœtida occurs in commerce in shapeless masses of waxy consistence, with small transparent brittle and white tears. The fracture is vitreous, at first white, and passing to red by contact with the air,—a property which distinguishes it from all other gum-resins.

Another and much more valuable kind of asafœtida is sometimes met with in the Bazars and druggist's shops. It is in tears, or semi-transparent whitish granulations, free from impurities, and of most powerful odour ; this kind is readily reduced to powder, and is much valued by European druggists. In India it is but rarely met with, and readily meets purchasers at a high price.

Medical uses. Asafœtida is a powerfully carminative and stimulant tonic, devoid of acrid and irritating properties. It produces a sensation of heat, and increased secretion in the alimentary canal, with eructation ; head-ache, and giddiness are often experienced, and the urinary and genital organs seem to be sometimes materially excited.

It is chiefly used in hysteria, hypochondriasis, flatulent colic proceeding from dyspepsia, in chronic catarrh, and in spasmodic asthma not connected with disease of the heart or lungs. In worm affections too it is often employed with benefit.

Dose, from 5 grs. to a scruple, in *pills,* or in *mixture, tincture,* or with ammonia in the *fœtid spirit* of *ammonia.* (See those preparations).

Sp. 2. Ferula persica.

Syn. F. Sagapenum. Feé, vol. ii. p. 201.

A native of Persia, stem about two feet high. According to some authorities it produces Sagapenum. Nees Von Essenbeck and Lindley consider it as one of many plants from which asafœtida is procured.

Sagapenum.

Vern. Sugbeenuj, *Arab.* Sugafioon, *Pers.* and *Greek.* Kundel, *Hind.*

Sagapenum is found in masses formed of soft, adhesive fragments, the size of the thumb or more, somewhat transparent, reddish yellow externally, pale within, of waxy or brittle consistence, often mixed with impurities and seeds. Its odour resembles that of garlic and asafœtida, its taste is hot, nauseous, and rather bitter. It is sometimes adulterated with Bdellium, gunda-birosa, and other similar gum resins or turpentines. Pelletier states that 100 parts contain resin 54, gum 31, volatile oil 11, the remainder being malate of lime and bassorine. Sagapenum is totally soluble in weak spirit. It softens under the fingers, becomes tenacious, and melts at a low temperature.

It is collected in the same manner as asafœtida; in the Bengal Bazars small quantities are procurable at the rate of four rupees the lb.

The medical uses of Sagapenum are the same as those of asafœtida, but it is considered less energetic, and is but little employed.

Sp. 3. *F. orientalis.* Feshook, *F. ammonifera.* Feé.

Asia Minor, Greece, and Morocco. In Morocco it is said to yield the gum resin called *ammoniacum.* (See that head.)

Sp. 4. *F. Hooshee.* Beloochistan.

Resembles the asafœtida in size and appearance, and yields a gum like the opoponax of the European shops, (*Mrs. M'Neil's letter,* 1833). Professor Royle alludes to this also as resembling opoponax.

Sp. 5. *F. ferulago.*

Syn. F. galbanifera, (Nees and Ebermaier.)

Coasts of the Mediterranean, the Caucasus, &c. yields copiously a secretion which dries into a gum resin, supposed to be galbanum. (See *Galbanum officinale.*)

Gen. 19.—Dorema.

Sp. D. Ammoniacum. (Don. *Linn. Trans.* xvi. 601.)

Vern. Oshak, *Pers.*

Persia, plains of Yerde Kaust, and Kumisha, in the province of Irak, and near the town of Jezud Khast, in very dry plains, and gravelly soil exposed to the sun. (*Lindley.*)

A glaucous green plant, looking like opoponax. Leaves large, 2 feet long, somewhat two pinnate, pinnæ in 3 pairs, petiole downy, very large, and sheathing at the base. Umbels proliferous, racemose. Flowers sessile, immersed in wool.

The stem and fruits yield abundance of Ammoniacum resin.

Ammoniacum.

This gum resin is obtained by incisions in the plant, and occurs in two forms,—first in voluminous masses of yellowish colour, enclosing white almond-like tears, the whole being of plastic consistence, and very impure;—secondly, in tears of irregular form, white or yellowish, opaque, rather solid, agglutinated or distinct, compact, brittle, of glassy fracture, and free from impurities. Its odour is faint and peculiar, taste sweetish and then bitter. Braconnot states 100 parts to contain gum 18, resin 70, bassorine 4, water 6. Its sp. gr. is 1,207. It is partially soluble in water, ether, alcohol, alkaline solutions and acetic acid.

Medical effects, similar to, but less powerful than asafœtida; for preparations, see Pharmacopœia. It is principally employed as an expectorant in the chronic catarrhs and asthmas of old persons. It is also applied externally as a warm and stimulating plaster. (See *plasters.*)

Gen. 20.—Peucedanum.

Sp. 1. *P. officinale.* Sulphur wort, hog's fennel.

Meadows and shady places throughout Europe, juice of the root dried before the sun, is deemed diuretic and antispasmodic. (*Lindley.*)

Sp. 2. *P. Oreoselinum,* middle of Europe and Caucasus. Leaves and stem bitter and aromatic, fruit still more so; considered powerful alimentary stimulants. *P. montanum,* north and middle of Europe; root abounds in a white, bitter, fœtid juice, which hardens into an acrid resin, employed by the Romans as ginger, and in Courland deemed a good remedy in epilepsy.

Gen. 21.—Imperatoria.

Sp. I. Ostruthium, (master-wort) Europe and Newfoundland.

Root acrid and bitter, used in toothache, and praised as a remedy in intermittent fevers, some writers affirming that it has cured agues in many cases after the cinchona bark had failed.

Gen. 22.—Anethum.

Calyx obsolete, petals roundish, entire, involute, with a square and retuse lobe, fruit lenticular, flattened from the back, surrounded by a flattened border, half fruits with equidistant filiform ridges, the three dorsal acutely keeled, the two lateral more obsolete, losing themselves in the border, vittæ broad, solitary, filling the whole channels, two on the commissure. Upright, smooth—annuals—leaves decompound, with setaceous linear segments, involucre none, flowers yellow. (*Lindley.*)

Sp. 1. *A. Sowa.*

Vern. Shubit, *Arab.* Soya, *Hind.* Cultivated in Bengal.

Root annual, but of a few months duration, stem flexuose, branched, smooth, striated with deeper and lighter green, and covered with a whitish bloom; from 2 to 3 feet high, leaves decompound and supradecompound, leaflets filiform, umbels terminal, convex with involucres or involucella, calyx scarcely any, petals ovate, oblong, inflected, stamens longer than the petals, styles scarcely any, fruit oval, compressed, half fruits with three ridges on the back, and surrounded by a membranous margin. (*Roxb. Fl. Ind.* ii. p. 96.)

Fruit aromatic and carminative, and used by the natives in their curries and for medicinal purposes, especially to relieve flatulence and colic. The best form for adults is probably that of a few drops of the essential oil on sugar, or dissolved in spirit. By distillation the fruits of this and the next species yield a pale yellow volatile oil, sp. gr. 881, soluble in alcohol, ether, and in 1441 parts of water.

Sp. 2. *A. graveolens,* Dill.

Syn. 'Ανηθον, Dioscor.

Europe, the Levant, Astrakan, Egypt, Cape of Good Hope, &c.

Closely allied to the preceding species. The seeds yield an essential oil, distilled water, &c. and are much employed as carminatives. It is supposed by some to promote the secretion of milk.

Gen. 23.—Heracleum.

Sp. 1. *H. Sphondylium,* Siberia and Unalashaka, (brankursine). Rind and root acrid, and capable of producing ulcers on the skin ; root contains sugar.

Sp. 2. *H. gummiferum,* is erroneously supposed to yield opoponax, and by Wildenow, Ammoniacum.

GEN. 24.—GALBANUM.

Sp. G. officinale.

Vern. Barzud, *Arab.* Bireeja, *Hind.* (kenneh and nafiel, the plant) γαλβανη, Dioscor.

Little is positively known about the plant which furnishes the galbanum of the druggists, but in the opinion of the best botanists it is not obtained from the Bubon galbanum or Ferula ferulago of most Pharmacopœiæ.

The gum resin is obtained by incisions in the root and stems; the juice is cream-coloured, and soon concretes into a solid mass.

GALBANUM.

Syn. Khelbenah, *Hebrew,* γαλβανη, *Greek.*

Vern. Bireja, *Hind.*

In agglutinated plastic masses, mixed with seeds and fragments of leaves, of greasy aspect, adhering strongly to the fingers, by which it is quickly softened; white, brittle tears occur in the mass resembling pine resin; in odour this drug is analogous to ammoniacum; its taste is hot, acrid, and bitter. Pelletier's analysis shews it to contain in 100 parts resin 66, gum 19, volatile oil 6, wood and impurity 8; its specific gr. is 1.212.

The essential oil is colourless, but becomes yellow by keeping if distilled from water; of a deep blue if distilled by direct heat.

Water dissolves about a fourth of this drug, but deposits the greater part again; weak alcohol dissolves it altogether.

Its properties are the same in kind as those of asafœtida, but it is much less powerful. For its preparations, see Pharmacopœia.

GEN. 25.—CUMINUM.

Sp. C. Cyminum, (Cumin) Κυμινον ημερον, Dioscor.

Vern. Kumoon, Zeera suffed—Upper Egypt, Ethiopia.

Fruits resemble others of this order in stimulant and stomachic properties, and are used in a stimulating plaster. They yield a large quantity of essential oil, of yellow colour, lighter than water.

GEN. 26.—THAPSIA.

Sp. 1. *T. villosa*—on hills and thickets in Spain, Portugal, south of France, &c.

Roots acrid and corrosive, once considered purgative, which property however is now disputed.

Sp. 2. *T. Silphion*—on the mountains of Cyrene.

"The *Laser Cyrenaicum,* or Asa dulcis of Cyrene, was a drug in high reputation among the ancients for its medical uses. It had miraculous powers assigned to it, as an antidote, a remedy for blindness, and restorer of youth," (*Lindley,*) &c. The plant was struck on the Cyrenean coins, and the drug was sold at its weight in gold. "It has been successively referred to several plants of this order, but the question as to its origin seems set at rest by the discovery in Cyrene of the umbelliferous plant now quoted." (*Lind.*)

Gen. 27.—Laserpitium.

Sp. L. glabrum. Feé, vol. ii. p. 209.

Mountains of Europe.

Root gorged with a gum-resinous juice, acrid, bitter, and somewhat caustic; a violent purgative; the "false herpeth" of the French.

Gen. 28.—Daucus.

Sp. D. Carota. Carrot.

Vern. Gajra, *Hind.* Europe, now cultivated in Bengal; fruit 1½ lines long, pale dull brown, oval, primary ridges filiform, bristly, three near the middle of the convex back, two on the plane of the commissure; of bitter and hot taste. Roots fusiform, about a foot long, of reddish yellow colour, parenchym fleshy; smell feebly aromatic, taste sugary and mucilaginous.

Poultices of the rasped root are much used for correcting fœtid discharges from sloughing sores. The seeds are stimulating, and reputed to be diuretic; like the fruits of most of this order they yield essential oil.

Gen. 29.—Anthriscus.

Sp. 1. *A. sylvestris.* All over Europe.

Recommended in an extract in syphilitic cases, and deemed similar to, but less powerful than hemlock.

Sp. 2. *A. vulgaris.* (Rough Chervil).

A common European weed; poisonous.

Sp. 3. *A. Cerefolium.* (Chervil.)

Cultivated all over Europe. A common pot-herb, with edible roots.

Gen. 30.—Cachrys.

Sp. C. odontalgica. Siberia, Crimea, Caucasus.

Root excites salivation, and is used accordingly to relieve tooth-ache.

Gen. 31.—Prangos.

Sp. P. pabularia.

Vern. Fiturasulioon, north of India, near Draz.

This plant constitutes excellent fodder for cattle, fattens quickly, and destroys the "liver fluke" of sheep. Mr. Royle considers this one of the plants which yielded the Silphium of Alexander's historians.

Gen. 32.—Conium.

Sp. C. maculatum. (Spotted Hemlock.) Κωνειον, Dios. Europe, east of Asia and America.

Fruit a line and a half long, ovate, compressed, pale sage green, primary ridges five, elevated, sharp, wavy, commissure and channels finely wrinkled, but no vittæ.

This plant is of great importance as a medicine, and derives additional celebrity from being considered to have been used as the Athenian state poison, by which Socrates and Phocion perished. In the form of fruit, in locality (Crete and Candia) in the effects as a poison, and in some properties as a remedy, our article corresponds exactly with the descriptions of Dioscorides and Nicander—one very strong fact is, that no other poisonous Umbelliferous plant is found in Greece but this, which grows plentifully in the localities from which historians state the Athenian poison was gathered.

The stem of the hemlock is 2 to 5 feet high, round, smooth, hollow, marked with dark purple spots, leaflets pinnatifid, very fœtid when bruised—ovarium ovate, 2-celled, striated; the general involucres consist of from 3 to 7 leaves, the partial involucres of 3 leaves. *Conia*, the active principle of this plant, was first obtained by Geiger in 1831, and its properties have since been studied by Dr. Christison and Boutron-Charlard. Conia exists in all parts of the plant, but most abundantly in the seeds, from 40 lbs. of which (green) Dr. Christison obtained 2½ ounces of this alkali. Dr. Christison prepared it by distilling the alcoholic extract of the seeds with its own weight of water and a little caustic potash; the natural salt of conia is thus decomposed, and the conia volatilized. It is an oily, transparent, colourless liquid, lighter than water, of strong acrid smell, described as resembling that of hemlock juice and tobacco combined, sparingly soluble in water, freely in alcohol, neutralizing acids; its vapour is inflammable. It boils at 370, but distils with water at 212°. According to Liebig 100 parts are composed of carbon 66.91, hydrogen 12, oxygen 8.28, nitrogen 12.8. Several of its salts are crystallizable, and all are decomposed by potash, the conia being set free, and at once detected by its smell.

Conia is a powerful narcotic poison, five drops killed a small dog in less than one minute; it first stimulates the part to which it is applied, but the local effect quickly ceases, and general paralysis soon follows, first affecting the voluntary muscles, then the respiratory muscles of the chest and abdomen, and lastly the diaphragm, causing death by asphyxia. The sensibility does not seem to be impaired.

The other constituents of hemlock are green starch, vegetable albumen, an odorous principle, extractive and resin, but these do not need particular notice.

The effects of hemlock on man in small or medicinal doses depend apparently on the character of the disease in which it is employed; in healthy persons small doses scarcely produce any marked physiological effect. In poisonous doses paralysis, coma, rarely convulsions and delirium, are the most prominent symptoms.

Medical uses. The extract of hemlock is chiefly employed as an anodyne in scrofulous or cancerous affections. Baron Stŏck of Vienna, and several other able and experienced writers, have borne strong testimony to the value of the remedy in many cases of this kind. Bayle has published accounts of 46 cases of cancerous diseases cured, and 28 improved by hemlock. Still, as Pereira observes, but little reliance is placed on it by practitioners generally, "except for the purpose of alleviating pain." Hemlock has also acquired great reputation in scrofula, but the preceding remarks apply to this, as well as to the preceding class of diseases.

In rheumatism, neuralgia, and painful ulcerations, especially those of a syphilitic character, hemlock is employed with decided benefit.

Doses, &c. The powdered leaves (which should be green, recent, and evolve the odour of conia when treated with potash) may be given in doses of from 2 to 3 grains twice or thrice daily. The extract met with in the shops is nearly always inert, the conia being destroyed either during the preparation, or by age. If recent and well prepared, 2 grain doses may be given every third or fourth hour, until a decided anodyne effect is produced.

An alcoholic extract of the bruised ripe fruit is proposed by Dr. Christison and Mr. Pereira, as the best form of preparation, 220 gr. of this alcoholic extract being equal to five grains of hydrate of conein.

Hemlock poultices, prepared in various ways, are often applied with great advantage to irritable sores, particularly those of a cancerous, scrofulous, or syphilitic character; 2ʒ of the extract with a pint of water thickened by linseed meal constitute the London form. The bruised leaves themselves are occasionally employed; an ointment is made according to the Dublin Pharmacopœia, by boiling the fresh leaves in prepared lard, and is much used in the cases above mentioned, and also as an application to painful piles.

GEN. 33.—SMYRNIUM.

Sp. S. Olusatrum, Europe, in wet places.

Formerly cultivated instead of celery, as the leaves are pleasantly aromatic. The fruit is stimulant and stomachic.

GEN. 34.—CORIANDRUM.

Sp. C. sativum, Coriander plant.

Vern. Duniya, *Beng.* Kushneez, *Pers.* Kuzeereh, *Arab.*

Levant, Tartary, and south of Europe, cultivated in all parts of India. Fruit pale brown, coriaceous, spherical, 1½ lines in diameter, all the ridges indistinctly shewn on account of their slight elevation; vittæ of the commisure short, lunate, just visible without dissection. *(Lindley.)*

Fruit carminative and aromatic, aroma proceeding from an essential oil. Cullen considered that it concealed the flavour of senna better than any other aromatic. During the unripe state the odour resembles that of bugs, but this changes rapidly as ripening proceeds. Feé derives coriandrum from χορις, *a bug*, on account of the fætor of the young seeds.

NAT. ORDER LXXII.—ARALIACEÆ.

A small order, remarkable however for containing the celebrated Chinese ginseng, the ivy, and the Aralia nudicaulis, used in America as a substitute for sarsaparilla.

Gen. 1.—Aralia.

Sp. Aralia nudicaulis.

A native of North America.

Roots (rhizomes) are clothed with a grey epidermis, much cracked, covering a cortical part of pale grey colour, soft, spongy, and sometimes glutinous. The ligneous system is white, and traversed towards its centre by a large medullary canal, without a ligneous meditullium, which distinguishes it from the tree; sarsaparilla in flavour is sweet and then bitter, odour weak. This root is often mixed with sarsaparilla; if however the assertions of some American writers are to be depended on, the medicinal effects of this Aralia are quite equal to those of sarsaparilla. The subject however demands additional investigation.

Gen. 2.—Hedera.

Sp. Hedera Helix. The ivy.

Syn. H. arborea. κιττος, Theoph. κισσος, Diosc. Hedera, Pliny, a kind of *lablab* of the Hakeems.

A native of Europe and the high lands of Asia.

This lovely climber, the theme of poets, and the favourite of every European who recollects it clasping the ruined abbeys and feudal castles of his native land, affords a resinous substance of some remarkable properties, and its leaves and berries are used in medicine in some countries.

The berries are nauseous, somewhat bitter to the taste, and aperient in action; the leaves are applied to cauterized sores to stimulate them gently, and in decoction are used to kill vermin.

Hederine.

This substance exudes from old ivy stumps, and may be obtained also by incision. It occurs in masses of reddish yellow colour, transparent, covered with yellow powder, odour strong, taste acrid and aromatic, fracture glassy, and of a pretty red tint, texture brittle. Partly soluble in alcohol, and affording an orange red solution; according to Pelletier's analysis Hederine is composed (in 100 parts) of gum 7, resin 23, malic acid 0.30 and finely divided ligneous fibre 69. It is used in several varnishes, and was once considered depilatory, emmenagogue, and resolvent.

GEN. 3.—PANAX.

Sp. P. quinquefolius. Ginseng.

Syn. Aureliana canadensis.

The roots are about the thickness of the finger, like those of parsley, of whitish yellow colour externally, white within, two to three inches long, wrinkled, or with rings, often divided into two branches, rarely into three or four, and these presenting a slight likeness to the human form, whence the Chinese name is derived; the parenchyme is formed of a horny and compact tissue, displaying some resinous points. Above the neck is a knotty twisted tissue formed by the remains of the old stalks.

The odour is sweet, and weakly aromatic, the taste saccharine, somewhat like that of liquorice, subsequently bitter, and rather aromatic.

The root of an Umbelliferous plant, the *Sium Ninsi*, is often mixed in the druggist's shops, or mistaken otherwise for the ginseng; the essential difference consists in the ginseng having the neck covered with fibrous threads, the remnants of the cortical part of the stalk.

The root abounds in gum and starch, and has a little resin and essential oil.

The plant is about a foot high, with glabrous, straight, simple stalks, terminating in three leaves, each composed of six uneven leaflets, a little pedicelled, oval, lanceolate, acute, and toothed at the edge. The flowers are borne on a central peduncle, and disposed in an umbel. The berries are kidney-shaped, red, compressed, crowned with the calyx and styles, and containing two semicircular seeds.

The ginseng root is one of the substances which, without any obvious cause, has attained the highest celebrity and esteem among mankind for its alleged medicinal virtues. The Dutch were the first nation who made it known in Europe, where they brought it from Japan in 1640. The Japanese themselves were indebted for it to China. The plant grows in the great forests of Tartary between the 39th and 47th degrees of north latitude; it is also found in abundance in Virginia and Canada, a circumstance which has rendered the roots so common that they are now cheap in China, where they once sold for their weight in gold.

It would be superfluous to follow M. Feé and other authorities in the details they afford regarding the cultivation and gathering of the ginseng. The Chinese in their hyperbolical phraseology name the root, "the pure spirit of the earth," the "recipe of immortality," the "queen of plants,"

&c., and in short regard it as a panacea for all the diseases to which they are liable.

Dr. Wallich has discovered in Nipal a species of Panax closely allied to our present article, and of which he has published an account in the 4th vol. of the Transactions of the Medical and Physical Society of Calcutta, and in his *Plantæ Abeat. Rarior.* vol. ii. p. 30, t. 137. Dr. Wallich names his species *P. Pseudoginseng.*

The next natural order *Hamamelideæ* contains no remarkable species.

NAT. ORDER LXXIII.—CORNEÆ.

A small order long associated with the *ivy* until separated by Decandolle; it occurs in Mexico and America, and from Europe spreads east as far as Sylhet in the Himalayan mountains. As some species of the genus *Cornus* have been much praised as remedies in intermittent fever, we deem it desirable to insert such details as may encourage the trial of the Sylhet kinds.

GEN.—CORNUS.

Calyx with a very small toothed limb, petals 4 oblong, sessile, stamens 4, style 1, drupe baccate, marked with the traces of a calyx, stone 2-celled, rarely 3-celled, seeds solitary, pendulous. Albumen fleshy, radicle of the embryo shorter than the cotyledons. (*Lindley.*)

Sp. 1. *C. florida,* moist forests in the United States.

Wood very compact. Bark a powerful bitter, with an astringent and rather aromatic taste; it acts as a tonic, astringent, and antiseptic, resembling cinchona in its effects. Many writers consider it not inferior to cinchona in the treatment of periodical fevers. The bark of the roots yields a good scarlet colour.

Sp. 2. *C. sericea,* a shrub.

Moist woods in United States, said to be one of the best tonics in North America, and the best substitute for Peruvian bark.

Sp. 3. *C. suecica,* is celebrated as a tonic in the highlands of Sweden and Norway.

Sp. 4. *C. mas.*

Remarkable for the hardness and durability of its wood, hence used for spear-shafts and pikes; the fruits are extremely rough when immature, but when ripe become acidulous and agreeable; the bark has been employed with great success in the treatment of intermittent fevers.

Sp. 5. *C. sanguinea,* common in Europe; the fruits contain fixed oil of very agreeable flavour, and a good substitute for olive oil.

Several species have been found in the Himalayas, in Sylhet, and Nipal by Drs. Wallich and Royle; these are the Cornus oblonga, in the Deyra Doon; C. macrophylla, and C. nervosa, Mussoorie; and Cornus capitata, Wall. (Benthamia fragifera, Lind.) at a still higher elevation. The fruit of *Benthamia* is eaten in the hills, and from the seeds of some species an oil is expressed.

NAT. ORDER LXXIV.—LORANTHACEÆ.

This family consists of parasites, which are not only sustained upon, but take root in the substance of other trees. The chief genera are Viscum and Loranthus, the former well known as the mistletoe of the Druids.

No medicinal properties of any importance had been observed in these plants until we accidentally discovered, in 1836, that the Viscum found on the nux vomica trees of Cuttack possessed all the properties of the supporting tree. As we believe the occurrence has attracted some attention, and is of considerable interest in botanical physiology, we deem it necessary to state the particulars in detail.

In 1837, Lieut. Kittoe, then with his regiment at Cuttack, received information of the existence of a parasite on the nux vomica trees, to which extraordinary medicinal powers were attributed by the natives. They called it *Kuchila ke mulung*, held it to be an extremely powerful *narcotic*, and poisonous in small doses, and they used it in the treatment of agues and rheumatism. Mr. Kittoe having procured specimens of the leaves sent them to the Editor for experiment.

Given in three grain doses to dogs and kids tetanic spasms set in, in the course of from five minutes to a quarter of an hour, recurring at intervals, and proving fatal by fixing the diaphragm, and causing asphyxia. The convulsive movements were precisely the same as those occasioned by strychnine, brucine, and the nux vomica seeds or bark. On analysis the powdered leaves yielded—

Green colouring matter and fibre, ...	64
Wax, ...	4
Strychnine, ...	1
Brucine, ...	3
Extract, ...	18
Saline matter and Resin, ...	10
	100

Specimens of the leaves were referred to Dr. Wallich, who supposes them to belong to the *Viscum monoicum;* but no fruit or flowers having been obtained this point is not yet clearly ascertained. Mr. Kittoe subsequently favoured us with a branch of the nux vomica tree in which the parasite was firmly rooted, but as neither fruit nor flowers were present the difficulty in identifying the species was not removed.

The powder of the dry leaf has been used with complete success as a substitute for strychnine and brucine in the Hospital of the Medical College, by Dr. Duncan Stewart, and by several other practitioners. The dose is one to three grains thrice daily. The precautions observed in using strychnine and nux vomica are equally necessary with this remedy; it should be remitted as soon as tingling or spasmodic contractions are observed.

The *Viscum album*, or white mistletoe, is generally supposed to be the parasite which held such an important part in the superstitious ceremonies of the Druids. It yields no medicinal product, but the berries are used for the manufacture of a kind of glue, of little importance even in the arts.

NAT. ORDER LXXV.—CAPRIFOLIACEÆ.

The plants of this family are possessed of but weak properties; the leaves of the elder tree are purgative, and the bark of some of the same genus astringent. Dr. Royle informs us that the shoots and young leaves of *Lonicera diversifolia* (woodbine) called *dandoo*, are used in medicine by the hill people.

Gen. 1.—Triosteum.

Sp. Triosteum perfoliatum.
United States; called 'fever root,' and 'wild ipecachuan.' "The bark of the root is emetic and purgative, leaves diaphoretic, their efficacy impaired by age; they should be preserved in closely stopped jars, and changed annually." (*Lindley, Fl. Med.* p. 445.)

A species of Triosteum, *T. himalayanum*, has been discovered by Dr. Wallich's people at Gossainthan in Nipal.

Gen. 2.—Sambucus.

Sp. 1. *Sambucus Ebulus*, (Dwarf-elder.) Europe, roots deemed cathartic.

Sp. 2. *S. nigra*, common elder; inspissated juice of the fruit said to be cooling, laxative, and diuretic; inner bark purgative, or in large doses emetic; flowers diaphoretic and expectorant.

S. adnata is found in the Himalayas.

NAT. ORDER LXXVI.—RUBIACEÆ OR CINCHONACEÆ.

This order, remarkable for embracing the renowned Peruvian bark trees, the ipecachuan, and the coffee plant, is composed of herbs, shrubs, and trees, almost exclusively natives of hot climates. The leaves are simple, with very entire edges, verticillated in the herbaceous species, sometimes opposite and stipulate. The flowers are usually terminal or sessile, forming sometimes, though rarely, tufts or whorls.

M. Feé divides the family, as regards its structure, into "herbaceous," and "woody," and also into the "indigenous," and "exotic."

The European herbaceous Rubiaceæ possess no energetic properties, being slightly bitter, and of weak astringency, while in warm climates some genera possess an active emetic principle in the roots; in Europe the only analogy in composition is the presence of rich colouring principles, much used in dyeing and painting.

The emetic principle *emetine*, has been found in the roots of the Cephælis, Richardsonia, and Psychotria; tannic acid abounds in almost every species, herbaceous or arborescent.

The bitter principles of the largest and most important genus are the celebrated alkalies *quinine, cinchonine*, and *aricine*, the discovery of which by MM. Pelletier and Caventou has proved such an extraordinary addition to the resources of medicine.

Caffeine is another crystalline principle of peculiar properties found in the berries of the coffee.

Gen. 1.—Rubia.*

Sp. 1. ***Rubia tinctorum***, Madder.

Sp. 2. ***R. manjista***, Roxb.
Vern. Menjithe, ***Hind.***

Natives of the south of Europe, the Levant, and Asia Minor, cultivated in India, and in many parts of Europe.

Sp. 1. Stem diffused, brittle, branched, angular, very rough with sharp hooks, leaves six in a whorl, lanceolate or oblong lanceolate, mucronate, somewhat membranous with pinnated veins, flowers small, white, limb of calyx hardly any, corolla volute, five-parted, lobes of corolla ovate, lanceolate, apiculate, stamens five short, styles two short, fruit didymous, globose, baccate, juicy, anthers ovate oblong, stigmas conical. *Lindley.*

The roots are creeping, the thickness of the little finger, very long and branching, provided with numerous articulations, and tough fibrils, epidermis thin, pale brown, bark and meditullium intensely red. The odour is weak and peculiar, taste bitter and styptic. According to Kuhlman's analysis the roots contain red colouring matter, (*Alizarin*, Robiquet,) yellow do, (*Xanthine*, Kuhl.) woody fibre, mucilage, gum, sugar, bitter matter, resin, salts, albumen, &c.

Alizarin occurs in orange red crystals, tasteless, inodorous, little soluble in cold, but soluble in boiling water, also in alcohol, ether, the fixed oils, and alkalies. The alcoholic solution is rose coloured, the etherial golden, the alkaline violet or blue. A solution of alum added to a solution of alizarin, and precipitated by potash, gives a rose lake of the most charming tint.

Xanthine is yellow, very soluble in water and alcohol, slightly in ether; the solution passes to orange-red by contact with alkalies, to lemon-yellow by acids. It is devoid of odour, but has a sweetish bitter taste.

The red colouring matter of madder tinges the bones, milk, and urine of animals if fed on the roots.

* Stellatæ or Galiaceæ of Lindley, a separate order.

The great consumption of madder is as a dye stuff for giving a red colour to wool, silk, and cotton.

In pharmacy the roots are sometimes used for colouring ointments. It was at one time, like saffron and turmeric, a favourite remedy in jaundice, on the ancient doctrine of signatures, which regarded the colour of the skin as the important point in this disease, and the colour of these substances as infallible indications of their value in its treatment. For a similar reason it was prescribed in suppression of the catamenia, as well as in too profuse menstrual discharges. It is now however altogether disused.

Gen. 2.—Asperula.*

Sp. A. odorata. Wood roof.

In woods throughout Europe.

The herb while drying has the scent of new hay, approaching to bitter almonds. It is deemed diuretic, and used as a substitute for tea.

Gen. 3.—Galium.*

Sp. G. verum. Resembles the preceding genus in smell. The flower stalks are used as a yellow dye, and employed for colouring Cheshire cheese.

Gen. 4.—Cephaelis.

Sp. C. Ipecachuana.

Off. The roots.

A native of New Granada in Brazil. Three modifications or varieties of these invaluable roots are found in commerce and pharmacy.

1. "*Grey*" *or annulated Ipecachuana.*

A wrinkled root, 3 to 4 inches long, twisted, strictured in various places, and forming rings on a continuous woody axis, thin towards its inferior extremity, the thickness of a quill in its general length. Simple and sometimes branched, with grey resinous, compact bark, readily broken at the strictures; the bark is thick, covered with a blackish grey epidermis, grey internally, hard, horny, and half transparent. The meditullium or ligneous centre is white, and very hard.

The odour is strong, irritating, and nauseous, taste acrid,

* See Note in preceding page.

aromatic, and bitter, powder grey. In preparing the powder the meditullium should be rejected as inert. It is easily separated by pounding the roots lightly. If ground entire the meditullium is last reduced to powder, and the separation may thus be accomplished, but with greater difficulty and loss.

M. Pelletier in the 3rd vol. *Journal de Pharmacie*, 148—151, gives an admirable analysis of these roots, with the subjoined results:—

	Bark and meditullum,		Meditullum alone.
Emetic principle,	16.0	...	1.15
Fatty matter,	2	...	a trace.
Wax,	6	Inert Extract.	2.45
Gum,	10	...	51
Starch,	42	...	20
Fibre,	20	...	66.60
Gallic acid,	traces.	...	traces.
Loss,	4	...	4.80

2. "*Grey-red*" *Ipecachuana.*

Root closely resembles the first variety, colour less deep, but reddish, horny, and half transparent, sometimes it is opaque and farinaceous, and is then inactive; the taste is decidedly bitter, odour stronger than in the former kind; on analysis it yields 14 per 100 of emetine.

3. "*Starchy or whitish grey*" *Ipecachuana.*

Root rather thick, rings less decided, more regular, tint whitish grey, in other respects like the preceding kinds; not yet analysed.—Feé and Pereira regard all these varieties however as merely the first kind, accidentally enlarged or altered in form.

EMETINE.

Emetine is white, pulverulent, unalterable in air, little soluble in cold water, very fusible, decomposed by heat, very soluble in alcohol, insoluble in ether and in the fixed oils; does not form neutral salts with acids, composed of carbon 64.57, azote 4, hydrogen 7.77, oxygen 22.95. Inodorous, of bitter and disagreeable taste.

The third of a grain of this emetine causes speedy vomiting, and also proves cathartic.

As generally employed in medicine, emetine is in brown or reddish transparent scales, deliquescent and crystallizable.

It is obtained by treating the powdered ipecachuan by ether in order to remove fatty matter. An alcoholic extract is then prepared, which is redissolved in cold water; wax and fat are thus removed, calcined magnesia now takes away some gallic acid, and the emetine is precipitated with magnesia; this must be washed with a little cold water to separate colouring matter, then dried and boiled in strong alcohol, which by evaporation affords the emetine. This may be further purified by solution in acidulated water, and by a second precipitation by an alkaline base.

The earliest works in which ipecachuana is mentioned are those of Pison on Brazilian medicine, and in Marcgrave's Natural History of Brazil. The emetic effects of the root were known to the Brazilians from time immemorial, and it received from the Portuguese the name of 'rais d'oro,' or golden root. The father of the celebrated Helvetius was the first to establish its utility after numerous experiments performed in the hospitals of Paris, for which he was rewarded by Louis XIV. with a thousand *louis d'or*.

The roots of the *Viola parviflora*, the *Psychotria emetica*, and several other plants, have been occasionally used to adulterate the ipecachuana.

The plant is not cultivated in Brazil, and as it only flourishes in the large forests daily falling before the planters' axe, the root is rapidly becoming scarce, and proportionally high priced.

Medical uses. Ipecachuana in doses of from 20 to 30 grains produces free and copious vomiting without much nausea, especially if the action of the medicine be promoted by draughts of tepid water; vomiting usually occurs in a period varying from 5 to 10 minutes.

In small doses, say one grain repeated every hour, nausea is induced, and the secretions and movements of the intestinal system so much augmented that purging ensues.

United with opium, each in small doses, the action of the remedy seems specially directed to the skin, and copious perspiration results; this is well exemplified in the action of the well known *Dover's powder*, (ipecachuan 1 gr., opium 1 gr. sulphate of potassa 8 grs. the last ingredient being added merely to give bulk and sub-division to the powder.) This remedy is one of the most powerful and certain of sudorifics when given in doses of from 10 to 20 grs. It is accordingly constantly employed in the treatment of rheumatism.

With blue pill and gentian, as well as with opium, it is very much employed in the treatment of the dysentery of warm climates. Referring to its use in this disease, Mr. Twining observes in the preface to the second edition of his valuable work on the diseases of Bengal, "this plan of treatment is confirmed by the practice of Mr. Geddes of the Madras European Regiment, who is well known as the author of a scientific work on the Seringapatam fever; he states that the employment of ipecachuana with the usual adjuvants generally precludes the necessity of having recourse to mercury in dysentery." Drs. Mortimer, Bakie, Egerton, and French, have strongly corroborated this opinion. At p. 92 of the 1st vol. full details of this system are recorded. Mr. Twining's observations are of the highest practical value. For this author's formula, see the Pharmacopœia.

In the pulmonary affections of young children ipecachuan is employed with great success, either as an emetic or nauseant remedy. A tea-spoonful of the ipecachuan wine (see that head) will act as a ready and easy emetic in infants of from one to four years.

GEN. 5.—PSYCHOTRIA.

Sp. P. emetica.

To this plant is attributed the "*striated* or *black ipecachuana.*—The striæ are long with indistinct intersections, but still penetrating to the woody axis. The rings are faint. The colour externally is grey, slightly reddish, the fracture resinous, deep black grey, especially when moistened, meditullium yellowish, and perforated with small holes.

On analysis these roots yield 9 per 100 of emetine.

In commerce this root is called the "ipecachuan of the gold mines," and is kept separate from the preceding articles.

GEN. 6.—RICHARDSONIA.

Sp. R. brasiliensis.

The roots of this plant are sold under the name of "*White or starchy Ipecachuana.*"

The root is wrinkled, twisted, with well marked rings, which however are but semicircular, instead of completely surrounding the axis as in the true species. The tint is whitish grey, thickness about that of a goose quill, fracture dull and in no respect resinous. Presented to the sun brilliant points of starch are at once seen.

It yields on analysis but 6 per 100 of emetine. It is little employed, it is nevertheless emetic in doses of 24 grains, and where abundant proves an efficient substitute for the genuine drug.

For Indian substitutes for ipecachuanha, see ASCLEPIAS, CRINUM, RANDIA, PÆDERIA &c. &c.

Tribe.—Cinchoneæ.

In this article we adopt M. Feé as our guide in arrangement, and in the history, geography, and general circumstances of the subject. In the botanical notices we have embodied the most important facts elicited by Professor Lindley in his recent researches on the specific characters of the barks of commerce. To Mr. Pereira we are also indebted for a very ample collection of interesting analytical facts, and lastly on the medicinal effects of bark and its preparations, we have consulted the most recent writers, and added the results of our own inquiries.

This sub-group has been formed by Kunth from the Rubiaceous family. It contains six genera, two of which only need occupy our attention. The barks are all rich in tannic acid, and also contain three alkaline principles—*quinine, cinchonine*, and *aricine*. These principles do not exist, however, in all the Cinchoneæ, being found only in those genera in which the stamens do not pass beyond the corolla; where the stamens are longer than the corolla these alkalies do not exist, a new and remarkable proof of the perfection of the theory of natural relations in the families of plants.

GEN.—CINCHONA. [*Cosmibuena*, Ruiz and Pav.]

This genus founded by Linnæus has long been deemed to consist of two species, of which one now makes part of the Exostema division. Vahl recognizes 9 species of cinchona, Gmelin 8, Lambert in his monograph describes 11, Ruiz and Pavon 13, Humboldt gives 18, Poiret 24, Stendel 22, which together with some Brazilian species made the number in 1825 to amount to 38. On this subject Lindley gives us the most recent and correct information. Of true Cinchonas Lindley describes 24, and under the heads of Lasionema, Cosmibuena, Remija, Hymenodictyon, Exostema, Manettia and Pinckneya, 11 articles are also mentioned.

The true Cinchonas are trees which thrive best at moderate elevations (1000 to 1300 toises), several attain a great height, and the trunk may become as thick as a man's body.

M. Feé presents us with a copious tabular view of the geographical distribution of the family. He assigns 18 to Peru, 4 to Brazil, 1 to Coromandel, and he enumerates also 15, the localities and characters of which were not perfectly ascertained at the time of the publication of his book. Under the head of *Exostema,* or those with the projecting stamina, 15 are mentioned, all of which are small trees or shrubs with opposite leaves, entire, and provided with stipules; they are all natives of South America, whence some have spread into Australia, and many are now known to exist in Africa and in the peninsula of India.

Historical notice. It is altogether unknown to whom is due the discovery of the medicinal virtues of the cinchona barks, but it is nearly certain that the Spanish colonists of Peru were the first to ascertain their nature. The Indians, who call the bark *Kinkin* and *Kina,* think that we use it merely as a dye stuff, and they scarcely ever employ it in the treatment of intermittent fever, on the contrary they regard it as a poison capable of causing gangrene. The introduction of the cinchona into Europe took place in 1640, and is attributed to the Countess of Cinchona, who had experienced its good effects in Peru, and after whom it has accordingly been named. The Jesuits were the first to import it on a large scale, and hence it was also long known as the "Jesuit's bark." All knowledge as to the source of the bark was however very uncertain until the voyage of De la Condamine in 1738.

The first cinchona trees were discovered in South America in the neighbourhood of Loxa, about the 4th degree of South latitude, and according to la Condamine furnished in 1738 the greater part of the Peruvian bark of commerce. The tree was observed first at Uritu Singa, and was subsequently named Cinchona condaminea. The same naturalist also spoke of the cinchonas of various parts of Peru, and especially of those of Cuenca, Agavaca, and Jëan de Bracamoros. About the same period Joseph de Jussieu, who visited these districts, brought back to France specimens of the Cinchona pubescens, a tree 15 to 20 feet high, and all parts of which are covered with down; it was found at Praya Granda, Cuenca, Loxa, and elsewhere. The attention of botanists having been thus attracted to these important trees, Jacquin, Swartz, and Desportes discovered in Cuba, the Antilles, and St. Domingo, a bark which since has been found to be an exostema, but which they described as a cinchona (floribunda?). Mutis also perseveringly explored the localities of Grenada, and discovered the species termed *lancifolia*, *cordifolia*, *oblongifolia*, and *ovalifolia*, the barks of which were speedily introduced into commerce under the names of orange-coloured, amarilla, rosy, white, &c. Ruiz and Pavon in 1777, and subsequent years, extended very much the state of knowledge on this subject; these botanists having traversed the provinces of Tarma and Zanca, and the mountains of Peru, and discovered many new and valuable species. Humboldt and Bonpland lastly added much to our knowledge not only of the botany but of the commerce and collection of these barks.

Several important monagraphs have been published on this subject, of which we may notice an excellent one by Lambert in English, and the article by M. Guibourt in the *Dictionnaire des Sciences Medicales*, and in the second edition of his *Historie des Drogues;* to this we should add the article by Lindley in his *Flora Medica*, from which we proceed to collate some remarks still further illustrative of the history of these important agents.

Professor Lindley attributes much of the confusion still existing regarding the sources of the commercial barks to "the false estimate usually formed of the botanical skill and consequent credibility of the most original writers on this subject." Don José Mutis, whose name we have already quoted as the discoverer of extensive bark forests in the neighbourhood of Santa Fé de Bogota, and whose species are still adopted by the British colleges as the sources of the officinal barks, is charged by Lindley with the utmost botanical incompetence, in consequence of which, and of his undue zeal for the interests of that province, a great quantity of inert or spurious barks found their way through Carthagena (the sea-port of the province of Santa Fé) into commerce. The proofs adduced by Dr. Lindley in support of these statements seem to us altogether conclusive.

The opinions and writings of Pavon and Ruiz, Lindley finds to be most accurate, and as far as they indicate deserving of perfect confidence; they are altogether opposed to those of Mutis and his follower Zea, and have been adopted by Guibourt, Pereira, and others, the most eminent pharmacologists of the present day.

The statements published by MM. Humboldt and Bonpland, Lindley shews to be unsatisfactory, as far as the synonymes are concerned, these eminent authorities having it seems been materially misled by Mutis, in whose house

Humboldt resided. Lambert, Romer, and Shultz, and even Decandolle, have it seems been similarly duped.

Among the authorities quoted with respect by Lindley is Mr. Poppig, from whose narrative of a journey in South America some interesting passages are quoted. He tells us that in cinchona forests the collectors attend closely to variations proceeding from locality, gathering the bark only from trees growing on steep declivities or on mountain tops, rejecting all situated on moist soil, or in ill ventilated situations. Wherever the valleys are close and warm the produce deteriorates so much in virtue as to be nearly worthless in the market.

The true cinchonas extend from 20° south to 11° north latitude, at elevations varying from 1200 to 10,800 feet, the mean temperature being estimated at 68°. The enormous consumption of these barks may be estimated by the fact that Pelletier has in one year consumed 200,000 lbs. of yellow bark, in the preparation of *sulphate of Quinine.*

Collection. The persons engaged in the collection are called *Cascarilleros.* They judge of the fitness of bark by slices of it rapidly reddening when exposed to the air; longitudinal incisions are made with sharp knives along the branches through the entire thickness of the bark, which is then removed by the back of the instrument. The harvest takes place during the dry season, the bark is then placed to dry before the sun. If the pieces are thin they roll up longitudinally into thin cylinders like quills. The larger pieces may retain their original form, shewing thus that the old distinction of *quill, round,* and *flat* barks, as characteristic of *species*, are altogether delusive. As the bark of moderately grown trees is the richest in the powerful alkalies, too great *quilling* or its total absence, are unfavourable characters of barks, as shewing that the branches were either too young or too old. The superior barks are also very heavy. The best colour is the orange, the worst white; and in proportion to the prevalent tint is the article esteemed by the dealers into whose hands it first passes.

We have next to notice the physical characters of the leading varieties of the barks found in the druggist's shops. These are denominated the *pale*, the *yellow*, and the *red.*

The first is now comparatively rare in commerce, and is also known as *Crown* bark; it reaches Europe in chests covered with skins, and containing about 200lbs.; the pieces are about 9 inches in length, smell trifling, slightly aromatic, taste acidulous, pleasantly bitter, rather astringent; some scarcely 1-10th inch in thickness, singly or doubly quilled; the epidermis is cracked, greyish coloured, covered often with lichens, the substance of pale fawn colour, when dry orange; when moistened, the powder is paler than the bark itself.

The *red* bark reaches Europe in chests of from 100 to 160 lbs.; the internal part is of a dark rust colour, and the powder a deeper colour still; the pieces are of various sizes, and usually flat, smell weak and peculiar, taste bitter, but more astringent and nauseous than in the *pale* bark.

The *yellow* bark is the most employed and esteemed in Europe. The tree grows at an altitude of about 7000 feet in the mountains of Loxa in Quito. The bark reaches Europe in chests of from 90 to 100 lbs., the bundles consisting of pieces about 10 inches long, some quilled, but the greater number flat. The epidermis is greyish brown, often as thick as the bark itself, (about ⅓ of an inch). The inner bark has a yellow colour passing into orange. In odour it resembles the pale variety. The taste is more bitter, and scarcely at all astringent or rough; when moistened the colour passes to a bright orange, the fracture is woody and fibrous; the colour of the powder is still brighter than the bark itself.

The first important examination of the chemical constituents of the cinchona barks was made by Pelletier and Caventou in 1820, in which year they made the memorable discovery of the two alkalies *Cinchonine* and *Quinine*. A third alkali, *Aricine*, has been detected by Pelletier in 1829, lately a substance named *Pitayna* has been obtained by MM. Folchi and Peretti from a bark of uncertain species sent to Pope Gregory the XVI. from the republic of Colombia. Besides these principles the barks also generally contain red or yellow colouring matter, resin, tannic and *kinic acid*, starch, fibre, and salts of lime.

Officinal Species.

The last edition of the London Pharmacopœia designates as the sources of the medicinal barks—

1. Cinchona *cordifolia*, ... Heart-leaved Cinchona, yielding the *Yellow* bark.

2. C. *lancifolia*, ... Lance-leaved C., yielding the *Pale* or *Quill* bark.

3. C. *oblongifolia*, ... Oblong-leaved C., yielding the *Red* bark.

It has been clearly shewn by Lindley that these specific names are all erroneously applied—that the *pale* barks are furnished by C. Condaminea and C. micrantha—the *yellow* bark chiefly by C. lanceolata—the source of the *red* bark is still doubtful, while those of the commercial varieties of white Loxa, Calisaya, Carthagena, Cusco, and many others, are yet altogether unknown.

The Edinburgh Pharmacopœia enumerates—1. *Cinchona Coronæ*, crown bark, referred to *C. Condaminea*; 2. *C. cinerea*, grey or silver bark, referred to *C. micrantha*; 3. *C. flava*, yellow bark, from an "unascertained species"; 4. and 5. *C. pallida*, pale bark, and *C. rubra*, red bark, "species also undetermined."

It would be quite misplaced to insert in our work a minute botanical account even of the ascertained Cinchona trees, which it is well known do not exist in India, and which our readers can have no opportunity of observing.

M. Feé in his excellent work also repudiates minute botanical descriptions, and arranges the known varieties of barks containing Cinchonine or Quinine under the heads of grey (equivalent to our pale), yellow, and red. As his account is the clearest we have met, we follow it in the remainder of this article.

Sect. I. CINCHONA BARKS AFFORDING QUININE OR CINCHONINE.

1. GREY, OR PALE BARKS.

a. *Of the grey or pale Loxa bark or Crown bark.*

This bark has long been known in Europe, and is admitted to belong to the Cin. condaminea; it occurs in solid pieces of variable thickness, 12 to 18 inches long, covered with clear or deep grey epidermis, with transverse fissures and wrinkled, between ¼ and 2 lines thick; light, fibrous, inner surface pale yellow or reddish, fracture clear or slightly fibrous; powder deep brown, odour peculiar, taste bitter and astringent, adulterated sometimes with willow bark, and with other kinds of cinchona. Imported in packages holding 60 to 90 lbs., or chests of 100 lbs.

This bark contains but very minute quantities of the active alkalies—but 28 grs. of Cinchonine in 16 ounces, and at most 11 ounces of Quinine in 100 lbs.

CINCHONINE.

This principle is white, transparent, soluble in 2500 times its weight of boiling water, soluble in cold alcohol, difficultly in fixed oils and ether, unites with acids and forms salts; unalterable in air.

It is composed of carbon, oxygen, hydrogen, and nitrogen. Its salts possess the property of curing intermittent fevers when administered in the intervals, but they are inferior in virtue to the preparations of Quinine.

b. *Of the grey Cinchona of Lima.*

Syn. "Silver," or "grey C." in England and Germany. "Huanuco, or Guanuco bark."

Of variable thickness, but seldom exceeding an inch; epidermis thin, cracked or flaky, variable in colour according to the parasitic plants by which it is covered, but generally pale grey, with transverse fissures, easily broken or cut, clean, resinous, and more or less compact; odour weak, taste astringent and bitter.

The chemical analysis, and the uses of the variety correspond closely to those of the preceding, or Loxa kind. The parent tree is most probably the *C. micrantha.* Fl. Peruv. ii. 52. t. 194, a native of the high, cool, and wooded mountains of Peru. Mutis erroneously attributed it to a species he termed the *C. lancifolia.*

In Mr. Pereira's lectures there are placed under this head two varieties which are called the "ash bark," and "dark ash" bark; the first is distinguished by the crookedness of the quills; they are rare in commerce, and but of little value.

---

2. YELLOW BARKS.

Royal yellow bark, Royal bark. Calisaya.

This bark was first brought to Spain in 1789, and was monopolized for the Royal family. The name Calisaya is that of a province in South Peru, where the tree prevails.

The pieces are very variable in size, sometimes 1½ feet long, more or less rolled and thick; the smaller wrinkled, with transverse cracks in the epidermis, which is thin, readily detached, fracture very fibrous; the larger with epidermis deeply chinked, covered with lichens, 2 to 4 lines thick, formed of numerous layers, of fibrous fracture, with brilliant points (plates of young wood) often adhering to the inner surface; nearly inodorous, very bitter and astringent; powder dun-yellow.

Feé regards the botanical origin of these barks as altogether hypothetical; Pereira agrees in this opinion. Lindley, from subsequent researches of the most elaborate kind, and from the examination of 33 specimens, refers it to the *C. lanceolata*, Fl. per. ii. t. 223, a native of the cold and mountainous situations on the Andes, about 15 leagues from the city of Huanuco.

Quinine.

1 lb. of Calisaya bark of good quality will yield from 154 to 286 grs. of *quinine*, difficultly crystallizable, soluble in boiling water in proportion of 5 parts to 1000; very soluble in hot alcohol and ether, also in some essential oils, unalterable by the air; it neutralizes acids to form crystalline salts, remarkable for their pearly aspect; inodorous, taste very bitter; composed of carbon 20, hydrogen 12, nitrogen 1, oxygen 2 eq. Quinine fuses when heated to 300° into a yellow resinous-like mass. It agrees with Cinchonine in many of its characters, but differs in being much more soluble in water, being very soluble in ether, in the form of its crystalline compounds, and in containing 1 atom more oxygen. A very remarkable effect is produced also on dilute solutions of sulphate of quinine by adding a small quantity of chlorine water and then weak ammonia, drop by drop; a splendid emerald colour is immediately produced.

Sulphates of Quinine.

Of these there are two—the neutral sulphate, and the sub- or di-sulphate.

Sub- or di-Sulphate of Quinine.

For an account of the manufacture of this most important salt the student will consult the Pharmacopœia.

The salt crystallizes in minute, fibrous, pearly, flexible needles, which melt at a high temperature; they are but little soluble in cold water, but are freely dissolved on adding a minute proportion of sulphuric acid; the solution has a blue tinge. Soluble in alcohol, but not in ether.

*Composition**		
	Quinine, 2 atoms, ...	40.50
	Sulphuric acid, 1 atom, ...	5.
	Water of crystallization, atoms,	2.25
	Total,	47.75

* According to Liebig's last analysis.

For an account of the adulterations of quinine, see the Pharmacopœia; for its medical uses consult the sequel of this article.

---

3. THE RED BARKS.

These barks stain the fingers red, contain both *Quinine* and *Cinchonine*, and are at the same time bitter and astringent to an extreme degree.

The common red bark, (*warty* or *plain*, Guibourt)—*China rubra* of Bergen.

Introduced into England in 1779; imported in chests, in quills or flat pieces; the bark is frequently warty, the colour of the fine quills is faint red brown, in thick pieces this darkens to chesnut, sometimes with a purple tinge, (Pereira); fracture of quills smooth, of larger pieces fibrous, taste strongly bitter, and rather aromatic.

Feé and Pereira deem the tree to be unknown, and the supposition of the bark belonging to the C. oblongifolia to be erroneous; Lindley participates in these opinions.

On analysis Santen found 1 lb. to yield, according to quality, from 20 to 184 grs. of cinchonine, and from 7 to 77 of quinine. 1 drachm of cinchonine, and 2 scruples of quinine may be deemed average results.

Under the head of *brown* barks Mr. Pereira describes one called the "Huamalies," its history, source, and properties are but little known. It contains both quinine and cinchonine, and yields usually from 12 to 34 of the former, and from 38 to 60 of the latter base.

It is ascribed by Lindley to *C. purpurea*. (*C. pubescens* of Fl. Per. ii. 52. t. 193.) A native of groves on the lower part of the Andes. The bark while fresh is extremely bitter, and has been used for adulterating beer.

All the preceding barks have naturally a *brown* epidermis. Besides these there is a class of barks having a whitish epidermis, but of which the cortical layers are yellow or red. Although they contain cinchonine and quinine, these bases are in such very minute proportions that the barks are nearly useless to the physician or to the manufacturing druggist. Their study is of importance, as they constitute the bulk of the kinds designated by Mutis and Zea as exported from Carthagena, and adopted by the British Pharmacopœiæ.

In appearance they so strongly resemble the valuable barks as to present also pale, yellow, and red varieties. The sources of these barks have not been very clearly made out, and many Pharmacologists are inclined to attribute them to genuine cinchonas which have deteriorated by an unsuitable climate or soil. Pereira considers them the produce of *Cinchona cordifolia*.

The variety which most resembles good yellow bark may be distinguished by a thin soft epidermis, of an appearance like mica, and by the taste, which is scarcely if at all bitter; 1 lb. of this bark will not yield more than 60 grs. of quinine and 40 of cinchonine.

CUSCO BARK.

This bark is remarkable for yielding the alkali *aricine*. It has been known no longer than seven years. Its epidermis is white, smooth, and uncracked; its cortical layers orange-red. It is very fibrous, and containing no lime its infusion is not precipitated by sulphate of soda.

Aricina.

In 1829 a quantity of bark was imported into Bourdeaux from Arica in Peru, as genuine yellow cinchona bark, which it exactly resembled. On analysis by Pelletier and Coriol instead of quinine it yielded the new alkali called *Aricina*, from the place of exportation. It is white, crystallizable, insoluble in water, forms with acids intensely bitter salts, melts like quinine, but cannot be volatilized like cinchonine. The sulphate of aricina dissolved in hot water on cooling forms a soft gelatinous coagulum, which dries like horn. With concentrated nitric acid aricina strikes a deep green colour. On analysis it yields one atom more oxygen than quinine. The three alkalies may thus be represented as the Protoxide, Binoxide, and Teroxide of a compound radical Quinogen, composed of C. 20. Hyd. 12, Az. 1:—thus—

Protoxide of Quinogen,	Cinchonia,	C. 20 H. 12, N. 1, Ox. 1.
Binoxide ...	do.	Quinine,	C. 20 H. 12, N. 1, Ox. 2.
Teroxide ...	do.	Aricine,	C. 20 H. 12, N. 1, Ox. 3.

There can be no doubt of the salts of aricina participating in the febrifuge properties of those of cinchonine and quinine; should the sources of the true yellow bark diminish, the Cusco article will become proportionately valuable.

SURINAM BARK

occurs in flat, or arched pieces or quills; epidermis smooth and whitish, with fissures, taste astringent, somewhat bitter; in general appearance it has however little or no resemblance to the other cinchona barks. It contains little if any alkaline principle. Lindley refers it to *C. magnifolia,* Fl. Peruv. ii. p. 53, t. 196. It is abundant in low lands near torrents, in sunny and ill ventilated places. Ruiz describes it as being of indifferent quality, and trifling value in the market. It is most used for the purpose of adulterating the genuine red bark of Lima.

FALSE CINCHONA BARKS.

These are barks not belonging to the group Cinchoneæ, and which contain neither quinine, cinchonine, aricine, nor pitayine.

Sp. 1. *Exostema caribæum,* a native of the West India islands and Mexico. The bark is febrifuge and emetic; excessively bitter and disagreeable.

Sp. 2. *Exostema floribundum.*
West Indies among woods. Bark similar to the last, but purgative also.

Sp. 3. *E. Souzanum,* (Brazil.)
Bark excessively bitter; has yielded an alkali erroneously named *Essenbeckia,* on the idea that the bark was that of Essenbeckia febrifuga.

Sp. 4. *E. peruvianum,* lower parts of Peru; bark very bitter, a little sweet, and with a nauseous smell.

Besides the species above described, there are several mentioned in Lindley under the genera of Lasionema, Cosmibuena, Remija, Pinckneya, and Manettia, natives of South America, the West Indies, and Carolina; some reputed to be possessed of febrifuge properties, others emetic or purgative. Too little is known regarding these articles to warrant our devoting to them any more extended notice.

The *Portlandia hexandra,* (*Coutarea speciosa,* Aublet's, Guiand) French Guiana bark, is reputed to be a very powerful febrifuge. An empirical preparation, "Warburg's fever drops," now very widely advertised, and on very high testimonials, is supposed to contain the active principle of this bark. Dr. Warburg is a German naturalist, resident in Guiana.

One genus however is indigenous in India, which was long considered by Roxburgh to be a true *Cinchona,* and which for various reasons deserves our careful attention.

Gen.—Hymenodictyon.

Sp. H. excelsum, Wallich, in Roxb. Fl. Ind. ii. 148. (ed. Carey.)

Syn. Cinchona excelsa, Roxb. Fl. Ind. i. 529. A native of the mountainous parts of the Circars of India.

Vern. Pundaroo, Bundaroo, Kala Buchnak, *Hind.*

Trunk straight, of considerable thickness and height; branches numerous, spreading, bark of the trunk pretty thick, exterior coating grey, light, spongy, cracking in various directions, and frequently falling off; the middle coat brown, of a farinaceous nature, and as thick as both the exterior and interior coats, the interior white; leaves opposite, oblong, entire, soft, downy, particularly on the under side; veins simple, and frequently opposite, from 6 to 12 inches long, and from 3 to 5 broad. Floral leaves at the lower part of the ramifications of the panicle in shape like the rest, but much smaller, coloured, more permanent and bullate, petioles round, downy, 2 or 3 inches long, stipules within the leaves, ovate, cordate, acutely serrate, erect, caducous; panicles terminal, large, generally with the lower ramifications decussating. Flowers fascicled, small, greenish white, exceedingly numerous, exquisitely fragrant; calyx superior, five-toothed; corolla funnel-formed, downy, tube long, border five-parted, with oval spreading divisions not half the length of the tube; filaments five, short, *inserted into the mouth of the tube;* anthers erect, *one-third within the tube,* style twice the length of the tube, stigma capitate. Capsule oblong, crowned with the remains of the calyx, about as thick as a field bean, but twice as long, four streaked, marked with small white elevated specks, two-celled, two-valved, opening from the top, placentæ slender, angular, the length of the capsule, affixed lengthwise to the suture of the partition, seeds from 6 to 12 in each cell, chesnut-coloured, imbricated, oblong, compressed, enlarged all round by a membranous ragged wing, which at the base is split up to the seed itself. (*Roxb.*)

The two inner leaves of the bark possess great bitterness and astringency; the bark is used by the tanners, and also as a medicine among the Hindoos, in cases requiring astringents.

We have analysed the bark of Cinchona excelsa from the Botanic Garden of Calcutta, but could detect no alkaline ingredient; nevertheless the trees of hilly regions may furnish the valuable desideratum. The stamina being contained within the tube affords much ground for expecting the discovery of a febrifuge alkaline in this species, and in that view we have quoted Roxburgh's description in full.

Medicinal Properties of the Cinchona Barks.

The medicinal uses of all the preceding articles, are referable to the effects produced on the living system by the febrifuge alkalies, by tannic acid, and the aromatic principle of some varieties of the barks.

Tannic acid is known to be in all its forms a powerful astringent, diminishing the secretions of the part to which it is applied, and in some tissues (those containing gelatine and albumen), causing actual contraction of the organ itself.

The febrifuge alkalies administered to individuals in the healthy state act as general and remote stimulants; their action is not speedy; its local nature is however often evinced by the occurrence of vomiting and purging. Its remote tendency seems chiefly towards the cerebral centre. Giddiness, singing in the ears, the apparition of sparks before the eyes, headache, and confusion of ideas being very common results.

These effects are the sequel of the absorption of the remedy into the circulation, as shewn by some curious experiments recently instituted by European chemists, who have succeeded in recovering quinine from the urine of patients taking large quantities of that remedy.

In the diseased state the most remarkable effect occasioned by quinine, cinchonine, and aricine is the suspension of the course of numerous periodic or intermittent affections, of which ague affords us the best example.

When ague is of recent date, and is unattended by inflammation or enlargement of any important organ, such as the liver or spleen, whatever be the period of recurrence, whether after one, two, or more days, it will be found in a very large proportion of cases that the use of bark in powder, infusion, extract, or tincture, or of the saline compounds of quinine, cinchonine, or aricine, will speedily and certainly prevent the return of the disease.

Even in remittent fevers in which the disease abates rather than ceases, and in which the interval is of uncertain duration, these remedies judiciously administered produce the same effect. Of the nature of the action of bark, and its preparations in thus averting the recurrence of febrile paroxysms, we are completely ignorant; a similar effect is produced by several other remedies, such as arsenic, anarcotina, nux vomica, muriate and sulphate of ammonia, &c.; of these, however, anarcotina alone approaches quinine in certainty, and speediness of effect.

The antiperiodic virtue is exercised not only in fevers, but in numerous other intermittent maladies, such as neuralgia, periodical hæmorrhages, spasmodic strictures, &c.

There are many circumstances, however, which limit the applicability of bark in its various forms; some of these we deem it necessary to point out.

In the opinion of the majority of practitioners bark is injurious in any form if administered to fever patients until all symptoms of fever have subsided, especially until the head and skin become cool and moist. Constipation of the bowels again is a condition which must be removed before these remedies can be employed with any certainty of success.

The presence of inflammation of the viscera, and of cerebral symptoms especially, is by many deemed prohibitory of the administration of bark or quinine. Dysenteric symptoms, especially when acute, seem to be much aggravated by all forms of these remedies.

In the treatment of fevers, remittent or intermittent, or in the latter stages of typhus, the sulphate of quinine must always be preferred to bark itself, from the smallness of the necessary dose, and its consequently remaining more certainly on the stomach. The requisite dose ranges from 2 to 10 grs. every third or fourth hour; on this point, however, considerable difference of opinion exists among practitioners, some prefer using small doses at short intervals, others recommend a large quantity, say 10 grs. a short time (from an hour to half an hour) before the period of the expected paroxysm; on this point we have collected the opinions of several highly experienced practitioners in India, of which we have the pleasure to give an adequate synopsis in the appendix to this work.

The antiperiodic virtues of quinine and its salts are not only experienced when the remedy is taken into the stomach, but even when applied to raw surfaces on the skin. This is called the "endermic" method.

Bark in substance is best given in the form of *powder*, in doses of 20 grs. to one or two drachms, or in *infusion* (see those heads); decoction renders the bark comparatively useless, apparently by the oxidation of its soluble parts, which are thus rendered insoluble and inert. For the same reason the extracts of bark, whether watery or alcoholic, however well prepared, are uncertain and feeble remedies, owing their virtue more to the tannic acid they may contain, than to the peculiar principles for which bark is really to be valued.

In all diseases of debility, in passive hæmorrhages, in convalescence from acute diseases, in dropsical effusions not dependent on inflammation or on mechanical obstruction, bark and its preparations are often most successfully employed.

In mortification proceeding from diminished action or obstruction, cold, the sequel of typhus fevers, or from pressure on soft parts, the use of bark or quinine with wine, and a generous diet, will in many cases accelerate the occurrence of healthy action in parts adjacent to the mortified tissues, and cause a separation to ensue. In all cases of mortification bark in powder is a favourite application to the dead parts, the decomposition of which it prevents by the influence of its tannic acid, thus moderating or destroying the abominable fætor.

In one disease of highly increased action, namely rheumatism in its most acute form, bark and quinine have been used in large doses with wonderful effect in multitudes of cases. The practice was introduced by the late celebrated Dr. Haygarth, of Cheltenham; 10 grain doses of quinine are given every two or three hours, with the effect of inducing profuse sweating, and very often of entirely and at once relieving the disease. We have too frequently witnessed the full success of this practice to allow us to doubt its great efficacy.

We cannot conclude this brief sketch of the effects and uses of the "bark" remedies, without alluding to the distressing nervous symptoms they often occasion, and especially in warm countries, amounting to intolerable headache, deafness, an indescribable degree of restlessness and agitation, &c. In many individuals these symptoms are so distressing that they have been compelled to abstain from quinine even when suffering from violent ague. In some, every symptom of remittent fever has been exasperated by the remedy which generally proves so successful. In these cases Anarcotine will usually succeed, though itself capable of producing exactly similar symptoms; and in the persons the latter affects, thus quinine, on the other hand, may often be used with impunity and success.

(Vide Sulphate of Quinine, Anarcotina, Sulphate of Ammonia, and Arsenious acid, Pharmacopœia.)

Gen.—Uncaria.

Sp. Uncaria Gambir.
Syn. Nauclea Gambir.
Vern. Gambir, *Malay.* (*Roxb. Fl. Ind.* i. 517. *As. Res.* xi. 187.)

A stout climber, a native of the islands of the Indian Archipelago, cultivated in the Calcutta Garden.

Bot. Desc. Leaves opposite, short stalked, from ovate oblong to ovate lanceolate, entire, acute, smooth on both sides, about four inches long, and two broad, stipules oblong, uniting the upper margin of the base of the petioles, deciduous, spines axillary, solitary or in opposite pairs, simple, recurved, hooked, peduncles axillary, solitary, about the middle jointed and bracted, supporting a single globular head of beautiful green and pink small florets. Bracts about the middle of the peduncle forming a 3—4 cleft annular involucre, calyx silky on the outside, with a five-cleft border, tube of corolla funnel-shaped, filiform, border of five obtuse divisions villous on the outside, and hairy in the centre of the inside. Filaments short, anthers large on the mouth of the tube, ovary turbinate, subsessile, sericeous, style as long as the tube of the corolla, stigma clavate, capsules stalked, clavate, longitudinally grooved, crowned with the five-cleft permanent calyx, two-celled, two-valved, seeds numerous, imbricated, winged.

Gambier.

Gambier is the Malay name of an extract prepared from the leaves of this plant; it is an important article in commerce, and was formerly called Japan earth in Europe. Roxburgh quotes a description of its preparation and properties by Dr. Campbell of Bencoolen, to the effect that the Malays use the gambier with betel and areca, as *kuth* or catechu is employed in India,—that the young roots and leaves are sliced and bruized in water for some hours until a feculum is deposited, this is inspissated before the sun to a proper consistence and cast in moulds of a circular form. Dr. Roxburgh adds, that in other parts the extract is made by decoction of the leaves, and evaporation by fuel and solar heat, the product dried being cut into small thin cakes.

Eight species of *Uncaria* are described by Roxburgh, and twelve of *Nauclea.*

The Gambier extract is described by M. Feé as the true or Indian kino. It is but little soluble in cold water or in boiling water; it is almost entirely dissolved by boiling spirit. It gives a rose-coloured precipitate with gelatine, and a deep permanent green with the salts of iron. It is rich in the tannic, but contains no gallic acid.

Its uses in the arts and in medicine depend altogether on the presence of the tannic acid.

Mr. Pereira on strong grounds denies that the gambier is one of the kinos of the druggists; Ainslie regards it as the *Cuttacamboo*, one of the varieties of catechu of the Indian Bazars. The *cashcuttee* he considers to be the produce of the betel nut tree.

In 1837—38, there were imported into Calcutta from Singapore, Penang, and Pegu, 3677 maunds of gambier, at a valuation of 15,916 rupees.

Gen.—Randia.

Limb of calyx five-lobed, corolla salver-shaped, with a short tube and five-parted limb, anthers enclosed, sessile within the throat, stigmas two, thick. Berry nearly dry, crowned by the calyx, corticated, two-celled, many-seeded. Seeds fixed to the central placenta imbedded in pulp and imbricated downward; spiney shrubs with conspicuous flowers.

Sp. R. dumetorum.

Syn. Gardenia dumet. *Retz.* Posoqueria dumet. *Roxb. Fl. Ind.* i. p. 714.

Vern. Jooz-ul-kueh, *Arab.* Muenphul, *Hind.*

A thorny branching shrub or small tree, common in Coromandel and Bengal; leaves oval, rather blunt, cuneate at the base, smooth, flowers very sweet-scented, sessile, solitary, mostly terminal, calyx with oblong lobes rather shorter than the villous corolla, fruit smooth, yellow, firm and fleshy (deep brown when dried) seeds oval, numerous, lying in mucus, when dry imbedded in the dried and brown pulp.

The fruit when bruized and thrown into water intoxicates and even poisons fish, which are still however deemed fit for food. Powdered it is deemed a powerful emetic, but this seems an undeserved attribute. The bark of the root is given in infusion as a nauseating remedy.

During our search for an efficient substitute for ipecachuana, the fruit of this article underwent careful examination; for specimens we were indebted to Drs. Wight and Wallich, and we found these identical with the *muen phul* of the Bazars. The results of our experiments shew that little or no dependence can be placed on the fruit as an emetic remedy.

Roxburgh describes 11 species of Gardenia, and 8 of Posoqueria. The fruits of G. turgida and P. uliginosa (Peeraloo, *Beng.*) were examined at the time of the experiments above alluded to, and with equally negative results. The Gardenia campanulata, a native of Chittagong, which flowers in March and ripens its fruit in November, is stated by Roxburgh to be used by the natives as a cathartic and anthelmintic, and also to wash out stains in silk.

Gen.—Condaminea.

Sp. Condaminea corymbosa.

Peruvian Andes; bark slightly bitter, collected chiefly for the purpose of adulterating the cinchona bark.

Gen.—Ophiorrhiza.

Sp. Ophiorrhiza Mungos.

Wal, eka, weriya, *Cing.* Lohech of Avicenna, *Roxb. Fl. Ind.* i. 701.

A native of Java, Ceylon, and Sumatra; all parts are intensely bitter; it has high reputation as a remedy for snake-bites. Roxburgh altogether discredits its supposed virtues.

This plant is often confounded with the Ophioxylum serpentinum, of the family of *Apocyneæ*, (*Chundra*, Bengalee,) described by Roxburgh (Fl. Ind. ii. p. 530, *ed. Carey*) and by Ainslie, vol. ii. 441.

Gen.—Oldenlandia.

Sp. Oldenlandia umbellata.

Vern. Imborel, *Tam.*

A native of Java, Coromandel, and Mexico; root long and orange-coloured, employed in Coromandel to dye an excellent red on cotton cloth; considered by the native doctors to be expectorant.

O. biflora is very common in Bengal, and called in Bengali *Khet-papŭra;* other species also occur and are called *Gunda badalee*, and *Poonkha.*

Gen.—Pæderia.

Sp. Pæderia fœtida.

Vern. Gundha-Badhalee, *Beng.* Gundale, *Hind.*

A native of the islands and continent of India, but rather a rare plant. *As. Res.* iv. p. 261.

Stem woody, twining when young, round and smooth, leaves opposite, long stalked, oblong cordate, pretty smooth, entire, stipules broad, cordate. Panicles axillary and terminal, brachiate ; flowers numerous, deep pink, bracts ovate, calyx five-toothed, corolla with the tube long, somewhat gibbous and woolly inside, the limb narrow, divided into five cordate crenulate segments. Filaments short, inserted irregularly about the middle of the tube, anthers erect within the tube, ovary turbinate, two-celled, cells containing one ovule, each attached to the bottom of the cell, style single, stigma two-cleft, with the lobes bent amongst the anthers, berry dry, compressed, smooth, with five lines on each side, one-celled, two-seeded, seeds compressed, smooth, enlarged with a somewhat membranous ring all round. *Roxb. Fl. Ind.* i. p. 683.

The leaves are very fœtid and alliaceous, are used in baths, and given internally in retention of urine and in some fevers. The root Roxburgh states is used as an emetic by the Hindoos.

Two other species are described by Roxburgh.

GEN.—CANTHIUM.

Sp. Canthium parviflorum.

Vern. Balusoo-kura, *Tamul.* Naga valli, *Sans.*

A common thorny bush through India, especially on the Coromandel coast.

A decoction of the leaves or root is prescribed in India in dysentery, and is also given in worm cases. About three ounces are given daily. The fruit and leaves are eaten.

GEN.—CHIOCOCCA.

Sp. 1. *C. anguifuga.*

A native of Cayenne, Brazil, Peru, and some of the West Indian islands.

Sp. 2. *C. densifolia.* Native of Brazil.

The roots of these two species are deemed in Brazil certain remedies in snake bites. The infusion of the bark of the root is a powerful emetic and cathartic, and these effects are followed by perspiration and sleep. This remedy has been used in dropsy by several regular and highly informed practitioners, and with excellent results.

GEN.—COFFEA.

Sp. Coffea arabica.

This celebrated plant is inserted here only to shew its place in classification.

GEN.—PALICOUREA.

Sp. Palicourea Marcgraavii.

A poisonous plant of Brazil, the properties of which are but little known.

Several other species are mentioned by Lindley, some of which are diuretic.

NAT. ORDER LXXVII.—VALERIANEÆ.

The valerians are herbaceous, with leaves opposite, entire, or divided; flowers in terminal bouquets. The order is found only in temperate climates, being absent from the plains of India, and one species only being found in Deyra-Doon.

Dr. Royle informs us that the valerians extend from Sylhet to Sirmore and Cashmere, the V. Hardwickii, villosa, and alata, being the prevailing species.

The annual valerians are devoid of smell in all their parts, while the perennial species have perfumed flowers and roots, which contain a very strongly scented volatile oil.

GEN. 1.—VALERIANA.

Sp. 1. *V. officinalis.* Valerian.

Off. The roots.

Found in wet places all over Europe. The roots are white, small, with a short truncated neck with long thick cylindrical filaments, covered with short hairs of brownish or olive colour; substance white. The odour is very strong and penetrating, and increased by drying the roots. The taste sweetish and bitter. Roots of various other species and of some poisonous Ranunculaceæ have been fraudulently mixed with this article.

According to Tromsdorff's experiments, 381 parts of valerian root contain 48 peculiar matter soluble in water, 24 black resin, 1 volatile oil, 36 gum, 6 fecula, and 266 woody fibre.

The volatile oil is pale yellow tinged slightly green, lighter than water, thickens considerably by the action of the air; its odour is camphor-like, and very penetrating; its taste acrid, and bitter. Cats are remarkably affected by, and attached to, the odour of this oil. It seems to intoxicate them with pleasure. Feé considers the odour to resemble that of the urine of the animal, and thus attempts to explain the effect produced on their system.

Valerian given in infusion has long been deemed a very valuable remedy in the treatment of the atonic forms of hysteria, hypochondriasis, chlorosis, and amenhorrea; it has also been used in epilepsy, but with very doubtful advantage. For formulæ for the infusion and tincture, see the Pharmacopœia.

Sp. 2. *V. celtica.* Ναρδος χελτιχη, Celtic valerian.

A native of Piedmont and the Tyrol, found also in other mountainous countries. The roots are cylindrical, the thickness of a goose quill, fibrous, surrounded with membranous, linear, oblong, smooth, and loosely imbricated scales. In odour and taste this root resembles, but is weaker than the first species. The aqueous infusion smells of saffron, and is rendered brown by the addition of salts of iron.

These roots are annually exported from the Austrian states to Egypt, to the amount of about 60 tons weight. They are much esteemed in the Levant as a perfume and cosmetic; in Europe they are no longer employed.

Gen. 2.—Nardostachys.

Sp. Nardostachys Jatamansi, (see Royle's Illust. p. 243. t. 54.)

Syn. Valeriana Jatamansi, (Jones As. Rs. ii. p. 405. iv. p. 109.) Patrinia Jatamansi, *Don.*

Ναρδος ινδικη. Dioscorides—*Indian spikenard.*

Vern. Sumbul Hindee. Sumbool-ul-teb, *Arab.* Balchur, *Hind.*

A native of the mountains of the north of India, at very great elevations.

A dwarf herbaceous plant, with a long hairy tap root, stems perennial, very short, simply divided into a number of shaggy scaly crowns from which the leaves proceed; branches erect, a few inches high, downy, leaves obovate, lanceolate, three ribbed, downy, those next the root acute, the upper obtuse. Flowers pale pink, clustered in the axils of the upper leaves, which serve as a kind of involucre. Limb of the calyx five-parted, lobes ovate oblong, acute, leafy, somewhat toothed, permanent, corolla regular, ecalcarate, obtusely five-lobed, bearded in the throat. Stamens four, attached to the bottom of the corolla, stigma capitate, capsule three-celled, crowned by the lobes of the calyx, and almost shorter than they are; not adnate to a bract. D. C.

The roots of the Jatamansi are brought down from the mountains in large quantities. Considerable discussion has arisen as to the true origin of the celebrated spikenard of the ancients, but the labours of Sir William Jones and Professor Royle leave no longer any reasonable doubt as to its being truly referrible to this article. The root is of blackish colour, and resembles the bushy tail of the ermine. Its odour is strong and fragrant, and is much esteemed by all Eastern nations.

For medicinal purposes our experience leads us to believe that this species is a perfect representative of the valerian of the English Pharmacopœia.

NAT. ORDER LXXVIII.—DIPSACEÆ.

The Dipsaceæ are generally herbaceous, with opposite and rarely verticillated leaves; the flowers are seldom distinct, but usually combined on a common receptacle. Their interest to the medical practitioner is but trifling; some are slightly bitter, and have been deemed antiherpetic, but apparently on inadequate grounds.

The *Dipsacus fullonum*, teasle, or fuller's thistle, is, according to Royle, the *Dunsakoos* of the Indian Materia Medica.

NAT. ORDER LXXIX.—SYNANTHEREÆ.

A great and very natural order, usually termed *Compositæ*, and named as above from their anthers being collected into one adherent mass. They have been also named *Syngeneseæ* from the same cause.

It is composed of herbaceous, rarely woody plants, with compound flowers, that is, bearing a variable number of flowers, sometimes unisexual, and sometimes hermaphrodite, united together on a common receptacle. They occur in all parts of the globe; in France they constitute as much as one-seventh of all the phanerogamic division; at the Cape one-sixth; in Germany one-eighth; in America one-sixth.

Dr. Wallich enumerates 426 Indian species from the plains and mountains.

The prevailing colour of the flowers is yellow, those which blossom in the spring are usually blue, white, or rose-coloured.

The order has been divided into 19 tribes by Cassini, and these have been adopted by Feé. Lindley has made three separate orders of it, namely, *Asteraceæ, Cynaraceæ,* and *Cichoraceæ.* We shall adopt Feé's arrangement of genera as most convenient for the purposes of this volume.

A bitter principle abounds in several of this order, for example in the Absinthiums, or wormwoods; essential oil exists plentifully in the camomiles and pellitory, and these species are at the same time exceedingly bitter; the seeds of many possess a fixed oil in such quantities as to render its manufacture economical; for example, the seeds of the sunflower, and ramtilla. The essential oil resides in the perisperm, the fixed oil in the almond.

The proper juice of some Synanthereæ is milky and rather narcotic, still but few are justly suspected of dangerous properties. Starch is but in very small proportion in any of the species, hence few can be deemed alimentary, though from the presence of mucilage, saccharine matters, and extractive or modified bitter principles, some are used as table vegetables, such as the artichoke, lettuce, and endive; no peculiar principle of much importance has been detected in the plants of this order.

In their medical uses these plants are tonic, febrifuge, vermifuge, or emollient. The properties of one species generally co-exist in all the congenerous individuals, and thus the research for substitutes is much facilitated.

Gen. 1.—Lactuca.

Europe produces a great number of lettuces, and a few occur in Asia. They are generally herbaceous plants containing a very abundant watery juice; they grow rapidly; the roots are fibrous. The roots and stalks often abound in a milky juice, which is rather astringent and sometimes slightly narcotic. The seeds contain fixed oil easily obtained by expression; no essential oil occurs in any of these plants hitherto examined. The Lactuceæ are generally innocent, by cultivation their tenderness is increased, and their bitterness diminished.

Sp. 1. *Lactuca virosa,* Strong scented lettuce.
θριδαξ αγρια, Diosc.

A native of Europe, of disagreeable and virose smell, acrid and bitter taste; on analysis yields a bitter principle and a peculiar acid, resin, caoutchouc, wax, gum, albumen, and salts.

The inspissated juice of this lettuce produces symptoms like those caused by opium, but it requires to be administered in at least a sixfold dose; neither morphia nor anarcotine have been detected in this substance.

Sp. 2. *Lactuca sativa.* Garden or Roman lettuce.
Vern. Kahoo, *Hind.*

A well known garden vegetable, inodorous, of scarcely sensible taste, or slightly bitter; at the flowering time it contains a milky juice, which has acquired some celebrity under the name of—

Lactucarium, or Thridace.

A resinous looking substance in irregular masses, colour brown, imperfectly soluble in water, destitute of morphine or anarcotine, containing resin, malate of lime, and an azotized extractive substance; odour strong and virose, taste bitter, analogous to the smell.

Lactucarium is obtained by cutting off the tops of the full grown lettuce, collecting the milky juice which exudes, and inspissating it by a moderate heat.

We are indebted to Dr. Cox of Philadelphia, Dr. Duncan of Edinburgh, and M. Francois for the first experiments on the sedative and anodyne influence of this preparation. It is stated to produce sleep without determining narcotism; to prove sedative without any previous stimulation, and thus to afford an excellent substitute for opium in many cases in which the latter drug is inadmissible.

In the Transactions of the Medical and Physical Society of Calcutta, Dr. Graham has published a valuable paper on this subject.

Dr. Graham's lactucarium was prepared under his own care. He describes the cultivation of the plant as being attended with no difficulty, and resembling that of the poppy. Eight or ten inches radius is given in all directions to the growing plants to permit them to grow large. When about to flower the juice is most abundant, and is to be collected by making a clean oblique division of the stem about an inch and a half from the top, when the milky secretion instantly exudes from both extremities, and is removed with a knife about two inches long and ¾ broad, with a blunt edge. The collected juice rapidly turns brown and granular, like opium. From four to twelve grains are recommended as a dose. Dr. Graham cites some interesting cases in proof of its valuable sedative action.

We are indebted to Mr. Porteous, of Calcutta, for a very fine specimen prepared in his own garden at Howrah. We could not detect in it the least vestige of morphia, anarcotine, or meconic acid, but found it distinctly sedative in six grain doses. It did not seem to affect the bowels in any degree either as an astringent or aperient.

In the Appendix to the Vol. of the Calcutta Transactions above quoted, the late Mr. Twining details the particulars of six cases in which lactucarium prepared by Dr. Graham was given to the extent of 12 grain doses. The remedy appeared to produce very little effect, except under circumstances rendering the results but doubtful. In a note it is added however that it was given in several cases in the European Insane Asylum with decided advantage; the dose was 12 grains at bed time, repeated daily till amendment was produced.

GEN. 2.—TARAXACUM.

Sp. T. officinale, Dandelion.

Syn. Leontodon Taraxacum.

A native of Europe and the Himalayas; root tap-shaped, very milky, externally black, difficult of extirpation, leaves numerous, spreading, of a bright shining green, quite smooth, tapering downwards, sessile, pinatifid with sharp unequally toothed lobes pointing downwards, or *runcinate* as it is termed by botanists. Scapes one or more, longer than the leaves, erect, smooth, brittle, naked. Flower heads 1½ inch wide, of a uniform golden yellow colour, expanded only in the morning and in fine weather; outer scales of the involucre several, linear, oblong, loosely recurved and wavy. As the fruit ripens the involucre becomes reflexed close to the stalk, leaving the light globe two inches in diameter formed by the radiating pappi, quite exposed till dispersed by the winds.

The inspissated juice of the plant, the infusion, decoction, and extract of the root, are strongly bitter, and prove tonic and diuretic, in large doses aperient. It is a favourite, and we believe useful remedy in the old hepatic diseases of persons who have long resided in India, and returned to a cold climate. The dose of the extract is 3 to 10 grains, thrice daily. For formulæ for infusion and decoction, *see Pharmacopœia.*

GEN. 3.—CICHORIUM.

Sp. C. Intybus. Wild succory, Κιχωριον, Diosc. Europe. Leaves radical, oblong, deep green, deeply lobed, lobes toothed, cauline leaves small, sessile, and very entire; inodorous, taste very bitter. Roots fusiform, cylindrical, the thickness of the finger, 8 to 10 inches long, descending, fibrous, whitish or yellowish externally, very white within. Bark of root fleshy and lactescent, root inodorous, taste at first sweetish and mucilaginous, then very bitter, the bitterness greater in summer than in spring.

An Indian species called *Kasni*, scarcely differs from this article.

The roots contain nitrate and sulphate of potash, mucilage, and some bitter extractive principle. An infusion of succory mixed with syrup causes a thickening of the liquid, and a substance is formed termed by the discoverer, M. Lacarteria—

SACCHO-CICHORINE GUM.

This substance is solid and elastic, grey, heavier than water, in which it is imperfectly soluble at common temperatures, but is dissolved at 212; it is destitute of smell, is of somewhat bitter taste, and is not applied to any useful purposes.

When succory is cultivated in a dark place it remains colourless, the root lengthens remarkably, loses its bitterness, and becomes very tender.

The roots roasted and ground have been proposed as a substitute for coffee, and were much employed in France during the suspension of the foreign trade of that country.

Under this group we find several plants noticed by Feé possessed of great bitterness, and probably deserving of further examination. The chief are the following genera:—

Hieracium,	Bitter and milky.
Sonchus,	Very bitter.
Lapsana,	Bitter and milky.
Picris, Picridium, Crepis, Barkhausia,	Bitter and milky.

The Picris repens is used in Cochin China as a bitter tonic.

GEN. 4.—CENTAUREA.

Bitter, not lactescent plants, the majority of which are European; they are distinguished by a peculiar, somewhat musky odour.

Sp. 1. *Centaurea benedicta.* Blessed thistle, south of Europe. *Ακορνα,* Theoph.

Stalks reddish, woody, branched, 12 to 18 inches high, elongated, toothed, velvety, having one nerve; the inferior leaves deeply lobed, flowers yellow, with a double calyx, the external one armed with yellow branching prickles, inodorous, leaves intensely bitter; the seeds contain an oily kernel. The entire plant by incineration yields a large proportion of carbonate of potash.

Sp. 2. *C. Cyanus,* Μηκων Ηεραχλεια, *Theoph.* Casse lunette, *French.*

Flowers a lovely azure blue, taste slightly bitter. The distilled water was once so esteemed as an application to weak eyes, that the plant received the popular name of *casse lunette,* or "*break your spectacles.*" A fine azure colour is prepared from the petals, and is much used by miniature painters.

In the French Codex, with the preceding species we find, as enumerated by M. Feé,

Sp. 3. *C. Centaurium,* or great centaury, common in the Alps, three to five feet high, root very bitter, and rather aromatic.

Sp. 4. *C. Jacea,* Europe, bitter and astringent.

Sp. 5. *C. Calcitrapa,* Star thistle, caltrop—bitter, and asserted to be febrifuge.

Sp. 6. *C. lanata,* (Carthamus lanatus, Lin.) bitter.

Sp. 7. *C. Behen,* white Behen, white Rhapontic, *Behmen Abiad* of the Arabs.

An annual plant which abounds on Mount Lebanon, with lyre-shaped radical leaves, and opposite lobes, the stem leaves amplexicaul, roots the thickness of the finger, rugose, grey externally, whitish within, with an agreeable aromatic odour, and glutinous, slightly styptic taste. It is a bitter tonic, and used for seasoning among the Persians.

Gen. 5.—Arctium.

Sp. A. Lappa, Burdock or Clit-bur. *Απαρινα, Theoph.* Αρκτειον, *Diosc.*

Syn. Lappa minor, D.C.

Common everywhere in Europe.

Root cylindrical and spindle-shaped, large, a foot and a half long, descending, with thready fibres, ash-brown externally, white and spongy within; near the neck there are traces of withered scales; odour weak and unpleasant, taste mucilaginous and bitter. The seeds are exceedingly bitter when fully ripe.

The leaves have been used as a local application in medicine, the seeds are deemed diuretic. The roots are given in decoction as a tonic and alterative in Ireland, where we have witnessed effects from the remedy quite equal to those of sarsaparilla.

The root deserves extensive trial; the seeds also are very likely to prove of value on further examination of their properties; in Ireland they are used as a popular remedy in ague.

Feé alludes to three varieties of this plant—the downy, great, and dwarf burdock. The generic name is derived from αρκτος, "a bear," on account of the thorny nature of the fruit.

A closely allied species is found in the Himalayas.

Gen. 6.—Carthamus.

Sp. C. tinctorius, Safflower, or Bastard saffron.

Κνηκος, Hippocr.

Vern. Koosumbha, *Sans.* Koosum, *Beng.*

A native of the south of Europe, of Egypt, and of India, cultivated especially in Behar and Dacca.

The Carthamus is an annual plant, with an upright, firm, smooth stem, of a colour approaching to white, and about 3 feet in height. Leaves oval, and edged with small spines; each branch bears a flower-head composed of several flowerets, all of which are furnished with stamens and pistils. The flowers are of a deep red colour.

The plant is propagated by seeds sown in drills at 1½ feet distance from each other. The young plants appear in about a month, and after the second month are hoed and thinned, each plant being left a foot from the other. The richer the land, the larger the proportion of colouring matter afforded by the flower.

On the opening of the flowerets they are rapidly gathered without being allowed to expand fully. They are then dried in the shade with great care.

The flowerets are red, funnel-shaped, with elongated filiform tube, and 5-parted limb; they are nearly tasteless, but have a strong saffron-like odour. The fruits are white, brilliant, conical, slightly incurved, sub-quadrangular with enlarged base, obtuse towards the summit, nucleus oily, covered with a cartilaginous episperm, taste sweetish and somewhat acrid.

According to the experiments of Dufour, Marchaco, and Dobereiner, the petals of the safflower contain in 100 parts moisture 6, dust 3, vegetable albumen 5, yellow colouring matter 24, extract and saline matter 5, resin 0.3, red colouring matter 5 (per 1000) with wax, fibre, oxide of iron, &c.

The yellow principle is worthless as a dye. It is soluble in water, is removed by washing, and thrown away as the first step, in the preparation of the valuable red product.

The red dye is an acid resinous substance of superb colour, insoluble in water and in acid solutions, little soluble in alcohol, and not at all in ether. It is dissolved freely by aqueous alkaline solutions, which it neutralizes. Its salts (carthamates) are crystallizable, and quite colourless; acids precipitate the carthamic acid from solutions of these salts. To obtain it on the large scale after the separation of the yellow matter, the dried flowers are treated by a solution of carbonate of soda, and lemon juice added; the carthamic acid precipitates, is collected by subsidence, washed, and carefully dried at a gentle heat.

The most lovely tints are imparted by this dye to silk and cotton; *rouge* is a mixture of the dry carthamic acid, and finely powdered talc. The *pink saucers* used for giving a flesh tint to silk are prepared from this dye with a small portion of soda. 8 oz. of the prepared petals, and 2 oz. carbonate of soda are acted on by 2 gallons of water, 4 lbs. of prepared chalk are added, and the colour precipitated upon this by citric or tartaric acid.

The Chinese card-rouge is a carthamate of soda, colourless when rubbed on, but the salt being decomposed by the acetic acid secreted by the skin itself, the carthamic acid separates in the most perfect rosy tint, which can be imagined.

The seeds are said to be purgative and emetic in moderate doses.

It is certain, however, that paroquets feed on them with great avidity, and without experiencing any ill effect. They yield abundance of fixed oil.

In 1837—38, the trade in safflower from Calcutta stood as follows :—

Exported to		Bazar Maunds.	Value.
			Rupees.
Safflower,	Great Britain,......	10,052½	2,01,349
	N. America,.........	288	5,760
	France,..............	456	8,750
	Pegu,...	6¼	120
	Singapore, ...	140¾	2,185
	Gulphs,...	12¼	248
	Total,................	10,956	2,18,412

Or 18 rs. 7 as. per Bazar Maund.

Gen. 7.—Anthemis.

This remarkable genus exists chiefly in the ancient continent. All its species are bitter and aromatic; they abound in essential oil, and the bitterness is accompanied by a nauseating principle which has not as yet been separated. From the essential oil crystals of camphor are deposited by long keeping. The taste of the roots is sometimes very pungent, and determines copious salivation.

Sp. 1. *Anthemis nobilis.* Camomile.
Vern. Baboone phool, *Pers.* and *Hind.*
Off. The flowers.
A native of Europe and Persia.

The flowers are radiated, receptacle nearly flat, paliaceous, florets tubular, yellow; demiflorets numerous, short, white, three-toothed, calyx composed of whitish sepals.

Odour strong, balsamic, agreeable, taste analogous to the smell, bitter and rather hot, both dissipated by time; cultivation causes the demiflorets to disappear, when the flower becomes globular and large, but its aroma and bitterness diminish.

Besides essential oil and bitter matter, camomile flowers contain gum, resin, and traces of tannic acid.

The essential oil is azure blue, passing to yellow by contact with the air, consistence rather thick, lighter than water, odour and taste like those of the flowers. By keeping it deposits camphor in crystals; 82 lbs. of the flowers afford only 13 drachms of the oil.

An extract and tincture of these flowers occur in most Pharmacopœiæ.

Medical uses. Camomile flowers afford in Europe a cheap and efficient antispasmodic and bitter tonic. They are much used in infusion as the vehicle for other medicines employed in the treatment of hysteria, colic, suppressed menstruation, &c. The warm infusion taken freely after tartrate of antimony and ipecachuana much facilitates the action of these emetics. The powder has been employed to the extent of two drachm doses as a preventative of ague, and it is stated, on good authority, with much success.

The essential oil is in proportion more powerful as an antispasmodic than the other preparations, but is destitute of tonic or emetic properties.

Sp. 2. Anthemis Pyrethrum, Pellitory.

Syn. Anacyclus Pyrethrum, D. C. Πυρεθρον, Diosc. iii. p. 86.

Vern. *Akurkura.*

A native of the south of France, Barbary, &c.

Off. The roots.

The roots are descending, the length of the finger, and the thickness of a swan quill, of ash-brown colour, with capillary scattered fibres; they terminate superiorly in silky filaments, or remains of leaf stalks. Internally the roots are white, a little fleshy while fresh, the medullary centre orbicular and starred. When dry they are hard and brittle, when recently collected the smell is heavy and disagreeable, but this ceases on perfect drying. The taste is peculiar and saline, tenacious, acrid, determining profuse and immediate salivation. It is worthy of remark, that like the blistering fly, notwithstanding its acridity this root is rapidly devoured by worms.

100 parts of the Pyrethrum root give traces of volatile oil, 5 of fixed oil, 14 yellow colouring matter, 11 gum, 33 inuline, 35 lignine, muriate of lime and loss 2. The stimulant principle appears to be a compound of the oil and resin.

Pyrethrum root is used as a masticatory to relieve toothache, enters into the composition of certain snuffs, and the powder is used in large quantities by the Mahommedans to excite transpiration, being rubbed upon the skin; it is used internally also as a cordial and stimulant in lethargy and palsy, and in certain stages of typhus fever. *Ainslie*, vol. i. p. 301.

We are acquainted with two remarkable cases of spontaneous salivation of the most obstinate form, which after resisting every other treatment for more than three months were effectually cured by this root.

Gen. 8.—Artemisia.

Sp. 1. *Artemisia Absinthium*, Wormwood, Αψινθιον, Hippocr. and Diosc.

A native of hilly and uncultivated situations in Europe. The stalk is erect, about 2 feet high, rather pubescent, the leaves inferior, tripinnate, with oval segments, lanceolate, silky, and sometimes confluent; the cauline leaves are twice pinnatifid, the floret ones simple. Flowers yellow, small, pedunculate, drooping, disposed in axillary clusters. The odour strong and disagreeable, taste so intensely bitter, that it has become proverbial.

According to Braconnot's analysis in the 5th vol. *Bul. de Pharmacie*, p. 549, the Absinthium contains a very bitter and azotized matter 18, insipid substance 8, resinous bitter 1.4, green volatile oil 0.09, chlorophyle a trace, albumen 7.5, fecula 1, salts of potash 7.5, ligneous fibre and water 55, in 599.3 parts.

The Absinthium is still much used in medicine, and affords an extract, a tincture, tonic syrup, &c. The volatile oil is green, camphoraceous, lighter than water, of repulsive bitterness; it has been used as a vermifuge, but requires to be employed with caution.

The flower is sometimes substituted for the hop in beer. A liqueur is prepared from it in Switzerland, which is a general favourite, despite of its bitter flavour. It has been remarked that the milk of animals under the influence of absinthium is nearly as bitter as the plant itself.

Sp. 2. *Artemisia indica.* Indian Absinth. Native of Nipal. *Vern.* Afsunteen, *Arab.* Mustaroo, *Duk.* Duna, and Murwa, *Hind.* Dana, *Sans.*

Substituted for the former, but weaker.

Sp. 3. *Artemisia Abrotanun*, Αβροτανον, Diosc. iii. p. 29. Abrotanum, *Pliny*.

A native of the south of France. Stalk woody, two to three feet high, the thickness of the finger, brittle, brown, branching, and resembling a little tree; leaves petioled, greenish, divided into linear leaflets. Flowers yellow, sessile, racemiform, thin and terminal, odour strongly that of the lemon, taste bitter, and very acrid.

Extravagant notions were once entertained of its virtues, which however do not surpass those of the other congenerous species.

Sp. 4. *Artemisia vulgaris.*

Vern. Nagdowna, *Hind.*

A native of Europe.

Stalks woody at their bases, channelled, vertical, 3 to 6 feet long, leaves whitish below, and green above, pinnatifid with linear incisions towards the summit of the stalk. Flowers in loose sheaths, lateral, small, and whitish. Inodorous, slightly bitter. Inferior in power, but of similar properties to the preceding species.

The Moxa of Japan is prepared with the leaves and stalks of a neighbouring species.

Sp. 5. *Artemisia Dracunculus.* Ταρχον. Diosc.

A native of Siberia, cultivated in gardens in Europe.

Stalks thin, branching, several feet in height, leaves simple, very entire, linear, lanceolate, the surface scattered over with an infinity of minute glandular pores containing essential oil. Flowers small, yellowish, and terminal.

Odour of the leaves smart, pungent, and agreeable; taste pungent, a little acrid and aromatic. The inspissated juice of the leaves is by many practitioners considered a powerful sudorific. It owes its name Dracunculus, or dragon, to the numerous snake-like twistings of its root.

Sp. 6. *Artemisia rupestris.*

A native of the rocks and ravines of Auvergne, Switzerland, Siberia, &c.

Stalk not higher than 4 or 5 inches, covered in common with the rest of the plant with a silky down. The flowers form terminal spikes, the leaves are divided and petioled. The whole plant evolves a sweet aroma; its taste is bitter and camphor-like. It is much esteemed as an application to injured parts, and also taken internally, and supposed to be tonic and diaphoretic.

Sp. 7. *Artemisia Contra.* Semen-contra of the Levant, Aleppo, and Alexandria. A native of Persia.

The unopened flowers and calices (worm-powder, semen-contra, semen-sanctum, &c.) are small, globular, turbinate, subaggregate, obtuse, greenish, very slightly pubescent, or smooth and scaly. The scales oval, obtuse, concave, very slightly ciliate, the lower smaller than the superior.

Floral peduncles short, stiff, and cylindrical. Leaves green, small, subulate, obtuse, compressed at both extremities, keeled, smooth.

Odour strong, nauseous, and balsamic, taste analogous, rather bitter, hot, durable, and very disagreeable; on chewing this substance a most distinct sensation of coolness is experienced.

The vermifuge properties of this celebrated medicine reside in a volatile oil, and resinous extract; 500 parts of *semen-contra* furnish two of essential oil, of light lemon-colour, of bitter and burning taste, of smell resembling that of peppermint.

Sp. 8. *Artemisia judaica*, worm seed. Saheba, *Avicenna*. Indian Semen-contra. A native of Judea, Arabia, Cochin-China. Undeveloped calices affecting two forms—linear, striated, obtuse at both extremities, or at one only, of yellowish white colour, and downy. Odour and taste as in preceding species.

The semen-contra of Barbary is more coloured than that of the East; it is cheaper, and of more certain origin. Both varieties resemble each other in quality; one only being smooth and green, the other downy and grey. Semen-contra was long attributed to the Zedoary plant.

M. Merat in his *Dictionnaire des Sciences Med.* p. 50, recognised three varieties of this drug. M. Feé believes that two of the sorts alluded to proceed from the same source. The *Artemisia palmata* has a similar taste and smell. According to Batké the *A. glomerulata* has equal virtues.

Sp. 9. *Artemisia moxa*, a native of China and Siberia. Stalks herbaceous, simple, about two feet high, straight, branching, covered with very thick leaves, the inferior obtuse, 3 lobed, superior, leaves lanceolate, linear, very entire, all are sessile and downy, flowers small, pale, terminal, and turned upwards; all parts of the plant are alike nearly inodorous and tasteless.

The moxa, a slow caustic, is prepared from the down of this plant. It is made into conical masses, and burns like tinder, when touched by a spark or any red hot body.

Besides the preceding species, Feé enumerates and gives very brief notices of the following :—

A. maritima, Bitter.

A. procera, like the last.

A. campestris, do. do.

A. zeylandica, or *biennis*, used in beer by the celebrated Captain Cook for his crew when labouring under scurvy.

A. annua, esteemed a febrifuge in Cochin China.

A. arborescens common in Italy and all the East; employed for the same purposes as the "greater absinth" of our article.

[*Medicinal uses of the Artemisiæ.*]

The *Semen-contra* is a well known, and much esteemed anthelmintic, especially in the round and long worm of children, (*lumbricus teres.*) The action is heating and stimulant, dose 10 grs. to ½ a drachm finely powdered, in electuary with honey, or diffused through milk, and taken when the stomach is empty. In infusion or decoction the bitterness is quite disgusting; cathartics should either follow or accompany its use.

The leaves and flowering heads of the common wormwood, or mugwort, are used chiefly as a stomachic tonic; a cold watery infusion is applied to bruises, but with very questionable benefit. The roots have been strongly recommended by Drs. Burdach, Hufeland, and Loewenhoeck in the treatment of epilepsy, the dose being from 50 to 70 grains given in warm beer half an hour before the expected paroxysm, and the patient put to bed, and warm diluents given so as to excite free perspiration. We are told that the remedy is to be persevered in as long as the disease remains.

The extract of wormwood is a mere bitter, and like many others used with great benefit in some forms of dyspepsia, intermittent fevers, dropsies proceeding from debility, scurvy, and similar diseased conditions. Hufeland prescribed it in ten cases of epilepsy, of which three were completely cured, three much relieved, and four received no benefit; the operation in these cases was tonic, diaphoretic, and diuretic; in plethoric cases its use should be preceded by cathartics and depletion of blood.

The use of moxa, or of actual fire, to the surface of the body is a favourite practice in all savage and even half civilized nations. In China the down of the Artemisia Chinensis is set on fire, and the burning end applied directly to the part. In India a red hot *gool*, or hookah pastille, is usually employed. In Italy a small flame of hydrogen has been lately tried, and in Germany it is a common practice to place a particle of phosphorus on the skin, and then ignite it. The object in all is to effect counter-irritation, and the usual cases in which it is applied are chronic rheumatism, sciatica, neuralgia, deep seated diseases of the bones, cartilages, or ligaments. In India *gools* are used by the native empirics for almost all diseases, especially for enlargements of the spleen and liver.

The most disastrous effects often succeed the application of the cautery in this or any other form to the tendinous parts, such as the wrist, back of the hand, temple, &c. We have witnessed three fatal cases of lockjaw induced by the cauterization of the wrist by an ignited gool.

To prepare an excellent substitute for Chinese moxa, take fine cotton, soak it in a solution of saltpetre in cold or tepid water, dry it before the sun, when dry press it into cones of various sizes from ½ an inch to 1½ inch in diameter at the base, and about two inches high. To apply these cones press one on the part by a wire ring or a pair of forceps, ignite the apex of the cone, and blow gently on it through a reed, to facilitate the combustion. The moxa should be removed before it has burned quite down to the skin; a blistered surface is thus at once formed which usually sloughs, leaving an open suppurating sore, rather difficult to heal.

Gen. 9.—Achillea.

Sp. A. Millefolium. Europe.

Contains a bitter principle and essential oil, is of very little value. The *A. herba-rota,* common in the Alps of Piedmont and Dauphiny is bitter, acrid, and aromatic, contains much essential oil, and deserves experimental trial.

Gen. 10.—Tanacetum.

Sp. T. vulgare. Tansy. Europe, everywhere.

An herb of very strong and fragrant odour, aromatic and bitterish taste, containing much essential oil with bitter extractive and resin. The leaves are generally employed for seasoning in Europe, and the whole plant enters into numerous popular receipts for producing sweating and curing colds.

Besides the preceding articles Feé quotes under the tribe of the Anthemideæ the *Santolina Chæmycyparissia* (*citronelle,*) as a powerful bitter and stimulant, and the *Diotis candidissima,* employed in the East as a diuretic; he also mentions others of no importance.

Gen. 11.—Inula.

Sp. Inula Helenium. Elecampane. Europe.

Off. The root.

Roots white, very large, branched superiorly, branches cylindrical, shortened, covered with filiform fibrils, parenchyma fleshy, a transverse section of which presents radiating streaks. Smell strong and camphor-like, taste bitter, disagreeable, and tenacious, not unlike the Acorus calamus, or *butch;* when chewed it excites copious salivation. Powder yellowish white. According to Finke's analysis these roots contain a white solid matter, apparently intermediate between essential oil and camphor, a bitter extractive, free acetic acid, crystallizable resin, albumen, fibrous matter, &c. also a variety of starch termed *inuline.*

Inuline is insoluble in cold water, or merely suspended and soon thrown down. Soluble in hot water, but deposited unaltered on cooling, insoluble in alcohol, decomposed by nitric acid, oxalic acid being formed. It is inodorous and insipid, and not rendered blue by iodine.

Although first detected in this root, inuline has subsequently been found in the pellitory, in gall nuts, and in many other vegetable substances.

A decoction of the root is much praised as an application in several cutaneous diseases, especially those in which itchiness is a troublesome symptom. In decoction, and applied externally, it is a gentle stimulant; the extract is merely a weak bitter.

I. dysenterica is astringent, and therefore used in some countries, as its name imports.

Gen. 12.—Conyza.

Sp. 1. *C. anthelmintica,* India.

Syn. Vernonia anthelmintica, D. C.

Vern. Bukchie, *Hind.*

All parts of this plant are bitter. The powdered seeds are used as a worm medicine.

Sp. 2. *C. balsamifera,* India. *Soomboong* of the Javanese.

Syn. Blumea balsamifera, D. C.

A substitute for sage.

Sp. 3. *C. alopecuroides.* Martinique, diuretic.

Syn. Pterocaulon alopecuroideum, D. C.

In this order is included by Feé and several other writers the tribe Asteraceæ, which has been separated by Decandolle into a distinct family. Though few are quite inert, none are of much value. Some are acrid, others afford considerable quantities of potash on incineration. The only species quoted by Feé is the *Solidago virga-aurea*, (golden rod) Europe, reputed to be astringent and diuretic.

The tribe SENECIONEÆ, are also generally unimportant. The following are specified by Feé :—

S. vulgaris, France, emollient, a popular but useless vermifuge.

S. Jacobaea, of the same qualities.

Feé however notices, though with extreme brevity, some species of Cacalia, which as well known, and we believe useful Indian remedies, we find it necessary to advert to.

GEN. 13.—CACALIA.

Sp. 1. *Cacalia sonchifolia.*

Syn. Emilia sonchifolia, D. C.

Vern. Shudimudi, *Beng.* Udiram panum, *Sans.* Palla camudie, *Malay.*

A decoction of this plant is deemed antifebrile on the Malabar coast.

Sp. 2. *C. Kleinia.*

Vern. Lisan ulsaur, *Arab.* Gao Zuban, *Pers.*

The leaves resemble the tongue of the buffalo, and the stalks are prickly and covered with white spots. While fresh the leaves have a strong smell like hemlock, they are given in decoction in rheumatism, syphilis, and lepra, indeed in the class of cases in which sarsaparilla is usually employed by European practitioners. In Bombay they seem to be highly esteemed (*see* Bombay Committee's report in the Journal of the Medical and Physical Society of Calcutta.) We find the article common in the Bazars, and think it deserving extensive trial from a few experiments we have made with it ourselves.

The tribe TUSSILAGINEÆ are European plants of little or no energy. The following seems the only article worth notice.

GEN. 14.—TUSSILAGO.

Sp. T. Farfara. Coltsfoot.

Βηχιον, Diosc.

Europe. Inodorous, slightly styptic and bitter. The leaves and flowers are bitter and mucilaginous. A popular remedy for cold as a sudorific in infusion or decoction; hence its name *tussilago*, or cough resolver.

The tribe ARNICEÆ are European plants, chiefly found in hilly regions, and having usually splendid yellow flowers. Their properties are very active, and they produce violent effects on the stomach and nervous centres. The roots of the *Doronica* are poisonous, and in the leaves of the Arnica has been detected the poisonous principle *cytisine*, first found in the *Cytisus Laburnum*.

GEN. 15.—ARNICA.

Sp. Arnica montana. Wolfsbane.

Syn. Doronicum montanum.

A native of mountainous pasturages in Europe. The stalks are cylindrical, velvety, about 15 inches high, simple and unifloral, or branched, and with several flowers. Roots horizontal, brownish, vivacious, the size of small quills, very fibrous. Leaves oval, entire, obtuse, sessile, or attenuated into linear petioles, very finely ciliated in the margin, smooth and trinerved above. Flowers terminal, solitary, pedunculated, erect, yellow and very large; calyx common, imbricated; scales linear, lanceolate, sessile, corolla radiated, florets ligulate, lanceolate, treble the length of the calyx, spread out, limb toothed.

The whole plant has a strong irritating smell, especially just before drying, and which causes violent sneezing. The taste is herbaceous, acrid, and rather bitter. Powder a violent sternutatory. The flowers are blanched by time, and attacked by insects. Other synanthereous plants afford flowers so like those of the arnica that they are often mixed in the druggist's shops in Europe.

According to Chevallier and Lassaigne (*Journ. de Pharmacie*, t. v. 248.) the flowers of the arnica contain odorous resin, *cytisine*, gallic acid, yellow colouring matter, albumen, gum, and saline and earthy matters of no importance. The medical properties of the article are due altogether to the presence of cytisine. This principle is nauseous, bitter, brownish yellow, neutral, and uncrystallizable. Small doses in Chevallier's experiments killed various animals with vomiting and convulsions. Eight grains taken by a man in four doses brought on giddiness, violent spasms, and frequency of the pulse, lasting for two hours, and followed by exhaustion, (Christison on Poisons, p. 842). The same principle exists in the seeds of Cytisus laburnum, and Dr. Christison details two very serious cases of poisoning produced thereby in boys who had swallowed the seeds.

An *unfiltered* infusion of the arnica flowers causes violent vomiting through the mechanical irritation of little particles of down suspended in the fluid. On filtering these are removed, and vomiting is no longer occasioned by moderate doses. The powdered root, in five to ten grain doses, almost certainly occasions vomiting.

In small doses the various parts of this plant, especially the flowers, are stimulating, and somewhat astringent. In paralytic cases the remedy is described as producing effects analogous to those of nux vomica. In excessive doses all the symptoms of acrid poisoning are induced, accompanied or followed by deep coma, or extreme anxiety, convulsions, and death. Vinegar is said, on doubtful grounds, to be the best remedy for these symptoms. In Dr. Trail's dangerous cases, quoted by Christison, emetics and stimulants were resorted to with success.

Paralysis, rheumatism, and amaurosis are the diseases in which the arnica has been most usefully employed. It has been given, but with very questionable results, in fevers, dysentery, uterine inaction, and many other diseases.

Dr. Duncan recommends the infusion of two scruples in a half pound of water, and taken in divided doses. For the reason above specified the infusion should be carefully filtered.

The *Doronicum Pardalianches*, or leopard's bane, produces very powerful effects, resembling those of the arnica. The *D. plantagineum* has similar properties. Both are natives of the Alps, but have not been employed in medicine in Europe.

Of the tribe, EUPATORIEÆ but one species has been found in Europe, the majority of the genus being American. In general they are odoriferous and bitter, especially the *E. Aya-pana* and *perfoliatum*; the latter much used at New York as a febrifuge remedy.

GEN. 16.—EUPATORIUM.

Sp. 1. *E. cannabinum*, a native of Europe. Taste bitter and aromatic, roots purgative.

Sp. 2. *E. Ayapana*—Brazil and Bengal.
Vern. Aya-pana, *Beng.*

Stalks straight, firm, nearly simple or slightly branched, brown, slender, about three feet high—leaves almost sessile, lanceolate, very entire, smooth, contracted into a petiole at the base, nerves little prominent, loosely reticular, nearly longitudinal, inferior leaves opposite, superior alternate. Flowers purple in a terminal corymb.

Odour slightly aromatic, agreeable, and balmy. Taste aromatic, astringent, and bitter. By Cadet de Gassicourt's analysis the stems and dried leaves appear to yield brown aromatic extract, volatile oil, gallic and benzoic acids.

The infusion is very agreeable, resembling that of the coarser varieties of tea. The plant has had immense celebrity, and has been used in fever, cholera, tetanus, snake bites, and other most dangerous cases. All the romances about its extraordinary virtues are now however exploded; and we know it only as an agreeable and useful diaphoretic and gentle tonic.

The *E. perfoliatum*, or *bone-set*, possessed of greater bitterness and less aroma, is stated to be employed with much success as an antiperiodic in the intermittent fevers of the United States of America.

NAT. ORDER LXXX.—CAMPANULACEÆ.

Includes only herbaceous plants of sweet taste, and destitute of medicinal properties.

NAT. ORDER LXXXI.—LOBELIACEÆ.

Some of this family are acrid and narcotic, especially those of warm and hilly climates. The juice sometimes yields caoutchouc of great purity.

GEN. 1.—LOBELIA.

Sp. 1. *Lobelia inflata*, Indian tobacco.

A native of the United States; an acrid narcotic, and violent emetic; in small doses diaphoretic and expectorant. A popular remedy in the United States, where from incautious use it has often proved fatal. Its chief employment is in asthma, and in the form of enema in strangulated hernia. It is emetic in doses of 10 grs. to 1 drachm of the powdered leaves and capsules; of the tincture 1 to 4 drachms; as an expectorant 1-10th of these doses is given, and repeated every second or third hour.

It is unquestionably a remedy of very great power, and though of recent introduction is now very generally used in Europe and America.

Sp. 2. *L. syphilitica,* United States.

Action similar to that of L. inflata. The root has been used in the treatment of syphilis, but its utility is not decidedly proved.

Two closely allied plants, the *Lobelia longifolia* of Linnæus (Hippobroma longif. Don) and the *Lobelia Tupa,* Lin. (Tupa Feuillæi, Don), are possessed of still more potent qualities, and may be classed among the most violent of acrid poisons. Both are natives of the West Indies.

Roxburgh describes three Indian Lobeliæ. The generic character is as follows:—

Calyx 5-cleft, corolla 1-petalled, irregular, anthers united, capsule inferior, 2 or 3-celled.

Sp. 1. *L. nicotianifolia.* Erect, leaves sub-sessile, lanceolar, acute, entire, raceme terminal. A stout tall species, occurring in the vicinity of Bangalore.

Sp. 2. *L. trigona.* Annual, base creeping, erect parts three-sided, leaves sessile, cordate, serrate, peduncles axillary, longer than the leaves, one-flowered. A small annual ramous plant which delights in wet pasture ground, and appears during the wet and cold seasons. Stems near the root creeping, above erect, ramous, three-sided, smooth, the whole plant is from six to twelve inches high, leaves sub-sessile, cordate, grossly serrate, smooth. Peduncles axillary, solitary, erect, the length of the leaves or longer, two bracted at the base. Flowers small, blue, corolla inserted in the mouth of the calyx.

Sp. 3. *L. radicans.* Annual, creeping, smooth. Leaves sessile, lanceolate, remotely serulate. Peduncles axillary, solitary, twice the length of the leaves, one-flowered. Accidentally introduced from China into the Calcutta Garden, where it flowers during the rains; small, much branched, spreading over the ground, and sending forth roots from each branchlet. Flowers large, pink coloured, segments of corolla unequal, unilateral and narrow, lanceolate, with two green glands under the two middle sinuses opposite to the long green two-lobed stigma.

We have instituted numerous experiments on the last species, but found it to be altogether inert.

NAT. ORDER LXXXII.—VACCINIEÆ.

Small shrubs with alternate leaves, simple and axillary flowers; stalks and flowers usually astringent, and rich in tannic acid. Fruits generally acidulous and agreeable. The leaves of some species are provided with glands secreting resin, and in these the leaves are also bitter.

NAT. ORDER LXXXIII.—RHODORACEÆ, OR RHODODENDRA.

Plants allied to the heaths (Ericeæ), shrubs, rarely trees, with simple, alternate, rarely opposite leaves, the edges of which are rolled up during immaturity. The family is suspected of possessing dangerous properties.

GEN. 1.—KALMIA.

Sp. K. latifolia. A poisonous plant, native of Virginia and Carolina. The flowers exude a secretion on which bees and wasps feed, and which renders the honey of the former powerfully intoxicating.

GEN. 2.—RHODODENDRON.

The *R. ferrugineum* is common in the Alps, where it often proves a poison to goats and sheep; several other species are enumerated. The leaves of all have been used in small doses in chronic rheumatism, gout, and syphilis. The effect is stimulant and narcotic. The *R. arboreum* of the Himalayas has doubtless similar properties.

The leaves of *R. campanulatum* are imported from Thibet and Cashmere, under the names *Burg-i-tibbut* and *Hoolas Cashmeree*, and used by the natives as a snuff. The leaves of *R. aromaticum* (of Royle), are highly fragrant and stimulating; they are brought from Cabul, and called *Talesfur*. (*Royle's Illustrations*, p. 259.)

The brown dust found adhering to the petioles and seeds of the kalmia and rhododendra of the United States is also used as a medicinal snuff.

GEN. 3.—AZALEA.

The *A. pontica* of Colchis and Mingrelia yields a dangerous honey, celebrated in Grecian history.

Gen. 4.—Ledum.

Sp. L. latifolium (Labrador tea) a little shrub, a native of the cold provinces of North America. Its odour is aromatic and resinous, the infusion of the leaves stomachic, but induces giddiness if too strong. The Ledum palustre has in every respect similar properties.

NAT. ORDER LXXXIV.—ERICACEÆ. (*Heaths.*)

Lovely shrubs, most abundant at the Cape. All seem inactive, or at most but of slightly astringent and diuretic properties. Still the following species are entitled to attention.

Erica vulgaris, common heath of the north of Europe, diuretic, and used in tanning leather.

Andromeda polifolia, used instead of gallnuts in the silk factories of St. Petersburgh.

Pyrola rotundifolia, astringent.

Pyrola umbellata, Winter-green.

Syn. Pipsissewa, Chimaphila corymbosa.

A perennial evergreen found from Canada to Georgia, taste bitter and astringent, contains tannic acid, gum, and resin. Astringent, tonic, sudorific, and diuretic.* It is described as especially active in the last named property, combining a speedy diuretic with much tonic power. It is given in the same mode as the plant next described.

Gen.—Arctostaphylos.

Sp. Arctostaphylos Uva ursi. Bear's whortle berry.

Syn. Arbutus Uva ursi.

Common in France and Ireland. The infusion is astringent and aromatic, and is used with excellent effect in the treatment of chronic gleet and catarrh of the bladder, in some kinds of gravel, and in diarrhœa. It is much used by British practitioners; the powdered leaves are also employed in doses of five grains to a scruple, every second or third hour, taken with water.

Under the head of "*doubtful,*" Feé here inserts the *Penæa Sarcocolla,* Lin. now of the (*Natural order* Penæaieæ.)

* See *Bigelow's American Botany,* ii. p. 15. t. 21. for an excellent account and figure of this plant.

A native of Ethiopia and of the Cape of Good Hope, which produces the peculiar substance called—

Sarcocolla.

Sarcocolla (Ungeroot, *Arab.* Runjudeb, *Pers.* Dioscor. lib. iii.) is yellow, or reddish, like gum arabic, in oblong globules, the size of a pea or of grains of sand, friable, opaque or demitransparent, softening, but not melting by heat; sp. gr. 1·268. According to Pelletier it contains pure sarcolline 65·30, gum 4·60, gelatinous matter 3·30, woody fibre 26·80 per 100. Sarcocolline is half transparent, crystalline, brittle, like gum, soluble in 40 parts of cold water and 25 of boiling water, soluble also in alcohol. Odour weak and peculiar, taste saccharine and slightly bitter; composition, carb. 22, hyd. 19, oxy. 10, atoms.

Sarcocolla was once deemed a powerful healer of wounds (σαρξ flesh, and κολλα glue), but this idea has been long abandoned.

It is rarely met with in India, and then only brought from Persia and Arabia. Mesue regarded it as cathartic.

We have now reached the third sub-class Corollifloræ, distinguished by the corolla being monopetalous, bearing the stamens, and inserted into the receptacle. The *Ternströmiaceæ* mentioned at page 224, should have been inserted in this subdivision.

Sub-class 3—Corollifloræ.

NAT. ORDER LXXXV.—SAPOTEÆ.

Trees or shrubs, with simple and alternate leaves, flowers solitary, or in fascicles at the axillæ of the leaves, gorged with a milky white juice.

No individual of this order is really dangerous, the juice being devoid of acrid or irritating properties. The barks of many species are astringent, the fruits pulpy, acidulous, and edible. The seeds contain an oil rich in stearine. The butter tree of India, and of Mungo Park, *Bassia butyracea*, is one of this family. It also contains the *Sideroxylon*, or iron wood. The *Achras Sapota*, Sapodilla plum, has delicious fruit with very bitter seeds, believed in Martinique to be powerfully diuretic. The bark is deemed a substitute for cinchona, (see Lindley Fl. Med. p. 388.)

Gen.—Bassia.

Sp. Bassia longifolia, (Illupei tree,) *Roxb. Fl. Ind.* ii. p. 523. The fruit by expression yields a large quantity of oil, much used in India.

B. butyracea, As. Res. viii. 477. *Fulwa,* or *Phulwara* of Nepal and Almora.

B. latifolia, Madooka, *Sans.* (Mowa tree, Roxburgh) both yield oil abundantly.

The petals of the Mowa contain sugar, and are much used for the manufacture of a very intoxicating spirit.

The products of the Bassia trees deserve further investigation. The Fulwa butter is a soft solid at 95°.

NAT. ORDER LXXXVI.—EBENACEÆ.

Trees devoid of milky juice or resin, with alternate, entire, often coriaceous and shining leaves, flowers solitary or united at the axillæ of the leaves, the central system of the stem is coloured, of a deep black.

Gen.—Diospyros.

Sp. 1. *Diospyros Embryopteris.*

Syn. Embryopteris glutinifera. D. glutinosa, *Kön.*

Vern. Sindica, *Sans.* Gaub, *Hind.* and *Bengalee.* Jumika, *Tel.* Toombikai, *Tamul.*

Fruit about two inches in diameter, green when ripe, and farinaceous externally. On being pressed, an excessively astringent juice exudes. This is so powerful that it generally yields on analysis 60 per 100 of pure tannic acid. It is used in medicine as a valuable astringent and styptic, and is employed in Bengal for paying the bottoms of boats. The bark has been given with doubtful results in the treatment of intermittent fevers. See "*Extracts,*" Pharmacopœia.

Sp. 2. *D. Melanoxylon,* ebony tree.

Vern. Kendoo, *Beng.*

Coromandel, Malabar, Ceylon, Midnapore jungles. Bark astringent, given by the native doctors with pepper in dysentery.

Sp. 3. *D. virginiana.* United States. Bark said to be powerfully astringent.

NAT. ORDER LXXXVII.—STYRACINEÆ.

Trees of variable elevation, with alternate, simple leaves without stipules, flowers axillary. The genus styrax is the only one in this order the medicinal properties of which have been duly examined. The species of *Symplocos* yield a valuable dye stuff called *lodh.*

Gen.—Styrax.

Sp. 1. *Styrax officinalis.* Storax tree.

Trunk 20 feet high, branches covered with short down, leaves alternate, petioled, oval, glabrous, green above, cottony and white below; flowers white, large, pedunculate, united in little clusters at the ends of the branches; fruit a drupe, coriaceous, containing one to two kernels.

Storax.—*Vern.* Ustoruk, *Hind.*

This product occurs in three different forms—1. in grains; 2. in soft masses; 3. in brittle masses.

1. *Storax in grains,* the rarest and purest of all, in transparent, yellowish-white or reddish-yellow grains, the size of a small bean, the consistence of wax, and capable of consolidating into a thick mass. Odour strong, penetrating, and very agreeable. Taste aromatic and bitter.

2. *Storax in soft mass,* or amygdaloid storax (*Storax calamite,* Lemery) softer than the preceding species, easily fusible, with brown fracture, displaying almond-like yellowish tears. Odour very sweet, like benzoin, taste sweet and perfumed.

3. *Massive hard storax.* Light brown, yellow, and reddish brown, friable, sometimes slightly tenacious, softens under the teeth. Odour less than that of the two preceding varieties, and resembling balsam of Tolu; flavour sweet. This variety is very impure, being usually adulterated with sawdust, &c.

The better kinds of storax burn with a white flame, and give a light, spongy, carbonaceous residue. It communicates to water a yellow colour and fragrant smell. It is soluble (except the impurities) in alcohol and ether. By analysis storax affords resin, benzoic acid, and empyreumatic oil; from 480 grs. Neumann obtained alcoholic extract 360, watery extract 90, and inversely watery extract 120, alcoholic 240.

Storax is brought to Europe from Turkey in Asia; formerly it was packed in bulrushes, at present it is sent in bladders. M. Feé deems the origin of this drug uncertain; the styrax tree, cultivated in the south of Europe, affords no balsam, but this may be because the soil and climate differ from those of its native country.

The strong resemblance between this product and the balsam copalm produced by the Liquidambar styraciflua, led to the idea that storax might probably be secreted by some congenerous tree, and Bernard de Jussieu pointed out the Liquidambar orientale, a tree common in Syria, as the most likely source of the article. It is now, however, ascertained that storax is in reality produced by the Styrax officinale, a native of the Levant, Syria, Palestine, Greece, and the Peloponesus. Storax or styrax, (Greek *στυραξ*, Arabic *estorak*,) is a word of unknown origin.

Sp. 2. Styrax Benzoin. Benjamin tree.

Sumatra, Borneo, Siam, and Java.

A lofty tree loaded with rounded branches with whitish and downy bark. Leaves alternate, borne on rounded, striated, and downy petioles, oblong, entire, and pointed, veined, smooth above and downy beneath, flowers in axillary parcels, displayed and velvety, calyx campanulate, short, corolla with 5 linear, obtuse petals, reunited at their base, ovary superior, oval, style thin, stigma double.

Benjamin, or Benzoin.

Vern. Looban.* *Hind.*

In dry and hard grey masses, rather shining, brittle, formed of ovoid, whitish tears, like stripped almonds, and placed as it were in a cement of a greenish red porous mass. Fracture resinous. Sp. gravity 1092.

Odour sweet, peculiar, very agreeable, increased by friction, taste sweetish, subresinous, balsamic, irritating, powder yellowish grey, disposed to cake.

The analysis by Brande represents the composition of 100 parts of benzoin as, benzoic acid 9, acidulous water 5.5, empyreumatic oil 60, carbon and carburetted compounds 25.5. Bucholz' examination of 1500 parts gave, benzoic acid 187, resin 1250, substance resembling Peruvian balsam 25, peculiar aromatic principle soluble in alcohol and water 8, ligneous fibre 3. Bucholz' results correspond as nearly as

* In Upper India this is the name given to the resin of *Boswellia thurifera*, see page 283.

could be anticipated with our own examination of fine specimens of this substance. Undervorben describes three different resins as existing in benzoin. The points of difference are not important in a pharmaceutical point of view. With the resin generally sulphuric acid strikes a deep red colour.

Benzoic Acid.

Benzoic acid is readily obtained from the crude benjamin by either of the following processes—sublimation, or boiling with an alkali.

1. By sublimation—coarsely powdered benzoin is strewed on an earthen pot, a second pot is inverted over the first, and luted on with clay, or a cone of paper is substituted for the second pot, and heat is gradually applied. The benjamin fuses, boils, and the acid sublimes and condenses in fine feathery crystals, soiled by a little empyreumatic oil.

2. By boiling powdered benjamin with lime or carbonate of soda in a large quantity of water, filtering, and adding an acid, benzoate of the base is first formed, and the benzoic acid subsequently precipitated in a pulverulent form. The impure acid given by either of the above methods may be refined by a second sublimation, or by four or five times its weight of sulphuric acid diluted with six times its weight of water; heat, and when the solution is boiling add a very small quantity of pure animal charcoal, filter and allow the liquid to cool. The benzoic acid is deposited in fine crystals, next washed on the filter with cold water, and then dried in the shade.

Benzoic acid when pure is inodorous, melts at 248°, boils at 473°, sublimes readily, and condenses in beautiful satin-like needles and feathers. According to Liebig's analysis benzoic acid contains carbon 14 at., hydrogen 6 at., and oxygen 4 at., the crystals containing one atom of water. Its taste is pungent, and rather bitter. It is soluble in alcohol, and slightly in water.

Benzoic acid is a stimulant and diaphoretic remedy, of considerable power. It is used in the paregoric elixir (*see Pharmacopœia,*) and in several formulæ for the treatment of chronic cough. It is also an ingredient in court plaster. Its principal consumption is for the manufacture of fumigating pastiles, and for incense in religious ceremonies.

The Styrax benzoin occurs chiefly in Java and Sumatra. The balsam is obtained by incisions practised in the trunk of the tree after it has attained the age of five or six years. The resin is white, and transparent at first. About 3 lbs.

are given by each tree, for six years. Benjamin is a word of Hebrew origin. It is most likely that the Hebrews applied the term to some other similar balsam, and that it has in the lapse of time been adopted for the present article.

NAT. ORDER LXXXVIII.—JASMINEÆ.

This order embraces three groups—the Olives, Jasmines, and Lilacs.

Olive Tribe—Oleineæ.

Trees or shrubs, with simple, thick, stiff leaves, flowers usually inodorous, with fleshy fruit saturated with a sweet fixed oil. Some of the trees also afford a peculiar resin; the leaves are rich in gallic acid. The bark of the root in some species is astringent and styptic.

Gen.—Olea.

Sp. Olea europea. The Olive.

A native of Spain, Italy, and Sicily, and generally cultivated extensively along the coasts of the Mediterranean.

The fruit is perfectly oval, rounded at both ends, about one inch long, smooth, shining green, its sarcocarp fleshy, succulent, covering an oval, oblong, rugose, pointed nut, marked with longitudinal furrows of ash colour; almond white, and compressed. Inodorous, taste rough, modified by salting.

Olive Oil.

Olive oil is of pale yellow colour, greenish in one variety (*virgin oil*), freezes some degrees below zero; composed of carbon 77.21, hydrogen 18.36, oxygen 9.43. Specific gravity 0.913; easily saponified, nearly inodorous. Taste sweet, analogous to that of the fruit, if the oil is extracted immediately after the fruit is gathered.

By long exposure to the air it absorbs oxygen, and rancid acids are formed.

Olive oil is often adulterated with the oil of poppies. Poutet describes a test by which he states the adulteration may be detected; 8 parts of liquid nitrate of mercury when mixed with 92 parts of *pure* olive oil solidify completely in a few hours; should the oil contain even one-twentieth of the oil of poppies a soft mass only is obtainable. These experiments are however only available in India during the nights of the cold season. M. Rousseau states that olive oil is inferior to all other bodies in its power of conducting electricity, and proposes an instrument he calls the Diagometer, to test the rapidity with which an electric current traverses the oil. We have frequently tried the method, and find it requires so much care, time, and dexterity, that we do not regard it as one of general utility.

The principal use of olive oil is as an aliment; it is consumed extensively too in soaps, cerates, liniments, plasters, &c.

According to the mode of expression, the quality of the oil varies considerably; *virgin oil,* the product of the perfectly recent fruit, is of greenish colour, and highly esteemed; *common olive oil* results from the expression of the fruits after they have undergone a slight fermentation. It is yellow, sweet, and well suited for culinary purposes. The oils inferior to this are consumed almost exclusively in the fabrication of soap, and are obtained by subjecting to the press a second time the crushed fruits which have already yielded the first and second qualities of oil.

The finest olives and the worst oil are produced in Spain.

The oil of the Sesamum orientale, of the arachis, and of the poppy, are perfect substitutes for the olive oil for medicinal and pharmaceutical uses.

Olive Resin,

occurs in tears, or rather large masses of reddish-brown colour, sometimes containing half-transparent nodules like those seen in benzoin, fracture resinous and conchoidal, becomes highly electric by friction, inodorous, but when burning diffuses an agreeable vanilla-like perfume. According to Pelletier it contains a peculiar substance which he calls *Olivine,* brown resin, and benzoic acid.

Olivine is a white, brilliant, starch-like, sometimes crystalline powder, fusible at 70 *centigr.* into a very transparent mass like resin, in this state it is electric; olivine is more soluble in cold than in hot water; nitric acid dissolves it, acquiring a deep red colour. Inodorous, taste bitter at first, then sweet, and slightly aromatic.

Theophrastus and Pliny state that the olive resin was the basis of an important medicine named Euhæmon.

Sp. 2. *Olea fragrans,* (Thunberg, Fl. Jap. t. 2,) a native of China and Japan; its flowers evolve a most delicious odour, and are sometimes used to perfume teas.

Tribe Lilaceæ—Lilacs.

Shrubs or trees with simple or compound leaves, dry fruits, flowers in thyrsi, or in parcels at the axillæ of the branches.

The genus Fraxinus (ash) which belongs to this sub-order, affords a saccharine juice which concretes in the air, and is called *manna*. The flowers are fragrant; the leaves of the *lilac* strongly bitter. The *Cantharis vesicatoria*, or blistering fly, finds its favourite pasture on the leaves of some species of this tribe.

Gen. Fraxinus.

Sp. 1. *Fraxinus rotundifolia.* (*Syn.* Ornus rotund :) round-leaved Manna ash tree, a native of Calabria and Sicily.

Sp. 2. *Fraxinus florifera.* (*Syn.* Ornus flor :) flowering ash, mountains of the south of France.

To these two trees, and probably to other species also, we owe the manna of the European druggists.

Manna.

Vern. Shirkisht, *Hind.*

Var. Manna in tears, Calabrian manna.

This occurs in fragments the length of a finger, uneven, wrinkled, brittle, resembling stalactites, light, porous, and pulverizable, white, with traces of bark on one side. Examined by the microscope it is seen to be composed of an assemblage of minute crystals.

Manna is devoid of odour, of sweet, mild, and rather heavy taste, dissolves entirely in the mouth, it becomes yellowish or red by time, is sometimes adulterated with sugar, soluble in thrice its weight of cold water and in an equal weight of boiling alcohol, from which there separate on cooling crystalline stars like flakes of snow. These crystals constitute the peculiar principle of this substance, and are termed *mannite;* manna also contains ordinary sugar, a yellow nauseous and purgative substance, with minute quantities of gum.

Mannite is solid, inodorous, highly crystalline, very soluble in water and in hot alcohol. The watery solution does not undergo the vinous fermentation. Composition—carbon 12 at., hydrogen 14 at., oxygen 12 atoms.

Manna is a mild purgative frequently employed, especially for children and delicate females. It is apt to gripe, however, and requires to be taken in large quantities.

Some authors divide mannas into the Oriental and European. The former are chiefly the produce of the *Alhagi Maurorum* (see Leguminosæ.) The latter include with the ash-manna of the present article another kind called Briançon manna, secreted on the larches and pines of that country by an insect. The ash-manna is called Italian or Calabrian, according to its local source. In commerce we find besides the kind described at the commencement two others, namely the manna in *sorts*, and *fatty* manna.

The manna *in sorts* is the produce of Sicily, and occurs in lumps or irregular masses of the same composition and properties as the first kind, but more liable to adulteration; it generally ferments and spoils in a year.

Fat manna, in soft adhesive impure masses, is of very little use or value.

Besides these the Calabrians specify several other varieties—the *spontaneous* and *forced*, and also manna of the *leaves* and of the *trunk*. The juice exudes from the trees in the hot weather, during June and July, the discharge commencing in the middle of the day, and continuing till evening. During the night the juice concretes, and in the morning the masses are detached. Towards the end of July the natural discharge ceases, and incisions are then practised. The syrup-like juice now flows with more abundance than ever, concretes as before, and constitutes the *forced* manna. The leaf manna is scarce, and resembles much the turunjabin of the alhagi. An ash tree may produce all the above varieties for more than 40 years.

Sp. 3. Fraxinus excelsior. Europe.

Bark bitter and astringent, once called European cinchona, but very undeservedly. Its leaves are purgative. A little manna sometimes exudes from the trunk.

The fruits are in England preserved in vinegar as a pickle. The blistering fly feeds with avidity on the leaves of this species.

The genus *Syringa* is remarkable for the beauty and fragrance of its flowers. The seeds are said to be astringent, and to contain also a bitter principle.

The genus *Ligustrum* has bitter and astringent leaves, and coloured berries, used in dyeing wines. The bluish colour they yield is very much admired.

Tribe—Jasmineæ.

These are shrubs with very flexible branches, flowers aromatic, leaves astringent. The perfume is very fugacious, and apparently does not depend on essential oil. It cannot be communicated to water or spirit, but the fixed oils imbibe it readily.

GEN.—JASMINUM.

Sp. Jasminum officinale.

The only use is for the preparation of a perfumed oil, with the fixed oil of the *moringa*, and of which Dr. Jackson has given an interesting account in a paper drawn up for this work, and published by the Editor in the Journal of the Asiatic Society for 1839.

The *Nyctanthes arbor tristis,* (*Vern.* Hursinghar) is well known for the delicious though evanescent perfume of its flowers.

NAT. ORDER LXXXIX.—STRYCHNEÆ.

This order contains but a few trees, but these of high importance, being amongst the most formidable of vegetable poisons; India and the Eastern Islands constitute the residence of the group. Their action on the system is marked by peculiar, and terrible symptoms. These effects are due to the presence of the vegetable alkalies—strychnine, and brucine, and of another substance hitherto not thoroughly examined.

GEN. 1.—STRYCHNOS.

Gen. character. Calyx 4—5 parted, corolla tubular, with a spreading 4—5 cleft limb, and valvate æstivation; stamens 4—5, inserted into the throat of the corolla, which is either naked or bearded; ovary 2-celled, with indefinite ovules attached to a central placenta; style one; stigma capitate; berry corticated, one-celled; many-seeded, or by abortion one-seeded; seeds undulant, and discoidal; albumen large, cartilaginous, almost divided into two plates, embryo with leafy cotyledons.

Sp. 1. *S. Nux-vomica.*

Vern. Yettie cotay, *Tam.* Musada, *Tel.* Culaka, Cutaka, also Veshamoostibeejum, *Sans.* Kuchila, *Beng.* Koodaka doruatta, *Cing.* Koochla, *Duk. Hind.* Khanek ul kelb, *Arab.*

Off. Bark and seeds.

A native of Coromandel, Ceylon, and the Bengal jungles, especially near Midnapore; trunk short, often crooked, but pretty thick. Branches irregular, covered with smooth ash-coloured bark, young shoots highly polished, deep green, wood white, hard, close grained, and bitter. Leaves opposite, short stalked, oval, shining, smooth on both sides, from 3 to 5 nerved, or rather between that, and triple or quadruple, differing in size from 1½ to 4 inches long, and from 1 to 3 broad. Flowers small, greenish white, collected in small terminal corymbs. Calyx 5-toothed, permanent; filaments scarcely any, or exceedingly short, inserted over the bottom of the divisions of the corolla; anthers oblong, half within the tube, and half out. Ovary 2-celled, with many ovules in each cell, attached to the thickened centre of the partition, style the length of the tube of the corolla, stigma capitate, berry round, size of a small orange, with a smooth, hard shell of a beautiful orange colour when ripe, filled with white, gelatinous pulp, in which the numerous seeds are immersed. All parts of the plant, except the pulp and flowers, are exceedingly bitter, especially the wood of the root, and the inner layers of the bark. *Roxb. Fl. Ind.* i. 475.

The *seeds* are plano-orbicular, about a line in thickness, 6 to 8 lines broad, somewhat arched, hard, leathery, marked with a prominent umbilicus on one side and a depression on the other; they are horny and white, and semitransparent, sometimes by age becoming dark and opaque; covered with fine ash-grey or yellowish-grey shining divergent and silky hairs. The seed is inodorous, but its taste insupportably acrid and bitter.

It is very difficult to reduce the seeds to powder; they must be first rasped, the raspings steeped in mucilage, then dried and powdered; or what is preferable, the raspings should be exposed to the steam of water for an hour, and then stove-dried, and powdered in a covered mortar.

The *bark* is of ash-grey colour while young, thin, compressed, inner surface black, outer surface of the larger pieces spotted with red rust-like patches. Fracture brittle, taste intensely bitter; nitric acid gives a blood-red stain to the black parts, and changes the red to a rich grass green. This bark is known to the European druggists under the name of the "*false augustura.*" Its nature was long suspected, but first clearly ascertained by the Editor of this work, (see the Journal of the Medical and Physical Society of Calcutta, Jan. 1837). The same bark is commonly sold in Calcutta, under the name of "*Rohun,*" and substituted for the harmless bark of the *Soymida febrifuga.*

According to Pelletier and Caventou's analysis the seeds of the S. N. vomica contain the alkali strychnine, with traces of brucine, an acid they termed the *igasuric*, since named the *strychnic*, a yellow colouring substance, concrete oil, gum, starch, wax, and bassorine.

Strychnine.

Strychnine crystallizes in minute four-sided prisms, terminating in pyramids with bevelled edges. It is unalterable in the air, neither fusible, nor volatile, carbonized at a comparatively low temperature; 6677 parts of water only dissolve 1 of strychnine at 60° Faht. and this even in this minute proportion renders the solution very bitter. With acids strychnine forms crystalline and neutral salts. By nitric acid it is decomposed, and a deep blood-red solution is formed. It is altogether devoid of odour.

Strychnine is so poisonous that half a grain destroys a rabbit in five minutes in violent paroxysms of tetanus. Dr. Christison has killed a dog in two minutes with the one-sixth part of a grain dissolved in spirit and injected into the chest, and he has seen a wild boar killed in the same manner with the third of a grain in ten minutes. It acts most energetically when injected into a vein.

Brucine.

Brucine occurs in scaly crystals, resembling talc flakes or boracic acid. It is contained in small quantities in the nut, but to the extent of about 2—3 per 100 in the full grown bark. It is soluble in 850 parts of water, combines with and neutralizes acids, forming crystalline salts. It is inodorous and very bitter, but not so much so as strychnine. In action on the living system they are identical in nature, although they differ so much in intensity that strychnine is twelve-fold more powerful than brucine. It is reddened by nitric acid, and the red colour changed to a beautiful violet by a little of the solution of the proto-chloride of tin.

100 parts contain

Strychnine,	C. =30.	H. = 2.	Az. =1.	Ox. =3.	ats.
Brucine,	C. =32.	H. =18.	Az. =1.	Ox. =7.	ats.

The *strychnic*, or *igasuric acid*, possesses no important properties.

Effects on the living system.

Strychnine, brucine, the nut, bark, and their extracts, with several of the like products of congenerous species agree in producing effects on the animal economy, which, when they amount to actual poisoning, Dr. Christison thus succinctly, but most accurately describes.

"The symptoms produced are very uniform and striking. The animal becomes agitated and trembles, and is then seized with stiffness and starting of the limbs. These symptoms increase till at length it is attacked with a fit of violent general spasm, in which the head is bent back, and the spine stiffened, the limbs extended and rigid, and the respiration checked by the fixing of the chest. The fit is then succeeded by an interval of calm, during which the senses are quite entire, or unnaturally acute. But another paroxysm soon sets in, and then another and another, till at length a fit takes place more violent than any before, and the animal perishes suffocated. The first symptoms appear in 60 or 90 seconds when the poison is applied to a wound; when it is injected into the pleura I have known them begin in 45 seconds, and Pelletier and Caventou have seen them begin in 15 seconds; M. Bouillaud has recently found that it had no effect when applied directly to the nerves." *Christison on Poisons*, p. 797, 798.

Death however does not always take place by tetanus, for in some cases the convulsions have totally ceased, and been succeeded by general and fatal collapse.

The chief action of all these poisons is manifestly on the spinal chord. The irritability of the heart seems also to be diminished by their influence.

When taken in very small or medicinal doses, all this class agree in proving at first stimulant and tonic, the appetite is remarkably improved, the powers of digestion increased. The secretions are rendered more copious and regular, sexual feelings are unusually excited, and cheerfulness of spirits often induced. After a variable period tremors, startings, and often cramps of the limbs occur, with a sensation of prickling or creeping, and should the remedy be any longer persisted in, fits of tetanic spasm take place. It is remarked moreover that in patients labouring under paralysis, general or local, that the paralysed parts are the first to experience these effects.

Habit will however enable persons to take very large doses of all these poisons. Mr. Baker, lately a surgeon on this establishment, has published an interesting paper on this subject in the Trans. of the Medical Society of Calcutta; he says—"The natives of Hindostan often take the kuchila nut morning and evening, continuously for many months, beginning with the eighth of a grain, and gradually increasing the dose to an entire nut, or about 20 grains. If taken immediately before or after meals no unpleasant effect is produced, but if this precaution be neglected spasms are apt to ensue."

The morbid appearances in fatal cases are variable and inconclusive. In some cases portions of the cerebellum and spinal chord have undergone softening. In others, these organs are unusually vascular, in many altogether unchanged. A few instances are on record in which the stomach and small intestines exhibited signs of violent irritation and inflammation. In some individuals the body becomes rigid immediately after death, and seems as it were fixed in the tetanic spasm.

The smallest doses known to have proved fatal to man are three grains of the alcoholic extract of the kuchila nut, and 30 grains of the powdered nut. But from the formidable symptoms occasioned both in man and animals by much smaller medicinal doses, it seems very likely that fatal effects might follow far inferior quantities to those now specified.

Medicinally, nux-vomica and its preparations have been chiefly employed in paralysis, local or general, in rheumatism, and neuralgia, in intermittent fever, in convalescence from acute diseases, as a stimulant in sexual impotency, and to prevent incontinence of urine. It has also been given, with alleged advantage, in atonic dyspepsia, and in amenorrhea.

Before we venture to administer any of the strychnine preparations in paralysis we must first ascertain the absence of inflammatory action in the cerebro-spinal system, and if possible convince ourselves of the non-existence of organic disease or change of structure in these organs. The conditions now alluded to are deemed by all experienced practitioners extremely unfavourable to the use of these agents.

In suitable cases we may commence the treatment with the following doses, repeated thrice daily :—

Powdered nut, (Koochila),...	one grain.
Alcoholic extract of Nut, ...	quarter grain.
Do. do. of Bark, ...	half grain.
Powdered leaf of Strychnos parasite,	one to two grs.
Muriate or other salt of Strychnine,...	one-tenth grain.
Do. do. of Brucine, ...	one quarter gr.

A gentle aperient of castor oil, or extract of kaladana may be advantageously given every third day. It generally happens that within a week twitchings or creepings of the paralysed parts supervene, when we must omit the remedy for two or three days, and then resume it as before. Under this treatment we have witnessed the perfect recovery of many cases of paralysis, some even of very long duration.

In the disease called amaurosis, or defective vision, proceeding from impaired functions of the retina, when independent of organic disease, much good has been accomplished in a few cases by the use of these preparations, according to what has been called the endermic method. This consists in applying a minute portion, say one-fourth of a grain of a salt of strychnine or brucine, or a grain of the alcoholic extract, with some inert and soft powder (flour) to a surface of the skin made raw by the action of a blister. This surface may be about the size of a rupee, and the dressing should be renewed daily.

The same precepts apply to the doses and use of these remedies in the other diseases we have mentioned. As a febrifuge the strychnine class is possessed of indisputably great power, being often known to cure obstinate agues where every other remedy had failed. But they can only be used with safety and advantage when the patient is free from organic disease, such as of the liver and spleen; they do decided mischief where the stomach and bowels are in an irritable or inflamed state. In the remittent form of fever with cerebral symptoms they have been but seldom tried, and we believe are dangerous in the extreme.

On the whole the physician possesses few remedies of greater value, none of superior power, and scarcely any so formidable, as this class affords. The utmost skill is required in deciding as to the cases in which they should be used at all, and the greatest care in the course of their administration. Should too violent symptoms appear, large doses of opium or extract of hemp, leeching of the temples and a blister to the spine, the warm bath with diluent drinks and aperient enemata are the measures to be most relied on. Emetics are only of use in case of too large doses having been taken, and symptoms of immediate poisoning being induced. In such cases the stomach-pump may sometimes be had recourse to with the best effects.

Sp. 2. S. Sancti Ignatii. St. Ignatius' bean.
Syn. Ignatia amara.
Vern. Papeeta.

A branching tree, a native of the Philippine islands. Flowers white, smelling like jasmine. Fruit large, pear-shaped, dry, one-celled, many seeded, covered with a very smooth, woody rind, rather like that of some of the gourds. It contains about 20 seeds, applied one to the other.

The seeds are an inch long, (the size of a large olive) irregularly flattened, convex at one side, angular at the other, marked with striæ or rays, usually ash-coloured and spotted, with a whitish, very adherent dust. By close examination they are found to be covered with a yellowish down. Internally they are horny, and remarkably hard, towards the summit they present an umbilicus shewing the point of attachment of the seed. Inodorous, extremely bitter, nevertheless readily attacked by worms.

According to the analysis of Pelletier and Caventou, these beans contain igasurate (strychnate) of strychnia, wax, concrete oil, yellow colouring matter, green starch, bassorine, and vegetable fibre. The strychine is present in three times the quantity of that in the kuchila nuts, but there is no brucine. Its activity is consequently very great, its uses the same as those already mentioned under the preceding head. Besides the symptoms therein described, the papeeta nut purges in small doses, and is hence deemed, and we believe correctly, to be an efficacious vermifuge medicine.

Sp. 3. *S. colubrina.*

Vern. Modira canoram, *Rheede.* Naga musada, *Tel.* Malabar and Ceylon.

Off. The wood, (lignum colubrinum.) Pao de Cobra.

A climber with stem of great size, often from 8 to 12 inches in diameter, wood hard, intensely bitter, and of light grey colour. Bark ash-coloured. Tendrils lateral and simple, leaves opposite, short, petioled, in shape ovate to oblong, entire, obtusely acuminate, triple nerved. Corymbs terminal, small, flowers small, greenish yellow. Bractes one under each division and sub-division of the corymb, tapering, villous, calyx 5-parted, with clammy, glandular pubescence; corolla infundibuliform, smooth, tube cylindrical, border 5-parted. Filaments five, short, ovary superior, ovate, smooth, two-celled, with ovules in each, attached to a fleshy ridge down the middle of the partition, style the length of the corolla. Stigma capitate, berry often as large as an orange, round, the rind hard and brittle, bright yellow to dull brown, pulp gelatinous and yellow, seeds 2 to 12, orbicular, shield-like, about an inch broad. Exterior integument of seed covered with soft short hairs like fine velvet. *Roxb.*

The wood of this plant is the true Pao de Cobra of the Portuguese. That of the root is deemed a powerful remedy for the bite of the cobra capella. Several species of wood have however received the appellation of *Bois de couleuvre*, (Lignum colubrinum) in different countries, viz. the Ophioxylum serpentinum in Amboyna, the Ophiorhiza mungos in Java, Polygala senega in North America, &c. &c. all for their supposed virtues as antidotes to snake poison.

A very large proportionate quantity of strychnine exists in the wood of this root.

Sp. 4. *Strychnos potatorum*, Clearing nut tree.

Vern. Nirmullee, Induga, Titancotta, *Beng*. and *Hind.*

A large tree found among the mountains of Bengal, flowers during the hot season, occurs in gardens in many parts of India. The leaves are opposite, from ovate to oval, smooth, pointed, corymbs small, in ternary order, with numerous small, erect, fragrant, greenish-yellow flowers; berry shining black when ripe, one-seeded. The wood is hard and durable, pulp when ripe eaten by the natives. The ripe seeds are sold in the Bazars for clearing water. The entire plant is destitute of the poisonous ingredients of the other species.

By rubbing the nuts round the inside of water-pots, the impurities very soon fall to the bottom. This effect is so generally known that the seeds are usually carried by travellers in India. The nature of the action has not been clearly ascertained. It probably depends on astringency in the fruit.

Ainslie informs us that the ripe fruit is deemed emetic by the Tamools of Southern India, when given in powder to the quantity of about half a tea spoonful.

Sp. 5. *Strychnos toxifera.*

A native of Guiana, ascertained to be the basis of the celebrated Woorara poison.

Sp. 6. *Strychnos Tieute.* (Tshellik or Tjettik.)

A native of Java, a large climbing shrub; an exceedingly violent poison, which acts exactly in the same manner as strychnine, is prepared from the bark of the root of this tree. The root is called Upas Radja, but does not belong to the true Upas tree of Java, which is the Antiaris toxicaria of the Nat. Order Urticaceæ.

Sp. 7. *S. ligustrina.*

Caju-alar, Caju-nassi, Caju-badaira pail of laut. Malayan archipelago.

A tree resembling the orange tree; berries globose, yellowish green, two to eight seeded. This yields the *Lignum colubrinum* of Timor, used for the objects already described.

Sp. 8. *S. pseudoquina.*
Brazil, considered by A. de St. Hilaire to be the best febrifuge in Brazil, all parts except the fruit being extremely bitter, and rather astringent. It is universally employed instead of cinchona. It contains neither strychnine, brucine, nor quinine.

Gen. 2.—Carissa.

Sp. Carissa Carandas.
Vern. Kurunda, *Hind.*
This species is a marked exception to the generally poisonous nature of this family, the acid fruits affording the well known and favourite caranda jelly of our tables.

NAT. ORDER XC.—APOCYNEÆ.

This important and very extensive order is composed of trees, shrubs, and even some herbaceous plants. The leaves are opposite or alternate, the inflorescence exceedingly variable. An acrid principle combined with a milky juice containing caoutchouc pervades the family; tannic and gallic acid are also occasionally present. A few species from which the acrid principle is absent or separable are used as articles of food.

While the stalks of the annual plants of this order have little or no activity, the roots of the perennial species, on the contrary, are of great energy. Their chief action is emetic, but the species contain no emetine. The woody stalks and the bark also frequently contain active principles; when the fruit is a berry, it is usually milky, and participates in the general properties of the plant. If the fruit be dry it is generally inert, or at least of inconsiderable energy.

The Apocyneæ usually occur in tropical countries. In India they are chiefly found in the peninsula, and the southern parts of Bengal as far as Sylhet, extending to Burmah and the Malayan peninsula.

Gen. 1.—Nerium.

Sp. 1. *N. Oleander.* The oleander, rose bay, or spurge laurel. Νηριον Ροδοδενδρον, Ροδοδαφνη. Diosc.

Vern. Karzahra, *Hind.*

A native of the warm parts of Europe, of Asia Minor, and the lower Himalayas, common in gardens in Bengal.

The stalks are numerous, 6 to 9 feet high, branches long, straight, leafy, smooth, with greenish bark, leaves ternate linear, lanceolate, pointed, entire, smooth, coriaceous, stiff, green, traversed by a medium, whitish, very decided nerve; flowers large, handsome, purple or bright red (or white) disposed in umbellate cymes. Corolla monopetalous and infundibuliform.

The whole plant is impregnated with a dangerous principle which has not as yet been insulated, though many attempts have been made to procure it. Its activity and volatility are very great; it is even a popular belief that the vapour of the flowers in a close apartment will prove poisonous.

Externally the leaves and bark have been used (and sometimes even internally) as a remedy in herpes and itch. The rasped wood is employed as ratsbane. The wood itself is used by some eastern nations as the best material for gunpowder charcoal.

Sp. 2. *N. odorum.*

Vern. Kurrubee. *Hind.* Common in gardens in every part of India.

Corolla hypocrateriform, the orifice surmounted by lacerated multifid processes, segments of the limb contorted, filaments inserted into the middle of the tubes, anthers sagittate, adhering by the middle to the stigma, ovaries 2, style filiform, dilated at the apex. Stigma obtuse, some teeth at the bottom of the calyx on the outside of the corolla, follicles cylindrical, leaves linear, lanceolate, three together, segments of the calyx erect, anthers bearded at the point, flowers white or red. (*Roxb. Fl. Ind.* ii. p. 2.)

The bark of the root, and the fragrant leaves are used by the native Indian practitioners as powerful repellents applied externally. The root is very poisonous.

The *N. piscidium* of Dr. Roxburgh is used for its tough fibres, and contains a narcotic principle which proves pernicious to fish inhabiting tanks in which the fibres are steeped.

Gen. 2.—Wrightia.

Sp. 1. *W. antidysenterica.*

Syn. Nerium antidys :—Echites antidys : *Roxb.*

Vern. Tiwaj and Lisan ul-asafeer, *Arab.* Anduraroon, *Greek.* Seeds called *Indurjuo shereen*, or the mild, to distinguish them from seeds of *Holarrhena pubescens*, and *Antidysenterica,* called *Indurjuo tulkh*, or the bitter.

A native of the coast of Malabar, of Ceylon, and the Isle of France, and common in many parts of India.

A small shrub, leaves ovate oblong, or exactly oblong, shortly acuminate, smooth, bright green on each side.

Corolla hypocrateriform, throat surmounted by ten lacerated scales, stamens projecting, inserted into the throat, anther 1, sagittate, adhering by the middle to the stigma, ovaries 2 adhering, style filiform, dilated at the apex, stigma narrower, follicles distinct or united, 5 to 10 scales at the base of the calyx on the outside of the corolla; corymb terminal, few flowerets, corolla white, very sweet-scented, with a slender tube $\frac{3}{4}$ of an inch long, limb spreading, flat, with obovate segments, follicles very long and slender. (*Lindley.*)

The bark (conessi bark) is astringent and bitter, and also deemed febrifuge. The seeds, *Indurjuo,* are intensely bitter, and used as a vermifuge.

Conessi bark has been given with much alleged advantage in chronic dysentery. The infusion seems the best form, 4 drachms of the dried and powdered bark being infused in 8 ounces of hot water for an hour :—dose one ounce thrice daily.

W. tinctoria is indigenous over a tract of 1000 miles, its leaves yield the finest indigo. Being perennial, hardy, and luxuriant, this is considered by Roxburgh the best for cultivation of all the indigo-bearing plants.

Gen. 3.—Cerbera.

Gen. char. Calyx permanent, five-parted, leafy, corolla hypocrateriform, tube clavate, throat five-angled, with five scales, limb five-parted, contorted, stamens five, short, in the middle of the tube, drupe with a hard, woody, fibrous half seeded putamen. (*Lindley.*)

Sp. 1. *C. Tanghin,* Madagascar.

Nut filamentous and woody, albumen none, the kernel said to be a formidable poison; it was used in Madagascar for the trial by ordeal, but the practice is now discontinued.

Sp. 2. *C. Manghas.*

A common plant in the East Indies, occurring in wet situations. The leaves are broad, lanceolate, stalked, smooth, entire, clustered at the ends of the branches. Racemes terminal, branched, unequal, calyx with lanceolate, coloured deciduous leaves, corolla white, with a tube longer than the calyx, and a limb shorter than the tube, anthers ovate, quadrangular, covered by the wool of the tube. Drupe as large as a goose's egg, ovate, green, marked with numerous white points, compressed, seeds two, an inch and a half long by ¾ in diameter. (*Lindley.*)

The kernels are described by Lindley as emetic and purgative. Waiz states that the leaves are used in Java as an excellent substitute for senna. The milky sap is also said to be purgative; the properties of all parts of the plant deserve most attentive investigation.

Sp. 3. *C. Ahovai*, properties as in the last species.

Sp. 4. *C. Thevetia*, milk poisonous, bark bitter and purgative, also said to be powerfully febrifuge, "two grains being affirmed to be equal to a common dose of cinchona." Perfectly naturalized in India, according to Royle.

GEN. 4.—OPHIOXYLON.

Calyx 5-cleft, permanent, corolla funnel-shaped, tube long, thickest in the middle, limb spreading, five-cleft, oblique, anthers subsessile, inserted into the middle of the tube, ovary double, each lobe with one ovule, style filiform, enclosed, stigma capitate, drupe berried, two, by abortion solitary, each with a wrinkled one-seeded nucleus. (*Lindley.*)

Sp. O. serpentinum.

Vern. Chandra, *Beng.* Chota Chand, *Hind.*

Various parts of India, see Roxb. Fl. Ind. i. p. 694.

The stems are woody, erect, climbing, and twining, leaves in threes or fives, short stalked, oblong, pointed, wavy, entire, smooth, 4-5 inches long. Fascicles axillary, peduncled, many flowered, peduncles long, smooth, round, sometimes nearly erect, sometimes drooping. Pedicels and calyces bright red, corolla white.

Root used as a febrifuge, as an antidote to snake poison, and to *promote delivery* in tedious cases. *Lindley*, p. 532.

GEN. 5.—ALYXIA.

Sp. A. stellata, Malay Archipelago, Society and Friendly islands.

Bark contains benzoic acid, and is possessed of properties analogous to those of canella and winter's bark; now used in Germany in chronic diarrhœa and nervous disorders. *Lindley.*

GEN. 6.—WILLOUGHBEIA.

Sp. W. edulis. Roxb. Fl. Ind. ii. p. 57. Forests of Chittagong and Sylhet.

Vern. Lutiam.

A very large climber; every part of the plant on being wounded discharges an abundance of fluid caoutchouc.

The fruit is pulpy, soft, and yellow, and esteemed by the natives.

GEN. 7.—ALLAMANDA.

Sp. A. cathartica. Cayenne, Guiana, and coasts of Brazil, introduced by Lord Auckland into the Botanic Garden, but previously naturalized, according to the statements of Royle. A climbing milky shrub, leaves in fours, subsessile, ovate oblong, ferruginous beneath, with white hairs on the veins, flowers fascicled, axillary, yellow, large and showy, with villous, dichotomous, rigid peduncles.

The leaves a valuable cathartic, used especially in painter's colic. In too large doses violently emetic and drastic.

GEN. 8.—VINCA.

Sp. V. pusilla.

Syn. V. parviflora. Roxb. Fl. Ind. ii. p. 1. Common in the East Indies.

A small erect annual, stem smooth, 4-sided, 6 to 12 inches high, leaves lanceolate, flowers small, white, axillary, in pairs, mouth of corolla closed with hairs.

Applied in India as an external stimulant in lumbago. *Royle.*

GEN. 9.—APOCYNUM.

Sp. A. androsæmifolium. Dogsbane.

United States. Milky, root bitter, while fresh emetic, when dried, tonic in small doses.

Sp. A. cannabinum, also emetic; in decoction diuretic and diaphoretic.

Gen. 10.—Ichnocarpus.

Sp. I. frutescens, Ceylon.

According to Royle, sometimes used in India as a substitute for sarsaparilla.

Gen. 11.—Hasseltia.

Sp. H. arborea, Java.

Milk mixed with honey used as a powerful drastic in tape worm. A dangerous remedy.

Gen. 12.—Vahea.

Sp. V. gummifera, Madagascar, yields caoutchouc.

Gen. 13.—Urceola

Sp. U. elastic, Roxb. As. Res. v. 169. Sumatra and Pulo Pinang. A large woody climber, yields caoutchouc of the finest quality in great abundance.

Gen. 14.—Plumieria.

Several species of this genus, natives of Jamaica, Surinam, Brazil, the Malayan Archipelago, and Cochin China, are used as drastic cathartics. *Plumieria acuminata* is abundant and luxuriant in the Pinjore valley. (*Royle.*)

Gen. 15.—Cameraria.

Sp. C. latifolia, Jamaica, Cuba, and St. Domingo (Bastard manchineel.)

Yields a great abundance of milk, is reputed to be very poisonous, but its properties are not distinctly ascertained.

Gen. 16.—Tabernaemontana.

Sp. T. utilis, Hya Hya, Demerara milk tree. Milk harmless. *Lindley.*

Gen. 17.—Holarrhena.

H. pubescens. Roora.

Wood light. This species and the *H. antidysenterica* yield the *Indurjuo tulk* of the bazar. (See *Wrightia*, p. 447.)

NAT. ORDER XCI.—ASCLEPIADEÆ.

This order has been recently separated from the Apocyneæ, to which it is nearly allied. They differ entirely in the sexual apparatus. In Asclepiadeæ the whole of the sexual apparatus is consolidated into a single body, the centre of which is occupied by a broad stigma like a gland, and the grains of pollen adhere in the shape of waxy bodies, attached to the five corners of this stigma by the intervention of particular glands. The pollen coalescing into masses fixed or applied to processes of the stigma in a determinate manner, constitutes the determinate character of this order. *Lindley Intr. to Nat. Syst.* p. 212.

The family chiefly abounds in the south of Africa, in India, and New Holland.

Their properties are generally active, all secrete a milky juice of an acrid stimulating kind; valuable emetic, cathartic, diuretic, diaphoretic, and alterative remedies are afforded by its numerous and abundant species.

Gen. 1.—Cynanchum.

Sp. 1. *C. monspeliacum.* Montpelier scammony.

A native of the south of France, having herbaceous, smooth, cylindrical, and creeping stalks, oval rounded leaves, deeply notched, whitish small flowers in corymbs, fruits follicular and single celled.

This species affords the Montpelier or French scammony, a black, hard, compact, resinous substance, of peculiar smell, and nauseous disagreeable taste. It is obtained by subjecting the recent plant to the press and inspissating the juice by heat. In action it resembles the true scammony, but requires to be given in much larger doses. Its chief consumption is for the adulteration of the valuable scammony of the East.

Sp. 2. *C. Argel.* Upper Egypt.

The leaves are elliptic, entire, pointed, an inch long, very smooth, thick, of pale green colour above and still paler below, nearly sessile, of nauseous odour, bitter, nauseous and acrid taste. In small doses these leaves are purgative, and they are much used in Egypt for adulterating senna. (see that article.) The Indian, or Tinnevelly senna is not liable to this adulteration, to which many practitioners attribute the severe griping which senna often occasions.

Sp. 3. *C. Ipecachuana*, Mauritius Ipecachuana.

A root procured from the Mauritius, and subjected to analysis by Pelletier. Its emetic properties are well established, but it requires to be given in double the dose of the true ipecachuana; great difference of opinion exists as to the plant by which it is supplied. The article does not occur in commerce, though it may probably be identical with the root of the next species.

Sp. 4. *C. Vincetoxicum.*

Syn. Asclepias Vincetox: *Feé.*

Sandy places in most parts of Europe. The roots are oblong, cylindrical, plane, horizontal, creeping, short, ash-coloured, covered with numerous fibres; odour strong, taste acrid and disagreeable. On analysis Feneuille found the roots to yield resin, mucilage, starch, jelly, fixed oil, malates of potash and lime, and an emetic extract differing from *emetine.*

In large doses the powder of the root is emetic, and it is said purgative also. The specific name of the plant refers to its supposed efficacy as an antidote to poisons.

The *C. ovalifolium* of Penang, yields abundance of very fine caoutchouc.

Feé here enumerates the Asclepias laniflora, curassavica, syriaca, asthmatica, lactifera, and spiralis. Some of these will be noticed under other heads.

Gen. 2.—Secamone.

Sp. 1. *S. emetica.*

Syn. Periploca emetica, *Retz.*

Southern parts of the peninsula of India at the foot of mountains; common; a smooth twining shrub, leaves short stalked, veinless, smooth, varying from elliptical to narrow lanceolate, cymes interaxillary, shorter than the leaves. Flowers very small, greenish; follicles slender, pointed, corolla rotate, coronet five-leaved, pollen masses 20 erect, attached by fours to the point of each unfurrowed corpuscle of the stigma. (*Lindley*, p. 544.)

Roots acrid and emetic.

Sp. 2. *S. Alpini.*

Syn. Secamone, (*Prosper Alpinus.*)

Stem twining, shrubby, smooth, leaves lanceolate, elliptical, stalked, smooth, paler beneath, with transverse veins. Panicles axillary, dichotomous, shorter than the leaves, flowers minute, white, hairy inside. A drastic purgative.

The *Smyrna* scammony has been attributed to this plant on very insufficient grounds.

Feé here notices briefly—*Periploca græca*, a rather violent poison—*P. esculenta* (the Asclepias rosea of Roxb. Fl. Ind. ii. p. 40,) common on the continent of India, said to be eaten by the natives—also *Periploca Mauritiana*, thought to yield the false ipecachuana of Bourbon, the *Katapal-valli* of Rheede.

Gen. 3.—Asclepias.

Calyx five-cleft, very small, corolla volute, with a short tube, and a five-parted or reflexed limb, coronet of appendages five-leaved, leaves cucullate, fleshy, erect, with a horn proceeding from within each; pollen masses attached by a taper point. Stigma depressed, not pointed. (*Lindley.*)

Sp. 1. *A. tuberosa.* Butterfly or pleurisy root, United States.

The root is expectorant and diaphoretic, used in catarrh, inflammation of the lungs, and pleura. Bigelow regards it as a mild tonic and stimulant.

Sp. 2. *A. decumbens.* Similar properties.

Sp. 3. *A. curassavica.* West Indies and tropical parts of American continent.

Stem about three feet high, corolla scarlet, herbage downy. This plant is called wild ipecachuan in the West Indies, where the negroes use it as an emetic; roots purgative. A decoction is given in fluor albus and gleet.

Gen. 4.—Calotropis.

Corolla somewhat campanulate, with angular tube, and a five-parted limb, the angles saccate internally, coronet of appendages five-leaved, leaflets carinate, attached vertically to their tube, revolute at base, anthers terminated by a membrane, pollen masses compressed, pendulous, attached by a narrow point. Stigma not pointed, follicles ventricose, smooth. (*Lindley.*)

Sp. 1. *C. gigantea.* Mudar.

Syn. Asclepias gigantea, *Linn.*

Vern. Madorius, *Rumph.* Ericu, *Rheede.* Arka, Akund, *Sans.* Ashur, *Arab.* Ak, Mudar, *Hind.* Jumakioos, *Greek.*

A large shrub common in many parts of India, and extensively cultivated in the Calcutta Botanic Garden. The stem is often as thick as a man's leg, nearly erect, branched, abounding in acrid milky juice, bark ash-coloured, young shoots downy. Leaves opposite, decussate, subsessile, embracing the stem, broad, cuneate, obovate, bearded on the upper side where they end in the petiole, upper surface pretty smooth, under one very woolly, leaf 4 to 6 inches long, 2 to 3 broad; umbels generally simple, sometimes compound, stalked, peduncles round, woolly, alternately coming from between the opposite leaves, nearly erect, half the length of the leaves, involucres several with oblong pointed scales, flowers large, beautiful, rose and purple coloured, calyx five-parted, corolla two inches in diameter, segments oblong, obtuse, revolute, reflexed at the point. (*Roxb.*)

The root, bark, and inspissated juice are used extensively for their emetic, diaphoretic, alterative, and purgative properties which have been known for many centuries to the Indian practitioners, and have of late attracted much notice from European physicians.

The milk when dried on the water bath loses 75 per 100. The residue yields to alcohol 17, and then to water 4 parts. The watery extract prepared previously to the action of alcohol is 11 grs. The alcoholic tincture is precipitated by water, yielding a white resin. The alcoholic extract in doses of 10 grs. acts as a powerful but uncertain cathartic, and frequently causes violent vomiting; we have used it in an extensive series of trials, and do not regard it as a remedy on which reliance can be placed.

The dried bark of the root is of greyish yellow colour; heavy and very peculiar smell, acrid, nauseous. It yields to water at 70° 15 per 100 of gummy saccharine matter, and a peculiar extractive principle, which has the singular property of gelatinizing as it is heated, then liquefying again, and as the solution cools gelatinizing as before. This principle is termed *mudarine* by its discoverer Dr. Duncan, at whose chemical and clinical experiments thereon the Editor was present.

The powdered bark of the root in doses of from ½ a drachm to one drachm proves emetic after an interval of from 20 minutes to an hour, generally causing much nausea, and in about one case in every three inducing a cathartic operation. In doses of from 2 to 5 grs. taken every half hour, it proves nauseant, powerfully diaphoretic, and after several doses gently cathartic. On the whole this preparation may be deemed one of our best substitutes for ipecachuana, producing similar emetic and diaphoretic results; combined with opium it affords a good representative of the Dover's powder of the British Pharmacopœiæ. In dysentery it may be very safely substituted for ipecachuan in Mr. Twining's, and other formulæ, about twice the quantity being used in each dose.

In Indian medicine the powdered root, bark, and the dried milk are used in small doses in a multitude of disorders, and enjoy high reputation as alteratives in the treatment of lepra, elephantiasis, secondary syphilis, and in several spasmodic diseases. The clinical experiments of Mr. Playfair, Dr. Duncan, and Dr. Royle, leave no doubt of the bark of the root being really efficacious in incipient leprosy, and in numerous diseases of the skin. Dr. Playfair's Essay occurs in the Transactions of the Med. Society of Calcutta. The results of Dr. Duncan's chemical experiments appear in the "Lancet," vol. 1829-30.

Sp. 2. *Calotropis procera.* Persia and Arabia.
Syn. Asclepias procera, *Hort. Kew.* Ascl. gigantea. *Bot. Rep.* Beid-el-sar. *Prosper Alp.*
Vern. (See next species.)

A shrub, much resembling the last, juice extremely acrid, used to remove hair from the skin, and as an external remedy in ring worm, and several other cutaneous diseases. A kind of manna named Shukr-ul-ashur is produced on this or some nearly allied species by the puncture of an insect called *Gultigul,* (Royle, Illustr. p. 275.)

Sp. 3. *C. Hamiltonii,* Wight.

This is the most common species in the upper provinces, and obtains the same native names as the true mudar. By Dr. Royle's experiments and those of the Editor of this work the bark of the root and the dried milk possess similar properties to those of the C. procera; we consider it however far inferior as an emetic remedy. According to Dr. Wallich this and C. procera are the same species.

Gen. 5.—Hoya.

Corolla rotate, five-cleft, coronet of appendages depressed, five-leaved leaflets, fleshy, spreading, with the inner angle extended into a tooth lying upon the anther, anthers terminated by a membrane, pollen masses fixed by the base, converging, compressed. Stigma not pointed, follicles smooth. (*Lindley.*)

Sp. H. viridiflora.
Syn. Asclepias volubilis, *Roxb. Fl. Ind.* ii. p. 36.
Vern. Nakchikni, *Hind.*

Coromandel, Sylhet, Neilgherries. Leaves opposite, stalked, ovato-cordate, pointed, membranous, smooth, 3 to 4 inches long. Petioles 1 to 2 inches long, umbels lateral or axillary, simple, many flowered. Flowers numerous and green, corolla flat, crown of appendages turbinate, truncate, anthers reflected over the stigma. Follicles horizontal, obtuse, 3 to 4 inches long, 4 in circumference; root and young shoots used as alteratives; leaves with oil form a popular cataplasm applied by the natives to boils in all stages.

Gen. 6.—Tylophora.

Sp. T. asthmatica.
Syn. Asclepias asthmatica.
Vern. Untamol, *Hind.*

We have noticed elsewhere the C. ipecachuana of Willdenow, which by many writers is supposed to be the same as the present species, and which is common in Bengal.

The root is of many long, thick, whitish, fleshy fibres, issuing from a small woody head, stems several, twining, slender, round, from 6 to 12 feet long, young parts downy; leaves opposite, petioled, linear, cordate, ovate, all entire, smooth above, downy below, 2 to 3 inches long, petioles about half an inch long, channelled, umbels solitary, axillary and alternate, generally compound, peduncles and pedicels twice the length of the petioles, round, downy. Involucres lanceolate, flowers numerous, small, colour orange yellow, corolla flat, divisions oval, follicles lanceolate, spreading, 3 or 4 inches long, about 2 in circumference. (*Roxb.*) The dried roots of this article are of very great value, and according to the experience of Drs. Roxburgh and Anderson, confirmed fully by our own trials, afford an excellent substitute for ipecachuana, if given in rather larger doses.

Gen. 7.—Sarcostemma.

Sp. S. glaucum. A milky twining plant, used in Venezuela instead of ipecachuana.

Gen. 8.—Hemidesmus.

Corolla rotate, with five pointless scales inserted below the sinuses. Filaments connate at the base, distinct at the upper end, inserted into the tube of the corolla, anthers cohering, separate from the stigma, beardless, simple at the point. Pollen masses 20, granular, attached in fours to a solitary reniform appendage of each corpuscule, stigma flattish, pointless, follicles cylindrical, very much divaricating, smooth. Seeds hairy. *W. A.*

Sp. H. indicus.

Syn. Periploca Indica, *Wild.* Asclepias Pseudosarsa, *Roxb. Fl. Ind.* ii. 39.

Vern. Ununtamul, *Hind.* and *Beng.*

Common all over the Indian peninsula.

The root is long and slender, with few ramifications, covered with rust-coloured very fragrant bark, the odour remaining after drying, and strongly resembling that of new mown hay. Stems twining, diffuse or climbing, woody, slender, the thickness of a quill, leaves opposite, short stalked, of variable shape, on the young shoots issuing from old roots, linear, acute, and striated; on the old, and superior branches, broad, lance-shaped, ovate or oval; all are entire, smooth, firm, and shining. Stipules four-fold, small on the side of each petiole, caducous. Racemes axillary, sessile, imbricated with flowers, and then with scales like bractes; flowers small, outside green, inside deep purple, calyx divisions acute, corolla flat, divisions oblong, pointed, inside rugose, follicles long, slender, spreading. (*Roxb.*)

The roots of this plant have been long employed on the Madras coast as a substitute for sarsaparilla, and have been also used in England, and very highly spoken of. Our trials here have been numerous and satisfactory. Its diuretic operation is very remarkable; two ounces infused in a pint of water, and allowed to cool, was the quantity usually employed daily, and by such doses the discharge of urine was generally trebled or quadrupled.

It also acted as a diaphoretic and tonic, and so increased the appetite that it became a most popular remedy in our hospital, the patients themselves entreating its administration and continuance. The taste and smell of the infusion are balmy and sweet; we have used it with the most decided benefit in numerous cases of the description in which sarsaparilla is generally given; indeed we consider the activity of this medicine to be much more decided than that of sarsaparilla itself.

The ununtamul can be purchased in Calcutta of good quality at from two to four annas the seer.

No good analysis has yet been made of this drug.

A volatile acid is described by Mr. Garden of London as having been obtained from the *Smilax aspera*, under which name it is thought our article became the subject of his experiments. This is however as yet doubtful.

Gen. 9.—Oxystelma.

Sp. O. esculentum.
Syn. Periploca esculenta.
Asclepias rosea. *Roxb. Fl. Ind.* ii. p. 40. Common in India on the banks of nullahs, used by the natives in decoction as a gargle in apthous ulcerations of the mouth, and in sore throat; cattle eat the roots. (*Royle.*)

NAT. ORDER XCII.—GENTIANEÆ.

This important order is formed of herbs or small shrubs, with opposite and entire leaves. In chemical composition the species correspond very closely, nearly all being powerful bitters, and many containing a large proportion of uncrystallizable sugar, from which alcohol may be manufactured. The gentians prevail in all climates and situations, especially in mountainous regions. The Indian species are about 60 in number.

Gen. 1.—Menyanthes.

Sp. Menyanthes trifoliata, water trefoil, buck bean, bog bean—common in Europe and North America, in marshes and peat bogs. All parts are intensely bitter, and are much used in popular medicine as a powerful bitter tonic and febrifuge. In some countries this plant is employed instead of hops as the bitter ingredient of beer.

Gen. 2.—Spigelia.

Sp. Spigelia marylandica. Indian pink.
A native of South America, of bitter, nauseous taste, and tea-like smell. Taken internally it causes vertigo and a kind of intoxication. The root is celebrated as a vermifuge, especially in cases of ascarides. It is given in doses of from 10 grains to a drachm, and also in infusion; in the larger doses it often proves purgative and emetic. It has also been recommended in irregular remittent fevers.

Feneuille has published an elaborate analysis of this plant, but his results are not of particular interest.

Gen. 3.—Chironia.

Sp. Chironia Centaurium. Lesser centaury.
A native of European meadows and pasturages, inodorous but intensely bitter, celebrated and very valuable where in-

digenous, as a tonic, vermifuge, and antiperiodic in the treatment of mild agues.

Gen. 4.—Gentiana.

Sp. 1. *G. lutea.* Gentian.

Off. The *roots.*

A native of the mountains of Europe, roots large, long, and branched, much wrinkled, or as it were withered after drying, of variable length and size, yellowish grey externally, decided yellowish red internally, and of spongy texture. Smell strong and peculiar, taste excessively bitter, powder yellowish. Sometimes the roots of congenerous species are substituted in commerce for the officinal article, but as all agree in their properties, this has no real disadvantage.

Several analyses of gentian root have been published; a yellow crystalline bitter principle has been described under the name of *gentianite;* but subsequent experiments have shewn that these crystals are an impure acid, and by careful management may be rendered quite tasteless. The acid is called the *gentisic.* The bitter principle has not yet been insulated. Gluten, oil, uncrystallizable sugar, a volatile odorous matter, gum, and fibre, constitute the ingredients of this root.

The gentisic acid is altogether devoid of any active properties. We mention the mode of its preparation for the guidance of those who may undertake experiments on any Indian plants of this order. The root is digested in successive portions of alcohol at 825°, until nothing more be taken up. Evaporate the tincture to an extract, treat this with water, which dissolves bitter extract, sugar, and an acid, and leaves a thick oil mixed with the acid and resin; act on this mixture with alcohol at 871°. This dissolves the gentisic acid with a little resin, and leaves the oil. By successive solutions and evaporations the acid is obtained pure. It is soluble only in 2000 times its weight of cold water, heat does not increase its solubility; with alkalies it forms very soluble yellow compounds, of which that with soda can be crystallized.

Boiling alcohol dissolves it, and minute yellow crystals are deposited as the solution cools.

In Switzerland a bitter liqueur is prepared by fermenting and distilling the sliced root, the alcohol being generated by the sugar it contains.

The distilled water is a strong narcotic, a table-spoonful being sufficient to occasion giddiness.

Gentian root is one of the most generally used bitter tonics, and is given in the form of infusion, tincture, and extract. Before the discovery of cinchona it held the first place among febrifuge remedies, and it is still deemed a very useful medicine in intermittent diseases. It is often added to remedies employed for other purposes, as to ipecachuana, and blue pill, in Mr. Twining's antidysenteric pills.

As well as the *Gentiana lutea*, several nearly allied species, possessed of the same properties, are used in various parts of the world. Lindley supplies us with notices regarding the following—

G. Catesbæi, ...	North America.
G. Amarella, ...	Chalky pastures in Europe.
G. campestris, ...	Do. do.
G. purpurea, ...	Norway, Switzerland, &c.
G. pannonica, ...	Alps of the Tyrol.
G. punctata, ...	European Alps.

Sp. 2. *G. Kurroo.*

Syn. Pneumonanthe Kurroo, *Don.* Royle's Illustrations, p. 278.

Mussooree, Simla, and other parts of the Himalayas.

Stems about one-flowered, leaves obtuse, the radical long, lanceolate, those on the stems linear. Teeth of calyx long, subulate, corolla funnel-shaped with an intense blue spreading 10-lobed limb, the principal lobes of which are ovate and acute, the intermediate ones have scale-like teeth.

The roots are used like the gentian in the north of India.

Gen. 5.—Agathotes.

Corolla withering, rotate, in œstivation twisted to the right, with glandular hollows protected by a fringed scale upon the segments. Anthers not changing, stigmas sessile, capsule conical, one-celled, with spongy placentæ upon the sutures, seeds indefinite, minute. (*Lindley.*)

Sp. A. Chirayta. (Don.) Chiretta.

Syn. Gentiana Chirayta, Flem. As. Res. xi. p. 167, Roxb. Fl. Ind. ii. p. 71. Wall. Pl. Rar. 3. p. 33. t. 252. Nepal and the North of India, Morung Hills.

Vern. Chirataka, *Sans.* Chirata, *Beng.* and *Hind.*

An annual, stems single, straight, round, smooth, jointed, branches generally decussated, nearly erect, with their extremities somewhat angular. Plant about 3 feet high, leaves opposite, amplexicaul, very acute, entire, smooth, 3 or 5 nerved; flowers very numerous, stalked, the whole upper part of the plant forming an elegant oblong leafy decussated panicle; bractes two at each division of the panicle, and like the leaves but smaller; calyx 4-cleft, divisions linear, acute, permanent, corolla yellow, the limb spreading and 4-parted, with divisions as long as those of the calyx, and also permanent, stamens 4, anthers cloven at the base, style single, as long as the ovary, stigma large, 2-lobed, capsules rather shorter than the permanent calyx and corolla, 1-celled, 2-valved, opening a little at the apex. Seeds numerous, affixed to two receptacles adhering to the side valves.

The plant is gathered when the flowers begin to decay, and is dried for use. All parts are extremely bitter, and are identical in composition with the common gentian, containing, according to Battley, malic acid, bitter extractive, resinous matter, gum, and salts, (*Royle*, p. 277.) It is highly esteemed as a tonic and febrifuge all over India. The cold infusion is the form best suited for its use.

M. Guibourt and other French chemists having advanced the opinion that the chiretta is identical with the *Calamus verus*, or *aromaticus* of the ancients, M. Feé has controverted the arguments of Guibourt with great address and conclusiveness; Mr. Royle has also investigated it with his usual research and ability, and come to the same conclusion with M. Feé. Mr. Royle regards the chiretta as identical with the *Kusb-al-durireh* of Mathiolus, and the Calamus with the *Andropogon Iwarancusa*, which yields the fragrant "grass oil," of Nemaur.

Ophelia augustifolia, Don, (*Swertia*, Royle) is called Puharee chiretta in the hills, and is substituted for the true kind. The *Exacum tetragonum* is similarly named *Ooda chiretta*, or purple chiretta.

Besides the preceding articles, Lindley enumerates the following:—

Frasera Walteri, or carolinensis, North America, the root of which while fresh is emetic and cathartic, when dry bitter and tonic, and the roots of which have been brought to England under the name of American Colombo. *Cicendia hyssopifolia* (*Syn.* Exacum hyssopif:) common in various parts of the East Indies, the whole plant bitter, and used by the natives as a stomachic, being also somewhat laxative. The *Chlora perfoliata*, Europe, the properties of which are comparatively weak. The *Sabbatia angularis* and *gracilis* of the United States, excellent simple bitters. The *Lisianthus pendulus* of Brazil. The *Cutubea spicata* and *racemosa* of Guiana, and the *Villarsia nymphæoides* of Europe, the properties of all of which are identical with those of the preceding species. The Villarsia indica, aristata, and nymphæoides occur in every part of India. The *Chironia centauroides* of Roxburgh (Erythræà Roxburghii, Don) is another and powerfully bitter species found in India.*

NAT. ORDER XCIII.—SOLANEÆ.

This is an order of very high interest, containing several of the most powerful and certain remedies in the Pharmacopœia. The plants of which it is formed are herbs, or small shrubs, with leaves alternate, simple, and rarely pinnate; the inflorescence is variable, flowers extra axillary, fruits capsules or berries. The properties of the order are variable, some species being alimentary, others formidable poisons, and from many of these active principles have been separated, which present, with slight chemical differences, the closest analogy of physiological and medicinal action, all being powerful narcotics, and producing a great degree of dilatation of the pupil. This principle may exist in various parts of the plant, as in the root of Atropa mandragora, the stalks of the Solanum dulcamara, the flowers and fruits of several Daturæ, and the seeds of the Hyosciamus.

When the roots are fibrous their activity is usually very great, if tuberculous they contain starch, and often prove alimentary. The woody stalks are usually of little activity, the herbaceous stalks however participate in the properties of the fruit. The leaves are generally narcotic, but vary much in power, according to circumstances of soil, climate, and cultivation. The fruits differ much in properties, all those which are dry or capsular are dangerous, the taste is nauseous, acrid, bitter, or pungent; while some of the berry fruits are very poisonous, others may be eaten with impunity.

Thus the Solaneæ may be considered to form three groups—1. that of which all the species are dangerous or suspicious; 2. that containing both poisonous and innocent species; 3. all the species of which are harmless or alimentary.

With reference to botanical affinities, the Solaneæ are closely allied to the Gentianeæ and the Scrophularineæ, in which the Digitalis occurs. They are chiefly found in the tropics, but many occur also in temperate or cold climates. The genera are very numerous, but the species of the genus "Solanum" exceed nearly all the rest in number.

* It is called "*Nye*," and much esteemed by the natives. For a small but characteristic specimen, we are indebted to Major Cox, 58th N. I.

Gen. 1.—Solanum.

Gen. character. Calyx permanent, 5—10 parted, corolla rotate, 4—5 or 6 divisions, anthers 4—6, converging into a cone opening by pores at the apex, fruit succulent, 2—6 celled. (*Lindley.*)

Sp. 1. *Solanum tuberosum,* Potatoe.

M. Feé devotes a long article to the history and consideration of this most important article of food. Our limits and objects do not permit us to follow him. It will suffice to say in confirmation of the analogies which pervade this order, that in the wild state the potatoe is bitter and acrid; that the leaves are generally very rich in potash, and that the roots even of the cultivated kind contain an acrid and narcotic principle dissipated by boiling. A very pure starch, resembling that of arrow-root, is readily obtainable from the rasped tubercles by the usual process of washing with cold water. This starch is easily convertible into sugar and alcohol by fermentation, and very large quantities of spirit are thus manufactured, especially in France.

Sp. 2. *S. Dulcamara.* Bitter sweet.

Off. Tops and twigs.

A native of temperate climates, a shrubby twining plant, with scarlet, oval, bitter and juicy berries. These are acrid narcotics, and poisonous in moderately large quantities.

The young stalks and tops have been much used in medicine as a diaphoretic and alterative, especially in the treatment of cutaneous diseases, and in asthma; in lepra, psoriasis, and similar affections, it is said to be employed externally with good effect. It is on the whole however an unimportant article, and not likely to be much prescribed in Indian practice.

An active principle, *Solanine,* has been discovered in the stalks of this plant by M. Desfosses. It is white, opaque, pulverulent, inodorous, unalterable in the air, not volatile nor fusible, insoluble in cold water, soluble in alcohol and ether, alkaline in reaction, but not producing crystallizable salts. In its physiological action it combines emetic and narcotic properties.

The Sol. Dulcamara, or a variety thereof, is found on the Choor mountain. (*Royle.*)

Sp. 3. *S. nigrum.* Waste places in most countries.

Vern. Arrub-ul-salib, employed as a narcotic by the Hakeems.

Stems herbaceous, 1 to 2 feet high, angular and branching, leaves solitary soft, oval, pointed, toothed, angular, green, smooth, rather decurrent, flowers in umbels, simple and pendant along the stalks. Corolla whitish, with a musky smell, 5-parted, berries black, round, shining, odour disagreeable, rather virose, taste herbaceous, insipid. (*Lind.*)

This species contains solanine united with malic acid, but is much less narcotic than has been generally supposed, indeed the leaves are in many countries eaten as salad. The fruits are very dangerous, and act in the same manner as those of the belladonna and mandrake. The extract of the whole plant, according to Orfila, acts like *lactucarium.*

M. Feé appends a brief notice of the following species :—

Sp. 4. *S. Lycopersicon.* Tomata, or love-apple, with large lobed, red berries, very succulent, containing much malic acid, and used in sauces.

Sp. 5. *S. Melongena,* (*Vern.* Begun) everywhere cultivated in India and Cashmere.

Fruits large, ovoid, firm, and innocent, insipid.

Sp. 6. *S. ovigenum,* or egg plant, is distinguished from *melongena* by its pulpy fruits, which are stated to be narcotic.

Sp. 7. *S. pseudoquina* of Brazil, having a bitter ingredient resembling that of colocynth, and as yet but imperfectly studied.

In Brazil, moreover, the fruits of *S. paniculatum, baccatum,* and *mammosum* are regarded as powerful diuretics, the bruised leaves, and unripe fruits of *S. paniculatum,* having much celebrity in the treatment of hepatic and visceral obstructions and in catarrh of the bladder. A decoction of the flowers and leaves of *S. cernuum* is also used in Brazil as a powerful and valuable sudorific in gonorrhœa and syphilis.

To these details we may add that the species of the genus Solanum are at least 400, of which about 30 occur in India, (*Royle*), and there chiefly in the southern parts.

GEN. 2.—ATROPA.

Calyx 5-parted, permanent, nearly equal, corolla campanulate, with a very short tube, limb with 5 shallow nearly unequal segments. Filaments nearly as long as the tube of the corolla, anthers cordate, 4-lobed, stigma capitate, berry

2-celled, many seeded, imbedded by the enlarged calyx. (*Lindley*.)

Sp. A. Belladonna. Deadly nightshade.

A native of waste places and ruins in Europe. The plant is about 3 feet high, cylindrical, and branched, leaves alternate, often in pairs, short petioled, soft, very entire, and marked with nerves, flowers solitary and axillary, of livid red or purple colour, corolla bell-shaped, with 5 obtuse segments. Berry shining black, $\frac{3}{4}$ of an inch in diameter, soft, 2-celled, with numerous kidney-shaped seeds.

Leaves nearly inodorous, taste of the whole plant herbaceous, acrid, and slightly narcotic, of the berries sweetish and slightly astringent.

The roots are long, woody, rounded, several inches in diameter, divided into fibrous, greyish white, soft, and succulent ramifications, odour disagreeable and nauseous, taste sweetish and astringent.

The effects produced by belladonna and its preparations on the animal system are powerful and peculiar; great agitation, violent delirium, with wild laughter, convulsions, succeeded by total insensibility, constitute the usual train of symptoms, all of which are accompanied by extreme dilatation of the pupil. The effects are due to the presence of the formidable alkali—

Atropia,

discovered by Brande in 1819, but the properties of which have only been very recently studied with success.

We subjoin Mein's process for the preparation of this alkali, since it contains some important practical directions applicable to the procural of the analogous principles found in other species of this order.

Take 80 parts of belladonna roots reduced to fine powder and digest in alcohol of 830° for some days—strain, press, and treat the powder with alcohol again. To the filtered tinctures add one part of slaked lime in powder, allow the mixture to rest for 24 hours, and then filter; now add sulphuric acid drop by drop to slight excess, sulphate of lime falls, and is separated by filtration.

Distil off rather more than one-half of the tincture, dilute with eight parts of water, distil off the spirit cautiously till the liquid is reduced to one-third, then add a solution of carbonate of potash drop by drop as long as a precipitate is obtained; filter. The atropia is thus obtained as a gelatinous, partially crystalline mass, by allowing this to dry, pressing and dissolving in five times its weight of alcohol.

Filter; on adding six times its volume of water the atropia is deposited by spontaneous evaporation in the course of 24 hours in light yellow crystals.

1000 parts of the root yield by this process about three of atropia.

Pure atropia is white, crystallizes in silky fibres, inodorous, soluble in alcohol and ether, epecially when heated, soluble in 500 parts of cold, and freely in hot water. The solutions are bitter, alkaline, and if dropped on the eye instantaneously dilate the pupil.

Atropia is not volatile at 212°, but evolves vapours at a higher temperature; with acids it combines in definite proportions, and forms salts. According to Liebig's analysis it contains carbon 22, hydrogen=15, azote=1, oxygen=3 eqs.

Several crystalline salts of atropia have been obtained in which the base exists in the proportion of 24.47 to the combining number of the acid. The chloride of gold gives a yellow crystalline precipitate with solutions of atropia and its compounds.

The great superiority in the process just described consists in its avoiding the use of caustic alkalies, by which it is found that atropia is very readily decomposed.

The uses of belladonna in medicine are almost limited to its external application. This is of advantage in painful nodes and neuralgic affections, in tic doloroux for instance; small quantities of the extract have been introduced into the rectum in cases of schirrus or cancer, with the effect of great alleviation of pain. The utmost caution is however essential in such applications of this most formidable substance.

The uniform and remarkable effects produced on the iris by belladonna render its preparations of great value to the oculist in the management of several serious affections of the eye. Before the operation for cataract, for example, it is the usual practice to dilate the pupil by these preparations so as protect its inner edge from the needle or other source of injury during the depression of the lens. Again, where the iris is inflamed, and coagulable lymph is effused into the anterior chamber of the eye, the total closure of the pupil by adhesion of the iris is often prevented by dilating the pupil by belladonna, while mercury is administered to cause the absorption of the lymph.

A solution of a drachm of the extract in an ounce of water may be employed for this purpose, being dropped into the eye, or as is the more usual practice, a paste of the extract is rubbed on the eye-lids and over the eye-brow; the action in the latter mode is slower, but as certain and effectual as when the remedy is more directly applied.

On a somewhat forced analogy the extract of belladonna has been recommended as an external and local application to the neck of the uterus when preternatural rigidity of the part opposes parturition, and also to the urethra for spasmodic stricture; cases are recorded of the alleged success of the latter practice, and it certainly merits repetition in careful hands.

Belladonna is in repute in Germany as an antidote against the contagion or virus of scarlet fevers, and some very striking proofs are adduced by Hufeland, and others, of its efficacy. The subject however is yet open to accurate investigation.

Diaphoretic and diuretic virtues are popularly ascribed to belladonna, but we possess so many powerful and safer remedies in these classes that we cannot recommend its use.

A. acuminata, (Royle) exists in Kunawur, on the northern face of the Himalayas. The *Mandragora,* or mandrake, the root of which was so celebrated in the magic rites and toxicology of the ancients, is known in the bazars of Central Asia and the north of India.* Its properties are identical in nature with those of the article above described, but weaker in consequence of drying and decomposition of the atropia.

Nicandra physalodes, Gaertn. (Atropa physalodes, Linn.) is also said to be diuretic.

Gen. 3.—Physalis.

Calyx 5-toothed, corolla campanulate rotate, plaited, 5-lobed. Anthers converging, opening longitudinally, stigma capitate, berry smooth, 2-celled, covered with the angular membranous inflated calyx. (*Lindley.*)

Sp. 1. *P. somnifera.*
Syn. P. flexuosa. Roxb. Fl. Ind. i.
Vern. Usgund, also Kaknuj, *Hind.*

A native of rocky places on the sea coast of the south of Europe, and the East.

Stems several, erect, shrubby, branching, and forked, round, downy, leaves in lateral pairs, short, stalked, ovate, a

* *Vern.* Ustrung, *Arab.* Merdum Seeah, *Pers.* Yebruj, *Beng.* Luckmuna, Luckmunee, *Hind.* These names are of very doubtful correctness, but are given on Ainslie's authority.

little scolloped, downy, 2 to 4 inches long. Flowers axillary, subsessile, crowded, small, greenish yellow or whitish, calyx ovate, pyramidal, greenish yellow or reddish. Corolla campanulate, berry red, smooth, size of pea. (*Roxb.*)

Supposed to be narcotic and diuretic, by some considered to be the *Strychnos hypnoticus* of Dioscorides; leaves steeped in oil are used as a poultice in India to inflamed tumors. (*Lindl.* p. 511.)

Sp. 2. *P. Alkekengi*, Winter cherry, Europe.

Berries red, shining, covered by the calyx, which is extremely bitter, taste of the berries acidulous, owing to the presence of malic acid. They are purgative and diuretic, and used in veterinary practice.

Gen. 4.—Capsicum.

Gen. character. Calyx 5-cleft, corolla rotate, equal. Filaments very short, equal, anthers converging, opening longitudinally. Fruit firm, succulent, 2-celled, containing numerous dry flat seeds not mixed with pulp. (*Lindley.*)

Sp. C. annuum.

Vern. Gach-mirich.

South America, Mexico, East Indies. Chillee, capsicum, cayenne pepper, red pepper.

An annual of dark green colour, almost smooth, 1 to 2 feet high, stem angular, furrowed, branched, leaves ovate or oblong, acuminate, long stalked, almost entire, sometimes hairy on the vein underneath. Flowers white, solitary, axillary, pendulous, with dark coloured anthers. Fruit of various forms, and either scarlet or yellow, in some scarcely pungent, in others intolerably hot.

Braconnot has shewn that capsicum contains the following ingredients:—

Starch, ...	9
Acrid oil, ...	1.9
Wax and red colouring matter, ...	0.9
Gum, ...	6.0
Azotized matter, ...	5
Salts of potash, ...	6
Lignin, ...	67.8
Muriate and phosphate of potash, ...	3.4
	100

The acrid oil has been called *Capsicin*, it melts when heated, and is then dissipated into fumes of such irritating properties that we are told "half a grain volatilized in a large room causes all who respire the air of the room to cough and sneeze." It is very soluble in alcohol, ether, and essential oils, and slightly in vinegar and in water.

Capsicum is of greater importance as a condiment than as a remedial agent. It possesses strong stimulating properties, and has been employed with success as a topical application to elongated uvula, and relaxation of the pendulous veil of the palate; made into a lozenge with sugar and tragacanth it is a favourite remedy for hoarseness with professional singers and public speakers. In putrid sore throat, whether symptomatic or strictly local, gargles of an infusion of red pepper are often very usefully employed.

In native formulæ we meet this ingredient constantly, especially in the prescriptions for gout, dyspepsia, cholera, and ague. The practice is doubtless good, and derived from long experience of the beneficial effects of this stimulant on the native of the East.

C. frutescens. Goat pepper, and bird pepper, (*lunka-mirich*,) has similar properties, but is more powerful. This species is extensively cultivated in Bengal.

Gen. 5.—Datura.

Gen. characters. Calyx oblong, tubular, five-angled, five-toothed, dropping from its base by a circular horizontal incision which remains permanently at the base of the ovary, corolla funnel-shaped, regular, angular, plaited with mucronate lobes, stigma thick, obtuse, two lobed, ovary four-celled, fruit dry, often prickly, half four-celled, with four valves and many seeds. (*Lindley.*)

Sp. 1. *D. Stramonium.* Thorn apple.

Vern. Datoora, *Beng.* (applied to other species.)

A native of waste places all over Europe.

A bushy, smooth, fœtid annual, 2 to 3 feet high, stem much branched, spreading, forked, leafy, leaves from the forks of the stem large, ovate, smooth, unequal at the base, variously and acutely sinuated and toothed, veiny and of a light dull green, flowers axillary, erect, white, sweet-scented, especially at night, about three inches long, fruit one-half inch in diameter, very prickly, seeds black. (*Lindley.*)

The narcotic properties of stramonium have been proved by Lindberger and others to correspond exactly with those of the belladonna and hyoscyamus; an alkaline principle has been separated from the seeds by Runge and other chemists, which so closely agrees with atropia in all its properties that the general opinion regards them as identical.

Sp. 2. *D. Tatula.* A native of North America, very nearly the same as D. Stramonium, but is a larger plant with purple stems, and the corolla similarly stained at its edges.

D. fatuosa (Kala dhatoora) and *alba* (Sâda dhatoora) are very common over the peninsula, of India, and are also called *Jowz maxil*, or methel, (Royle) the seeds being frequently used as a poison.

For the purpose of facilitating theft, and other criminal designs, the seeds are very commonly given in Bengal with sweetmeats to stupify merely, but not with the intention of killing; intoxication or delirium is seldom produced, the individual sinks into profound lethargy resembling coma, with dilated pupils, but natural respiration. These symptoms have been known to continue even for two days, and still recovery take place; cold affusion and strong stimulant emetics constitute the most effectual treatment. The vision often continues obscured long after the general recovery takes place. This state is best remedied by blisters to the temples or nape of the neck, and by cold affusion.

If given while the stomach is empty a much smaller dose may induce all the preceding symptoms, and prove fatal. This is well known to the Indian poisoners, who suit the time of administration according to the purpose they mean to serve.

Medicinal uses. The alcoholic extract of the seeds of the stramonium is a perfect substitute for belladonna for many of the purposes described under that head.

We are indebted to the native practitioners of India for a method of using stramonium in spasmodic asthma, which is certainly found of great benefit in numerous cases—we allude to the practice of smoking the leaves or dried stems. A drachm of the dried leaf or stem smoked like tobacco will often stop a paroxysm of asthma almost immediately. The practice however must be resorted to with great caution, and if carried to excess may prove exceedingly dangerous.

It has been resorted to also in mania, epilepsy, and chorea, and with alleged benefit.

Gen. 6.—Hyoscyamus.

Gen. characters. Calyx tubular, inflated at the base, five toothed, permanent, corolla funnel-shaped, irregular, with a spreading, unequal limb, divided into five obtuse segments;

filaments nearly equal, stigma capitate, capsule opening transversely by a convex lid, two-celled, many seeded. (*Lindley*.)

Sp. H. niger. Henbane.

A native of Europe and Asia Minor, now extensively cultivated in Seharunpore, in the neighbourhood of Agra and Ajmere, and also in the Botanic Garden of Calcutta. The seeds are sold in all the Bazars under the name of "*Khorasanee ajwain.*"

The henbane is biennial, from six inches to two feet high, of fœtid smell, taper, scarcely branched, hairy, the hairs tipped with a minute black gland, leaves sessile, amplexicaul, oblong-acute, coarsely and unequally slashed, pale dull green, slightly downy, with long glandular hairs in the midst, flowers axillary, sub-solitary nearly sessile, imbosomed in the uppermost leaves, than which they are shorter, calyx funnel-shaped, villous, five-lobed, regular, wider than the corolla to whose tube it is equal in length, each lobe acute, ovate, with an open œstivation, corolla dull dirty yellow, strongly netted with purple veins, and deep purple at the surface, funnel-shaped, five-lobed, lobes rounded, stamens five, shorter than the corolla, ovary nearly round, shining, pale green, two-celled, with numerous ovules adhering to the dissepiment, style purple at the apex, stigma capitate, fruit an ovate, many-seeded pyxis. (*Lindley*.)

In physiological action this plant and its preparations seem intermediate between belladonna and opium, combining great soothing and anodyne power with the property of dilating the pupil. Over opium hyoscyamus possesses the advantage of relaxing rather than constipating the bowels, and being less apt to occasion headache; in excessive doses however delirium, coma, and convulsions (the latter but rarely) supervene, and not uncommonly terminate in death.

The chemical properties of the leaves and seeds have been carefully investigated, and an alkali has been obtained by a slight modification of Mein's process for daturia. This alkali has been termed *Hyosciamia*, but it differs little, if at all, from atropia.

An excellent dry inspissated juice of the leaf has been prepared by Mr. Superintending-Surgeon Ludlow at Agra and Ajmere, by exposing the juice in thin layers on a shallow earthen vessel to the intense heat of the sun in April and May; we have used this extract very frequently, and deem it far superior to any imported from Europe or prepared in this country by other processes. In three grain doses its soporific and anodyne effects are most decisive, and its use rarely, if ever, followed by any headache or other unpleasant symptoms.

Gen. 7.—Nicotiana.

Gen. char. Calyx tubular, 5-cleft, corolla funnel-shaped or hypocrateriform, with a 5-cleft, plaited, spreading limb. Stamens declinate, stigma capitate, capsule 2 or many celled, 2-valved, opening by 4 points. (*Lindley.*)

Tobacco, though of such infinite commercial importance, is but of little interest to the medical practitioner; we shall therefore confine our notice to one or two species.

Sp. N. Tabacum. This remarkable plant we are informed by Mr. Royle, on the authority of the Persian works on Materia Medica, was introduced into India in A. H. 1014 (A. D. 1605) towards the end of the reign of Jelaladeen Akbar Padshaw; from India tobacco probably found its way to the Malayan Peninsula and China, though Royle quotes the authority of Pallas, Loureiro, and Rumphius, who think tobacco was used in China at a period anterior to the discovery of the new world.

The species of our article is a native of the warmer parts of America; the root is long and fibrous, stem 4 to 6 feet high, erect, round, hairy and viscid, branching at top, leaves sessile, very large, ovate or lanceolate, acuminate, viscid, pale green, bracts linear acute. Flowers panicled on the ends of the stem and branches, calyx swelling, hairy, glutinous, half as long as the corolla, ending in five acute segments, corolla funnel-shaped, swelling towards the top, border dull red, expanding, with 5 acute lobes, filaments enclosed, anthers oblong, ovary ovate, style long and slender, stigma cloven, capsule ovate, invested with the calyx, 2-celled, 2-valved, but opening crosswise at top, loculicidal. Seeds very numerous, small, somewhat reniform, attached to a fleshy receptacle. (*Lindley.*)

Tobacco leaves when properly dried have a greenish yellow colour, a strong pleasant smell, and acrid taste; taken into the stomach by persons not habituated to its effects violent vomiting, diarrhœa, and collapse are occasioned. The effects of smoking the leaf are too well known to require notice in our pages.

Posselt and Reimman have published a most elaborate analysis of tobacco. Together with extractive, gum, gluten, resin, albumen, lignin, starch, and several salts of malic and phosphoric acids, with lime, potash, &c. they describe the presence of two peculiar substances, which they term *nicotina* and *nicotianin.*

NICOTINA.

Nicotina is a vegetable alkali, of well marked properties, and is thus extracted. Boil 12 lbs. of dried tobacco leaves in water acidulated with sulphuric acid. Evaporate to dryness by a gentle heat, digest the residue in alcohol, sp. gr. 847, distil off the greater part, and mix the residue with hydrate of magnesia or slaked lime. Distil again, the product is water containing nicotina and ammonia in solution; agitate with ether which dissolves a portion of the nicotina; by repetitions of the distillation and agitation with ether a solution of nicotina in this liquid is obtained.

The etherial tincture is deprived of water by chloride of calcium; by a gentle heat the ether may be separated while the nicotina does not rise before 212°. Obtained in this way nicotina is of the consistence of honey, of acrid taste, and brown colour; to purify it, it is distilled from an oil bath at 284°.

For the preceding details we are indebted to Dr. Thomson's Organic Chemistry, p. 284. The original work in which the process is published we have not had the opportunity of referring to. In the *Journal de Pharmacie,* 1 vol. xxiv. MM. Boutron, Charlard, and Henry, give the following different and simpler process, one however which is less productive than that we have above described.

Mix 1 lb. avoirdupois of tobacco with 332 cubic inches of water and $6\frac{4}{10}$ ounces of caustic soda in a distilling apparatus. Distil into a receiver containing rather more than an ounce of sulphuric acid diluted with thrice its weight of water; distil over 150 cubic inches, evaporate the product to 1500 grains. Cool, filter, mix with excess of caustic soda, and distil in a small retort. A colourless volatile liquid is obtained, which if concentrated in vacuô deposits crystals of nicotina. These crystals are deliquescent, the solution of acrid caustic taste, the vapor of the smell of tobacco, it boils at 375. Reaction—alkaline, readily converted into resin by contact with oxygen or atmospheric air, inflammable, soluble in water, in ether, in several oils, and in acetic acid, sp. gr. 1043, atomic weight, 26.25.

Nicotina is a virulent poison, a single drop being sufficient to kill a full grown dog. Its salts are crystallizable, have the taste of tobacco, are soluble in water and alcohol, but apparently insoluble in ether.

The best tobacco yields about 1 per 100 of this principle.

Nicotianin is a concrete oily substance of the nature of the volatile oils, obtained by repeatedly distilling tobacco leaf with water.

The powerfully sedative and relaxing effects of tobacco have led to its employment chiefly in the form of enema in the treatment of strangulated hernia, ileus, spasmodic colic and cholera, and in obstinate constipation. During the deadly sickness which succeeds its administration all spasmodic action is indisputably suspended, and in hernia and ileus relief, or even a cure, may be effected. But it appears to us from a perusal of the cases in which the tobacco injection has been used in cholera, that the practice is most dangerous, and cannot be too strongly deprecated.

But a few years have passed since the injection of tobacco smoke into the rectum was recommended even by official authorities as a prominent part of the treatment of persons apparently drowned. We can scarcely conceive a more certain mode of destroying all chances of recovery than having recourse to tobacco under such circumstances.

Besides the *Nicotiana persica* we find several other species mentioned by botanical and pharmacological writers. The Nicotiana persica gives the esteemed tobacco of Turkey and Syria. The celebrated Shiraz tobacco is also the produce of this species.

Gen. 8.—Crescentia.

We have only to notice one species of this genus, the *C. Cujete*, or Calabash tree of the West Indian Islands and the Spanish Main. From the pulp and the fruit a syrup is prepared in the West Indies, much used as a pectoral medicine, and as a poultice for bruises and inflammations.

Gen. 9.—Cestrum.

Cestrum has been recently separated from the Solaneæ, and made a separate order. One remarkable species, the Cestrum venenatum occurs at the Cape, at Houtniqua land, and elsewhere. A decoction of the bark is used by the Hottentots to poison their missiles, and to destroy wild beasts.

M. Feé includes under the Solaneæ the Verbascum Thapsus, or Mullein, and its congenerous species. These we follow Lindley in treating of under the next order, with which they seem to be much more closely allied.

NAT. ORDER XCIV.—SCROPHULARINEÆ.

These are plants with herbaceous stems, rarely reaching the state of shrubs; their mode of inflorescence is very variable; some are very energetic narcotics, but the majority are devoid of any activity.

The most important botanical characters are the corolla being monopetalous, ovarium superior, seeds albuminous, stamens irregularly diandrous or didynamous. The fruit is capsular, with two to four valves, and numerous seeds.

They are found in abundance in all parts of the world. About 160 species are enumerated in the Indian Flora. (*Royle.*)

Gen. 1.—Scrophularia.

Sp. Scrophularia nodosa.

An insignificant plant, still however officinal in the British Pharmacopœia. It derived its name from its reputed antiscrophulous virtues, but it is now known to be quite useless.

Gen. 2.—Digitalis.

Gen. char. Sepals five, rounded or acute, permanent, much shorter than the corolla, the uppermost narrowest, corolla ventricose, contracted at the base, with an oblique limb, upper lip emarginate, lower three-lobed, with the middle lobe the largest, stamens didynamous, inserted into the base of the corolla, anthers acute, naked stigma, capsule ovate with a septicidal dehiscence. (*Lindley.*)

Sp. Digitalis purpurea. Purple foxglove.

A common plant by road sides and in waste places in Europe. Biennial, roots fibrous, stem straight, slender, with several very slight angles, three or four feet high, leaves alternate, ovate, or elliptic, oblong, crenate, downy, rugged and veiny, dull-green, tapering at the base into winged footstalks, radical ones largest. Raceme terminal, one-sided, erect, simple, of very numerous large hanging scentless crimson flowers, elegantly spotted and hairy within. The seeds are small, oblong, pale brown, and pitted.

The leaves, which are most extensively employed in medicine as a sedative and diuretic, are gathered while the plant is in flower, and dried by exposure to the sun, or suspension in a warm room. While fresh they are inodorous, when dry the smell is faintly narcotic, taste bitter and nauseous, they evolve ammonia if treated with lime, and communicate their properties to water and alcohol. The analysis of the leaves presents very discordant results. It is certain that they contain astringent matter, chlorophylle, and mucus, resin, starch, gum, fibre, and volatile oil. Hare considers the resin to be the active principle, Le Royer however ascribes it to a principle he names *Digitaline*. The existence of this substance has not however been satisfactorily proved.

Digitalis produces two remarkable effects on the animal economy, proving directly *sedative*, and also *diuretic*.

As a *sedative* it diminishes the activity of the circulation, abates morbid heat, and allays pain, at the same time that the activity of the absorbent vessels is increased, and the discharge of urine thereby promoted.

The pulse has been reduced from 110 to 40 beats in a minute in one case, in another from 130 to 60 in six hours, in a third from 125 to 45 in forty-eight hours; any sudden exercise, change of posture, or mental excitement however again accelerates the pulse, renders it fluttering, induces nausea and fainting, and has in more than one instance ended in sudden death. Such alarming symptoms are best met by ether, ammonia, brandy, and similar stimulants.

The dose necessary to produce these effects varies remarkable in different individuals. A servant girl, aged 17, in the family of the Editor, was thrown into almost fatal collapse by 20 drops of the tincture, given during an attack of peritonitis. In many cases the remedy accumulates in the system before it displays its effects. These may occur at an interval even of some days after the medicine has been remitted; together with the symptoms above described convulsions often occur in such cases.

In very large doses, vomiting, purging, and deadly collapse are induced, and death takes place in a period of usually from 6 to 24 hours, under many of the symptoms of malignant cholera.

No marked appearances of importance are observed in the bodies of persons poisoned by this substance.

The diuretic effects of digitalis are chiefly evident while its sedative influence exists; at this time also the system seems more sensitive to the influence of other diuretic remedies, such as squill and mercurial preparations. Formulæ for such preparations will be found in the Pharmacopœia.

Digitalis is chiefly used in hypertrophy of the heart, acute inflammation, and rheumatism, and in inflammation of the membranes of the brain, inflammatory dropsies, &c. The utmost caution is necessary in its administration, for the reasons above stated.

The powder, tincture, and infusion are the forms in which digitalis is most employed. The powder is given at first in half grain doses thrice daily, and carried on with great caution to two or three grains.

GEN. 3.—HERPESTES.

Calyx 5-parted, upper sepal very large, ovate, 2 lowest sepals narrower, lateral, linear, and covered by the rest. Corolla tubular, somewhat 2-lipped, upper lip bifid, lower trifid, with flat equal segments. Stamens didynamous, enclosed, anthers approximated in pairs, with diverging segments, capsule 4-valved. (*Lindley.*)

Sp. 1. *H. Monnieria.*

Vern. Jala brimmi, *Sans.* Adha Birni, *Beng.*

A native of tropical countries, stems several, annual, creeping, round, jointed, branching, smooth, succulent, leaves opposite, sessile, obovate, wedge-shaped, or oblong, smooth, entire, obtuse, fleshy, dotted with minute spots. Peduncles axillary, alternate, solitary, round, smooth, one-flowered. Flowers blue, bractes 2-awled, pressing on the calyx laterally. Calyx 5-leaved, corolla campanulate, border 5-parted, anthers 2-cleft, blue, stigma large, capsule ovate, 2-celled, 2-valved. Seeds very numerous. (*Roxb.*)

The natives use the expressed juice mixed with petroleum as a local remedy in rheumatism.

Sp. 2. *H. amara.*

Syn. Caranga amara, *Vahl.* Gratiola amara. *Roxb. Fl. Ind.* i. 135.

The leaves are described as excessively bitter, the plant is a native of the Moluccas, and was accidentally introduced into the Botanical Garden of Calcutta.

In this family also occur *Gratiola*, a separate genus, under which writers describe the Gratiola officinalis, or hedge hyssop of Europe, a bitter cathartic and emetic, also diuretic, and a violent poison—and *Scoparia dulcis*, a Spanish American, mucilaginous, laxative, by some thought febrifuge.

Roxburgh describes 18 species of Gratiola in the Flora Indica, of which three are natives of Molucca, the rest of continental India. They have however all been referred to other genera. Those mentioned above are the only species to which he assigns any remarkable properties.

Gen. 4.—Verbascum.

Verbascum nigrum and *V. Thapsus* or Mullein, are supposed to be narcotic, the seeds were used to poison fish. Feé gives a separate article to the Verbascums which they are too insignificant to deserve.

Gen. 5.—Calceolaria.

Lindley describes two species, C. trifida, and C. pinnata, natives of Peru, the former a tonic febrifuge, the latter emetic and purgative.

Gen. 6.—Linaria.

Calyx five-parted, corolla personate, stamens hairy at the base, capsule opening by pores or opercular valves or teeth.

Sp. 1. Linaria vulgaris. *Antirrhinum Linaria.* Toad flax, Europe.

Bitter, supposed to be purgative and diuretic, and employed in a lotion for some cutaneous diseases.

Sp. 2. *L. Cymbalaria*, Ivy-leaved snap-dragon.
Vern. Karamba, *Sans.*

Stems long, pendulous, filiform, very much tangled, smooth, hanging from old walls, leaves cordate, five-lobed, alternate, smooth. Flowers solitary on long axillary stalks, variegated with violet and blue, palate yellow, spur short and pointed, capsule roundish, irregularly torn at top, seeds black and wrinkled. Taste warm, and rather aromatic.

Given in India with sugar for the cure of diabetes. Lindley observes that Hamilton's remarks to this effect are probably applicable to the *Lin. ramosisimus* of Wallich, a nearly allied species.

Gen. 7.—Vandellia.

Lindley describes V. diffusa of the Isle of France, Brazil, and Yuagana, where it is considered of great value as an emetic and febrifuge, and in the treatment of dysentery.

Torenia asiatica, Linn. (Caela dola, *Sans.*) the juice of the leaves is considered in Malabar a remedy for gonorrhœa.

GEN. 8.—PICRORRHIZA. (Royle.)

Calyx leafy, campanulate, almost equally five-cleft. Corolla campanulate, shorter than the calyx, nearly equally four-cleft, with the segments entire. Stamens four, inserted into the throat of the corolla, nearly equal, diverging, projecting some distance; anthers two-celled with cells confluent at the apex, valves of the capsule septiferous, in the middle bipartite, with a double dissepiment, seeds enclosed in a bladdery arillus-like membrane. (*Bentham.*)

P. Kurrooa. (*Syn.* Veronica? Lindleyana, Wal. Cat.) Gosainthan, Kemaon, Kedarkanta. A fleshy rooted perennial, stems very short, ascending, leaves obovate, tapering to the base, serrated, smooth or nearly so, scape erect, naked. Flowers sessile, deep blue, in dense spikes.

The root is intensely bitter, and used as a medicine in India.

GEN. 9.—EUPHRASIA.

Lindley cites the *E. officinalis* (eye-bright) a pretty plant found in Europe, the Himalayas, and Cashmere. Slightly bitter and aromatic, once celebrated as an application to weak eyes, but now seldom or never employed.

GEN. 10.—VERONICA.

Sp. 1. *V. Beccabunga.* Speedwell.

A favourite popular remedy in Europe in coughs, chronic visceral affections, and dyspepsia. It contains a little tannic acid and mucilage, but no more remarkable ingredient. It is no longer employed in regular medical practice.

Sp. 2. *V. officinalis.* A similar plant, officinal in the French Codex.

There are several Indian species.

NAT. ORDER XCV.—CYRTANDRACEÆ.

The plants of this order are watery, and possess little sensible properties. *Didymocarpus aromaticus* is stated by Dr. Wallich to be used as a perfume and aromatic drug, called by the natives *Kumkuma* and *Ranigovindhi* (*Royle*, p. 294.)

NAT. ORDER XCVI.—PEDALINEÆ.

An order of some importance, identical with the Sesameæ of Brown. The genus Sesamum furnishes a valuable oil. Lindley merely makes the following note of the order:—

Sesamum indicum, *Linn.* } have mucilaginous seeds like lin-
Pedalium murex, *Linn.* } seed,
and yield a mucilaginous meal used in India for poultices.

GEN. 1.—SESAMUM.

Sesamum orientale, Schitchi, *Rheede.* *Σησαμον*, Hippocrates.

Vern. Black seeds, *Kala til,* white seeds, *Suffed til.* Oil, *meetha til, til ke tel,* gingilie oil, &c.

The sesamum plant is universally cultivated in the East for the oil expressed from the seeds.

The stalks are straight, herbaceous, nearly cylindrical, hairy, about 2 feet high, leaves oval oblong, with long petioles, entire, toothed, the upper leaves alternate, flowers solitary, axillary, with short peduncles and linear bractes, capsules oblong, rather compressed, marked with rather deep furrows. Seeds slightly oval, small, yellow or black, tasteless and inodorous.

A very sweet oil (siritch, *Arab.*) is obtained by expression from the seeds; this oil is much used as an article of diet, for frictions, and lighting. The oil-cake mixed with honey and preserved citron is esteemed an oriental luxury. The leaves of the plant are used as poultices.

Nine pounds of the seed yield two quarts of perfectly sweet oil, which will keep many years without becoming rancid; the oil made in Persia, and thence largely exported, is called *Kurit schuk.*

Sesamum oil is of the sp. gr. 911, insoluble in alcohol, readily saponifies with the alkalies, and combines with the oxide of lead. For all purposes of medicine and pharmacy it is when well prepared quite equal to the best olive oil.

GEN. 2.—PEDALIUM.

Gen. characters. Calyx 5-parted, corolla sub-equal, with 5-cleft border, nut corky, 4-cornered, thorny on the angles, 2-celled, seeds 2-fold.

Sp. P. Murex.
Vern. Gokeroo, *Hind.*

A pretty large plant, succulent, ramous, annual, growing generally over the country, but chiefly on the Coromandel coast, in a moist sandy soil; flowers in the rainy and cold seasons. Root annual, ramous, of deep orange colour, stem scarcely any, branches nearly opposite, spreading, with their extremity erect, round, and smooth, from 6 to 24 inches long, leaves opposite, petioled, oval, irregularly toothed, truncate, three-nerved, pretty smooth, two to three inches long, by one and a half or two inches broad, petioles channelled, about two inches long. Flowers axillary, short, peduncled, single, pretty large, yellow, erect, on each side of their insertion is a small round brown gland.

The fresh plant renders water or milk very mucilaginous without altering the taste, colour, or smell of the liquid. This thickening disappears in a few hours. A watery infusion of this kind sweetened with sugar is a favourite and excellent native demulcent in acute gonorrhœa. Butter milk is often fraudulently thickened by the use of this leaf. *Roxb. Fl. Ind.* iii. p. 114.

NAT. ORDER XCVII.—BIGNONIACEÆ.

The leaves of Bignonia Chica yield red colouring matter. The bark and capsules of B. indica are astringent, and used in tanning and dyeing. The pleasant tasted and fragrant flowers of B. chelonoides (suaveolens?) are described as being used as a cooling drink in fevers. Lindley quotes two species, B. catalpa and B. antisyphilitica, the former a native of the southern parts of the United States; leaves and bark extremely bitter, a decoction of the pods used in asthma, and the leaves employed for fomentations.

Sp. Bignonia antisyphilitica. The bark of the younger branches of this tree is considered in Brazil one of the most powerful remedies against malignant syphilitic swellings. The bark is used both internally and externally in decoction and powder.

NAT. ORDER XCVIII.—ACANTHACEÆ.

This order resembles the last in structure and distribution. Its species are extremely numerous, are found in India every where on the plains, and also at considerable elevations. Numerous as is the order, it still contains but few plants of much medicinal value; some are demulcent, a few others bitter and acrid.

Gen. 1.—Rhinacanthus.

Calyx regularly 5-parted, with small subulate bracts and bractlets, corolla hypocrateriform, 2-lipped, with a long slender tube, the upper lip narrow, the lower trifid with equal segments, stamens two, inserted in the throat of the corolla, anthers 2-celled, capsule clavate at the base, much compressed and seedless, in upper part 4-seeded, or by abortion 2-seeded. Dissepiment complete, adnate. Seeds ovate, biconvex with hooks, which are concave and obtuse. (*Lindley.*)

Sp. R. communis.

Syn. Justicia nasuta, Linn. *Roxb. Flora Indica*, i. p. 120. *Rheede*, ix. t. 69.

Vern. Pulcolli, *Rheede.* Kabooter ke jur, *Hind.* Jooi panee, *Beng.* Naga mulli, *Tel.* and *Tam.*

A native of the continent of India.

Leaves opposite, stalked, broad, lanceolate, obtuse, above smooth, below a little downy, entire, from 2 to 4 inches long, and from 1 to 2 broad, panicles corymbose, axillary, and terminal, always 3-cleft, bracts minute, flowers small and white, corolla with a long slender compressed tube, under lip broad, 3-cleft, upper lip erect, linear, sides reflected, apex bifid, anthers projecting beyond the tube, twin. *Roxb.*

Milk boiled on the roots is deemed aphrodisiac; with lime-juice and pepper it is used for the cure of ringworm, also for the bites of venomous snakes, hence the Telinga and Tamul name Naga mulli, or jasmine of the cobra capella. "Naga," as Roxburgh informs us, is prefixed to most of the native antidotes, and occurs very often in their writings. Roxburgh's further observations we esteem it our duty to quote most prominently, agreeing as we fully do with their import:—"like the ancient physicians of Greece and Rome those of India at this day make poisons and their antidotes a very chief part of their studies, but from the seeming inactivity of a very large share of them, we may safely conclude that their practice is equally frivolous with that of the ancients, and ought to be discouraged as much as possible, because at least they prevent the application of more efficacious remedies."

Gen. 2.—Justicia.

Sp. Justicia Ecbolium, Roxb. Fl. Ind. i. 114.

Vern. Jati, *Hind.* A native of the Indian forests, said to be diuretic.

Flowers pale blue, tube very long and slender.

Lindley also quotes *J. pectoralis*, a stomachic, *J. biflora*, and *Acanthus mollis*, having emollient leaves used for poultices.

Gen. 3.—Andrographis.

Calyx deeply five-parted with narrow segments, corolla bilabiate, the upper lip entire or bifid, when resupinate appearing to be divided in the contrary way. Stamens two, anthers two-celled, cells parallel, bearded at the base, four or many seeded, dissepiment adnate, seeds oval, obtuse, tapering obliquely, truncate at the base, pitted with a deep hilum, hooks stalked, dilated, scaly, deciduous. (*Lindley.*)

Sp. A. paniculata.

Syn. Justicia panic. *Roxb. Fl. Ind.* i. p. 118.

Vern. Kalamegh, *Beng.* Kalupnath, or Muha tita, (great bitter), *Hind.* Kreat of *Malabar.*

A native of dry ground under the shade of trees; flowers in the wet and cold seasons.

Stem erect, generally annual, at least down to the root, branchy, slender, four-sided, pointed, smooth, one to two feet high, branches opposite, cross armed, four-sided, spreading, leaves opposite, short, petiolate, lanceolate, entire, smooth two to three inches long. Racemes terminal, and from the exterior axils horizontal, long, secund, four-sided. Flowers remote, rose-coloured, long pedicelled, alternate, erect, downy. Bracts, a large exterior opposite pair, within the flower-bearing one; there are two smaller embracing the base of the pedicels, corolla bilabiate, tube recurved, lips linear and reflected, the superior broadest, three-toothed, the inferior two-toothed, filaments as long as the lips of the corolla, projecting, hairy. Anthers very flat, obovate, firmly united at the base and there bearded, capsule erect, subcylindric, seeds three or four in each cell, cylindrical. *Roxb.*

Celebrated as a stomachic bitter, and used in cholera and dysentery. It is the basis of the celebrated "*Drogue amere;*" this is a compound of mastic, frankincense, resin, myrrh, aloes, and creat root, steeped in brandy for a month, and the tincture strained and bottled.

Gen. 4.—Gendarussa.

Calyx regular, 5-parted, furnished at the base with small bracts, corolla bilabiate, upper top arched, tube short. Stamens 2, inserted below the throat of the corolla, connective rhomboidal, lanceolate, oblique cells of the anthers placed obliquely one above the other, valves half ovate, the lower calcarate, capsule sterile below, and little narrowed, four-seeded at upper end. (*Lindley.*)

Sp. G. vulgaris.

Syn. Justicia Gendarussa, Linn. *Roxb. Fl. Ind.* i. p. 128.

Vern. Caroo noochie, *Tam.* Kali shumbli, *Duk.* Jugut mudun, *Beng.* Nela nirganda, *Sans.*

Common in gardens in India, and supposed by Roxburgh to be a native of the Malay islands. Flowers during the wet season. It is a shrub with dark purple or green smooth shoots, leaves short stalked, lanceolate, obtuse, smooth, with the rib and veins dark purple. Spikes terminal, somewhat whorled, leafy at base, flowers reddish purple. Leaves and stalks when rubbed have a strong, rather aromatic odour. After being roasted they are given in chronic rheumatism by the native practitioners. The plant is also said to be emetic.

Adhatoda Vasica, (Nees.) Uroos or Utarusha, *Sans.* Justicia Adhatoda, *Linn.* All parts of the plant are bitterish and slightly aromatic, and supposed to be antispasmodic; the wood is soft, and much esteemed for making charcoal for gunpowder.

Thirty-two species of Justicia are described by Dr. Roxburgh. Those only which we have quoted have any medicinal virtues attributed to them, and all but one are now referred to other genera.

NAT. ORDER XCIX.—VERBENACEÆ.

This order contains forest trees, herbs, and shrubs of elegant aspect, with opposite or verticillated leaves. It is nearly connected with the following family. Many of the species are somewhat bitter or astringent, some aromatic or fœtid; an acrid pungent principle resembling pepper is secreted by the fruits of several of the vitex genus. The order is distinguished for including the magnificent teak tree, (*Tectona grandis,*) now widely cultivated over India.

Gen. 1.—Verbena.

Sp. 1. ***Verbena officinalis.*** Vervein, ιερα βοτανη, *Dioscorides.*

A native of the warm parts of Europe, this plant is described as astringent, febrifuge, &c. but has fallen into just neglect. Still among the ancient Greeks and Gauls it held the highest place in popular estimation; it was used to purify the altars, and formed the crowns of heralds and ambassadors. The Druids gathered it with the same marks of veneration as the misseltoe. Employed extensively as a medicine it was also the base of numerous philters, or love portions, and hence derived its name of *Veneris vena*, or source of love.

Sp. 2. *V. jamaicensis*, Linn.

Syn. Stachytarpha Jam. *Lindley.* The expressed juice of the leaves in doses of one to two table spoonsful is used in the French West India Islands as a cooling purgative for children, and in clysters.

Gen. 2.—Vitex.

Gen. char. Calyx campanulate, five-toothed, corolla bilabiate, the upper lip bifid, lower trifid, middle segment largest. Stamens somewhat protruding, anthers oval, erect, style filiform, stigma bifid, drupe globose, four-celled, four-seeded. (*Lindley.*)

Sp. 1. ***Vitex trifolia.*** Roxb. Fl. Ind. iii. p. 69.

Vern. Neer nochie, *Tam.* Panee ke shumbalie, *Duk.* Ussel ke abee, *Arab.* Nisindha, *Hind.* also Seduaree. Neela vavilie, *Tel.* Caranosi, *Rheede.* Jala nergundi and Sinduvara, *Sans.*

Young shoots round and villous, leaves opposite, ternate, leaflets all sessile, ovate, oblong, entire, hoary underneath, the pair from one to two inches long, the terminal one much longer, petioles about an inch long and hoary. Panicles terminal, linear oblong, composed of brachiate and dichotomous ramifications, every part hoary. Flowers small, of lively light blue colour, bracts minute, calyx campanulate, hoary, mouth slightly five-toothed, stamens as long as the corolla, ovary round, two-celled, style as long as the corolla, stigma of two filiform spreading lobes, drupe round, smooth, when ripe black, size of a small pea, stone of the same shape as the drupe, four-celled. Seed solitary, albumen when seeds are ripe none. (*Roxb.*)

Leaves slightly bitter, but of delightfully aromatic taste and smell; are deemed powerful external applications in rheumatism, sprains, &c. The powdered leaves are said to cure intermittent fevers. The fruit in powder is given usually in electuary, or decoction, for amenorrhœa and several other diseases. It is a common Indian plant. Sir William Jones in the 4th. vol. Asiatic Researches, p. 293, states that the leaves are used to stuff pillows, to cure catarrh and headache. The flowers, according to Dr. Hamilton, are prescribed in Behar with honey in fevers attended with vomiting and much thirst. (*Ainslie*, ii. p. 238.)

Sp. 2. *Vitex Agnus castus*—seeds globular, obtuse, mucronate, smooth, brownish grey, four-celled, half enclosed in the persistent and downy calyx. The leaves are digitate, having five or seven segments.

The seeds are inodorous when entire but when bruised their odour is acrid and disagreeable. The taste acrid and pepperish, very persistent. They are very rich in essential oil, and possess powerful stimulating properties. At Smyrna the powder strewed over a sliced onion and applied to the stomach is deemed a certain remedy in colic. (*Lindley.*)

Sp. 3. *Vitex Negundo.*

Vern. Noochie, *Tam.* Nergundi, *Beng.* Shumbali, *Duk.* Fenjengisht, *Arab.* Nisinda, *Hind.* Wayalakoo, *Tel.* Sinduya and Sindhooka, *Sans.*

Trunk irregular, often as thick as a man's thigh, branches three, opposite, young shoots downy, slightly 4-sided, leaves opposite, petioled, ternate and quinate. Flowers small, numerous, a beautiful bluish purple, corolla with the lower lip large, entire, upper lip shorter, four parted.

In India a decoction of the aromatic leaves is used as the warm bath for women after delivery. (*Roxb.*)

In medicinal qualities it is similar to, but weaker than the preceding species. The decoction of the root is a pleasant bitter, and is given in cases of intermittent fever. The warm leaves are stated by Mr. Sherwood to be a useful application in rheumatism or sprains. The Mahomedans are in the habit of smoking the dried leaves in cases of head-ache and catarrh. Fruit considered vermifuge in Behar.

To the fruits of all the preceding species the native name *Filfil burree*, or wild pepper, is applied.

Gen. 3.—Gmelina.

Sp. Gmelina asiatica.

Vern. Bidari, *Sans.* Goomodoo, *Tel.*

A very common bush on the Coromandel Coast. The root is mucilaginous and demulcent.

G. parviflora. Sheeri goomoodoo—a tree much resembling the last. Its leaves slightly bruised under water renders it mucilaginous, which property the water retains till the mucilage is decomposed by fermentation.

Roxburgh has five species of Gmelina—the G. arborea, (Gumar, or goombur of Bengal, Joogam, Chookur, *Hind.*) is a very large timber tree, the wood of which much resembles teak, and is very little affected by worms or the ordinary causes of decay. (*Fl. Ind.* vol. iii. p. 85.)

Besides the preceding we may notice,

Callicarpa lanata; (Roxb.) bitterish, and rather aromatic. *Congea villosa* has leaves of heavy smell, and is used by the natives in medicine.

Premna integrifolia (Agnimantha, *Sans.*) root warm and bitterish, given in decoction as a cordial and stomachic, decoction of the leaves used in colic and flatulence. (*Rheede.*)

Gen. 4.—Volkameria.

Sp. Volkameria inermis.

Vern. Shangam coopy, *Tam.* Sangkoopee, *Hind.* Nalla Opie, *Tel.* Kundali, *Sans.* Bunjoma, *Beng.*

The juice of the root and leaves is bitter, and given as an alterative in venereal, and scrofula. Dose a table spoonful. The plant is common in the jungles, and is very beautiful.

Nine species are described by Roxburgh, but he gives no account of their supposed medicinal virtues.

NAT. ORDER C.—LABIATÆ.

A very extensive order, containing chiefly herbs, rarely shrubs. The stalks are branching, with opposite and quadrangular branches, the leaves opposite, sometimes verticillate, in sets of three. Flowers naked and opposite, have bracteæ, and are disposed in spikes, corymbs, or panicles.

The flowers are irregular, ovary 4-lobed, and style arising from the base of the ovules.

The characters of this family are so uniform that Jussieu said they might be considered as one large genus; this extends to their chemical as well as botanical peculiarities; all are odoriferous, a few fœtid; their odour depends on an essential oil containing camphor, or its basis camphene. This oil is yellow, of pungent taste and smell, and is lighter than water. It adheres so strongly to the plants, that most of these will retain their peculiar smell for years after being sun or stove dried.

Besides this oil several of these plants contain a bitter principle. This is strongly developed in the Germanders, which have consequently been regarded as febrifuge.

All the Labiatæ are innocent, none however alimentary, with the exception perhaps, M. Feé observes, of the Ocymum tuberosum of India, a species regarding which he suggests additional investigations.

In medicine this family supplies us with tonics, febrifuges, stimulants, and anthelmintics; their chief use is in cookery and by the perfumer, as they yield several highly esteemed essential oils. Their geographical distribution is most extensive, extreme cold seeming to be the only limit to their diffusion.

Lindley in his *Flora Medica*, p. 485, introduces this order by stating, that "a great number of different plants have from time to time been introduced into medicine as aromatics or stimulants, or for imaginary virtues. It would be only encumbering the pages of this work to notice any thing like all such cases in detail, as the greater part are abandoned in modern practice, and appear to be of little or no consequence except in the kitchen." These remarks are especially applicable to the Indian plants of this order.

Gen. 1.—Salvia.

Sp. 1. *Salvia officinalis.* Sage.
Vern. Salbia, *Hind.*

A slightly aromatic, shrubby, but dwarfish plant, of somewhat bitter and very hot, aromatic, and slightly astringent flavour. These qualities are retained on drying. It affords on distillation with water a large quantity of essential oil, containing 26 per cent. of camphor. The oil is used by the perfumers, and the plant is a very favourite seasoner in Europe; it is but little employed in medicine.

Sp. 2. *Salvia bengalensis*, Roxb. Fl. Ind. i. p. 146. (Murtoo) *Meriandra bengalensis* (Bentham). Common in Bengal and Coromandel, much stronger than the officinal sage,—a straggling shrub with a trunk often as thick as a man's arm.

There are very numerous species of this genus, which correspond very closely in their properties; one, the *S. amarissima,* is excessively bitter.

GEN. 2.—ROSMARINUS.

Sp. R. officinalis. Rosemary, Europe, Asia Minor.

Vern. Ukleel ul jilbal. Hasalban achsir, *Arab.*

In many properties similar to the last, odour and flavour differ. The essential ingredient in the well known *Eau de la reine d' Hongrie* is the essential oil of this plant.

A shrub three to four feet high, densely leafy. The oil is stated most positively to possess the power of encouraging the growth of hair and of curing baldness. It is the colouring ingredient of green pomatums.

GEN. 3.—TEUCRIUM.

Sp. T. Chamædrys. Common germander, European thickets.

Taste more bitter than the preceding articles; an ingredient in the celebrated Theriaca andromachi, or *treak farook.*

GEN. 4.—HYSSOPUS.

Sp. H. officinalis. Hyssop.

Vern. Zoofáè gabis, *Arab.*

This owes its celebrity to a passage in Josephus, who used the hyssop as a term of comparison with the cedar to give an idea of Solomon's botanical knowledge, (*Feé* p. 455). In the Old Testament we meet its name in several of the sacred texts: "Purge me with hyssop, and I shall be clean;" and again—"The hyssop which groweth on the wall."

The dried plant is brought to India from Syria. The Arabians place it among their anthelmintics and stimulants. Pliny thought it useful in diseases of the chest. It is cultivated in the Calcutta Garden. Celsus regarded it as diuretic.

GEN. 5.—LAVANDULA. (*Lavenders.*)

Sp. L. vera and *Spica* of Decandolle.

Syn. L. Spica of Linn., and its variety. Europe.

Flowers small, bluish, calyx tubular, cylindrical, streaked, tomentose, corolla infundibuliform, pubescent, tube rather longer than the calyx, limb with five unequal divisions, upper lip large, obcordate, bifid, lower lip trifid.

Odour agreeable and penetrating, taste aromatic, acrid, rather hot.

The volatile oil is limpid, very transparent, yellowish white; four parts contain nearly two of camphor. Often adulterated with the oil of turpentine, and of a species of lavender of superior aromatic power, though more acrid.

The variety *b.* (spica) yields an oil much used by porcelain painters, and called "oil of spike."

L. Stœchas, (æstakhoodus,) is different in some botanical characters, in other respects nearly the same as the last. It is much prized as an expectorant and antispasmodic by the Arabs.

Gen. 6.—Mentha.

Sp. M. piperita. Peppermint. Europe.

The odour is strong and camphor-like, taste aromatic, hot, and camphoraceous, producing a sensation of cold on the tongue; the aroma of this plant is almost destroyed by drying.

The essential oil is greenish yellow, and very liquid; after long keeping it deposits crystals of camphor; it is often adulterated, especially with the oils of congenerous species, a fraud almost impossible to detect.

The essential oil is a very valuable stimulant, and is especially useful in flatulent diseases, and in the early stage of the malignant cholera. It is a deservedly great favourite in the nursery.

Dissolved in spirit it constitutes the tincture or essence, distilled with water it affords the Aqua menthæ piperitæ of the shops.

M. sativa. Widdelilam, *Tam.* Poodina, *Duk.* Nana, *Arab.* Hibbuk, *Arab.*

Prescribed by the Mahomedans in dyspeptic complaints, and to stop vomiting.

M. viridis. Spearmint.

Vern. Pahari Podeena. This species is a native of Cashmere, and cultivated in the plains for its essential oil and distilled water (see Pharmacopœia.)

M. Royleana is much used by the hill people of the Himalayas.

All the mints possess analogous properties. M. Feé mentions briefly,—

—*M. arvensis.* Field mint.

—*M. hirsuta.* Hairy mint, or water mint, acrid, bitter, and aromatic, reputed to be diuretic; an ingredient in the celebrated " thieves vinegar," the " baume tranquille," &c.

—*M. Pulegium,* Pennyroyal; the distilled water much used as a vehicle for medicines for children, and in flatulent colics—a popular emmenagogue.

—*M. rotundifolia,* or round leaved. Bitter, acrid, and astringent, acts as a rubefacient when applied to the skin; said to be anthelmintic.

—*M. rubra,* (red) abounds in essential oil; one of the best substitutes for peppermint.

—*M. sylvestris,* (wild) less powerful than the preceding kinds.

Gen. 7.—Glechoma.

Sp. G. hederacea, (ground ivy.) Europe.

Aromatic and rather bitter, has had a great reputation in the treatment of pulmonary diseases.

Gen. 8.—Lamium.

L. album, or white nettle, supposed to be astringent, but altogether inert.

Gen. 9.—Betonica.

Sp. Betonica officinalis.

Dried leaves in powder cause sneezing, the roots were once deemed emetic, but this supposition is disproved by recent experiments.

Gen. 10.—Marrubium.

Sp. M. vulgare. Horehound. Europe. Odour very agreeable but strong, taste bitter and durable; an ingredient in the *Theriac,* and a very celebrated popular remedy in the treatment of colds, consumption, and such diseases. It is said also to be febrifuge and emmenagogue. (See art. *Pucha Pat.* p. 493.)

Gen. 11.—Origanum. Marjoram.

Sp. O. vulgare. O. Dictamnus. Dittany.

Analogous in their properties to mint.

Buklukt ul gezal, *Arab.*—still much esteemed by the Arabs and Persians as a tonic and stimulant; Celsus deemed it an emmenagogue. The leaves are given in doses of from half a drachm to one drachm.

O. creticum, or Dictamnus creticus, the oil of which is of blood red colour. The virtues of the latter plant have been celebrated by Pliny, Theophrastus, and Dioscorides; it grows on Mount Ida, and is the plant alluded to by Virgil in the 12th book of the Æneid, l. 412. *Feé.*

O. Majorana, Marroo, *Tam.* Murwa, *Duk.* Αμαραχον *Greek.* Cultivated in some parts of lower India, is supposed to be the σαμφυχον of the ancients.

Gen. 12.—Thymus.

Sp. T. vulgaris.

A pretty, though very dwarfish shrub, of agreeable strong and penetrating odour, yielding a volatile oil, and much used for seasoning food by Europeans. Another species, the *T. Serpyllum* is similarly employed

---

Additional articles noted by M. Fee.

Ajuga reptans, Bugle, ...	Slightly astringent and bitter.
Leonurus cardiacus, ...	Tonic.
Satureia hortensis, ...	Stimulant.
——— capitata, ...	Stomachic and emmenagogue.
——— Thymbra, ...	Ditto, ditto.
Nepeta cataria, ...	Antithysteric, a powerful aphrodisiac to cats.
Ocymum basilicum, ...	Very rich in essential oil, see *Ocymum.*
Prunella vulgaris, ...	Little used, weakly aromatic.
Plectranthus suaveolens, ...	Patchouley of Virey, a dried plant from Bourbon, the odour resembles valerian. It is placed among clothes to keep away insects.

Dr. Royle very appropriately sums up his account of this family by stating that many which are indigenous in the Himalayas, and the native names of some of which we have quoted, continue to be imported from the Red Sea "to be prescribed at the foot of mountains, where the fresh and genuine articles may be had in any quantity." Dr Royle especially recommends the introduction of the peppermint, with the essential oil of which the natives are well acquainted from its common use in cholera. He informs us that species of Anisomeles, Dyospita, Elscholtzia, and Pogostemon are however used as substitutes for their European allies. The *Ocymum sanctum* is sacred among the Hindoos—*Plectranthus cordifolius* and *Coleus barbatus* very aromatic. The *Meriandra strobilifera* (*murtoo*) from its strong fragrance is considered by Royle to be very promising, the *M. bengalensis* being already in use, and called Kafoor-ke-putta. *Roylea elegans* (Putkuroo) is deemed a febrifuge by the hill people, like some species of Teucrium in Europe.

The only plant of this family much cultivated in India is the Dracocephalum Royleanum, or Balungoo, the seeds of which, *Tukm balungoo,* are very generally used in India for the preparation of mucilaginous drinks. *Royle. p.* 303.

In Lindley's Flora Medica besides the species we have already noticed we find the following—

Gen. 13.—Anisomeles.

Sp. Anisomeles malabarica. (Malabar cat mint.)

Ajuga fruticosa, *Roxb. Fl. Ind.* iii. p. 1. East Indies and Isle of France. Nepeta malabarica, *Ainslie,* vol. ii. p. 294.

Vern. Pemayrutie, *Tam.* Moga beerakoo, *Tel.* Bootan kooshum, *Sans.*

The stem is erect, 2 to 5 feet high, 4-sided, with obtuse angles, branches numerous, axillary, ascending. Leaves petiolate, ovate lanceolate, obtuse, crenate, except at the base, which is entire, strongly reticulated with prominent veins, below wrinkled, above downy, flowers in axillary clusters, forming whorls, bractes filiform, pubescent, 1 or 2 to each flower, calyx 5-cleft, 10-angled, corolla, 2-lipped, upper lip entire, under one large, 3-cleft, lateral divisions reflexed, middle one orbicular, the root hairy, spotted with purple, anthers deep purple, stigma 2-cleft with divaricated lobes. *Wight.*

Ague patients are made to inhale the vapour arising from an infusion of this plant; this causes copious sweating. The leaves are bitter, astringent, and somewhat aromatic; they are given in infusion in the latter stages of dysentery and in intermitting fevers to the quantity of an ounce and a half twice daily *(Ainslie.)* The juice expressed from the slightly warmed leaves is prescribed for children in fever, from dentition. The entire plant is deemed emmenagogue in the West Indies.

Gen. 14.—Ocymum.

Sp. 1. *O. Basilicum.* Sweet bazil.

Vern. Tirnoot patchie verie, *Tam.* Subze ke beenge, *Duk.* Vepoodipatsa vittiloo, *Tel.* Deban shab, *Pers.* Kalee tulsee, *Hind.* Manjirika, *Sans.*

The small seeds deemed cooling and mucilaginous, and consequently given in gonorrhœa, ardor urinæ, and affections of the kidneys.

Sp. 2. O. pilosum, common in Upper India. *Arabic*, Habak; *Persian*, Rihan and Nazboo. Seeds aromatic, used by women to relieve after-pains.

Sp. 3. O. sanctum. Toolsi kejur, *Duk.* Toolasee vayr, *Tam.* The root is given in decoction in fevers, half a tea-cupful twice daily. In Hindostanee and Bengalee the plant is called Kalatoolsee, in Sanscrit *Arjaka* and *Parnasa*, (Nalla tirtava, *Rheede.*) The Brahmins regard it as sacred to Vishnu, and use it in their funeral ceremonies. The Malays also strew it over the graves of their dead.

Sp. 4. O. hirsutum. Koolimitan, *Tam.*
Whole plant slightly aromatic, prescribed by the Hindoos in decoction in the bowel complaints of teething children.

Sp. 5. O. album. (White basil.)
Suffaid toolsee, *Duk.* Badrooge abeeg, *Arab.* Kookatolasie, *Tel.* Viswa tulasi, *Sans.*
A shrub about a foot high, leaves have a most pleasant aromatic taste and smell. The juice is given to children in colds to the extent of a tea-spoonful twice daily. The dried leaves are used as a substitute for tea.

Pucha Pat.

This is a well known article in Bengal. Its source is still doubtful. We extract the following notice regarding it by Dr. Wallich, from the Transactions of the Medical and Physical Society of Calcutta for 1835. Dr. Wallich has also kindly favoured us with an additional note on the subject.

"I shall now advert to another vegetable substance which, although most extensively used by the natives of this country, has hitherto continued one of the problems in our Indian Materia Medica. The drug to which I allude, is called in Bengallee as well as in Hindee, *Puchá Pát*, and is found in every bazar, almost throughout Hindustán. My esteemed friend Baboo Radhakant Deb informs me, that "there exists no Sanscrita name for this leaf, which is largely imported by Mogul merchants; that it is used as an ingredient in tobacco for smoking, and for scenting the hair of women, and that the essential oil is in common use for imparting the peculiar fragrance of the leaf to clothes among the superior classes of natives." I believe that the people of the peninsula are peculiarly fond of this perfume, as are also the Roman Catholic inhabitants of this country generally.

"Having ascertained, on my return from Europe two years ago, that a large quantity of what appeared to be the same drug as that commonly sold in the bazars under the name of Puchá Pát had been imported from Penang, I requested Mr. George Porter, late of that Island, and formerly in charge of the Botanical establishment there, to favour me with an account of the article, and also, if possible, with some growing plants of it. In February last year (1834), I had the pleasure to receive from him several plants, which I have succeeded in multiplying by cuttings, and which appear to thrive remarkably well in this Garden. Mr. Porter has furnished me with the following memorandum: 'The Puchá Pát grows perfectly wild at Penang, and on the opposite shore of the Malay Peninsula, in Wellesley province. The Arabs use and export it more than any other nation. Their annual pilgrim ship takes up an immense quantity of the leaf. They use it principally for stuffing matrasses and pillows, and assert, that it is very efficacious in preventing contagion and prolonging life. It requires no sort of preparation, being simply gathered and dried in the sun; too much drying, however, is hurtful, in as much as it renders the leaf liable to crumble to dust in packing and stowing on board. In Penang it sells at the rate of a dollar and a quarter, to a dollar and a half, per pekul. In Bengal, some which was sent from thence several years ago, sold at 11 rupees 8 annas per maund. At times the price is much higher. The last investment sold so low as six rupees only per maund. It has not been seen in flower.' So far Mr. Porter's memorandum.

"The Puchá Pát plant is evidently of the family of Labiatæ. It forms a shrub (in the Botanical Garden) of two to three feet in height. The obtusely four-cornered branches and the leaves are juicy, and somewhat fleshy, and covered, especially the inferior surface of the latter, with a great deal of soft, pallid pubescence, which gives the plant a greyish appearance. All the young parts are densely villous. The leaves are opposite, petioled, ovate, obtuse, grossly and obtusely lobato-crenate, measuring from two to four inches; the lowermost on the branches are subcordate, all the others are cuneate, and entire at the base; the upper surface slightly rugose; under surface pallid, with very thick rib and nerves, and largely reticulated veins.

"None of the individuals in this Garden have hitherto shown any disposition to blossom; owing perhaps to the plant being so easily multiplied by division. All the green parts, on being rubbed, emit the peculiar smell of the drug sold under the name of Pucha Pát, which is also very like our shrub in the form, margins, and surface of the leaves.

"I should have mentioned above, that the Baron Hügel informs me that he has found a plant growing wild at Canton, which closely resembles that from Penang cultivated in this Garden.

"Whether *Marrubium odoratissimum Betonicæ folio*. J. Burm. Thesaur. Zeylan, p. 153, tab. 71, fig. 1, (*Marrubium Indicum*, N. L. Burman, Flor. Ind. p. 127,) be our plant or not, it is difficult to say; but it strikes me that there is at least a considerable affinity between them.

H. C. Botanic Garden, 6th June, 1835.

The plant has not to this time (April 1841) shewn any disposition to produce blossoms in the Calcutta Garden. Dr. Wallich has been informed by Major Jenkins, the Commissioner in Assam, that there is a similar plant, probably a different species, in the lofty range of hills to the northward of Gowhatti.

NAT. ORDER CI.—BORAGINEÆ.

These plants have alternate leaves, generally covered with rigid hairs, and are nearly allied to the Labiatæ, by their 4-lobed fruits. The flowers occur in unilateral spikes; a few of the species are ligneous or arborescent. They abound in the warmer parts of Europe, and in Asia. No important remedy is found in this family, which is usually watery, inodorous, and insipid. Some have been eaten by the ancients, and the borage is to this time deemed alimentary in France; one or two species are rather astringent. A peculiar colouring matter, of some commercial importance, exists in the cortical part of the roots of some species.

GEN. 1.—BORAGO.

Sp. Borago officinalis, Borage. Mucilaginous and watery, now obsolete.

GEN. 2.—ANCHUSA.

Sp. 1. *Anchusa italica*, (Bugloss.)

This plant is mentioned by Nicander v. 5, 38, and is called Bugloss, from the supposed resemblance of its leaves to a cow's tongue (Βος γλοσσα.) There is some doubt however as to the actual plant to which this term is applied. In India the Greek synonyms *bugloozun* and *fooghulus* are assigned to *Onosma bracheatum* (Royle.) In the Bombay Bazars the *Cacalia Kleinia* is similarly termed *Gao zuban*, or cow's tongue. The confusion however is but of little importance, as the article is destitute of any real medicinal value, being simply emollient, mucilaginous, and perhaps slightly diuretic.

Sp. 2. *A. tinctoria*. (Alkanet.)

A native of Europe, the root extensively used in dyeing. The plant is about two feet high, the roots cylindrical, 4 to 5 inches long, rather twisted, thick as the finger, hairy, covered with a foliaceous and wrinkled envelope, of deep violet red colour. Beneath this is a woody substance, red externally, whitish within, formed of three cylindrical fibres, distinct from each other, and as if soldered together. Destitute of odour, taste slightly saccharine and bitter.

For this root those of the *Onosma echioides*, and *tinctoria* have been substituted. The *Onosma emodi* (Wall.) of the

Himalayas is closely allied to this, and is called *Maharunga* from the intensity of its colour.

The alkanet of Constantinople is produced by a different order of plants altogether, being the root of the Alcanna vera, (Natural order, *Salicariæ.*) *Feé.*

RED PRINCIPLE.

In masses of brown colour, resinous fracture, melting at a low heat, soluble in alcohol, ether, and the fatty oils, which assume a red colour, remaining still transparent; less soluble in water, forming blue compounds with potash, soda, baryta, and with lime, decomposed by hot sulphuric acid, changed into oxalic acid by the nitric acid. The alcoholic solutions treated by several metallic re-agents afford some beautiful lakes.

Orcanet is only employed in pharmacy as a colouring matter for ointments and pomatums. Its chief use is as a dye stuff, and for colouring sugared sweetmeats for confectioners.

GEN. 3.—CYNOGLOSSUM, Dog's tongue.

Sp. C. officinale.

Syn. Κυνογλοσσον Dioscorides.

Of no medicinal importance. The root yields a colouring matter of very little value.

GEN. 4.—SYMPHYTUM.

Sp. S. officinale.

Συμφυτον, Diosc. iv. p. 9. *Vern.* Sunkootun.

Roots large, externally black, and branching, about a foot long, the thickness of the finger, fleshy, brittle, succulent, and pulpy. Inodorous, taste sweetish and mucilaginous.

The plant is highly mucilaginous, and rather astringent, it also contains sugar and albumen. The recent root is in popular use in France in cases of rupture and bruises. Indeed the plant derives its name from its supposed virtue in consolidating wounds.

GEN. 5.—HELIOTROPIUM.

Sp. Heliotropium indicum. (Indian turnsole.)

Vern. Hatee shoora, *Beng.* Siriari, *Hind.* Srihastini, *Sans.* also Bhooroomdi.

Plant slighly bitter, juice of the leaves applied to painful gum-boils and to repel pimples on the face—also used in inflamed or excoriated tarsi. A very common plant. In Jamaica it is used with castor oil to relieve the pain of scorpion stings, and in the treatment of hydrophobia.

Besides these, M. Feé mentions,

1. *Heliotropium peruvianum* and *grandiflorum*, these are distinguished, the first by the odour of vanilla, the second by that of honey.

2. *H. europæum*, commonly supposed to have the power of destroying warts.

3. *Pulmonaria officinalis*, and *angustifolia*—plants used in popular cough medicines on account of the supposed resemblance between the white spots on their leaves and ulcerated lungs.

4. *Lithospermum officinale.* The seeds are long, very white, and like small stones or pearls, on which account they have been popularly used as a remedy for stone. They are known in India by the name of Lubisfirmun. (*Royle.*)

Royle states that the species of Trichodesma are deemed diuretic, and are supposed cures for snake bites.

NAT. ORDER CII.—CORDIACEÆ.

A small order, formerly included in the Boragineæ, it chiefly inhabits tropical climates. Cordia is the only Indian genus, of which there are four or five Indian species.

GEN.—CORDIA.

Calyx tubular 4, 5-toothed, corolla funnel-shaped, or campanulate with a flat five or seven cleft limb, and a hairy or naked throat, stamens five, short, inserted into the throat of the corolla, style protruding, bifid, with four stigmas, ovary three-celled, drupe containing one stone with three cells, two usually abortive. (*Lindley.*)

Sp. 1. *C. latifolia.* Roxb. Fl. Ind. i. p. 588. Hindostan, confined to the southern parts of India. (*Royle.*)

Vern. Buhooari, *Beng.* Burra lesoora, *Hind.*

Branches numerous, spreading, and drooping, young shoots angular and smooth, trees usually 20 feet high at 10 or 12 years old. Leaves alternate, petioled, round, cordate, and ovate, often slightly repand, three-nerved, hard, smooth above, scabrous and pale beneath, from three to seven or even eight inches long, and rather less broad, petioles nearly round and smooth, panicles short, terminal, and lateral, roundish. The branches alternate, diverging, and once or more frequently dichotomous; flowers numerous, small, white; bracts minute, villous; calyx villous, campanulate, leathery; mouth unequally toothed; corolla short, campanulate; segments five, linear, oblong; filaments as long as the segments of the corolla, and inserted immediately under their fissures. Anthers incumbent, ovary ovate, four-celled, with one ovule in each, attached to the upper end of the axis. Style short, stigma four-cleft, segments long, rugose, and recurved, drupe oblate, spheroidal, about 1 or 1¼ inch in diameter, smooth, when ripe straw-coloured, covered with a whitish bloom, pulp in large quantity, soft, clear, and very clammy, nut nearly circular, laterally compressed, rugose on the outside, with a cavity at each end, the lower one deeper than the other, exceedingly hard, four-celled, though rarely with all the cells fertile, integument single, white, soft, and oily, plumule very small, radicle conical, superior. (*Roxb.*)

Sp. 2. *Cordia Myxa.* Roxb. Fl. Ind. i. p. 590.
Syn. Sebestena officinalis.
Vern. Vidimaram, *Tam.* Kendal, *Jav.* Lebuck, *Avicenna.* Mochayet, *Forskal.* Lolu, *Cyng.* Buhooarie, *Beng.* Lesura, *Hind.* Nekra, *Tel.* Bukampadáruka, *Sans.*

A native of many parts of India, Persia, Arabia, and Egypt.

Trunk generally crooked, 8 to 10 feet high, and as thick or thicker than a man's body. Bark grey and cracked, branches numerous, spreading, and forming a dense shady head. Leaves ovate, oval, or obovate, 2 to 3 inches long, 1½ to 2 broad, exterior half slightly scolloped or toothed. Panicles terminal, lateral, globular, dichotomous. Flowers numerous, small, white, many barren, calyx smooth, tubular, widening towards the mouth, and there as if torn into two or three divisions, corolla with revolute lobes, drupe globular, smooth, ¾ of an inch in diameter, sitting in the enlarged calyx; when ripe yellow, pulp almost transparent, very tough and viscid, nut cordate, at both ends bidentate and perforated, rugose, somewhat four-celled, seeds solitary. *Roxb.* The wood is soft, one of the best for affording fire by friction; supposed to be the material for the Egyptian mummy cases.

The fruit of *Cordia Myxa* has been long used as a medicine under the name of Sebistans or Lobestens. *C. latifolia* is supposed to produce the larger, *C. Myxa* the smaller variety of this article. The bark is deemed a mild tonic. That of

C. angustifolia, Roxb. (Goondnee) is much used for making astringent gargles.

The dried fruits are very glutinous in the fresh state. They are slightly laxative, but it is especially as a pectoral that they are esteemed in India. In Java the fruit is used in gonorrhœa and ardor urinæ; 12 drachms of the pulp are said to be equally in aperient effect to the same quantity of cassia pulp.

The seeds of Cordia Myxa, are called *Chakoon ke beenge*, and deemed an infallible remedy in ringworm, the powder mixed with oil being applied to the eruption.

NAT. ORDER CIII.—CONVOLVULACEÆ.

This extensive order is made up of herbaceous plants and shrubs with twining stalks, generally alternate leaves, and axillary flowers, usually borne on unifloral or multifloral peduncles; the species are mostly lactescent.

The stalks, leaves, flowers, and fruits of the annual convolvulaceæ are inert, and very slightly active. The roots are vivaceous, gorged with a milky juice, almost entirely resinous, and generally possessing purgative properties. The bark in the woody species, though not equal in power to the root, is still acrid, and acts as a stimulant, and purgative. Lindley in his Flora Medica distributes the medical plants of this order into the following genera—species of all of which occur in the plains of India, and a few on the Himalayas.

GEN. 1.—ARGYREIA.

Sepals five, corolla campanulate, style one, stigma capitate, two-lobed, ovary two-celled, four-seeded, capsule baccate. (*Lindley.*)

Sp. A. bracteata. Wall. Cat. 1419, common near Madras.

(Sanscrit) *Samudra patta.* ?

A large twining, branched, milky shrub. Leaves alternate on long petioles, limb broadly cordate, ovate, beneath hairy and rather silky, peduncles axillary, dividing at the extremity into two or three branches, with a sessile ebracteated flower in the fork, each branch divides again: the solitary flower in the second, and all succeeding divisions furnished with a long lanceolate-leaved pale green hairy bractea, calyx of five ovate and mucronate hairy sepals, corolla campanulate, externally hairy, colour purple white within, near the bottom deep purple, paler near the throat, limb spreading, cream-coloured, stamens five, unequal, enlarged at base, ovary superior in a glandular cup-shaped disk, style as long as the stamens, stigma two-lobed, pericarp a three to four seeded berry, deep orange when ripe. *(Wight.)*

A decoction of the leaves is used in fomentations to the joints in scrofulous affections, and the boiled leaves are applied as a poultice.

Argyreia speciosa, is found wild in the Dhoon.

Gen. 2.—Convolvulus.

Sp. 1. *C. Scammonia.*

A native of Syria and the Levant, recently discovered by Dr. Burn in Kaira in Guzerat.

The stalk is cylindrical, thin, rather velvety, climbing, leaves alternate, smooth, triangular, hastate, supported on petioles 8 or 10 lines long, flowers large, bell-shaped, of whitish purple colour. Roots long, thick, fleshy and succulent. The proper juice when dried is called *Scammony.*

Aleppo Scammony. (Sugmoonia, *Arab.*)

Fragments voluminous, dry, light, spongy, friable, pulverulent, with dull fracture of blackish grey, but covered with grey powder resulting from the reciprocal friction of the pieces, slightly transparent in small flakes, which become white and rather adherent when rubbed with a wet finger, odour disagreeable, taste weak, acrid, bitter, and repulsive, powder greyish white.

This species of scammony is often adulterated with concrete juices of a similar kind, with flour, chalk, sand, and earth. According to the analysis of Boutron La Grange and Vogel, good scammony consists of resin 60, gum 3, extract 2, and earthy and vegetable impurities 25 per 100.

The most abundant harvest of scammony is in Smyrna and Aleppo. There are several modes of collection, which give rise to corresponding commercial varieties. The neck of the root being laid bare is divided transversely, and shells placed around the edges to receive the juice as it exudes. This subsequently thickens in the air. The drug collected in this mode, is called shell scammony.

This occurs in small porous masses, sometimes smooth, of reddish or whitish grey colour; of waxy fracture, yellowish and half transparent, in thin layers, of disagreeable taste and smell; on drying it becomes adhesive.

Instead of shells the leaves of the chesnut tree are sometimes used, and a flattened scammony of good quality collected. If the roots be cut in successive layers, the scammony is inferior, but still esteemed. It is dried either over a slow fire or before the sun, and then moulded into stamped pastiles, of a whitish colour. This variety is very rare in commerce.

Lastly, an extract is prepared from the expressed juice of the roots and stalks, this is moulded into round masses, of black, vitreous, and resinous fracture.

The Arab name of this drug, Ul Sugmoonia, signifies the *purgative*. Several old preparations called "diagredium" (διακρηδιον) are mixtures of scammony with sulphur and liquorice, and are now no longer used.

Scammony is one of our most valuable cathartics, especially for children—dose from 2 to 20 grs. It is usually given with cream of tartar, and it enters into the composition of the well known compound Colocynth pill.

Sp. 2. *C. scoparius*, Canary Islands.

To this climber is attributed the well known wood perfumed like the rose.

The root is knotty, woody, heavy, sometimes branched, 1 to 4 inches in diameter, with a fungous, wrinkled, reddish grey bark. The wood is hard, heavy, deep dun yellow, veined with red, takes fire readily at the candle flame. On being rasped or worked it evolves a strong smell of roses; its taste is bitter and balsamic. By distillation from salt water it yields an essential of the following characters:—

Colour golden-yellow passing to ruddy red by age, heavier than water, rose-like odour, bitter and balsamic taste. Often adulterated with fixed oil.

This substance has been long attributed erroneously to the *Genista canariensis*.

M. Feé also enumerates the following species:—

C. sepium, hedge weed, common in Europe, believed to be purgative.

C. arvensis, field-bind, the same as C. sepium. Vauquelin analysed both, and found them to yield about 5 per 100 of cathartic resin.

C. Soldanella, (golden rod) root contains 24 per 100 of purgative resin.

C. althæoides, South of France.

C. Batatas, Sweet potatoe. (Batatas edulis, *Choisy.*)

Gen. 3.—Ipomæa.

Sp. 1. *I. Jalapa.* Jalap plant.

Syn. Convolvulus Jalapa, *Linn.* Ipomæa Purga, *Wenderoth.*

Leaves stalked, the first hastate, succeeding ones cordate, acuminate, mucronate, smooth. Peduncles axillary or flowered, twisted, the length of the corolla. Sepals obtuse mucronate, smooth, corolla purple, with a long, somewhat clavate tube, and an undulated limb with 5-plaits, filaments smooth, unequal, anthers linear, projecting, stigma capitate, deeply furrowed, capsule 2-celled, cells 2-seeded. (*Lindley.*)

A native of South America, Xalappa, and on the Eastern declivity of the Mexican Andes. The roots are fleshy, large, oval oblong, rugose, and blackish externally, while recent; in the dry state, and as sold in the shops, they are cut in flakes of variable diameter, sometimes cleft lengthwise and pyriform. If entire they are usually small, wrinkled, heavy, unequal, hard, brittle, deep brown grey externally, of a dirty grey within, fracture smooth and wavy, shewing a great number of resinous points, visible to the lens, and often to the naked eye.

The odour is peculiarly nauseous, though weak. The taste acrid and disgusting. A brisk cathartic.

The powder is of brown grey colour, and must be prepared with caution, as it is exceedingly irritating. The worm-eaten roots are much more active than the sound, as the worms only attack the amylaceous and sweet parts.

According to Cadet's analysis the jalap of the shops contains water 24, resin 50, gummy extract 220, fecula and albumen 25, fibre 145, salts, silica, and loss 35 in 500 parts; jalap of good quality will however yield 10 per cent. of resin, in which principle the purgative virtues reside. Mr. Hume having brought this resin to an unusually pure state supposed it to be a new alkali, and termed it *jalapine.*

The resin of jalap is dry, brittle, readily reduced to powder, in rolls of elongated or spiral form, the size at most of the little finger, greyish yellow, dull, unequal, and chinked externally, of brilliant fracture, and yellowish brown while recent. Totally soluble in alcohol, insoluble in ether, inodorous until rubbed, when the peculiar smell of jalap is evolved; its taste is nauseous and very acrid.

This resin is exposed to numerous adulterations, especially with other resins, of which that of the Guaiac is most used; the perfect insolubility of the jalap resin in ether will lead to the detection of numerous frauds of this description.

Jalap root was first brought to Europe about the year 1610, but its origin was long uncertain. The size to which it attains varies very much. Thierry de Menonville describes roots 20 lbs. in weight, and Michaud sent from Charlestown to the Jardin des Plantes at Paris a root which weighed over 50 lbs.

In 1834, Lord Auckland introduced into the Calcutta Garden, a plant supposed to be the Linnæan Convolv. Jalapa, but which is a very distinct species, called *Ipomæa macrorrhiza*, a native of Georgia and Carolina. It perfectly succeeded, and the roots attained such an enormous size that we have seen a cluster belonging to one plant which weighed 79 lbs.; while recent it was fleshy, white, juicy, of mild flavour, and altogether devoid of the acrid resin. It had a sweetish taste, and has been eaten by several persons without any ill effect being experienced.

We should add, however, that to test the applicability of the root as fodder, we had seven sheep fed on it, six of which died suffering from diarrhœa within a month.

According to Humboldt 400,000 lbs. weight of jalap roots are annually exported from Vera Cruz. The plant thrives best on cool shady hills, about 2000 feet above the level of the sea.

Med. use. A most valuable purgative, dose 10 to 30 grs. usually given with twice its weight of cream of tartar and a little ginger.

Sp. 2. Ipomæa Mechoacanha, Mexico and Brazil.

This is now referred by Lindley to some variety of the Ipomæa orizabensis, a native of the temperate parts of the state of Oaxaca. An account of the root has been published by Pelletier in the Journal de Pharmacie, vol. x. p. 1. The experiments made with it in the French Hospitals have not been satisfactory.

The roots are divided in fragments of variable form, or in whitish slices, fibrous, softish, covered with a grey, wrinkled bark, solid white, and yellowish white internally, inodorous; at first insipid, then nauseous to the taste, almost always worm-eaten as sold in the shops, said to be frequently adulterated with the bryony root; no good analysis is on record of this root. It is said to be devoid of resin, but to contain an acrid principle of an oily character, soluble in alcohol, and exceedingly bitter. The purgative properties of the root are however comparatively trifling. It was known in Europe before the true jalap, Monard having described it in his history of American remedies, published in Seville, in 1595.

Sp. 3. *Ipomœa Turpethum.*

Vern. Teoree, Doodh-kulmee, &c. *Hind.* and *Beng.*

Syn. Convolvulus Turp:—a native of Bengal, Ceylon, and India generally. *Roxb. Fl. Ind.* i. p. 476.

Root perennial, stems twining, several fathoms long, 3 to 4 sided, a little downy, with winged angles, leaves stalked, varying in form from cordate to linear, all pointed and lobed, or angular and downy. Peduncles axillary and many flowered, flowers large, white, bractes oval, concave, velvety, deciduous, ovary on a glandular disk, stigma 2-lobed, capsules involved in the dry calyx, 4-sided, 2-celled, opening by an operculum, seeds round, black, one in each cell.

The recent roots are very long, cylindrical, bent, branched, gorged with acrid milky juice, the dried roots are in broken pieces the thickness of the finger, and 4 or 5 inches long. They are separated from the ligneous part, and consist of a grey or slightly reddish cortical system, composed of parallel longitudinal fibres, and of proper vessels in which particles of resin are observed; inodorous, tasteless at first, subsequently nauseous and acrid.

Boutron-Charlard's analysis shews that this root contains resin, fatty matter, volatile oil, albumen, starch, yellow colouring matter, fibre, free malic acid, and various salts.

The natives of Bengal use this root as a purgative, rubbing up a slip of the bark with water on a stone and swallowing the emulsion thus formed.

A strip six inches in length from a root as thick as the little finger is deemed a sufficient dose.

Mr. Gordon, Dr. Glass, and Dr. Wallich have published several notices of its effects in Carey's edition of Dr. Roxburgh's Fl. Ind. ii. p. 57. We have also subjected its properties to careful clinical experiment, and we feel warranted in asserting that the action of the medicine is so extremely uncertain that it does not deserve a place in our Pharmacopœia.

Gen. 4.—Batatas.

Sp. B. paniculata. (*Convolvulus paniculatus,* Roxb. Fl. Ind. i. 478.) East Indies generally.

Vern. Bhoomi koomra, *Beng.*

Root perennial, tuberous, young shoots round and smooth, stem and branches perennial, leaves stalked, palmate, three to six inches long, generally five-lobed, entire, smooth, peduncles axillary, erect, pedunculate, flowers numerous, large, beautiful reddish purple, capsules four-celled, seeds woolly all round. The large tuberous root is cathartic.

Gen. 5.—Pharbitis.

Sepals five, corolla campanulate, or campanulate funnel-shaped, style 1, stigma capitate, granular, ovary three-celled, or rarely four-celled, cells two-seeded. (*Lindley.*)

Sp. 1. *Pharbitis cærulea.* Wall.

Syn. Ipomæa cærulea. *Kön. Roxb. Fl. Ind.* i. p. 501. Nearly allied to Pharbitis Nil; but probably a distinct species.

Vern. Hub ul nil, *Arab.* Kaladana and Mirchai, *Hind.* and *Beng.*

Common all over the tropics every where, and in India even ascends the mountains to 5000 feet elevation.

Stems and branches twining, annual, round, hairy, 6 to 12 feet long, as thick as a crow's quill, leaves stalked, broad, cordate, three-lobed, downy, two to four inches long, acute, peduncles axillary, round, hairy, two to three flowrets, bracts and sepals linear, flowers large, beautiful bright blue, stigma sub-globose, large, glandular, three-lobed, capsule much shorter than the calyx, smooth, three-celled, with two seeds in each cell. (*Roxb.*)

Seeds, Hub ul nil, Kaladana, Mirchai.

Black, angular, weighing on an average ½ a grain each, in powder of a grey colour, of sweetish, and subsequently rather acrid taste, and heavy smell. On analysis yields resin, gum, starch, fixed bland oil, fibre, and colouring matter.

The powdered seeds in doses of 30 to 40 grains act as a quick, safe, and pleasant cathartic. We have made this seed the subject of numerous experiments. In 100 cases in which it was given under our direction in the Police Hospital of Calcutta it proved purgative in 94, occasioned vomiting in 5, and griping but in 15, and produced on an average 5 stools within 2½ hours; the operation generally commenced in an hour, and in these experiments was never delayed beyond four hours.

The alcoholic extract, which consists of resin and oil, is deep brown, ductile, of excellent pillular consistence, and keeps for several months. In 10 grain doses it produces all the effects of jalap with certainty and speed; the taste is scarcely perceptible. Dr. Chapman has used it in several cases at the General Hospital, and reported on it most favourably to the Medical Board; Dr. Leckie of Bhagulpore, Dr. Green of Howrah, Drs. Martin, Stewart and Goodeve, have given similar accounts of its efficacy.

The seeds sell for four seers (8 lbs.) for the rupee; these will yield from 15 to 20 per 100 of alcoholic extract, and the whole of the alcohol may be recovered by distillation. We have thus a remedy of unparalled cheapness, perfectly equal to jalap as a cathartic, superior to it in portability and flavour, and occurring in all parts of India. We are consequently independent in every respect of the South American article.

Besides the plants above described, Lindley quotes others of less importance, which we do not deem it necessary to include in our notice.

In Ainslie and other writers we find notices of the following:—

— *Convolvulus grandiflorus*. (Ainslie, vol. ii. 219.)

Nagha mooghatei kai, *Tam.* Munda Valli, *Rheede.*— Puthmapoo todemie, *Sans.* Alanga, *Cyng.*

Moonflower. Common on the Coromandel coast.

Capsule or pericarp containing four seeds the size of kidney beans, when dried used in snake-bites; dose three daily in powder.

— *Convolvulus reptans*, Mandavalli, *Rheede*, common in India, affords a milky juice which when dried is nearly equal to scammony in purgative efficacy. (*Ainslie*, on the authority of Plumier and the Hortus Malabaricus.) This plant is the Olus vagum of *Rumph.* Kulmi shak, *Beng.* Tootu kura, *Tel.* a native of standing sweet waters, very common. The tops and leaves are eaten in stews by the natives.

— *C. malabaricus*. Paymoostee, *Tam.* Kattu kelungu, *Rheede*, a native of the Malabar coast and of Cochin China, considered by the farriers in India a good horse medicine.

Roxburgh in his *Flora Indica*, pp. 466 to 487, describes 34 species of Convolvulus, and pp. 497 to 504, eleven species of Ipomæa.

NAT. ORDER CIV.—HYDROLEACEÆ.

Gen.—Hydrolea.

Sp. H. zeylanica. Vahl. Wight and Arnott in Hooker's Comp. 2. t. 26.

Water and marshy ground in East Indies. Herbaceous.

The leaves beaten into a pulp and applied as a poultice are in India deemed useful in cleaning and healing ill conditioned ulcers in which maggots have formed. *Lind. Fl. Med.* p. 401.

NAT. ORDER CV.—PRIMULACEÆ.

Lindley describes three species. The *Cyclamen hederæfolium*, or sow bread, a drastic purgative, common in Europe, but uncertain, and little used. The acrid principle has been called *Arthanitine;* the *Primula veris*, or cowslip, a native of European pastures, and having several allied species in India, the flowers possessing well marked sedative properties; the *Anagallis arvensis*, or pimpernel, common in Europe and in India in the cold season, an acrid drastic cathartic which was once much prescribed in madness, epilepsy, and dropsy; now disused.

NAT. ORDER CVI.—GLOBULARIACEÆ.

Herbs and under shrubs, of bitter taste and acrid purgative properties.

Gen. Globularia.

Gl. Alypum. South of France.

Frutex terribilis, (Bauhin.) Leaves alternate, obovate, lanceolate, very entire, narrowed like a petiole at the base, very acute at the apex, smooth, coriaceous, persistent, and of a lively green colour.

M. Loiseleur des Longchamps states that the decoction of 4 to 8 drachms of the leaves acts as a gentle but certain purgative without griping, and he recommends their use in preference to senna. The natives of Morocco use it as a popular cathartic.

NAT. ORDER CVII.—PLUMBAGINEÆ.

Herbaceous or woody plants, simple or branching, with simple leaves sometimes opposite, at other times cauline and then alternate. Inflorescence variable. Astringency and acridity are the prevailing qualities. The order is limited, chiefly occurs in temperate regions, but species are known which inhabit countries of extreme heat or cold.

GEN.—PLUMBAGO.

Calyx tubular, pentagonal, 5-toothed, covered with stalked glands, corolla hypocrateriform, with 5-cleft limb. Stamens hypogynous, dilated at the base, style simple, stigma 5-cleft, fruit seed-like, enclosed in the valve-like bases of the filaments, crowned by the conical base of the style. (*Lindley.*)

Sp. 1. *P. europaea*, South of Europe.
Vern. Chitra vani, *Sans.*

An erect, branching, smooth, herbaceous shrub, stems slender, angular, rather flexuose, with spreading rigid branches, leaves obovate, lanceolate, sessile, rather scabrous, amplexicaul, slightly toothed at the edge, the uppermost much narrowed and more linear. Flowers in terminal capitated uninterrupted spikes, calyx naked at the base, covered with stalked glands towards the upper end, corolla funnel-shaped, twice as long as the calyx, lilac coloured, striped.

The whole plant, especially the root, is very acrid, and applied as paste to the skin acts as a powerful vesicatory. Given internally in small doses, it is said to be a very efficacious emetic, but we would deem its administration as dangerous as that of cantharides.

The bruised root has been employed in Europe as an application to cancer, as a counter-irritant in toothache, and as a remedy for the itch.

Sp. 2. *P. rosea.*
Vern. Lal chitra, Chitraca, *Sans.* Cittra molum and Kodivaylee, *Tam.* Chitturmol, *Duk.* Chita, *Hind.* Chitra, *Beng.* Shiturridge, *Arab.* Tumbe codiveli, *Hort. malab.*

A native of various parts of the East Indies, an erect, herbaceous plant with a round striated stem, and ascending or erect branches. Leaves ovate, lanceolate, flat, rather obtuse, or apiculate, stalked, slightly toothed and ciliated, with the petiole clasping the stem, flowers distant, in long slender spikes, calyx closely covered with numerous spreading stalked glands, corolla hypocrateriform, bright reddish pink, with a slender tube, much longer than the calyx, lobes of the limb oblong, obtuse, flat, apiculate.

The properties of this species and of the P. scandens and zeylanica are nearly identical.

A paste made with rice congie and the bruised bark is applied by the natives to buboes in the incipient state; it acts as a vesicatory.

Plumbagin.

A peculiar and interesting principle, *Plumbagin*, was discovered in these plants by M. Dulong in 1824. It abounds chiefly in the bark of the root, and is thus prepared—

The bark of the root, is acted on by ether, the etherial tincture mixed with water, and the ether recovered by distillation. The watery liquid is then boiled and filtered while hot; on cooling, crystals of *Plumbagin* are deposited; the process is to be repeated as long as crystals are procured.

Plumbagin occurs in brilliant yellow crystals, of sweetish, but acrid and hot taste, easily fusible, partially volatile, scantily soluble in cold, freely in boiling water, very soluble in alcohol and ether, in the concentrated acids, and in alkaline solutions, with which it strikes a deep red colour; with hydrate of alumina or subacetate of lead a crimson red coloured precipitate is formed, which constitutes a very valuable and delicate test, available in many medico-legal inquiries.

[*Uses as a blister.*]

We have made numerous clinical experiments with the bark of the plumbago root of various species, especially the *P. rosea*, rubbed into a paste with water and a little flour, or congie; it occasions pain in about five minutes, which increases in severity till in a quarter of an hour it is equal to that of a cantharides blister or mustard sinapism. If the paste be removed in half an hour the pain is soon allayed, and in a period of 12 to 18 hours a large uniform blister, full of serum, is occasioned. The blistered surfaces heal readily, without unpleasant ulceration.

In the native the skin in a few minutes is intensely blackened; in white-skinned persons a deep redness is occasioned.

In all chronic cases and in many acute diseases this blister will prove an effectual and very cheap substitute for cantharides, over which it possesses the peculiar advantage of never producing strangury or any other form of irritation of the urinary organs. We speak from the experience of from 3 to 400 cases.

Our experiments lead us to believe that the blistering quality resides in the Plumbagin, but on this we are as yet unable to speak in positive terms.

The root, in various forms, is much employed as a poison in India; and as an irritant to occasion abortion it is introduced into the vagina and applied directly to the neck of the uterus. In a criminal case of the former kind, in 1837, the Editor succeeded in detecting the poison by acting on the contents of the stomach with alcohol, concentrating the tincture, re-dissolving in a small quantity of boiling water, and adding the sub-acetate of lead, by which the very characteristic red colour was immediately occasioned. By a modification of this process two grains of the powdered bark may be detected in a pint of a mixture of milk, blood, and various articles of food. For minute details of this process, see Appendix, *Art. Poisons.*

NAT. ORDER CVIII.—PLANTAGINEÆ.

Herbaceous plants with branched stems, leaves usually radical, undivided flowers in spikes or crowded heads, natives of temperate climates, or cultivated in the tropics in cold seasons. The leaves, herb, and root, are slightly bitter, the seeds mucilaginous, and a little acrid.

GEN.—PLANTAGO.

Sp. 1. *Plantago Psyllium.*

Seeds very small, oval oblong, obtuse at both ends, concave on one side, convex on the other, brown, brilliant, and not unlike the "petites pouces" (little fleas) to which M. Feé gives the origin of their name, ψυλλις, pulex, *a flea.* Inodorous, mucilaginous, one part being sufficient to render 48 of water as thick as the white of eggs. In the North of Europe they are used for scouring muslins.

Sp. 2. *Plantago Ispaghula.*

Vern. Ispagool, *Pers.* Buzr kaloona, *Arab.* Fuslioon, *Greek.*

Annual, stem short, dividing into 3 or 4 ascending round villous branches a few inches in length, leaves alternate, linear, lanceolate, 3-nerved, somewhat toothed, woolly, channelled at the base and amplexicaul, peduncles axillary, solitary, naked, erect, round, a little villous, spikes solitary, terminal, when in seed about 1 inch to 1½ inch long. Flowers numerous, small, white, bracts 1-flowered, ovate, concave, calyx 4-leaved, sepals with broad membranous margins, corolla hypocrateriform, limb 4-parted, spreading, stamens 4-long and flaccid, style simple, stigma unilateral, capsule 2-celled, few or many seeded. *Roxb. Fl. Ind.* i. p. 404.

In India the Plantago Ispaghula is cultivated during the cold season for the seeds, which are used as an emollient and light article of diet for convalescents.

Feé also describes the *Plantago major*, a native of Europe, a plant of slightly bitter and astringent qualities, and the roots and leaves of which tinge the saliva red—formerly much used as a febrifuge, now justly neglected.

NAT. ORDER CIX.—MYRSINEÆ.

This order should have been inserted after the *Sapotaceæ*, with which it is nearly allied; 36 species are found in India.

One of the most remarkable genera is the Embelia; the berries of *E. Ribes* (*Vern.* Baiberung) are of pungent pepper-like taste, and are used as an adulteration for black pepper. They are also used in medicine by the native physicians as a vermifuge cathartic. The same name is applied to the fruit of E. robusta. *Myrsine bifaria*, (Manus rohunee, *Hind.*) is also deemed cathartic. (*Royle.*)

SUB-CLASS 4—MONOCHLAMYDEÆ.

Corolla wanting, or united with calyx, staminiferous.

NAT. ORDER CX.—NYCTAGINEÆ.

Ligneous or herbaceous plants, with alternate or generally opposite leaves, with axillary or terminal flowers; there is no important remedy derived from this class.

GEN. 1.—MIRABILIS.

Sp. Mirabilis Jalapa, Marvel of Peru. *Belle de nuit.*

Vern. Patrash, *Tam.* Reso, *Japan.* Gulabbas, *Hind.* and *Duk.* Krishna keli, *Beng.*

Cultivated as an ornament in all the gardens of Bengal. Considered an aperient by the native doctors. Drs. Hunter and Shoolbred tried it without satisfactory results, and our own experiments lead us to believe it destitute of any efficacy. It is at best an uncertain cathartic.

The roots of this plant were long regarded as the source of the true Jalap. They are considered purgative, their taste is acrid and nauseous, and they abound in starch; the seeds also contain this principle in such abundance that they have been proposed as an alimentary article.

The Mirabilis dichotoma and longiflora are reputed to possess similar properties.

Gen. 2.—Boerhaavia.

Sp. 1. *B. decumbens.* Guiana-root—stated to be emetic and astringent, and given in decoction in dysentery.

Sp. 2. *B. tuberosa,* of Persia—said to be emetic, and purgative.

Vern. Mookaratty vayr, *Tam.* Tikrie ke jur, *Duk.* Attika mamedie varysoo, *Tel.* Sindika and Punarnava, *Sans.* East Indies. *Spreading hogweed.* Root deemed laxative, and given by the natives in powder, a tea spoonful twice daily. It is single, oblong, hard within, bark soft and thin, of a dusky colour outside, slightly bitter, and somewhat nauseous taste.

Horsfield says that in Java the Bœrhaavia diandria is deemed emetic.

Sp. 3. *B. diffusa.*

Vern. Gadha poorna, *Beng.*—has probably similar properties.

NAT. ORDER CXI.—POLYGONEÆ.

A very important family containing rhubarb, one of the most valuable remedies employed in medicine, and several other plants interesting as articles of food, as dye stuffs, &c.

The distribution of Polygoneæ is very extensive; the valuable species of rhubarb and fagopyrum (buck-wheat) flourish most however in cold or temperate regions.

The medicinal Polygoneæ are divided by Lindley into the genera Coccoloba, Rheum, Rumex, and Polygonum; these are herbaceous plants, rarely shrubs,

All these agree in being apetalous dicotyledons, with definite, erect ovula, ochreate stipulæ, and a radicle remote from the hilum. The calyx is divided, inferior, imbricated in œstivation, stamens definite, inserted in the bottom of the calyx, anthers dehiscing lengthwise, ovarium superior, with a single erect ovulum, styles or stigmas several, nut usually triangular, seed with farinaceous albumen, embryo inverted, generally on one side, radicle at the end, remote from the hilum, plumula inconspicuous. (*Lindley.*)

The leaves are alternate, stipulæ cohering round the stem in the form of an ochrea, when young rolled backwards; flowers occasionally unisexual, often in racemes.

The presence of oxalic and malic acid in the stems and leaves—of a purgative bitter principle in the roots—and of astringent matter, constitute the leading chemical properties of this order. In some we find moreover a peculiar yellow colouring substance, and in others an acrid principle, capable of inflaming and even of blistering the skin.

Gen.—Coccoloba.

Sp. 1. *C. uvifera.* Seaside grape.

West India Islands, and American Coast. A tree 20 feet in height, leaves very beautiful, orbicular, cordate, of a bright glossy green. Flowers fragrant, stamens 5, styles 3.

The leaves, wood, and bark are extremely astringent, and afford an extract termed Jamaica kino, which consists chiefly of tannic and gallic acid, with colouring matter.

The wood gives a red dye.

Gen. 2.—Rheum.—Rhubarb.

Off. The roots of several species.

Vern. Rewund Chinee, *Hind.* Rawund, *Arab.*

Calyx petaloid, 6-parted, withering, stamens about 9 inserted into the base of the calyx, styles 3, reflexed, stigmas peltate, entire; achenium 3-cornered, winged, with the withered calyx at the base, embryo in the centre of the albumen.

This genus embraces many species, and it is still uncertain which afford the true rhubarb roots of commerce. Lindley, the most recent writer on medical botany, quotes Mr. Royle's observations as affording a good summary of what is exactly known on the subject; these we find are derived chiefly from M. Feé's work. The rhubarb of commerce is brought by the Chinese to the Siberian frontier town of Kiachta, from Kansu in the province of Shensee, between NE. 35° and 40°, and also from the Snowy mountains from N. lat. 26° to 33°, E. long. 99° to 105°. The trade is in the hands of a Bucharian family, who farm the monopoly from the Chinese, and reside at Sining on the frontiers of Thibet. All other Chinese are restricted from the commerce on the penalty of death, and even the Canton traffic is in the hands of these proprietors. These purchase the rhubarb in the Tangutian towns of Kian Sin and Schan Sin, from which their place of abode is about 20 days' journey. The rhubarb country would accordingly be placed within 95° E. long. and in 35° N. latitude, or in the heart of Thibet.

At least four varieties of roots are known in commerce.

The first, purchased at Kiachta by the agent of the Russian government, is brought overland to Moscow and St. Petersburgh, and exported by the Baltic to various parts of the world.

The second, or Chinese rhubarb, is of inferior quality, is purchased at Canton, and imported into Calcutta or sent directly to Europe. The inferiority is attributable to the great care in selection observed by the Russian officers at Kiachta.

The third, or Turkey, is purchased from the Chinese Tartars by the Bucharians, who bring it to Bokhara, Samarcand, and other cities of central Asia, whence in the ordinary course of commerce it passes to the Levant and Constantinople.

The fourth, the produce of the Himalayan mountains, is brought in small quantities to Almorah, Katmandhu, and other mountain cities, and thence finds its way to the Indian Bazars.

Besides these, several other sorts have been distinguished, such as those produced by cultivation of different species in Europe. The best of all is however the first variety above described.

Cultivation. According to the statements of the Bucharians—" Muscovy or the Russian Rhubarb plant" thrives best in a light and sandy soil, and the finest roots proceed from plants grown in shady places, at the base of the mountain chain (Feé). The Siberian rhubarb is, on the contrary, of better quality in proportion to its exposure to the sun. The roots are gathered twice yearly, in spring and autumn, and they must be between six and nine years old. On being gathered the root is immediately cleaned, barked, strung on cords and dried in the shade. Saunders states, that in Bootan a kind of stove is employed for the purpose; other authorities inform us that the roots are cut into thick short junks, and hung round the horns of the sheep, and thus undergo drying during the wanderings of the Tartar shepherds.

According to the best writers, and information, it seems that the recent root loses during drying four-fifths of its weight; the cutting and stringing are described by some as operations subsequent to the drying process.

The cultivation of various species of rhubarb has been carried on in many parts of Europe with considerable success. The *Rheum rhaponticum* is grown in large quantities at Rheumpole, near L'Orient, in France, and the *R. undulatum* is also cultivated in other parts of that country.

The *R. palmatum*, the roots of which exactly resemble the Chinese article in colour, taste, and smell, is grown extensively near Banbury in England for the supply of the London market; and in the Botanical Garden of Chelsea the *R. crassinervium* (sent from St. Petersburgh) has produced roots of the colour and smell of the best Turkey rhubarb.

Some peculiarities in the cultivation and preparation of the European root demand our attention, as they seem deserving of imitation in the attempts to improve the Himalayan article.

The seed is sown in spring in a light soil, transplanted the following year at the same season, and the plants placed at three feet distance. The third year some plants flower, but the roots are only collected in the autumn of the fifth year, when they weigh 15 to 25 pounds. They are then more spongy than fibrous, of difficult desiccation, on account of the tenacity of the extractive matter, which is very abundant. The roots are first washed, and the fibres and small roots separated; a second steeping is performed, and then the roots are cut into pieces of suitable size; the brown bark is then rasped off, and the pieces steeped again in fresh water for three or four hours, during which time they give out a large quantity of gummy, transparent matter, resembling jelly; they are then placed in a stove heated to 120° or 140° centigrade, and dried, during which operation they lose 70 to 72 per cent. in weight; after perfect drying they are lastly introduced into a barrel mounted on an axis, to which a brisk rotatory motion is communicated for half an hour, when they are found to be covered with a fine powder formed by their mutual attrition.

Thus prepared, European rhubarb has all the characters of the Chinese article, and may be powdered under the pestle without flattening. Its physical characters indeed are all the same as those of the kind we have to describe under the head of Russian rhubarb.

Varieties of Rhubarb.

Russian Rhubarb, is in flattish, irregular, angular pieces, pierced with a hole the size of the finger, lively yellow exteriorly, veined with dark brown very delicate streaks, scarcely perceptible to casual inspection; internally it is mottled, red, yellow, and white, spongy, and rather difficultly cut; odour aromatic, taste slightly astringent, bitter, and peculiar, gritty between the teeth, tinges the saliva yellow, is easily powdered, powder bright yellow.

Canton Rhubarb, is in cylindrical compact pieces, sometimes but rarely pierced with small holes, simply for a cord, colour dull yellow, interior marbling deep red, taste and odour stronger than in the first kind, the saliva is tinged orange-red when it is chewed, heavier than the first variety, powder between fawn and orange yellow.

Himalayan Rhubarb is in irregular, dirty brown pieces, having a strong rhubarb smell and taste, but devoid of yellow colour or marbling, difficultly pulverized, powder deep brown colour.

Chemical composition.

Dr. A. T. Thomson has given us a useful contrast of the chemical properties of the Indo-Russian and Canton Rhubarbs.

Water at 212 takes up 24 parts in 60 of Russian, 30 in 60 of Canton Rhubarb. The infusion of the former is of deeper colour, and is less turbid than the latter; both redden litmus paper, owing to their containing a large proportion of super-oxalate of lime, both are precipitated by gelatine and sulphate of iron, but the precipitates differ somewhat in colour.

According to Henry's analysis rhubarb contains—1. a yellow colouring principle; 2. a bland oil; 3. fecula; 4. gum; 5. tannin; 6. one-third its weight of super-oxalate of lime; 7. malates and sulphates of lime, potassa, and iron. Henry also mentions vegetable jelly (Pectin and Pectic acid) as constituting nearly one-half the weight of the *recent* roots of the Rheum australe, or Himalayan species. A German chemist, Hornemann, has recently described a substance which he names *Rhaponticin*, detected in all the varieties of rhubarb. This is destitute of taste and smell, insoluble in cold water, ether, and volatile oils, soluble in 24 times its weight of boiling absolute alcohol, from which it crystallizes on cooling in yellow plates or needles. It seems destitute of any medicinal virtues, and bears but a small proportion to the other constituents of the root.

Rhein is another substance obtained by acting on rhubarb by moderately strong nitric acid, and precipitating with water. Its properties have not been accurately ascertained, but it seems to be little else than the bitter principle generated by the action of nitric acid on numerous other organic substances, such as silk, indigo, and aloes.

Other processes of analysis have separated a crystalline principle, termed indiscriminately *rhein*, *caphopicrite*, and *rhabarbarin*. The simplest process is by agitating powdered rhubarb with ether, distilling off two-thirds, allowing the remainder to evaporate spontaneously and to crystallize. These crystals are intensely yellow, but tasteless and inodorous, easily fusible, and volatile in a yellow smoke. The crystals seem to possess acid properties, combining with and forming beautiful red compounds with the saline bases.

Further details on these principles would be misplaced in this work. Their nature is not yet accurately ascertained, and the experiments on their medicinal properties have hitherto led only to negative results.

The acid so abundant in the stalks of the young rhubarbs was formerly regarded as peculiar, and named the *rheumic;* it is now deemed to be a mixture of malic and oxalic acids. It is so abundant that the stalks make a very agreeable tart, much esteemed at European tables.

Alcohol takes up from powdered rhubarb all its active constituents, leaving an inert mass. When taken into the stomach the colouring matter enters the circulation, and speedily appears in the urine, which assumes a deep yellow colour, and is changed to blood-red by alkalies. It also passes into the perspiration and milk.

Medicinal effects.

Rhubarb in any form is a gentle purgative. The dose of the powder is ½ a drachm to ʒ i.—that of the infusion (made with ʒ iij. of the bruised root and ℥viij. of water) ℥ i. to ℥ ij. The operation is generally accompanied with griping. In small doses the astringent acids it contains overpower the purgative principle, and a slight constipating or tonic action is induced. This action is even felt from larger doses, so that rhubarb is often known to strengthen the tone of the digestive organs, even when employed as a purgative.

From the mildness of its action it is deservedly popular in the management of diseases of children.

Rhubarb powder is generally given with calomel, scammony, jalap, sulphate of potash or with magnesia. This last adjunct lessens its griping tendency.

The purgative property of rhubarb is destroyed by roasting, boiling, or the process of forming the extract.

The *compound tincture* made with powdered rhubarb 2½

ounces, proof spirit two pints, with liquorice, ginger, and saffron is a useful stomachic aperient in doses of from two to four drachms—(see *Pharmacopœia.*)

Species of RHEUM *which yield the rhubarb of commerce.*

The difficulty of arriving at the truth regarding this question, is occasioned by the jealous vigilance with which the Chinese endeavour to guard the monopoly we have described, and by which they have baffled all the efforts of the Russian government to obtain indisputable specimens of the plant. The doubt however is solely of importance in a botanical point of view, since several species of rheum are now known, which by cultivation afford some of the finest qualities, both physical and medicinal.

We now proceed to notice succinctly the facts ascertained regarding the particular species of Rheum affording the articles we have described.

Sp. 1. ***Rheum Emodi,*** Wall. R. australe, *Don.*

Mountains of Gosain Than, Kemaon, &c.

Stems 6 to 10 feet high, much branched and furrowed, very thick below, gradually attenuated upwards into large panicles, and there rough with minute warts and excrescences, colour yellow, streaked with rust brown. Leaves very large, panicles or rather compound racemes terminal, very long, branches erect, virgate, round, pedicels solitary or clustered, somewhat verticillate, short, spreading, in fruit deflexed. Flowers very small, of a deep blood-red colour, calyces 6, small, spreading, ovate, deep segments, three alternate ones smaller. Stamens 9, shorter than the perianth, filaments subulate, monadelphous at the base. Ovary short, triquetrous, often abortive. Styles 3, spreading. Stigmas large, warty, fruit pendent, dark, blood-coloured, shining, cordate, triangular, the angles sharply winged and covered at the base with the persistent perianth, of which the three smaller segments are applied to the three-winged angles; leaves cordate, acute, dull green, but little wavy, flattish, very much wrinkled, distinctly rough with coarse short hairs on each side, sinus of the base distinctly open, not wedge-shaped, but diverging at an obtuse angle, with the lobes nearly turned upwards. Petioles very rough, rounded, angular, furrowed, with the upper side depressed, bordered by an elevated edge, and very much narrower at the upper than the lower end. *(Don and Hooker.)*

Sp. 2. *R. Webbianum*, Royle's Illustr. 318.
Gosain Than, Niti.

Root leaves large, long stalked, cordate, acute, cauline, obtuse, rather downy above, veiny beneath, and margin hairy, petioles rounded, upper branches and peduncles round, smooth, slightly striated. Axillary racemes clustered, terminal, panicled, pedicels in threes, sepals entire, broadly oval obtuse. Achenium somewhat cordate at the base, entire, or a little emarginate at the point. *Royle.*

Possibly what Mr. Moorcroft found at Niti, 12,000 feet above the level of the sea.

Sp. 3. *R. spiciforme*, Royle, 318. t. 78.
Northern face of the Himalayas at and beyond the Kerang pass.

Leaves thick, leathery, cordate, blunt, red and netted beneath, downy, petioles and peduncles smooth, pedicels numerous, clustered, racemes arising from the very root, spicate, sepals oblong, obtuse, the alternate ones narrower and petaloid, fruit rounded at the base and apex.

Lindley thinks it likely that this species, which grows 16,000 feet above the level of the sea, produced the fine roots sent to Dr. Royle by Moorcroft.

Sp. 4. *R. Moorcroftianum*, Royle 318. (*Small stalked Rhubarb.*) Roots called *Dooloo* in Bootan.

The fruits larger, and angles broader and more winged than the last, with other slight differences; root said to be more purgative than the last.

Several experiments were made by the late Mr. Twining on the medicinal qualities of the Himalayan rhubarb, produced by the *R. Emodi and Webbianum.* It was given in 43 cases with the following results—Mr. T. states that—" it has less aroma, and more astringency, than the best Turkey rhubarb; in doses of 2 or 3 drs. it has a good purgative effect, operating 3 or 4 times nearly as freely as the best Turkey rhubarb. It is not apt to gripe, is less disagreeable than the best Turkey rhubarb, nearly equally efficacious as a purge, and very superior in small doses as a tonic and astringent in profluvia." *Trans. Med. and Phys. Soc. Calcutta*, v. iii. p. 441.

Sp. 5. *R. leucorrhizum.* White-rooted rhubarb.
Stony places in the Kirghis desert. A small plant. Considered the source of a white rhubarb brought to Pallas at

Kiachta by the Bucharian merchants, and equal in effects to the best kinds.

Sp. 6. *R. rhaponticum.* Borders of the Euxine sea, in the deserts between the Volga and the Yaik, also in Siberia; cultivated in France at Rheumpole.

Sp. 7. *R. undulatum,* or *waved.* China and Siberia.

The leaves are oval, obtuse, extremely wavy, deep green with purple veins, petiole blood-red. This was once regarded as the real officinal plant, because this and the R. Palmatum were produced by seed given by a Tartarian rhubarb dealer to the Emperor of Russia's physician in 1750. But all attempts at its successful cultivation have failed in Europe, in the production of a good drug for medicinal uses.

Sp. 8. *R. caspicum.* Stony places on lower part of Altai mountains.

Sp. 9. *R. compactum.* Tartary and China.

Leaves heart-shaped, obtuse, wavy, deep green, petiole hardly tinged with red.

According to Guiboûrt this root nearly resembles the Chinese rhubarb, it scarcely however tinges the saliva, and is not gritty when chewed, the colour moreover is much darker.

Sp. 10. *R. palmatum.*

Mountains of Chinese Tartary to Lake Kokonor near Thibet.

Leaves half palmate, lobes pinnatifid, very much wrinkled, petiole pale green, flowering stems taller than in any other species.

This is generally considered the source of the best rhubarb, it was one of the species raised from the seed obtained frŏm the Tartar merchant. It is officinal in the last London Pharmacopœia, and M. Guibourt, one of the best living authorities on all pharmaceutical subjects, states, that of all the cultivated kinds this alone in Europe resembles exactly in taste, smell, and colour the best rhubarb obtained from China. We have already mentioned that it is cultivated extensively in England for the London market.

Sp. 11. *R. crassinervium.*

Distinct from any other species; sent from St. Petersburgh to the Chelsea Garden, where the roots when three years old were as thick as the wrist, brittle, and found to possess the smell and taste of the best rhubarb.

The preceding details constitute a sufficient epitome for the Indian student, of all that is clearly ascertained regarding the most important points in the history of this drug.

We find on reference to the records of the Company's Dispensary, that during the last three years there have been consumed annually 175 lbs. of rhubarb, and 20 lbs. of the extract, the former 15*s.*, the latter 1*l.* 10*s.* per pound. The inferior rhubarb found in the Bengal Bazars, and named Rewund chinee, (Rivend chinee, *Persian*) Rawund, *Arab*, ῥηον, Greek, sells for four Rupees the seer. Three kinds are usually found—Chinee, Khorassanee, and Hindee; the second is probably the root of the plants observed by Sir Alexander Burnes in Bokhara and Cabul.

Dr. Royle has very clearly shewn the practicability and advantages of undertaking the cultivation of rhubarb in the Himalayas. Species, as we have already seen, are common on Choor, near Jumnotree, on Jacho in Kemaon, Gossainthan in Nepal, and Tassesudan in Bootan; on the northern face is the *Rheum spiciforme,* discovered on the Kherang Pass; while Dr. Gerard describes the table land of Tartary as covered with rhubarb at the elevation of 16,000 feet; lastly, Mr. Moorcroft found specimens of unrivalled excellence near Ludak, in N. lat. 34°. and E. long. 77½°.

Kunawur and the Bhoteah pergunnahs of Kemaon are named by Mr. Royle as the most suitable localities for the cultivation. He attaches, we think, too much importance to the difficulty of procuring specimens or seeds of the true rhubarb, as we consider that most of the species already indigenous need only careful management to yield a drug perfectly equal to the best yet sent to the Siberian frontier. Mr. Royle however suggests that the seed and roots could be readily obtained in Kunawur, and Assam (upper), or a trade in rhubarb established with Thibet or western Mongolia by means of the Tartars who resort to the hill fairs. Mr. Royle observes that "the trade might be encouraged by the government purchasing all the rhubarb it required, which might thus be employed for hospital use after crossing the frontiers, instead of as now after making a journey of 20,000 miles, or nearly the circuit of the globe."

As however the government consumption of rhubarb in Bengal amounts annually only to 175 lbs. weight, valued at 15*s.* the pound, and 20 lbs. extract, valued at 1*l.* 10*s.* per lb. this extent of encouragement, even though it were doubled for the other presidencies, would we fear scarcely induce a trade in the article; we think it would be far preferable to cultivate and prepare the roots in a special farm, and sell the surplus in the Bazar, whence it would find its way to Europe, and doubtless meet extensive consumption.

The extract of Rhubarb is prepared by the natives in the Hills, where it is called *Ossara rewund*. See page 237.

GEN. 3.—RUMEX.

This genus comprehends several species, which prevail as common weeds all over Europe. The docks and sorrels are familiar to all the natives of temperate Northern latitudes.

The *Docks*, (Rumex crispus, and obtusifolius,) have astringent roots, which are used as an external application for the cure of some cutaneous diseases. The *Rumex acetosa*, or sorrel, contains the quadroxalate of potassa, and hence is of peculiarly pleasant acid flavour, and much used as a table vegetable in Europe, especially in France.

The *Rumex alpinus*, or Monk's rhubarb, is found on the European Alps, the Crimea, and Mount Caucasus. The roots are large and purgative like rhubarb, and the whole plant so resembles the Rheum that Linnæus himself mistook one for the other.

GEN. 4.—POLYGONUM.

Sp. P. Hydropiper. Water pepper.

Common in wet places in Europe, root fibrous, whorled, smooth, stem erect, two feet high, more or less red and shining, and swelled above each fruit. Leaves alternate, lanceolate, acute, calyx covered with glandular dots, which are very acrid; the leaves are so much so as to produce blisters when applied to the skin.

Reputed to be a powerful diuretic, but to lose its activity by drying. It gives wool a yellow colour.

Sp. P. Bistorta. Bistort. Pastures and woods in Europe.

Roots creeping, often bent in a double zig-zag, whence its name, powerfully astringent, owing to its containing a large quantity of tannic and gallic acids, hence it has been used in the treatment of diarrhœa, leucorrhœa, gleet, &c. It has also been given with gentian in intermittent fevers.

Sp. P. aviculare. Knot grass. Considered medicinal in Behar. Nisomali, *Sans*. Machooti, *Hind*. Fruit said to be emetic and cathartic.

Sp. P. barbatum. China, East Indies. Aatalari, *Tam*. Kunda mallier, *Tel*.

Considered diuretic at the Cape of Good Hope, and given in infusion by the native doctors in India in cases of colic.

Sp. P. amphibium.
Root-like stems of this polygonum, resemble sarsaparilla, as a substitute for which it has been used with alleged success.

Sp. P. tinctorium, chinense, and *barbatum,* yield a blue dye like indigo in China and Japan.

GEN. 5.—FAGOPYRUM.

Sp. F. esculentum.
Frumentum Sarracenicum, or *Buck wheat*—cultivated in many parts of Europe and in the Himalayas, and in all the mountainous countries north of Bengal, Oude, &c. *Phapra* and *Kooltoo* of the natives.

Seeds oval, acute, nearly triangular, with acute, smooth, brilliant angles, the size of a hemp seed, of ash-brown colour. Parenchyme white, farinaceous, covered with a brittle pericarp, inodorous, and nearly insipid.

A valuable article of diet in many countries where wheat will not succeed.

Roxburgh in his second volume, p. 285 et seq. (Octandria trigynia) gives 15 species of Polygonum, but no information as to their properties. His *P. lanatum,* common round Calcutta, is called *Swet panee merich,* or white water pepper; *P. pilosum; burra panee merich,* or great water pepper, is also common near Calcutta, and flowers at the beginning of the wet season. The name denotes its analogy in properties to the P. Hydropiper of our previous article; *P. flaccidum* is also called *Panee merich* in Calcutta.

NAT. ORDER CXII.—CHENOPODEÆ.

This order contains no very important medicinal species, although some are of interest in an economical light, as sources of alkali and articles of food.

GEN. 1.—CHENOPODIUM.

Sp. Chenopodium olidum.
Vern. Bhutwa, *Hind.* Several species in India used as food.

Roxburgh in vol. ii. p. 58 and 59, describes 3 species—the *C. albmu* (Betu sag) used by the natives as a pot-herb, and common in Bengal—*C. viride,* of which there are two varieties, one entirely green, the other with the angles of the stems and branches of a beautiful purple colour, and the leaves and panicles somewhat reddish—*C. laciniatum,* an erect annual, 3 or 4 feet high, leaves long-petioled, multifid, mealy, panicles terminal, erect, contracted.

The *Chenopodium olidum,* stinking goose-foot, smells like putrid salt fish, and exhales ammoniacal gas; herb employed as an emmenagogue and antispasmodic.

C. Baryosmon. (Salsola fœtida,) Upper Egypt, excessively fœtid, used for the same purposes as the last plant.

C. Botrys, (Jerusalem oak.)
South of Europe, and Siberia, and Upper India; whole plant very fragrant, said to be a powerful expectorant, and very useful in catarrh and humoral asthma.

C. anthelminticum, worm seed, United States.
Heavy disagreeable smell, seeds yield an abundant essential oil of powerful vermifuge properties. The expressed juice of the leaves and the powdered seeds have similar virtues.

C. ambrosioides.
Smell agreeable, plant used in chorea, and similar nervous diseases.

Beta bengalensis (palung), *Spinacia tetrandra* (Ispanack), and *Basella rubra* (poee) are cultivated by the natives as articles of food. Of Basella, Roxburgh describes three wild, and two cultivated varieties.

The *red beet* and *mangel wurzil* also afford abundance of amylaceous and saccharine matter.

Gen. 2.—Atriplex.

A. angustifolia, Europe, seed said to be emetic. *A. hortensis,* Tartary, (orache) is of the same reputed properties.

Gen. 3.—Salsola.

Flowers hermaphrodite, bracteate, sepals 5, stamens 5, inserted into a hypogynous ring or cup. Stigmas 2, usually combined at the base, subsessile and capitate, utricle depressed, somewhat papery. Seed horizontal, without albumen, with membranous integuments, embryo spiral, radicle dorsal, leafy or leafless, herbaceous plants or shrubs, with succulent sub-cylindrical leaves. Flowers axillary and sessile, dorsal appendages of the sepals wing-like, utricle occasionally slightly baccate. (*Lindley.*)

Sp. S. Kali, Europe, and colder parts of Asia; mostly found on sandy shores, or arid deserts; an annual bushy plant, with stiff thorny channelled leaves. Flowers solitary, each with three leaf-like bractes, calyx dilated, membranous, reddish, converging over the fruit; each sepal with small leafy appendage. Fruit turbinate, winged.

The dried plant when reduced to ashes yields 25 to 30 per cent. of carbonate of soda.

Sp. S. sativa. Spain. Equal to the last species.

Roxburgh describes two species, the S. nudiflora, and indica.

The *S. nudiflora* (Rawacada, *Tel.*) is a native of salt barren lands near the sea, and flowers during the greater part of the year. The stems are perennial, many-spreading, close upon the ground, and often striking root, ramous, extremities of the branches ascending. Young parts smooth, and coloured reddish. Leaves alternate, sessile, linear, fleshy, obtuse, smooth, generally about half an inch long. Spikes terminal, erect, very long, compound, leafless. Flowers very numerous, in little fascicles, filaments inserted into the bottom of the division of the calyx. Styles 3, spreading, seeds smooth, horizontal, oval, beaked, covered by a thin membrane, and partly by the permanent calyx. (*Roxb.*)

The plant is only used for fuel, but Roxburgh believes would doubtless yield excellent soda.

S. indica (*Tel.* Ella-kura), with Salicorneæ, and others, are natives of the salt marshes and grounds near the sea, flowering the greater part of the year. The green leaves are universally eaten by all classes of natives who live near the sea, and are reckoned very wholesome. The leaves of this plant alone saved many thousand lives during the famine of 1791-2-3. *Roxb.* vol. ii. p. 63.

S. Soda, South of Europe, Africa, America.

An annual, often three or four feet high, and frequently prostrated by its own weight. Ashes highly alkaline.

S. Tragus, same localities and properties.

Gen. 4.—Salicornia.

S. indica, Jidoo Palung, *Beng.*

A plant very common on such salt grounds as are inundated by the spring tides. It is especially plentiful on the coast of Coromandel, and would doubtless yield a fine and cheap carbonate of soda. But the probable value of this article as an Indian export has been much depreciated by the progress of chemical science in Europe. The purest alkali is now manufactured in England by decomposing common salt by sulphuric acid, and at the low rate of 10*l.* the ton of 30 maunds.

The coarse kind of barilla (*Saji mati*) to which Dr. Royle alludes, p. 319, as the produce of the incineration of some unknown plants, is a mineral product very abundant near Monghyr and in the Dooab. We describe it fully in our account of mineral remedies.

NAT. ORDER CXIII.—SALVADOREÆ.*

GEN.—SALVADORA.

Calyx small, quadrifid, with ovate, rather obtuse segments, corolla quadripartite, with revolute segments, styles short, with a simple obtuse, umbilicated stigma, berry globose, 1-celled, with a spherical seed, enwrapped in a callous tunic. (*Lindley.*)

Sp. Salvadora persica.
Syn. Cissus arborea, *Forskäl.*
Vern. Piloo-Kurjal, *Hind.*

Most part of the Circars of India, Arabia, and the Persian Gulf. Thrives well in every soil, and is in flower and fruit all the year round.

Trunk generally crooked, from eight to ten feet high to the branches, and one foot in diameter. Bark very scabrous and deeply cracked, branches exceedingly numerous, spreading, with their extremities pendulous like the weeping willow.

Leaves opposite, stalked, oval or oblong, entire, very smooth and shining on both sides, without veins, one to two inches long, and about one broad, stipules none, panicles terminal, and from the exterior axils. Flowers minute, calyx inferior, 4-toothed, permanent, corolla monopetalous, tube short, border 4-cleft, segments oblong, revolute, filaments 4, inserted into the tube of the corolla, under its fissures, and rather shorter than the border, anthers oval, ovary globular, style none, stigma scabrous, berry very minute, smooth, red, and juicy, seed single, strongly aromatic in smell and taste.

* This order properly belongs to the Third Sub-division, *Corolliflorae.*

The bark of the root is very acrid, and if applied to the skin soon raises blisters; it promises to be a stimulant of very great power. (*Roxb.*)

It is supposed to be the mustard tree of scripture (*Lind.*); a decoction of the bark of the stem is said to be tonic, and the red berries eatable.

Sp. 2. *Salvadora indica.* Royle, p. 319.

Vern. Jal, *Hind.* Irak, *Persian,* also *Miswak,* or tooth brush tree; leaves, *Rasuna.* Found on the banks of the Jumna, and from Dehli to Saharunpore.

The leaves resemble the lanceolate senna, and are also purgative; the fruit is called *Peel* and *Pinjoo.*

It is not known whether the root bark possesses the same acrid properties as in the preceding species. We deem both the plants highly deserving of further investigation.

NAT. ORDER CXIV.—PHYTOLACCEÆ.

A small order, allied to Chenopodeæ, chiefly natives of America; two species are found in India. One of the American species is a very valuable medicine.

GEN.—PHYTOLACCA.

Gen. char. Calyx 5-parted, coloured, permanent, stamens and styles 10 or more, fruit depressed, furrowed, 10 or more celled, covered with a succulent flesh, seeds solitary. *Lind.*

Sp. P. decandra. Poke weed, North America.

The root is very large and fleshy, with concentric rings, stem 6 to 9 feet high, of a fine purple colour after the berries have ripened, leaves scattered, ovate oblong. Flowers on long pedunculed racemes, calyx whitish, of 5 sepals, ovary round, depressed, 10 furrowed. Styles 10, short, removed, berries in long clusters, dark purple, depressed or flattened.

Bigelow states that in emetic properties the root is very nearly equal to Ipecachuana, its use is however sometimes attended with slight narcotic symptoms. It is also used as an external application in itch, and tinea capitis.

Roxburgh describes a *Phytolacca acinosa* obtained from Nipal, where the leaves are eaten after boiling, as is the case with the American species above described. It flowers in the Botanic Garden of Calcutta about the end of the cold season, and certainly demands careful trial.

NAT. ORDER CXV.—AMARANTACEÆ.

An order of some importance in an alimentary point of view, though affording no medicinal species of any value. We subjoin an epitome of the valuable facts regarding the chief species, accumulated by the late Dr. Roxburgh.

GEN. 1.—AMARANTUS.

Male calyx 3 to 5 leaved, corolla none, stamens 3 to 5. Female flower, styles 3, capsule membranous, one-celled, one-seeded, opening horizontally, embryo annular, furnished with a perisperm.

Sp. A. tenuifolius.
Vern. Jeel chumli, *Beng.* Cultivated grounds near Calcutta. Stem none; a spreading plant close to the ground.

Sp. A. polygonoides.
Vern. Cheeloo nuteeya, *Beng.* Chirakura, *Tel.* very small, and a common garden weed, used as a pot-herb, and deemed so wholesome that convalescents are ordered it in preference to all the other kinds.

Sp. A. polygamus.
Vern. Chumli sag, *Hind.* Chumpa Nuteeya, (var. *lal*) *Beng.* Annual, extensively cultivated.

Sp. A. tristis.
Quoi-tota-kura, *Tel.* Annual, and cultivated; held in great esteem by the natives. It may be cut down several times without destroying the plants, which are much used for food.

A. viridis, lividus (Gobura nuteeya, *Beng.*) and *A. oleraceous* (Sada nuteeya) are cultivated for the same purposes; the tops of the young stems and branches of the last were formerly brought to table in India as a substitute for asparagus.

A. gangeticus, is the *lall sag* of the Bengalees.

A. lanceolatus.
Vern. Banspata nuteeya, bamboo-leaved amaranth, the leaves and tender tops eaten by natives in their curries.

A. atropurpureus.
Vern. Banspata lall nuteeya.

A frumentaceus, (called *kiery.*) Hills between Mysore and Coimbatore, seeds ground into flour. In the Botanic

Garden 40 square yards, sown in June, yielded 21 lbs. of clean seed in September, the plant also grows from October to February, inclusive.

A. spinosus.

Vern. Kanta nuteeya, thorny amaranth.

Sharp spines in the axils of the leaves; a very troublesome weed during the rainy and cold seasons.

Nearly all of the preceding species may be used as emollients for enemata, cataplasms, diluents, drinks, &c.

Gen. 2.—Achyranthes.

Sp. A. aspera.

Vern. Agareh ke jur, *Duk.* Lal chirchiri, *Hind.* Apamarga, *Sans.*

An infusion of the root is given as a mild astringent in bowel complaints. The flowering spike made into pills with a little sugar is a popular preventive medicine in Behar for persons bitten by rabid dogs.

The root is used by the natives as a tooth-brush, the whole plant when macerated yields a considerable quantity of potash.

NAT. ORDER CXVI.—THYMELEÆ.

This order is very uniform in character, and is formed of shrubs or herbs with simple and alternate leaves, axillary or terminal flowers. Its most remarkable genera are the Daphne, Lagetta, and Dirca, from which some valuable medicines, and the celebrated Nipal paper are derived. Plants of this order are common in the central parts of temperate latitudes, and abound in the mountainous regions of Asia.

A few are found in tropical latitudes, as Linostoma in Southern India. On the other hand species of Daphne are common in the coldest latitudes.

An acrid stimulant principle abounds in most of the species hitherto examined, and which possesses very valuable medicinal properties, though not devoid of dangerous powers if taken in excessive doses. A crystalline substance named *Daphnine* has also been separated from the bark of some species of Daphne.

Gen. 1.—Daphne.

Calyx tubular, withering, tube cylindrical, coriaceous, longer than the limb, imperforate at the base containing the stamens, limb in 4 deep, spreading, ovate, coloured segments, filaments short, in two rows, from about the middle of the tube, anthers roundish, oblong, of 2 cells, simple, enclosed within the tube. Ovary ovate, style short, terminal, stigma capitate, depressed, entire, berry oval, one-celled, seed solitary, suspended, oval, large, with a thin brittle skin. (*Lind.*)

Sp. 1. *D. Mezereum.* Mezereon.

Mazrioon, *Persian.* Kameela, *Greek.* Europe.

Stem bushy, 3 or 4 feet high, flowers fragrant, seated on naked branches, and appearing before the leaves. Berries scarlet, bark greyish externally, easily separable into layers, whitish or yellowish within, tenaceous and fibrous, beneath the epidermis is silky white tissue. The odour of the bark is disagreeable, its taste acrid, corrosive, and very enduring, but both these properties are diminished by time. Applied to the skin while recent the bark speedily occasions considerable pain, increased vascularity, redness or blackness, and finally vesication. It is not exactly known to which of the constituents of the bark these effects are attributable.

The best analysis known is that by Gmelin and Baer, published at Tubingen in 1822. These chemists detected wax, resin, *Daphnine,* red colouring matter, incrystallizable but fermentable sugar, azotized gum, woody fibre, brown colouring matter, malic acid, with malates of lime, magnesia, and potash.

Daphnine is crystalline, colourless, transparent, brilliant, soluble in water, alcohol, and ether, coloured golden yellow by potash and lime, precipitated by acetate of lead, and changed into oxalic acid by nitric acid. Inodorous, but of acrid and persistent taste.

Its effects on the animal economy are not ascertained, but deserve accurate trial. It has been found in every species of Daphne yet analysed.

The berries of Mezereon have been also examined, but the analyses present no remarkable results. They are brisk but unsafe cathartics.

Fresh Mezereon bark is much used as a counter-irritant and external stimulant; the dried bark is given internally in small doses as a stimulant alterative in syphilitic, rheumatic, and scrofulous maladies. The usual dose is 10 grs. infused in 2℥ of water. It is more frequently combined with sarsaparilla, as in the Lisbon diet drink (for which see "compound decoction of sarsaparilla.")

Sp. 2. *D. Laureola.* Spurge laurel, Europe, (δαφνοιδες, Zaknodeedus,) every part very acrid.

Sp. 3. *D. Gnidium.* Garou, *French.* Κνεωρον, Theophr. and Dioscor.

Properties as in the other species, used in France for making a depilatory and caustic ointment called *Pommade a garou.* Macerated in vinegar it makes a good blister. M. Coldefy Dorly has separated its resin, which he finds to act with very great activity as a stimulant, and which he proposes as a cheap and efficient blister.

Sp. 4. *D. cannabina,* Loureiro? Wall. in Asiat. Research, xiii. p. 385, c. tab. Sikkim, Nipal, Kemaon, &c. 5000 to 9000 feet elevation. From this shrub the Nipal paper is prepared.

*** A very interesting account of the manufacture of this remarkable paper is given by Mr. Hodgson, the British resident at Nipal, in the 1st vol. of the Journal of the Asiatic Society, page 8. The bark is boiled in a metallic pot, with oak ashes, which of course are highly alkaline.

The softened bark is then pounded with a mallet in a stone mortar till reduced to a pulp, like dough. This pulp is churned with water into a very thin paste, until it loses all traces of fibre, and will diffuse and settle smoothly. In this state it is poured through a coarse sieve, placed over a frame with a cloth bottom floating on water. The sieve stops the coarse pieces, allows the fine emulsion to pass through, and then by agitation this is smoothly deposited over the cloth. Removing the frame the water filters away, and the pulp dries rapidly by placing the frame before a fire.

The paper is subsequently polished by friction with a shell or piece of hard wood. Sheets have been made many yards square; it may be purchased in Katmandhu for 17 annas sicca for 3 seers. Bricks of the pulp are sold at 8 to 10 annas for 3 seers. The greater part of the paper is made by the Cis-Himalayan Bhoteas, east of the Kali river. The manufacture seems to have been introduced from China, about 500 years ago. (For the uses of this paper in Pharmacy, see *Filtration*, p. 7.)

Gen. 2.—Lagetta.

Sp. L. lintearia. Lace bark tree.

Jamaica, Mexico, St. Domingo; properties same as Mezereon, remarkable for the inner bark splitting into three whole layers, with delicate transverse fibres, exactly resembling beautiful lace, and capable of being washed with soap.

Gen. 3.—Dirca.

Sp. D. palustris. United States.

Bark acrid, cathartic, and vesicatory like the Mezereon, fruit narcotic, and in action resembling stramonium.

NAT. ORDER CXVII.—SANTALACEÆ.

The celebrated sandal wood tree is the only species of this family which demands our notice.

Gen. char. Calyx urceolate, 5-parted, stamens 4, alternate with the sepals, ovary occupying the whole tube of the calyx; ovules solitary, erect, drupe with a rim at the apex. (*Lindley.*)

Lindley enumerates three species.

GEN.—SANTALUM.

Sp. 1. *S. myrtifolium.*

Synonymous with the S. album of Roxburgh's Coromandel plants, a native of the continent of India, Timor, &c.

A small tree, with yellow flowers in stalked, trifid, axillary cymes, leaves narrow and oval.

This species affords the sandal wood of Malabar.

Sp. 2. *S. paniculatum.* Owhyhee on the volcano, also yields a sandal wood.

Sp. 3. *S. Freycinetianum;* this species was discovered by M. Gaudichaud in the Sandwich Islands.

Roxburgh makes the Santalum album and S. myrtifolium two distinct species. His S. album thrives luxuriantly in the Calcutta Garden, and is in flower and seed nearly the whole year.

SANDAL WOOD.*

Two species of this article are known in commerce—the *white* and the *yellow*. Ainslie states, and his opinion is generally received, that both are from the same tree, the former being the outer layers of the wood.

The *white* sandal-wood is coated with thick, compact bark, having a grey and brownish epidermis; the wood is very hard, heavy, susceptible of a fine polish. It occurs in billets of middling size, is nearly inodorous, its taste being slightly bitter.

The *yellow*, or citron sandal-wood, is straight or twisted, lighter than water when taken from the trunk, heavier if

* Chandanum and Shandana cuttay, *Tam.* Sundel, *Duk.* Sandoon, *Cing.* Sundel abiez, *Arab.* Sundul suffed, *Pers.* Chunden, *Hind.* Chandana, *Hind.* and *Beng.* Srigunda, *Can.* Tsjendana, *Mal.* Chendanum, *Tel.* Chandana, *Sans.* Malayaja, *Sans.* Aikamenil, *Timor.* Ayasra, *Amboin.* Katchundan, *Hind.* Tan Muh, *Chin.* Cayhundahn, *Cochin Chinese.* (*Ainslie*, vol. i. p. 376.)

from the roots in yellow, fawn-coloured, or reddish billets, slightly shining, of middling hardness, taking a fine polish, and being very easily cleft.

The odour of this wood is very strong, rose-like, and enduring, its taste slightly bitter. The wood of the *Plumeria alba* is occasionally substituted for the true sandal. The odour is due to the presence of an essential oil, heavier than water, readily congealed, and having a peculiar sweet smell. Sandal-wood is extensively used by cabinet-makers for the fabrication of various articles of ornamental furniture. The oil is employed by the European perfumers, and in India is very extensively used for the adulteration of attar of roses. The wood in powder is given by the native physicians in ardent remitting fevers, and supposed to be sedative and cooling, with milk it is also prescribed in gonorrhœa. (*Ainslie.*)

The powder is rubbed on the skin to allay the irritation of musquito bites, of prickly heat, and other cutaneous disorders.

NAT. ORDER CXVIII.—PROTEACEÆ.

Chiefly natives of the Cape, and remarkable for the extraordinary variety of their foliage and appearance. Two species are used medicinally at the Cape, *P. grandiflora* as an astringent in diarrhœa, *P. melliflora*, yielding from its flowers a saccharine liquid, employed in diseases of the chest; several species are used in tanning leather. (*Feé.*)

NAT. ORDER CXIX.—MYRISTICEÆ. (*Nutmegs.*)

The best account we have met with of this interesting family is the article by M. Feé, in his excellent work already referred to, and quoted so frequently. We follow M. Feé throughout in the subsequent account, incorporating with his descriptions the more recent information contained in the writings of Royle, Lindley, and others.

The Myristiceæ are trees bearing the appearance of the laurels; their leaves are alternate, devoid of dots, without stipules, entire, petioled, coriaceous, often downy below; they are not numerous, and are exclusively inhabitants of the tropics of India and America.

From the bark there exudes a reddish or yellow acrid

viscous juice, which gives linen a durable stain. The bark is not odorous, and the leaves but very faintly aromatic.

The fruit is the important part of these trees; the arillus, the sarcocarp, and the perisperm contain two oils, one volatile and the other fixed, and in variable proportions. The arillus, or mace, gives less volatile oil than the almond; the fixed oil found in the perisperm of several Myristaceous seeds is of more or less butter-like consistence; from the *Virola sebifera* for example, it is so abundant as to be prepared for numerous economical uses, and has nearly the firmness of suet. The fixed oil of Hernandia seed is purgative.

Gen.—Myristica.

The flowers diœcious, calyx urceolate, three-toothed, ♂ filaments monadelphous, anthers 6, 10 connate, ♀ ovary simple, styles none, stigma 2-lobed, pericarp fleshy, 2-valved, 1-seeded, seed enveloped in a fleshy arillus. (*Lindley.*)

Sp. 1. *M. officinalis.* Nutmeg tree.
Syn. Myristica moschata.

A diœcious tree, 20 to 25 feet high, a native of the Moluccas, especially of Banda. Leaves oblong, glabrous, and acuminate, with simple veins, and solitary smooth fruit.

The fruit is fleshy, nearly spherical, the size and shape of a small pear, flesh astringent, almost white within, 4 or 5 lines thick, opening into two nearly equal longitudinal valves.

The arillus or Mace, (*Vern.* Jawatri, *Hind.**) is thick, between horny and fleshy, much lacerated, folded and anastomosing towards the extremity, almost enveloping the nut; when fresh brilliant scarlet, when dry more horny, yellowish brown and brittle. The smell and taste of the arillus are peculiarly fragrant and agreeable. It softens, but does not dissolve in the mouth.

Beneath the arillus is found a bony shell, which covers the almond or kernel; this shell is thin, hard, brittle, brown and shining above, pale grey within, insipid and inodorous.

The Nutmeg.

Vern. Juephul, *Hind.* Jatiphali, *Sans.*

The kernel (*nutmeg, muscade*) is large, rounded, obtuse at both ends, the size of a small Myrobalon nut, smooth, marked with reticulated chinks, those transversely placed

* Jatipatri, *Sans.* Bezbaz, *Pers.* Talzuffur, *Arab.*

being less evident than the longitudinal; grey externally. In the chinks occurs a whitish powder, apparently chalk; internally the almond is traversed by branching, reddish, irregular greasy veins, giving it a marbled appearance,

The nut is hard, and easily cut, scraped, or grated, very inflammable, but the smoke is devoid of the fragrance of the acid.

The odour of the nutmeg is most agreeably aromatic, its taste hot, and analogous to the smell. The nut readily divides under the teeth, and is partially soluble in the saliva.

Nutmegs are much injured by time, becoming the prey of insects, which perforate them in every direction; sometimes good nutmegs are adulterated with others from which the valuable principles have been extracted by alcohol. Worm-eaten nuts are also fraudulently repaired by the introduction of a paste of flour and nutmeg oil into the holes.

Analysis of Mace.

According to M. Henry's analysis, mace contains essential oil in small quantities, a fixed, fragrant red oil, very soluble in alcohol and ether, a peculiar gummy principle, in about the proportion of one-third, woody fibre to a very small amount.

The decoction of mace contains a portion of both these oils in suspension in the gummy solution; ether is the best solvent for procuring all the oily matters.

The *volatile oil* obtained by distillation is a yellow liquid, lighter than water, of the fragrance and flavour of the mace.

Traces of an oil heavier than water can also be procured by distillation. The fixed oil is obtained by expression; 750 parts of mace afford 48 of this principle, which is of butyraceous consistence, brown colour, and highly fragrant. The natives call it Jadiputrie telum, *Tam.* Jawatri ke tel, *Duk.* It is very stimulant, brought to India from Banda, and much employed as a liniment and embrocation in rheumatism.

Essential oil of Nutmegs.

White, lighter than water, acrid, pungent taste, and very powerful nutmeg odour.

Fixed oil, or Butter of Nutmegs.

This occurs in commerce (in Europe) in flattened masses, of square form, yellowish, solid, internally marbled, 500 parts containing about 60 of essential oil. This substance is much adulterated, particularly with suet, spermaceti, marrow, wax, the oil of the Moringa pterygosperma coloured with alkanet or *rocou*, &c. &c.

The fixed oil is obtained by bruising the nutmegs into a paste, which is compressed in bags between hot metallic plates.

Two kinds are found in commerce—one in small earthen pots, of mace colour, and very agreeable smell, is exported from the Moluccas to Holland chiefly; the second kind is obtained from Holland, occurs in flat cakes, is far inferior to the first, and is usually adulterated with spermaceti.

The chief use of nutmegs is as a spice, and for the preparation of perfumes, and scented soaps. The tree, according to M. Feé, was altogether unknown to the ancients, and the *κωμακον* of Theophrastus and the *Cinnamomum* of Pliny have been erroneously regarded as identical with this. Avicenna seems to have been the first who described it under the name "*Jauzboa.*" The tree itself however has only been identified clearly within the last few years.

The nutmeg tree is chiefly cultivated in the Banda islands, but plantations are now numerous at the Mauritius, Bourbon, Cayenne, Martinique, and in the English possessions to the Eastward, especially in Province Wellesley of Penang—also in the Tinnevelly district of Southern India.

The natives of the Moluccas gather the nutmeg fruit by the hand, strip off and reject the pulpy pericarp, detach the mace carefully, and expose it to the sun, which soon changes its blood-red colour to a light brown, it is then sprinkled with sea-water to render it flexible, and to preserve it. The nuts are first sun-dried, and then smoked, until the kernel rattles against the shell. This envelope is then broken, and the kernels dipped twice or thrice in lime water. They are then heaped together for two or three days, wiped, and packed in bales or barrels.

The nutmegs thus prepared have been long termed, "female," or "cultivated," in commerce, to distinguish them from a kind named the "wild" or male, which is less esteemed, and seldom found in European trade.

The medicinal uses of the nutmeg are not very important, nevertheless the natives of India deem it very valuable in dyspeptic complaints, and give it to children suffering during weaning (*Ainslie*). It is doubtless a good cardiac stimulant, but in certain constitutions is apt to produce much cerebral disturbance, inducing decidedly narcotic symptoms. Dose 3 grs. to ℈i,—of the volatile oil, 2 to 8 drops in emulsion.

Sp. 2. *Myristica tomentosa.* "Male" nutmeg tree. Also a native of the Moluccas.

The fruit is larger than in the preceding species, downy, its substance fleshy, more solid, and firm. The kernel is covered by a hard shell provided with a pale arillus, the kernel is 1½ to 2 inches long, elliptical, the parenchyme devoid of marbling. Its odour is weak, flavour disagreeable. The mace of this nutmeg is distinguished from the true mace by being formed of three or four regular bands united at the summit.

The chemical composition of the article is analogous to that of the true nutmeg, but the oils are so inferior in proportion, that the "male" nutmeg is but of little commercial value.

Sp. 3. *M. Otoba* in Santa Fé, also yields aromatic nuts.

Syn. Virola sebifera, Lamarck. *Myristica sebifera.*

A large tree of Cayenne and Guiana, the seeds of which when boiled with water give out a large quantity of a fixed oil, used for making candles. An acrid juice also exudes from incisions in the bark, and is employed as a popular medicine.

NAT. ORDER CXX.—HERNANDIACEÆ.

GEN.—HERNANDIA.

Sp. Hernandia sonora.

Bongko, *Jav.* (Ainslie.)

A native of various parts of the East and West Indies.

A tall erect tree, fruit a dry drupe, calyx very large, inflated, with a small roundish mouth. The wind blowing over this aperture causes a whistling sound, whence the specific name is derived; the kernel is oily and purgative. The bark, seed, and young leaves are indeed all aperient; the fibrous roots are reputed to be an antidote to the Macassar poison. The juice of the leaves is described as a powerful depilatory, (*Lindley*). Rumphius says that in Java the root is deemed a certain antidote to poison. This of course is but an imaginary property.

NAT. ORDER CXXI.—LAURINEÆ.

This very celebrated family is much more important in a commercial and literary than in a medicinal light.

Numerous genera of this family occur in British India, especially along the base of the Himalayas.

The best account of the distinctions between its species is perhaps to be found in Lindley's analysis of the monographs by Blume and Essenbeek. But Feé, with his usual skill, gives a view of the entire, which we think it more conformable to our objects to adopt.

The laurels are trees with simple, alternate, or subalternate leaves, solitary, alternate, or tuft-like flowers, either axillary or terminal.

Volatile oil is the predominant principle in this order. It occurs in the bark, leaves, flowers, and always in the fruit, in which a fixed oil is also often present, heavier than water, and perfumed by admixture with the volatile oil. Camphor also abounds in many species; tannin, resin, and a complex proper juice are also to be enumerated as occasional constituents. The medicinal action of the laurels is generally tonic or stimulant. The elements of hydrocyanic acid exist occasionally in the leaves. The fruits of some species are edible, the pulp surrounding the seed being fleshy, and imbued with oil, as in the avocado pear.

GEN. 1.—LAURUS.

Sp. 1. *Laurus nobilis.* Sweet bay.

Δαφνη, Homer, Hesiod, Dioscorides, 1, 106. A native of the south of Europe and Asia Minor.

The leaves are dry, deep green, 1 to 2 inches long, smooth, decrepitating when burned, odour agreeable, taste rather bitter, astringent, and aromatic.

The berries are oblong, small, deep blue while fresh, brown when dry; the epidermis is very brittle; they contain two discoloured, oval, fatty seeds, odour aromatic, taste aromatic, pungent, and bitter. They also contain two oils, volatile, and fixed. The former is fragrant, very hot, and pungent to the taste; the other is greenish, and concrete, of sweet and agreeable smell.

Hub-ool-ghar is the Arabic name of the berries, which are still used in medicine in India, with the Greek name Daphne corrupted into *Zaknee* and *Zafnee*. *Royle*, p. 326.

The mythological importance of the laurel is universally known. In the religious and civic ceremonies of the Greeks and Romans, it served as an instrument of divination, and formed the crown of the warrior and poet. The title *Baccalaureatus*, or bachelor, applied in our own times to young graduates of medicine, refers to the ancient custom of crowning the successful candidate for professional honours with a chaplet of laurel leaves and berries.

Sp. 2. *Laurus Malabathrum.* (Feé.)

Syn. Cinnamonum Malabathrum, (Nees and Ebermaier.) Folia malabathri of the ancients.

Vern. Leaves, Tej pata, *Beng.* bark Sadrus, Putruj, *Hind.*

A native of the Malabar and Coromandel hills, and of the mountain ranges from Sylhet to Missouri.

A stout tall tree, the branches nearly round, the younger rough and downy, leaves oblong, lanceolate, acuminate, acute at the base, smooth, triple nerved, midrib without any lateral veins at the apex. Panicle somewhat terminating and axillary, stalked, divaricating, calyx campanulate, segments obovate, rather sharp-pointed, hoary and silky on each side, deciduous below the middle.

The leaves are oblong-pointed, 5 to 7, shining, marked with three strong nerves, pale green, the nerves run from the insertion of the petiole. The odour resembles that of cloves. The flavour is aromatic and hot.

Sp. 3. *Laurus Culilawan.*

Syn. Cinnamomum Culilawan. *Blume.*

Vern. Telakal, or Sindoc, bark Suleekhe, *Arab.* Seleeka *Mathiolus.* Selechacha, *Avicenna.* Islioos assigned as Greek name. *Royle*, p. 325.

Amboyna and the Moluccas.

The bark of this tree is an aromatic stimulant like Cassia, with some astringency and a flavour of cloves. It contains resin, volatile oil, and bitter extractive. Dose 10 grs. to ½ a drachm. The oil is used in Amboyna as a stimulating liniment.

Sp. 4. *Laurus Cinnamomum.* Cinnamon tree.

Syn. Cinnamomum zeylanicum. *Blume.*

Ceylon, Java, cultivated in various parts of the world.

Branches somewhat 4-cornered, smooth, leaves ovate or ovato-oblong, 3-nerved, flowers hoary or silky, segments oblong, deciduous in the middle, fertile stamens 9 in 3 rows, anthers 4-celled, 3 capitate, abortive stamens next the centre. Trunk 15 to 20 feet high, by 1½ feet in diameter.

This is the source of the true cinnamon, and indeed nearly all parts of the tree are of value and importance.

Off. The *bark*.

CINNAMON BARK. *Vern*. Darchinee, *Hind*.

The bark is thin like paper in the superior qualities, thick and hard when inferior, more or less cylindrical, pale-brown or russet-coloured; in the parcels sold in the shops each consists of several pieces, the smaller being enclosed within the larger cylinders.

The odour and taste of cinnamon are too well known to render any attempt at description necessary. The powder is of dun colour.

The parcels are sometimes mixed with cinnamon from which the volatile oil has been removed by distillation; barks of allied but inferior species are also mixed with the true kind.

On analysis the best bark yields a very acrid and caustic volatile oil, tannic acid in large quantity, azotized colouring matter, a peculiar acid, mucilage, and starch.

Essential Oil.

Colour yellowish, white while fresh, soon however passing to a ruddy yellow; fluid, excessively hot and pungent, heavier than water, sp. gr. 1,035. On keeping it deposits crystals of camphor.

The pieces of bark too small to be packed are collected carefully for the distillation of the essential oil, so highly valued in Europe. For this purpose two alembics are employed, one of 800, the other of 360 lbs. The bark is powdered, macerated for 24 hours, and then 125 seers of the powder are distilled with 15 seers of common salt for the large apparatus; 125 seers of bark yield about 700 scruples of oil.

According to the Ceylon distillers, one part of the distilled oil sinks, and the other floats on water; both products are in equal quantity, and are mixed; about 400 bottles of oil are thus prepared annually for the European market.

From the leaves an oil is obtained which more resembles that of cloves than of cinnamon, and which is sold by traders as "oil of cloves."

Cinnamon bark is very much used in pharmacy as a gentle stimulant, and to communicate an agreeable flavour to numerous medicinal preparations; its dietetic and popular uses require no comment.

Cinnamon constitutes the chief object of commerce for Ceylon, the produce of which still surpasses in excellence the growth of any other locality. The tree occurs only in the South and East of Ceylon between Matura and Negambo, in a space of about 14 leagues, called the *Cinnamon Gardens*. The soil is of fine quartzose sand, the tree springing up more quickly, but the bark degenerating in quality in soils of a richer kind. The trees flower in February or March, but continue in verdure all the year. At the age of seven years they are about seven feet high, and may then be barked, but this operation should not be performed before the young tree is half an inch in diameter, and not after it has surpassed 1½ inch.

According to Thunberg, the *barkers* constitute a distinct caste called Chalias.* They enjoy peculiar immunities, and to them is intrusted the decision on the fit state of the tree; they test this by dividing the bark with a knife. If readily removed, the tree is then cut down. The trees from which the bark is not freely removeable are used for the distillation of the volatile oil.

The decortication takes place after the rains, and occurs twice annually from April to August, and from November to January. According to the size of the branches two or three longitudinal incisions are made, by which the strips of bark are easily removed. The strips are placed one above the other in parcels eight or ten inches thick, and allowed to remain for 24 hours. A slight fermentation ensues, which facilitates the separation of the external pellicle, or epidermis, and of the green part of the bark, of which the first layer of the liber is preserved. This is finally rolled longitudinally into cylinders, about three feet long, the pieces are arranged one within the other, and they are then dried on clay, first in the shade, subsequently before the sun. The barks when quite dry are sorted and packed in bales of about 80lbs. each. The entire harvest is stated not to exceed 5000 bales; when embarked, the bales are packed with black pepper in the interstices, by which it is said that damp is absorbed, and the flavour of the cinnamon preserved.

The Ceylonese distinguish several kinds of cinnamon trees under the following names:—

Kasse Couroundou, Honey cinnamon; Nai Cour, serpent cin.; Capoor Cor,; Camphor cin.; Canatta coround, or astringent cinnamon. These are merely casual varieties, and do not constitute separate species.

* From *Chawl*, bark, *Sans*.

The name of cinnamon is also applied in Ceylon to—1. a mucilaginous, soft, thready, rough, difficultly separable bark, called Souvel Couroundou; 2. to a flat bark, Davoul Couroundou; 3. to a hard fibrous bark, Nica Couroundou.

The wood is used for fuel, and for some articles of furniture; the roots are said to contain a large quantity of camphor.

The cinnamon tree has been introduced into Sicily, the Cape de Verd Islands, Brazil, the Mauritius, Pondicherry, Guadaloupe, St. Vincents, and Cayenne; the produce of the last localty being deemed superior to all the others, except the Ceylon. Loureiro states that cinnamon is also a product of Cochin China, and that it is superior to the Ceylonese kind. It has likewise been grown in Cairo with success.

Two varieties of cinnamon are known in commerce.

The 1st. embraces that of Ceylon and Cayenne, to which the preceding description applies.

The 2d. Chinese cinnamon, of far inferior value, and often smelling most distinctly of bugs.

A third species should be perhaps mentioned, the Mato cinnamon of the Portuguese, (Canella mata or plata) the wild canella of the Dutch, and Kapoor Couroundou of the Ceylonese. This Feé considers to be the bark of the large branches and trunk of the cinnamon tree, grown in all sorts of soils and localities.

In French the terms *Canelle* or *Canella* are applied to cinnamon, as well as to the—

Canella alba, Nat. Order, ...	Guttiferæ.
Canella caryophyllata, ...	Myrteæ.
Canella piperita, and / Canella falsa, ... }	Euphorbiaceæ.

Fruit. Cinnamon Wax.

The fruit is an ovoid drupe, like a small gland, half an inch long, containing a greenish pulp, and a nut with a reddish kernel; this yields essential oil, and by strong decoction a concrete oil called cinnamon wax, which is used for candles, and which exhales while burning a most delicious odour.

In addition to all these products the roots yields a pure, very volatile camphor, highly esteemed in Ceylon.

Medical uses. These are of but little importance. Cinnamon and cassia in small quantities yield to water infusions of very grateful flavour, and much used to cover the taste of disagreeable remedies. The distilled water of cinnamon is much used for the same object, (see essential oil and distilled water, *Pharmacopœia.*)

Sp. 5. ***Laurus Cassia.***

Syn. Cinnamomum albiflorum, Nees. Cassia lignea. Κιναμωμον and Κασσια, Hip. Κασσια, Dioscorid.

Malabar, Sumatra, Java, bark red brown, in fragments of a foot and longer, sometimes in plane pieces a line in thickness, and of variable width, or in rolled smooth pieces with a greyish epidermis covered with lichens, chiefly *graphides* and *lecanora.* Hard, inflexible, and with plane fracture.

Odour aromatic, agreeable, but weaker than the true cinnamon. Taste sweetish, mucilaginous, rather acrid, bitterish, and tenacious; powder of chamois leather colour.

The valuable properties of this bark, depend on its essential oil.

Cassia bark is much used for adulterating true cinnamon; it may be distinguished at once, by its very mucilaginous character when chewed.

Although we have followed M. Feé in placing the name of a separate species to this article, we agree with the opinion of Mr. Marshall, that cassia bark is merely an inferior kind of cinnamon, obtained from the larger branches and trunk of the true tree. Mr. Marshall's long residence in Ceylon, and his close habits of observation, entitle us to regard his opinion with full confidence.

Under this article M. Feé enters into a long and interesting discussion as to the nature of the plants yielding the Κασσια and Κιννᾳμωμον of Dioscorides, Pliny, and Theophrastus. All these writers describe the tree alleged to yield these products, and assign Ethiopia and Arabia as their localities. M. Feé shews that the descriptions do not correspond to any of the proved cinnamons, and that the localities are equally inapplicable. He therefore inclines to the belief that the cassia and cinnamon of these old writers refer to the products of an *Amyris.* We believe however that the actual barks were known to Theophrastus, but that he described the trees and localities on the deceptive data collected from the Syrian merchants, by whom the traffic in drugs was then nearly monopolized.

Lindley in his analysis of Nees and Blume's monographs, gives Cin. zeylanicum, *var.* Cassia, as the synonyme of Cassia lignea, and states it is naturalized on the continent of India. We have been favoured by Dr. Wallich with specimens of bark from Upper Assam, which in all physical characters correspond exactly with the cassia of the shops.

Lindley includes all these articles in the genus Cinnamomum, of which he gives twelve species.

C. zeylanicum,	.. Ceylon, ..	.. True cinnamon.
C. zeylan var. Cassia,	India, ..	.. Cassia lignea.
C. aromaticum,	.. China, ..	.. Source of Chinese cinnamon according to Nees.
C. Tamala, ..	.. India, ..	.. Tej-pat leaves, or Folia Malabathri of Indian shops.
C. Loureirii,	.. Cochin China,	.. Flowers of Cassia, and a very inferior cinnamon.
C. Kiamis, ..	.. Ditto, ..	.. Said to produce one kind of Massoy bark.
C. Culilawan,	.. Amboyna, ..	.. Culilawan bark.
C. rubrum,	.. Cochin China,	.. Similar to last.
C. Sintoc, ..	.. Neelgherries,	.. Similar, but more bitter.
C. xanthoneuron,	Moluccas, ..	.. Similar, but extremely like Massoy bark.
C. nitidum,	.. India, Java, Ceylon,	Furnished the greater part of the old "Folia Malabathri."
C. javanicum,	.. Java and Borneo,	Bitter and aromatic bark, strongly recommended by Blume in spasmodic colic, and the after-pains of labour.

Sp. Laurus Sassafras. Sassafras.
Syn. Sassafras officinale, *Nees.*
Off. Wood.

A native of North America, from Canada to Florida. The wood and roots occur in billets, the size of the arm or thigh, covered with a bark grey externally, rust-coloured within, substance yellowish, porous, light, and brittle. The dried leaves contain so much mucilage that they are used for thickening soup.

Odour strong, agreeable, resembling fennel seed, flavour aromatic, powder pale yellow. Sassafras owes its properties to the essential oil, which is yellow, highly fragrant, limpid, acrid, heavier than water; 125 parts of the wood yield one of the oil; by time the colour reddens, and crystals of camphor are deposited.

The infusion of sassafras is intensely red, and this and the decoction are blackened by the sulphate of iron.

The bark is far preferable to the wood, being richer in essential oil; it occurs in fragments, sometimes in thick pieces, covered with grey epidermis, sometimes as if rusted, with little crystals in its substance, highly aromatic both to smell and taste.

M. Guibourt mentions two other kinds of sassafras, one the *Massoy*, of which we will speak under the head of the *Ocotea Pichurim;* the second, a sassafras of Orinoco, produced by the *Ocotea Cymbarum.*

We are indebted to Dr. Wallich for specimens of the bark of the Nipal sassafras, described in the Transactions of the Medical and Physical Society.

This bark corresponds precisely in appearance, chemical properties, odour, and stimulating effects, with the sassafras bark of European pharmacy.

This is perhaps the bark of the Camphora glandulifera, Nipal. (*Royle*, p. 324).

Sp. 7. *Laurus Camphora.*

Syn. Camphora officinarum, *Nees.* Japan.

Trunk lofty, wood white, damasked with reddish waves, of aromatic odour, leaves alternate, oval, acute, shining, entire, 3-nerved, flowers small and white, disposed in small axillary clusters, fruit a drupe, the size of a pea, single seeded, blackish, surrounded at its base by the truncated calyx.

To this tree it is that the camphor of European commerce is chiefly due.

JAPAN OR FORMOSA CAMPHOR.

Impure camphor of the shops. *Vern.* Kupoor, *Hind.*

Concrete, grey, granular, moist, more or less impure, full of heterogeneous particles.

Or in white, transparent, homogeneous, brittle, smooth, compressible, crystalline loaves. Sp. gr. 0.9887.

The odour of this camphor is very penetrating, taste hot and bitter like peppermint. The weight sensibly decreases by keeping, owing to evaporation.

This camphor is insoluble in water, soluble in alcohol, ether, fixed and volatile oils, and several acids, readily volatile and very inflammable, and burns without residue or blackening, though it emits dense smoke.

Camphor has been manufactured in Spain from several Labiatæ, and has been prepared artificially by passing a current of muriatic acid gas through turpentine; this last variety however has not been used in medicine.

Camphor is not mentioned by the ancient writers; it was introduced into Europe about six centuries since, but it was previously known to the Arabs. The camphor tree has been successfully cultivated in Europe, and Feé mentions one at Malmaison, which we have ourselves seen, over 20 feet high by 6 inches in diameter.

To obtain the camphor, the wood is cut into billets and boiled in water, in iron pots covered with earthenware heads filled with straw; the camphor volatilizes and concretes on the straw. This process is followed in Japan, Sumatra, Borneo, and Malacca.

To purify the camphor it is introduced into a subliming vessel with one-fiftieth its weight of quicklime, to retain some oil with which it is contaminated, and heat is gently applied by a sand bath. Two Kedgeree pots luted together answer perfectly, a very small aperture being left for the escape of air on the first application of heat.

Camphor wood is considered valuable for the construction of chests and almirahs, as its powerful odour protects the contents from the ravages of white ants and other insects.

Medical properties. A valuable stimulant, especially in typhoid fevers—in large doses narcotic,—also much used as an external application. (See *Camphor mixture* and *liniment*, Pharmacopœia.)

Feé here describes the *Dryabalanops camphora*, which is not a *laurel*, but belongs to the Dipterocarpi. (See page 220.)

Gen. 2.—Ocotea.

Sp. O. Pichurim.

Species of Ocotea extend from Sylhet to Deyra Dhoon, and ascend to 7000 feet. The fruit would be worth examination.

The isolated lobes of the drupe (*sassafras nuts* or *pichurim beans* of the shops) are oval, oblong, obtuse at both ends, concave at one side, convex at the other, entirely glabrous, a little wrinkled, olive-brown, an inch long; two of these placed together constitute the entire fruit, except the pericarpial envelope. The substance is solid, flesh-coloured, and marbled, the odour is strong, resembling a mixture of pepper and camphor, taste aromatic, slightly bitter; the volatile principle often sublimes from the nut, and concretes on the interior of the containing vessel. This principle seems to be of an acrid nature.

500 parts of the kernel, according to Bonastre, afford concrete volatile 15, fixed oil 50, stearine 110, glutinous resin 15, brown colouring matter 40, fecula 55, soluble gum 60, gum like tragacanth 6, acid and sugar 6, parenchyme, 100, moisture 36, loss 6, saline matter 7.

In Venezuela and Portugal the pichurim bean is deemed febrifuge and astringent, the oil is said to be converted into a pleasant substitute for chocolate. A pichurim bark has been described by Murray, but its source is not accurately known; it is described as being of most delicious flavour, and a valuable febrifuge and tonic.

Bark of Doubtful Origin.

Massoy Bark.

This bark is light, soft to the touch, in long, convex fragments, covered with an epidermis of whitish grey colour, with numerous lichens, internally reddish, tissue rather spongy, brittle, fracture irregular, thickness not surpassing two lines.

Taste pungent, bitter, and peppery, odour strongly that of sassafras, with a trace of nutmeg.

The Indians attribute tonic properties to this bark; it is rich in essential oil, and proceeds from a lofty and robust tree, very common in New Guinea and in Java. M. Guibourt has detected in this bark the volatile substance previously observed in the Pichurim bean.

Feé adds to the preceding articles brief notices of two more species of *Ocotea*, and three of *Litsea*, but their properties are not of material importance.

Gen. 3.—Caryodaphne.

C. densiflora, Blume. Java.

Kiteja. A tree 60 to 80 feet high, leaves gratefully aromatic, used in infusion like tea against spasms of the bowels, and in puerperal convulsions.

Gen. 4.—Mespilodaphne.

M. pretiosa. Woods near Para.

Inner bark and rind of the calyx very fragrant, resembling cinnamon and bergamot.

Gen. 5.—Nectandra.

N. cymbarum. Nees. Oronoko sassafras.

A tree 100 feet high, bark aromatic, bitter, and stomachic.

N. cinnamoides. Bark resembles cinnamon. New Grenada.

N. Pachury major. Nees.

See *Ocotea*, in preceding page.

Martius assigns the pichurim beans to this plant. They are used in dysentery, diarrhœa, strangury, &c. The *N. Pachury minor*, according to Humboldt, is the source of the sassafras nuts of the London shops.

GEN. 6.—OREODAPHNE.

O. opifera, Nees. Para.
Yields a volatile oil, smelling of orange peel and rosemary, used as a stimulating liniment.

O. cupularis, is the cinnamon of the Mauritius.

GEN. 7.—BENZOIN.

B. odoriferum. Nees.
Syn. Laurus Benzoin, *Linn.*
Oil of the berries aromatic, bark highly stimulant, and tonic.

B. neesianum. Nipal berries, smell of cajeput oil.
A bush 8—10 feet high, bark highly aromatic and tonic, infusion of twigs vermifuge, berries yield aromatic oil. The name Benzoin has been applied to this genus from its strong odour of Benjamin, but it is not to be mistaken for a source of that article.

GEN. 8.—TETRANTHERA.

Flowers diœcious, some hermaphrodite, involucrated calyx 6-parted, segments nearly equal, deciduous, or wanting, or only 3—4—5, and those small and petaloid, fertile stamens in the 6-cleft flowers 9, in 3 rows, in the petaloid or naked flowers, 12, 15, 21, anthers ovate, 4-celled, sterile stamens 6 glandlike, attached in pairs to the three interior stamens, stigma peltate. Fruit a berry, leaves variable, with pinnate veins. (*Lindley.*)

Sp. T. Roxburghii, Nees.
Syn. Sebifera glutinosa, *Loureiro.* Litsea sebifera, *Pers.* Tetranthera apetala, Roxb. Corom. Pl. t. 147. and Fl. Ind. iii. p. 819.
Mountains of India.
A variable plant, leaves oval oblong, smooth above, downy beneath, umbels white, fruit globose, black, size of a pea, yields a greasy concrete oil used for making candles by the Chinese, also for ointments. Leaves and branches glutinous, and communicate this property by bruising to water.
The wood is the *mueda lukree* of the Hindostanee druggists, and a favourite application to bruises and wounds. It is somewhat fragrant, and slightly balsamic and sweet.

NAT. ORDER CXXII.—EUPHORBIACEÆ.

The Euphorbiaceæ are herbaceous, frutescent, or arborescent plants, generally milky, with alternate or opposite leaves, stipulate or naked. The order is exceedingly numerous in species; it conforms fully to analogical laws; with few exceptions its species are violent poisons, owing their irritating properties to the presence of an acrid, and generally volatile principle existing abundantly in all parts of the vegetable. This principle is combined with starch in the roots of the Tapioca plant, *(Jatropha Manihot)* with fixed oil in the seeds of the Euphorbia, Crotons *(Jumalgotta)*, and Ricini (castor oil plants), with caoutchouc in the proper juice of the stems of many species, with essential oil in some barks, and in the wood of cascarilla and aloes wood. A few seeds are edible, but still unwholesome or dangerous.

The active principle is very volatile; it was once supposed to reside only in the embryo of the seed, but conclusive experiments have disproved this idea, at least as to the seeds which furnish the castor oil. Still the volatile matter has not yet been procured in a state of perfect purity.

The important principle *Caoutchouc* will demand a special notice, in the sequel of this article.

The essential oil and resin are but rare in this order, and gum still less frequent. The "Euphorbium" of pharmacy is not, as it is commonly termed, a gum resin, but a peculiar substance, the nature of which we shall subsequently explain.

On the whole the group is perhaps the most formidable of the vegetable kingdom, considering the immense number of its species, and the virulence of their effects. Even in the smallest doses many of these vegetables produce frightful purging and vomiting; six drops of croton oil, or 35 drops of the juice of the tapioca root, suffice to occasion fatal symptoms, indeed the last poison has in the dose above mentioned destroyed a robust man in five minutes. The Euphorbium and the Manchineel are equally powerful. Hence in administering the products of this family for medicinal purposes, the utmost caution is essential.

The general history of the order has been most successfully investigated by Adrien de Jussieu and Feé, the former of whom in arrangement Lindley pretty closely follows.

With respect to geographical distribution, the Euphorbiaceæ are chiefly found in tropical countries, especially in America and Asia. The Indian species are understood to be over 400 in number, several being found in lofty mountainous situations. The whole family certainly includes over 1500 species.

The general aspect of the order is exceedingly variable, from lofty trees to diminutive herbs, and occasionally presenting "deformed, leafless, succulent plants resembling the cacti, but in appearance only. (*Lindley*.)"

Gen. Char.—Flowers monœcious or diœcious, calyx lobed, inferior, with glandular or scaly internal appendages (sometimes wanting). *Male*—stamens indefinite or definite, distinct or monadelphous, anthers 2-celled. *Female*—ovarium superior, sessile or stalked, 2, 3, or more celled, ovules solitary or twin, suspended from the inner angle of the cell. Styles equal in number to the cells, distinct, combined, or even absent. Stigma compound or simple, with several lobes, fruit consisting of two, three, or more dehiscent cells, separating with elasticity from their common axis, seeds solitary or twin, suspended, with an arillus, embryo enclosed in a fleshy albumen, cotyledons flat, radicles superior. (*Lindley*.)

GEN. 1.—BUXUS.

Sp. Buxus sempervirens. Evergreen box. Πυξος, Theophrastus. South of Europe.

Leaves opposite, oval, oblong, smooth, and coriaceous, single nerved, of decided odour, especially after rain.

Wood solid, hard, heavy, of pale yellow colour, insipid and inodorous. Distilled by the open fire it affords an empyreumatic oil. The alcoholic extract is slightly bitter, and has been used as a substitute for guaiacum without satisfactory results. The tincture has long been a popular febrifuge in Germany. The secret of its preparation was purchased from a quack by Joseph II., for 1500 florins.

The leaves are sometimes used for the adulteration of senna, but are readily detected by their thickness. They are said to prove poisonous to camels.

Box is chiefly important however as affording the best wood for blocks for the wood engraver, whose art is now brought to such exquisite perfection. Box is also preferred for scales, and supports for mathematical instruments, on account of its being but little affected by change of temperature, or the degree of moisture and dryness of the air.

Mr. Royle states that a true species of box is common in the Himalayas, found chiefly in vallies as at Mugra, near Khalsee, and in Kemaon.*

* We have seen large blocks of excellent box wood brought by Captain Vicary from Kemnour, in the possession of Dr. Wallich.

Gen. 2.—Cicca.

Sp. C. disticha, Linn.

Syn. Phyllanthus longifolia, Jacquin. *Roxb. Fl. Ind.* iii. p. 672.

Vern. Cheramella, or Huriphul, *Beng.* Hurfarori, Chelmeri, *Hind.*

Fruit subacid, universally used as an article of food, raw or cooked, or in pickles or preserves.

Leaves sudorific, seeds cathartic.

Gen. 3.—Emblica.

Sp. E. officinalis, Gaertner.

Syn. Phyllanthus Emblica, *Linn.*

Μυραβαλανος εμβλικα. Arctuar, 1. 24.

Nilicamaram, *Rheede.*

Vern. Amlaki, Umriti, *Sans.* Amla, Anola, *Beng.*, *Hind.* Nellie-kai, *Tam.* Userekee, *Tel.*

Tree crooked, thick as a man's body, leaves pinnate, flower-bearing, flowers minute, greenish yellow; male flowers very numerous in axils of lower leaves, anthers 3 to 5; female flowers few, solitary, sessile, stigmas 3, 2, cleft.

Bark strongly astringent, used for tanning, and in diarrhœa.

Fruits while fresh round, the size of a gall nut, with six valves projecting externally, pulp fleshy, enveloping white and angular seeds. When dry roundish, blackish grey, very wrinkled, sub-hexagonal; the dried pericarp is applied to a trilocular nut, and each cell contains two red shining seeds. Odour slightly aromatic; taste acidulous, acid, astringent; in the recent state this myrobalon is very acid and somewhat purgative; when dry chiefly astringent. It is used for tanning leather, and as a remedy in diarrhœas.

An interesting account of its efficacy in the treatment of the Nusseerabad scurvy is given by Dr. McNab, in the Quarterly Journal of the Medical Society of Calcutta.

Gen. 4.—Phyllanthus.

Sp. 1. *P. Niruri.* Native of the East Indies.

Vern. Sadee hazur munee, *Hind.* and *Beng.* Nella userekee, *Tel.* a common weed.

Annual, erect, leaflets oval, flowers axillary, capsules smooth, 3-celled, 6-seeded.

According to many writers the root is bitter and astringent, and a powerful diuretic. *P. urinaria*, (hazar munee, yerra userekee,) East Indies and Bourbon, is of similar properties, and used in several maladies; flowers sessile, capsules dull, scabrous, young plants deeply dark red.

Sp. 2. *P. simplex*, Retz. Roxb. iii. p. 654.
Oochie userekee, *Tel.*

Fresh leaves, flowers, and fruit, with cummin seeds and sugar are made into an electuary, and given by the natives as a remedy for gonorrhœa; fresh leaves bruised with buttermilk are used to cure the itch. *Roxb.*

Gen. 5.—Flüggea.

Sp. F. virosa, Hamilton.
Syn. Phyllanthus virosus, *Roxb.* p. 659.

A middle sized tree in the Circar mountains, a large shrub in the plains; bark a strong astringent, intoxicates fish if thrown into the waters they inhabit.

Gen. 6.—Cluytia.

Sp. C. collina, Roxb.
Vern. Kadishen, *Tel.* Flowers in hot season, seed ripens in December and January.

Flowers diœcious, calyx five-parted, petals five, stamens five, capsule three-celled, three-seeded. *Roxb.* p. 732.

Bark or outer crust of capsule said to be exceedingly poisonous.

Gen. 7.—Briedelia.

Sp. B. spinosa. Roxb. p. 735.
Vern. Kora man, *Tel.* Large tree, a native of the Circars, and Bengal. Berry small and globular. Bark a strong astringent, said to be vermifuge for cattle.

Gen. 8.—Croton.

Sp. 1. *Croton Cascarilla.* Cascarilla.
Off. The *bark.*

Bahama, Saint Domingo, Brazil. Aromatic Peruvian bark, Cortex eleutherii.

In short, rolled fragments, thin, very hard, brittle, of resinous brown fracture, with an ash-grey epidermis, or whitish according to the lichens which occupy it, colour deeper internally, odour aromatic and agreeable, especially on burning, when it resembles musk; taste aromatic, hot, acrid, and bitter, powder brown grey.

According to Tromsdorf this bark contains mucilage and bitter principle 108, resin 86, ethereal oil 9, fibre 383, water 6 in 592 parts. Benzoic acid has been traced in the bark by other chemists, but the analysis of Tromsdorf is generally considered to be incomplete.

The cascarilla bark is an important tonic, aromatic, and febrifuge, and is used with decided benefit in intermittents, and in all fevers during the collapse or typhoid state—*dose* 10 grs. to ʒi. It is burned as a perfume.

Cascarilla is imported from America, especially from Paraguay. The bark was known in Germany in 1690. Linnæus considered the tree to be a Cluytia; it is now placed in the genus Croton under the specific name of Eleuthera, from that of the island where the tree is very common. At a later date, Linnæus believed the tree to be the Croton cascarilla.

Sp. 2. *C. lacciferum.*

Syn. Aleuritis laccifera, *Willd.*

Trunk arborescent, with rude and angular branches, oval, dentate, petioled, downy leaves; with flowers disposed in terminal spikes, fruits small, round, and velvety, seeds solitary in each cell.

A lac of very superior quality is formed on this tree in Ceylon.

Sp. 3. *C. Tiglium.* Croton oil tree. *Roxb.* iii. p. 583.

Vern. Jamalghota, *Hind.* Jayapala, *Sans.* Dund, *Pers. Arab.*

Off. The seeds and oil.

A small tree from 15 to 20 feet high, flowers in the Botanic Garden the greater part of the year.

Trunk crooked, as thick as a man's thigh, bark smooth, ash-coloured, wood white and hard, branches rather thin, leaves alternate, petioled, ovate, cordate, slightly serrate, quilly, smooth, three to five inches long, two to three broad, racemes terminal, erect; male flowers above and numerous; female flowers single, situated on lower part of the raceme. Male calyx five-parted, petals five oblong, very woolly on one side and margin, filaments 15 to 20 distinct, woolly towards the base; female calyx as the male; corolla none.

The seeds have scarcely any sensible odour, the taste is acrid, burning, and nauseous.

Seeds subquadrangular, with yellowish epidermis dappled with brown; if of one colour they are black and smooth; the umbilical side has several longitudinal nerves, the lateral nerves form two projections near the base of the seed. In length these seeds do not exceed half an inch. When one of the three seeds happens to be abortive, the two fruitful seeds pressed against each other have the form of coffee, and present in the middle a distinct lateral impression.

Several analyses have been made of these formidable seeds. That by Brande is most conformable to the results of our own experiments; he detected volatile oil, a peculiar volatile acid (crotonic), an alkaline matter, crotonine, colouring principle, stearine, wax, resin, inulin, gum, gluten, albumen, starch, and inorganic saline matters.

All parts of this croton are drastic and dangerous cathartics. The wood is used in minute doses in the Moluccas, as a powerful purgative, (Lignum Panave or Pavane). It is light pale, covered with a greyish bark.

The acid is acrid and volatile, still it is not the only active principle in the oil. It is volatile below zero, emitting an intensely acrid vapour. When the oil is saponified, an additional quantity of this acid is formed.

Besides this another volatile matter is disengaged by heat, which cannot be acid as it passes through a solution of potash.

Crotonine is considered by Soubeiran to be a compound of magnesia with a fatty acid.

Croton Oil.

This oil is an exceedingly powerful cathartic, a single drop generally producing liquid evacuations within an hour.

The oil is orange yellow, is soluble in alcohol, and reddens litmus paper powerfully. It contains 45 parts of acrid acid, combined with 55 of bland oil.

During the preparation of the oil, it is very difficult to avoid the irritating effects of the acrid volatile matter, which causes an eruption of large painful pustules.

Croton oil is prepared by grinding the seeds, placing the powder in bags, and pressing between plates of iron; allow the oil to stand for 15 days—then filter. The residue of the expression is triturated with twice its weight of alcohol and heated on the sand bath from 120° to 140° Faht. and the mixture pressed again. In this step the utmost caution is necessary in avoiding the acrid fumes. The alcohol is distilled off, the oil allowed to settle, and filtered after a fortnight.

One seer of seed furnished Soubeiran by this process rather more than eleven fluid ounces of oil, six by the first step, and five by alcohol.

The oil obtained in the second step, contains resin, but Piedagnel has proved that in medicinal effects both products are alike.

Med. effects. Croton oil is one of the most violent cathartics we possess, one to two drops often causing within half an hour copious watery evacuations. It is an invaluable remedy in apoplexy and similar disorders where immediate cathartic action is requisite, and the swallowing of bulky medicines impracticable. Applied externally to the skin it causes an eruption of very painful pustules like those caused by tartar emetic ointment.

Sp. 4. *C. tinctorium,* Turnsol.
Syn. Crozophora tinctoria, *Jussieu* and *Lind.*
Ηηλιοτροπον μικρον. Dioscor. Europe.
Plant acrid, with emetic and drastic properties; powdered seeds mixed with oil used as a cathartic.
The summits of this plant and the fruits serve for the preparation of the dye named turnsol, used for giving a blue and red tint.

Sp. 5. *Croton Roxburghii,* Wall.
Syn. Croton polyandrum.* *Roxb.* iii. p. 682.
Vern. Hakoon, *Hind.* Konda amadum, *Tel.*
Perennial, native of Circar hills, seeds exactly like those of the castor oil plant, but much smaller.
Esteemed by the natives to be a good purgative, one seed bruised with water being given for each evacuation desired. (*Roxb.*)
It is very common on the banks of the Jumna, where it is called Jamalghota. (*Royle.*)
Feé also enumerates the following species—
1. *Cr. balsamiferum,* a Jamaica shrub, very aromatic, affording on distillation the liqueur termed " Eau de mantes". A thick yellowish and balsamic juice flows from the branches.
2. *C. sebiferum.* (Stillingia sebifera, *Michaux.* Sapium sebiferum. *Roxb.* vol. iii. p. 693), seeds covered with a waxy substance used in China for making candles; now common in gardens round Calcutta.
3. *C. thuriferum,* South America, affords a balsamic juic like frankincense.
4. *C. sanguifluum,* furnishes a product strongly resembling Dragon's blood (Damulukwain.)
5. *C. coriaceum.* Bark very aromatic when burned, alcoholic extract also exhales while burning a delicious odour.

Gen. 9.—Ricinus.

Flowers monœcious, calyx 3, 5-parted, valvate, petals none, ♀-filaments numerous, unequally polyadelphous, cells of the

* Not the *Cr. polyandrum* of Sprengel.

anthers distinct, below the apex of the filaments—style short, stigmas 3, deeply bipartite, oblong, coloured, feathery, ovary globose, 3-celled, with an ovule in each cell. Fruit generally milky, capsular, tricoccous. Trees, shrubs, or herbaceous plants, sometimes becoming arborescent, leaves alternate, stipulate, palmate, peltate, with glands at the apex of the petiole. Flowers in terminal panicles; lower male, upper female, all articulated with their peduncles, and sometimes augmented by biglandular bracts. (*Lindley.*)

Several varieties are cultivated in India; some attain the size of a pretty large tree, and are of many years' duration.

Sp. Ricinus communis. Castor oil plant. *Roxb.* iii. 689.

Vern. Eranda, *Sans.* Amadum. *Tel.* Arendi, *Hind.* Arindi, Bherenda, *Beng.*

Syn. Palma Christi, Cataputia Major, Αλχερνα, *Arab.* Κροτων, Hippocr. Κικι, Egyptian.

Fruits glaucous, capsules partially rounded, thorny, of middling hardness, with 3-monospermous cells, indicated by three projections externally.

Seeds oval, obtuse at both ends, the size of a large haricot, compressed, shining, convex superiorly, more flattened below, marked with an evident ridge, rather angular, marbled with little brown points, or incomplete and interrupted red lines, the seed is moreover carunculate, the kernel is covered with a sheath and a separable integument, the former being dry, brittle, insipid, of middling thickness; on removing these integuments we find a very oily and beautifully foliaceous kernel. The seeds are inodorous, taste sweetish at first, then acrid; the seed grows very speedily rancid, and then yields an acrid irritating oil.

CASTOR OIL. (*Vern.* Arendi-ke-tel, *Hind.*)

White or slightly yellowish, thick, viscous, difficultly congealable, specific gravity greater than that of any other fixed oil, soluble in alcohol. Taste and smell like those of the seeds, becomes readily rancid; the oil is then considered dangerous; often adulterated with other fixed oils, which may be detected by their insolubility in alcohol.

On distillation castor oil gives two-thirds its weight of solid residue—a volatile oil very transparent and colourless, and liable to crystallize on cooling—and three fatty acids which are very acrid and soluble in alcohol, and called the ricinic, oleo-ricinic, and stearo-ricinic acids.

Castor oil is very commonly used as a purgative, and is employed in lamps in America and many parts of India.

Three modes of extraction are particularly employed—1. boiling in water; 2. expression; 3. extraction by alcohol.

In the 1st, the seeds are slightly toasted to coagulate the albumen, cleaned of the integuments, bruised in a mortar, and the paste boiled in pure water. The oil which occurs on the surface is removed and treated with an additional quantity of fresh water; 10,000 parts of clean seeds give by this process (in Jamaica) 3.250 of oil of good quality, though amber coloured.

2. Expression is the simplest and most usually adopted process; the cleaned kernels are well bruised, placed in cloth bags, and compressed in a powerful lever and screw press. A thick oil is obtained, which must be filtered through cloth and paper to separate its mucilage. In Bengal the manufacturers boil the oil with water which coagulates some albumen, and they subsequently filter through cloth, charcoal, and paper.

3. The extraction by alcohol is practised by some druggists. Each pound of paste is triturated with 4 pounds of alcohol, sp. gr. 835°, and the mixture subjected to pressure. The oil dissolved by the alcohol escapes very freely, one-half is recovered by the distillation of the spirit. The residue of the distillation is boiled in a large quantity of water. The oil separates and is removed, and gently heated to expel any adherent moisture, then filtered at the temperature of 90° Fahr.—1000 parts of paste have by this process given 625 of colourless and exceedingly sweet oil. M. Feé describes this process as the easiest of all, and as giving more satisfactory results than any other.

It was long believed that the embryo was the source of the acridity of the oil. M. Guibourt contends however that the embryo possesses no distinct properties, and the experiments of M. Henry and Charlard are indeed quite conclusive on the point. Boiling is however universally believed to increase the acridity of the oil.

Several species of Ricinus are mentioned by Feé as yielding a castor oil of excellent quality.

Castor oil is an admirable purgative, especially in old persons or very young children; the dose is from a tea spoonful to an ounce, according to circumstances of age, disease, &c. It is often prescribed with laudanum in colics. With half its weight of turpentine it makes a very brisk but mild cathartic, especially suitable for apoplectic cases, and those of obstinate constipation.

GEN. 10.—JATROPHA.

Gen. character. Flowers monœcious, calyx 5-parted or lobed, corolla 5-parted or none. ♂ stamens 8 to 10, with unequal monadelphous filaments. ♀ styles two, bifid, or dichotomous, capsule tricoccous. *Roxb. Fl. Ind.* iii. 686.

Sp. Jatropha Curcas. Physic nut.

Vern. Bag Barendee, *Beng.* Napatain, *Tel.*

New Andalusia, Havanna, India. Fruit oval, size of a small nut, yellow or blackish, containing three whitish bivalve, monospermous seeds.

Seeds oval, size of a small bean (about eight lines long) smooth, blackish, convex on one side and plane on the other, both faces shewing a slight prominence. The lorica and tegmen separable; the internal tegmen is hard, brittle, with resinous and brownish fracture; the almond is white, foliaceous, covered with a thin membrane. Inodorous, taste agreeable, almond-like, afterwards acrid. It renders the saliva emulsive, and irritates the fauces extremely.

Leaves warmed and rubbed with castor oil are used as a poultice to hasten suppuration. The oil is chiefly used for lamps; seed excessively drastic.

The milky juice boiled with oxide of iron makes a fine black varnish.

The same idea exists as to the acridity of the castor oil, namely, that the embryo is the source of this quality, and that by removing the embryo the nut becomes bland and alimentary; MM. Feé and Humboldt support this opinion. The physic nut is a powerful cathartic, one seed, or three or four drops of the expressed oil, being a sufficient dose.

Curcas is an Indian name. Nearly all the Jatrophæ are powerful cathartics. Feé cites *J. gossypifolia*, America, *J. glandulosa*, Arabia, and the *J. multifida*, or coral plant, (Avellana purgatrix, *grand ben purgatif)* a native of America and India, a shrub 8 or 10 feet high, replete with acrid bitter juice, with large pinnatifid glabrous leaves, the fruits slightly pyriform, about the size of a nutmeg; a single seed is said to be purgative. Lindley says it is "one of the best of the emetics and purgatives, acting briskly without inconvenience, and the effects readily allayed by a glass of white wine." We still consider it a very dangerous article.

Jatropha glauca, (Ainslie); seeds yield a stimulating oil, used as an external counter-irritant.

J. glandulifera. Stipules bushy, many-cleft, each ending in a glandular head. Common in gardens about Calcutta;

a pale juice exudes from wounds in the bark, which is employed by the Hindus to remove opacities or specks from the cornea. *Roxb.*

Gen. 11.—Janipha.

Sp. Janipha Manihot. Tapioca plant.

Tapioca and Moussache are the fecula of the root of the Janipha manihot. The juice of the root deposits a white fecula, which after being well washed and dried constitutes what is called "*moussache.*" This is formed of rounded grains having a central dark point, and of remarkably equal size, the density of moussache to arrow root is as 14 to 16.

When the moussache is dried on hot plates the grains partly burst, and the fecula agglomerates in irregular semi-opaque gumlike masses, and is then called Tapioca.

Both these substances constitute excellent articles of diet, especially for convalescents. The Messrs. Speed cultivate the Janipha in the vicinity of Calcutta, and produce a *tapioca* of admirable quality.

To prepare *Tapioca* take one ounce of the grains, steep in soft water for an hour. Pour off the superfluous water, and boil with a pound of water for an hour. A transparent uniform syrup-like fluid is obtained, which jellies on cooling, and has a peculiarly rich and agreeable flavour.

The juice of the Janipha root from which the fecula has separated is a very formidable poison.

Cassava bread is made of the tapioca root, from which the acrid juice and fecula have been removed by washing.

Gen. 12.—Hevea.

Sp. H. guianensis. Caoutchouc plant.

Syn. Siphonia elastica.

Trunk 17 to 20 yards high, scaly like a pine apple, very straight, branched at the summit, leaves scattered at the extremities of the branches, and composed of three thick, and very smooth leaflets, flowers in numerous panicles, unisexual, and with monadelphous stamina.

Incisions in the bark cause the discharge of a juice which concretes into the well known and very valuable *caoutchouc* of commerce, a product however of many other trees in this and allied families, for example of Jatropha elastica, Ficus Indica, Artocarpus integrifolia, Urceola elastica, &c.

The juice when first obtained is white and milky, spec. gr. 1,011; spread in thin layers it quickly dries into a colourless and often transparent solid substance.

Pure caoutchouc is pale yellow, inodorous, tasteless. The ordinary black colour is attributed by some writers to its being smoke-dried, but we have prepared specimens by mere exposure to the air, which have assumed the black colour. At 32° caoutchouc is hard, at 60° to 100° flexible like leather, and exceedingly elastic and adhesive. Sp. gr. 0,933.

Caoutchouc is inalterable in the air, insoluble in water, though softened by it if heated, insoluble also in acids, alkalies, and alcohol. Soluble in ether, if previously well washed with water to free it of alcohol. The etherial solution on evaporation leaves the caoutchouc unchanged; it is also soluble in volatile oils, but the solutions usually leave the caoutchouc in a somewhat glutinous state; coal naptha, rectified oil of turpentine (free from water), the essential oils of gurjun and copaiba, and generally all the liquid carburets of hydrogen effect its solution, and leave it on evaporation in an elastic condition.

The fixed oils dissolve it by heat, but alter its properties, rendering it sticky.

At 248° caoutchouc melts, and on cooling remains in a semifluid state like tar, or thick turpentine. Heated in the open air it takes fire, and burns with a yellow flame and much smoke; distilled in close vessels it furnishes 83⅓ per 100 of volatile oil, at first dark, when rectified colourless and limpid; sp. gr. only 640; boils at 108°; one volume of its vapour contains 4 vols. of carbon and 4 of hydrogen condensed into 1 volume. It is isomeric with 2 vols. of olefiant gas in the liquid state; it contains in 100 parts, carbon 85,71, hydrogen 14.29.

According to Faraday's analysis caoutchouc milk contains water 56.37, caoutchouc 31.70, albumen 1.90, wax a trace, an azotic body 7.13, a gummy body 2.90. Caoutchouc itself Mr. Faraday found to be composed of carbon 8=hydrogen 7=or per cent. carbon 87.27, hydrogen 12.73.

The uses of caoutchouc are daily becoming more numerous and important. Its inalterability by chemical agents, its flexibility, elasticity, strength, impermeability to moisture, the infinity of forms into which it can be moulded, its great cheapness, and the abundance and low price of its solvents combine to render it one of the most practically useful substances produced by nature. To the chemist it gives tubes, joints, balloons, and blow-pipes; the mechanist obtains from it bands and straps of unequalled efficacy for communicating motion. Introduced into the interstices of cloth it renders it impervious to water, and thus gives us invaluable articles of wearing apparel, as well as tent cloths, mail bags, &c. For the protection of ammunition in rainy countries it is quite unrivalled. It is available for roofing houses, for constructing boats, and other light vessels. It enables us to enclose air in them, and use them as soft, elastic seats and pillows, and placed over water it gives an hydraulic bed, of inestimable value to patients suffering from ulcers on parts liable to pressure, the person literally floating on the water without coming in contact with its surface.

We might enumerate a catalogue of tenfold length of the useful applications of caoutchouc. It is produced in inexhaustible abundance in Assam, and owing to the exertions of Captain Jenkins is manufactured now of excellent quality.

In 1838 several maunds of caoutchouc, manufactured in Assam, were exported from Calcutta. The price they brought was comparatively low, but owing to improvements in the manufacture it is now rapidly reaching a remunerating rate.

In the preceding account of caoutchouc we have chiefly had recourse to the excellent article on the subject by Dr. Thomson, published in his "Organic Chemistry."

Gen. 13.—Alchornea.

Sp. A. latifolia.

A Jamaica tree, to which has been ascribed the *alcornoco* bark, the cause of so much discussion; this occurs in large thick, wrinkled fragments, the cortical layers being reddish or rosy, the liber yellowish, thin, fibrous, and readily separated in flakes, inodorous, taste bitter and astringent; the liber colours the saliva yellow. It contains gum, resin, extractive, moisture, fibre, and a trace of tartaric acid.

The bark derives its celebrity from having been long a reputed specific in pthisis. It is said to be emetic, but is now never employed in practice.

Gen. 14.—Caturus.

Sp. Caturus spiciflorus. Linn. *Roxb. Fl. Ind.* iii. p. 760.

A shrub with diœcious flowers, calyx trifid, stamens 3, calyx 3-parted, styles three, lacerated, capsules tricoccous, flowers axillary, pendulous; flowers said to be specific in diarrhœa and similar disorders.

GEN. 15.—ACALYPHA.

Sp. Acalypha indica. Roxb. iii. p. 675.

Vern. Shwet Busunda, *Beng.* Moorkanta, *Tel.* Cupameni, *Rheede.*

A common annual in Indian gardens. Root bruised in water cathartic, decoction of leaves laxative. *Lindley.*

GEN. 16.—TRAGIA.

Sp. T. involucrata. Roxb. iii. p. 576.

Vern. Bichittee, *Beng.*

Hairs sting violently; roots given by the Vaidas as alteratives in cachexia and venereal diseases. *Ainslie.*

GEN. 17.—SAPIUM.

Sp. S. indicum, Roxb. iii. p. 692.

Vern. Hooroos, *Beng.* Delta of Ganges.

Capsule or nut globular, size of a nutmeg, 3-celled, 6-valved, thick and exceedingly hard, seed solitary, fixed by apex, smooth, juice very poisonous, taste exceedingly nauseous, seeds used for intoxicating fish. *Roxb.*

GEN. 18.—MERCURIALIS.

Sp. M. annua. Αινωζοστις, Diosc. iv. p. 191. Europe.

Odour strong and very fœtid, taste disagreeable, bitter, and slightly saline; unworthy of further notice in a medicinal point of view.

GEN. 19.—HIPPOMANE.

Sp. H. Mancinella. Manchineel, South America.

Trunk rather lofty, with numerous branches, with grey bark, leaves petioled, alternate, green, shining, cordate at the base, flowers small, monœcious. Fruits in all respects resemble a small apple externally, but contain a white milky pulp, and a nut deeply grooved, with seven valves and seven monospermous cells. The taste is at first dull and unpleasant, then acrid and irritating.

All parts of this tree discharge, on being cut or punctured, abundance of very white caustic and poisonous juice, which acts as an immediate vesicatory, and is used by the Indians to poison their arrows.

It was long supposed that sleeping under the shade of the manchineel was destructive to life, but this has been disproved by numerous and conclusive experiments; it is equally hurtful to sleep under any tree in the climates and localities where the manchineel abounds.

Gen. 20.—Excœcaria.

Sp. Excœcaria Agallocha. Aloes wood?
Arbor excœcans, *Rumph.* Amb. ii. t. 79, 80. East Indies.
Vern. Ugooroo, Sunderbunds of Bengal.

Wood knotty, grey or blackish, smooth, and resinous; transverse sections shew the orifices of its proper vessels; odour agreeable on combustion. Taste bitter, powder brown.

A question has arisen as to whether this tree is the source of the "aloes wood" of the Greeks and Arabs. Three different genera of plants appear to yield the woods known by the above designation, viz. the Aloexylon, Excœcaria, and Aquilaria; Sprengel quotes the second, and traces the wood to China. The Arabian writers refer it to Java.

The name Excœcaria is derived from two Latin words signifying "producing blindness," on account of the terrible effects said to be produced by the juice coming in contact with the eyes.

See art. Agallochum, (*Leguminoseæ*) and Aquilaria (*Aquilarineæ.*)

Gen. 21.—Euphorbia.

Gen. characters. Monœcious, flowers in heads with an involucrum, consisting of one leaf with five divisions, having five alternating glands; ♂ naked, monandrous, surrounding the female; ♀ naked, solitary, ovarium stalked, stigmas 3-forked, fruit hanging out of involucrum, consisting of three cells, bursting at the bark with elasticity, and each containing one suspended seed. (*Lindley.*)

Sp. 1. *E. Tirucalli.* Milk hedge, *Roxb. Fl. Ind.* ii. p. 370.
Vern. Lunka sij, *Beng.*

Branches erect, naked, round, succulent, polished, very lactescent, leaves small, linear, sessile at ends of twigs. Flowers crowded, subsessile, terminal and axillary, lobes of involucre five, roundish, smooth, peltate, tube woolly on the inside. Capsule villous.

Milk mixed with flour, in doses of a drachm daily, an Indian specific in syphilis. The inspissated milk is a violent emetic and purgative.

Sp. 2. *E. antiquorum.* Common in India.
Vern. Nara sij, *Beng.*

Branches triangular or quadrangular, angles waved, and having double spines at the protuberances. Peduncles solitary or in pairs, 3-flowered, stamens five; bark of root given with water as a purgative.

No Euphorbium resin is obtained from this species in India.

Sp. 3. *E. officinarum.* Arabia and Africa. Mr. Pereira considers the Mogadore Euphorbium resin to be produced by this species, which has a bright crimson flower.

Euphorbium Resin.

Euphorbium is the proper juice of the Euphorbia antiquorum, cannariense, and officinarum. It is exceedingly acrid, and scarcely used except as an external rubefacient or blister. According to the experiments of Braconnot, Pelletier, and Brande, it is composed of resin, wax, malate of lime and of potassa, woody fibre, bassorine and volatile oil. It contains no gum soluble in water.

The resin is reddish brown, of weak odour, burning taste, mostly soluble in alcohol, and in the fatty oils; soluble with difficulty in the alkalies, but freely in acid menstrua, especially in the nitric and sulphuric acids. The resin obtained by hot alcohol if washed by cold alcohol leaves a residue which crystallizes from its solution in that fluid at a boiling heat.

In reducing Euphorbium to powder the utmost caution must be observed, as the particles of dust, if inhaled or introduced into the mouth or eyes, would cause dangerous inflammation. A tincture, an oil, and a plaster, are described by Soubeiran, but we do not consider them of much importance.

The smallest quantity of Euphorbium introduced into the nostrils occasions the most violent and continued sneezing.

Sp. 4. *E. Ligularia, Bengal,* Roxb. ii. p. 465.
Vern. Munsa sij, *Beng.*

A plant sacred to Munsa, the goddess of Serpents. The root of the tree mixed with black pepper is employed for the cure of snake bites, both internally and externally.

The trunk when old is about 20 feet high, branches succulent, 5-sided, angled, angles toothed, and armed with sharp black spines set in couples, flowers greenish yellow.

Sp. 5. *E. neriifolia.* Roxb. ii. p. 467.
Syn. E. Nivulia, *Hamilton.*
Vern. Patteoon, *Duk.* Pattakarie, *Sans.*
Branches round, otherwise like last species, juice used by the natives as a purgative, externally as a stimulant in rheumatism and contracted limbs; leaves diuretic.

Sp. 6. *E. thymifolia.* All over India.
Vern. Shwet Keerooi, *Beng.* Racta vinda chada, *Sans.*
A little annual plant, flowers white and red, juice of stalks and flowers a violent purgative, fresh plant applied to wounds by the Arabs, leaves and seeds given by the Tamools in worm cases, and in the bowel affections of children.

Besides the articles above quoted, M. Fee describes, under the head of Euphorbium —

Sp. 7. *E. Cyparissias.*
Syn. Tithymalus Cyparissias. Τιφυμαλος, Diosc. iv. 165. Europe.
Root excessively acrid. Des Longchamps considers the bark of the root a good emetic in doses of 12 to 18 grains.

E. Peplus, Purgative and emetic in dose of 24 gr.
E. Gerardiana, }
E. Pithyusa, } Same effect, dose 15 to 24 gr.
E. sylvatica, }

Sp. 8. *E. Ipecachuana.* Action of root exactly like that of Ipecachuana, but more violent. It only requires to be given in proportionally small doses to be a perfect substitute for the best ipecachuan.

Sp. 9. *E. Lathyris.* Spurge.
The seed of this Euphorbium contains yellow fixed oil, stearine, acrid brown oil, crystalline matter, brown resin, an extractive colouring matter, and vegetable albumen.
The stearine is white and insipid, the yellow oil purgative, owing however to the presence of other matters. The acrid brown oil seems to be the active principle. Its odour and taste are disagreeable, and very similar to the croton oil. It is easily soluble in alcohol and ether; the crystalline matter is tasteless and inodorous, crystallizes in needles, and is dissolved by alcohol and ether; the brown resin is nearly black, insipid, fusible, insoluble even in boiling alcohol, slightly soluble in ether, freely in the fixed oils.

These seeds are used for the extraction of the purgative oil, which is obtained either by expression, by alcohol, or by ether.

The 2d process consists in grinding the seeds, mixing them with twice their weight of alcohol, and heating on the sand bath to 90° to 110° Fahr. While hot, expression is performed, the expressed liquor is distilled to recover the alcohol, and after the oil has remained at rest for some days it is filtered. The expressed liquid from the first separates into two layers; the superior is the alcoholic solution of oil and resin, the inferior of the oil insoluble in alcohol, mixed with substances dissolved by that menstruum.

The product is a yellowish brown oil of thick consistence; after some days it deposits a thick matter, it is then filtered, still it is thicker and browner than the oil obtained by simple expression. It is also stronger; in the dose of a scruple to half a drachm, it produces nausea, colic, and abundant evacuations, but not more than five drops should be given at first.

To extract the oil by ether the seeds are powdered, introduced into the displacement apparatus of Robiquet, and ether poured on; the ether is then displaced by water, the ethereal liquors distilled, the oil allowed to rest for some days, and filtered. This oil is inferior in quality to the simple expressed kind, but preferable to that prepared by alcohol. It does not nauseate so much; in doses of a drachm to 1½ drachm it is emetic and cathartic.

Soubeiran gives the following formula for purgative "tablettes," prepared with this oil:—

Chocolate paste, ...	2	one scruple each.
Sugar,...	1	
Starch,...	1	
Canella powder, ...	10 grains.	
Lathyris oil, ...	30 drops.	

Triturate the oil with the sugar and starch, incorporate all with the chocolate, divide into 30 pills, which are to be subsequently flattened by a heated iron; each lozenge contains 1 drop of the oil.

Gen. 22.—Pedilanthus.

Sp. P. tithymaloides, Jew bush. West Indies.

Introduced into the Calcutta Garden, and now common every where about Calcutta in hedges. A shrub about 6 feet high, abounding in white bitter milk, known and used in America as ipecachuana. We regret to say that in numerous trials we obtained no proof of its efficacy; this is probably the result of deterioration of properties through the influence of the climate of Bengal.

See also mentions under EUPHORBIACEÆ—

Adelia venenata, ..	Africa, a blistering plant.
Aleurites trilobata,	Friendly islands, purgative.
Elaeococcus Vernicia,	Japan, seeds yield oil for burning.
Sapium aucuparium,	South America, affords a bird lime.
Stillingia sylvatica,	Florida, used as an antisyphylic.
Hura crepitans, ..	S. America, an acrid poison.
Omphalea diandra,	Jamaica and Guiana, fruits eatable and oily, when stale acrid.

NAT. ORDER CXXIII.—ARISTOLOCHIÆ.

Herbaceous or subfrutescent plants, trailing or climbing, with alternate, simple, and petiolate leaves. The properties of these plants are due to essential oil, and a yellow bitter principle soluble in water and alcohol; but still imperfectly examined. The odour of some is penetrating and camphor-like, one or two species are fœtid.

The *asarabacca*, one of this family, is powerfully purgative and emetic.

GEN. 1.—ARISTOLOCHIA.

Sp. 1. *Aristolochia Serpentaria,* North America.

Off. The roots.

Roots composed of a long thin body, surrounded by a multitude of radical fibres, thin, interlaced, several inches long, yellowish grey externally, internally white. The neck of the root often retains the remnants of the stalks.

Odour very powerful, resembling that of valerian and camphor; taste hot and bitter, powder grey. The roots of the common asarum are sometimes mixed with the true serpentaria; the false roots are black, and devoid of the characteristic smell and taste.

Chevallier's analysis shews the serpentaria root to contain essential oil, yellow bitter matter, resin, green albumen, starch, fibre, and salts.

Serpentaria is a valuable tonic, stimulant, and diaphoretic. It has also been used as a febrifuge with considerable success—dose 10 to 30 grs.

Sp. 2. *A. longa.* Αριστολοκια, of Diosc. South of France.

Roots cylindrical, obtuse, ash coloured, hard, very brittle, a foot long, often as thick as the arm, parenchyme brown, odour nauseous, taste very bitter, powder ash grey, analogous in composition and properties to preceding species.

The *A. longa* and *rotunda,* natives of the south of Europe, are found in the medicine bazars, under the names of *Zurawund tuweel* (Pers. *duraz,* long) and *Zurawund mooderuj* (Pers. *gird,* round,) with *aristolokia* as the Greek name.

Feé adds a notice of three European species—*A. rotunda, clematitis,* and *pistolochia,* all of which are bitter, stimulant, and sudorific. He also mentions several West Indian and American species. In the West Indies many of these are celebrated for their reputed efficacy in preventing the attacks of snakes, and in curing the effects of their bites; very little certainty exists however as to the existence of these alleged virtues.

Aristolochia is derived from αριστος and λοχος, significative of the supposed power of facilitating the lochial discharge of parturient women.

Sp. 3. *Aristolochia bracteata.* Roxb. Fl. Ind. iii. p. 490.
Vern. Cattrabunga. *Sans.*

Cultivated ground on the Coromandel coast.

Root perennial, long, slender, simple, perpendicular, waved, with many small fibres from every part. Stems or branches several, weak, resting on the ground, waved, streaked, 12 to 18 inches long, leaves alternate, petioled, kidney formed, beautifully curled round the margin, petioles channelled.

Flowers axillary, single, peduncled. Peduncles drooped with a kidney-shaped bract near the base. Calyx a very beautiful dark purple, anthers 6 pairs, capsules ovate.

Every part is extremely and very disagreeably bitter; two of the leaves bruised with water are given as a remedy in diarrhœa with colic; an infusion of the dried leaves is deemed anthelmintic.

Sp. 4. *A. indica.*
Vern. Isarmel, *Hind.* Hari, *Sans.*

A native of Bengal every where, the root is like that of sarsaparilla, perennial, stem twining, woody below, leaves stalked, wedge-shaped or obovate, 3-nerved, pointed, waved, scolloped, smooth, 2—4 inches long, 1—2 broad, racemes axillary, shorter than the leaves, with bracts, flowers erect, anthers in 6 pairs, oblong, pendulous.

The root is nauseously bitter, and is given as an emmenagogue, and in paroxysms of gout.

It is considered also by the native practitioners to be a valuable remedy in the diarrhœa of children proceeding from dentition.

The dose given in India, to an adult, of the decoction of the root, is an ounce to an ounce and a half twice daily.

The Guaco of the Caraccas, so celebrated as an antidote to snake poison, and the trials of which in hydrophobia by Dr. Elliotson attracted such notice some years since in London, is asserted by Dr. Hancock to belong to this family.

Gen. 2.—Asarum.

Sp. A. europæum, Asarabacca.

Leaves remarkably kidney-shaped. Roots quadrangular, thickness of a goose quill, knotted, contorted, and having usually white fibres at each knot. Odour of the leaf none, of the roots pepper-like, especially when bruised, taste of the leaves acrid, of the roots less so. Thé acridity diminishes by age, and finally disappears.

Feneuille and Lagrange have subjected the roots of this plant to analysis, and found it to contain concrete volatile oil, very acrid fatty matter, a yellow substance resembling cytisin, fecula, mucus, albumen, citric acid, citrate of lime, and other salts.

The leaves and roots of the asarum are emetic in doses of from 40 to 60 grs. infused in eight ounces of water. It only acts well while fresh. In larger doses it is cathartic; the powder of the leaves used as snuff causes violent sneezing.

Until the introduction of ipecachuana into Europe, the asarum was used for most of the purposes for which the South American drug is now employed.

The dried plant is sold in the Indian bazars under the name of *Asaroon*. Royle states however that a hill plant, called *Tuggur*, is generally substituted for it.

NAT. ORDER CXXIV.—BALANOPHOREÆ.

This order contains several parasitic plants, such as the extraordinary Rafflesia, and the Cytinus hypocistus, a small plant found on cisti trees in Europe, and which yields the substance long known in medicine as hypocistus juice. This is supposed to be an extract of the plant, and owes all its properties to the presence of an abundance of gallic acid. Balanophora gigantica is a favourite astringent remedy in Burma. From Dr. Wallich's naming it *Neerbees*, it is conjectured to be one of the kinds of Nirbisi,—see *Ranunculaceæ*.

NAT. ORDER CXXV.—CHLORANTHEÆ.

Royle states that many of these plants are fragrant and aromatic, and the leaves and roots of some species are said to resemble snake root in properties and uses. They are found in Goalpara, Assam, and on the Khassea hills. According to the statement of Blume, the root of the *Chloranthus officinalis* of Java is one of the most efficacious of all known remedial agents as a stimulant tonic and diaphoretic; its efficacy in the treatment of the Java fevers is attested on the strongest authority.

The flowers of the order are spiked each with a bract, calyx none, anther solitary and 2-celled, or triple and 4-celled, with a thick fleshy connective seated in the exterior of the ovary, stigma sessile, drupe baccate, one-seeded.

The Java officinal species is a shrub about five feet high, branches opposite, straggling, tumid at the articulations, fistular when young. Leaves spreading, opposite, stalked, oblong, acuminated at each end, with glandular serratures, thin, shining, and somewhat blistered, petioles short, sheathed, sheaths having two teeth at each side, spikes terminal, branched, bracts glandular, drupes straw coloured.

NAT. ORDER CXXVI.—SAURUREÆ.

An order allied to the pepper family. Royle mentions one species of interest, the *Aponogeton monostachyon*, the roots of which Roxburgh says are nearly as good as potatoes, and are much liked by the natives.

Vern. Kakangi, *Sans.* Pania kalanga, *Rheede.* Ghetchoo, *Hind.* Nama, *Tel.* Nama dumpha, the root.

NAT. ORDER CXXVII.—PIPERACEÆ.

This important order is formed chiefly of shrubs; their branches are more or less flexuose, generally climbing, articulated and knotty. All have alternate leaves, very entire, and sometimes nerved. About 150 species are described; the flowers are axillary to the leaves, and sometimes opposite to the alternate leaves; the order is nearly allied to the *Arums*, remarkable plants of which we will have subsequently to treat.

This order is remarkably uniform in chemical composition. The seeds are all of burning taste, owing to the presence of a volatile oil and acrid resin, which abound especially in the perisperm. Oersted discovered in the black pepper a principle named *piperin,* which has since been found in several of the species.

GEN.—PIPER.

Stamens one to ten, stigma three-lobed, fruit baccate.

The numerous species of this group inhabit Asia and America. Mr. Crawford states, the pepper countries extend from about the longitude of 96° to that of 115° E. and from 5° to 12° N. Within these limits we have Sumatra, Borneo, the Malayan Peninsula, and the countries to the east of the gulf of Siam.

Sp. 1. *Piper nigrum.* Black pepper, Πιπερι Hip.

Vern. Mellaghoo, *Tam.* Gammiris, *Cing.* Merialoo, *Tel.* Marichu, *Sans.* Gol murch, *Hind.* Kali murichu, *Duk.* Filfil uswud, *Arab.* Filfil seeah, *Pers.*

A native of Malacca, Java, and Sumatra, cultivated all along the Malabar Coast. Dr. Roxburgh describes it as being found wild among the hills of the Rajamundry district.

The stem is trailing or climbing, shrubby, flexuose and dichotomously branched, jointed, swelling at the joints, and often throwing out radicles which adhere to adjacent plants, or strike into the ground; leaves from 4 to 6 inches long, alternate, distichous, broadly ovate, acuminated, very green and glossy, paler beneath, 5 to 7 nerved, nerves connected by transverse veins. Petioles rounded, short, spikes opposite the leaves, stalked, 3 to 6 inches long, drooping, some female, others hermaphrodite. Stamens 3, fruit ripens irregularly all the year round, sessile, the size of a pea, first green, then red, subsequently black, covered by pulp. The black pepper of commerce is the berry dried with the pulp.

By Pelletier's analysis of black pepper contains *Piperin,* concrete acrid oil, volatile oil, gummy matter, extractive, malic and tartaric acids, starch, and bassorin.

PIPERIN.

Discovered by Oersted, is according to the analysis of Liebig a compound of 40 carbon, 20 hydrogen, 8 oxygen, 1 azote. It crystallizes in 4-angled prisms, is transparent, tasteless, melts about 212°, is insoluble in cold water, very soluble in hot alcohol, from which it partly separates on cooling; soluble in acetic acid, difficultly in ether. The best process for obtaining it is that by M. Poutet. Make an alcoholic extract, and act upon it with a weak solution of caustic potash, dilute with water and filter, wash the matter on the filter, and dissolve it in boiling alcohol, which by evaporation yields Piperin in fine crystals; about two per cent is the usual product; the use of the potash in this process is to dissolve the resin and oils with which the Piperin is associated in the extract.

The acrid concrete matter of the pepper is excessively pungent, very soluble in alcohol, ether, and oils. It is in this that the stimulant property of the pepper resides. The volatile oil is more balsamic than acrid.

Piperin has been much praised as a febrifuge remedy. Were any such virtues confirmed by cautious trials the discovery would be of the utmost importance, considering the cheapness and ease with which the substance may be prepared. We have carefully examined all the evidence on the subject, and tried the substance ourselves in numerous cases; we regret however that in no one instance have we ever found it of the least utility. If impure, that is to say mixed with the acrid resin, it acts as a general stimulant, and as such, like all other stimulants such as wine, serpentaria, musk, &c. will in a few trifling cases moderate a paroxysm of ague, if taken immediately before its occurrence. Such we apprehend is the nature of the cases which have been adduced by some writers in proof of its efficacy. Common black pepper bruised and mixed with water, has long been a popular stimulant in ague.

The dose of piperin is from 6 to 8 grs.; we have given it in all doses from 1 to 30 grains without the least general or febrifuge effect. In confirmation of our opinion on this subject, we may adduce the very recent and eminent authority of Soubeiran, who states in his *Traite de Pharmacie*, 1837, t. ii. p. 46, that experience has not confirmed its reputed febrifuge virtues. Pelletier, perhaps the greatest authority in existence on all pharmaceutical matters, pronounces it altogether devoid of action on the animal economy.

Pepper is much more valuable as an external application; Ward's paste, so celebrated in the cure of chronic piles, is a compound of pepper and simple ointment.

If dried black pepper be macerated in water the pericarp swells, bursts, and readily separates. White pepper is thus prepared, and being less acrid than the "black," is preferred for culinary purposes, and by some chemists for the preparation of piperin.

Sp. 2. *P. Cubeba.*

Vern. Val mellaghoo, *Tam.* Kubabchinie, *Hind.* Dumke mirchie, *Duk.* Komoon koos, *Malay.* Salava mirrialoo, *Tel.* Kababah, *Arab.* Suganda marichi, *Sans.*

Κουβεβα, modern Greek.

A native of Java.

Berries sub-rounded, the size of a small pea, brown, pedunculate, marked with a prominent network of veins, peduncle sharp. By softening in water they are found to have a quadruple envelope—1st. external, fleshy, greyish; the 2d. grey, almost transparent; the 3d. thin like an onion peel, yellow and brownish; the 4th. and last, is a white membranous pellicle, closely applied to the seed. The parenchyme is white and oily, its odour aromatic, taste acrid, hot, powder greasy and nearly black. Vauquelin's analysis shews cubebs to contain volatile oil, resin, colouring matter, gum, extractive and saline matter. 12½ lbs. of cubebs gave Baume over two ounces of oil. In our experiments, using cubebs recently imported, we obtained 10 per 100, and on one occasion 13½ per cent.

There has lately been described a crystalline substance, *Cubebin*, apparently identical with *Piperin.*

The volatile oil congeals at a moderate temperature. By long keeping, at 60, it deposits crystals of stearoptene, commonly termed "cubeb camphor." The oil is lighter than water. The flavour is very fragrant and agreeable.

Powdered cubebs are employed with almost certain success in gonorrhœa, unless when extremely violent; one to two drachms may be given at a dose. It may be taken thrice daily. The usual effect is to abate the sensation of scalding, and to increase the secretion of urine, to which it communicates a peculiar odour. Some difference of opinion exists as to the propriety of giving cubebs in the height of inflammatory gonorrhœa. This stage we think should be treated with diluents, purgatives, and antimonials; but as soon as the severity of the very acute stage abates the cubebs may then be advantageously given.

The powder may be taken in water or in milk.

According to Blume the *Piper caninum*, which corresponds with the P. Cubeba of Roxburgh, Fl. Ind. i. p. 161, is also a native of Java, and the chief source of the cubebs of commerce.

In Sierra Leone *P. Afzelii*, a plant resembling the cubeb, produces a similar berry, but its qualities have not been accurately ascertained. A kind of cubeb is also said to be obtained from the Mauritius and Bourbon, and to occur in very minute grains. Its source and properties are alike uncertain.

The following preparations are advantageous forms for administering this remedy.

Oleo-resinous extract. Take 6 lbs of bruised cubebs, distil with 12 parts of water, and collect six pints, separate the volatile oil which floats on the surface. Replace the distilled water, and add six lbs. more cubebs, distil again and separate the oil as before.

Express the marc, exhaust it by alcohol, and distil the tinctures to the consistence of honey; about 12 ounces are obtained, which mix with the essential oil.

This is M. Dublanc's excellent preparation. It combines all the active principles of the cubebs, and rejects the inert. Its odour is aromatic and agreeable, its taste hot, leaving an after-sensation of coolness like peppermint. It can be taken with great ease in pills, or wrapped up in a morsel of bread.

Concentrated essence of Cubebs.

Alcohol, 12 ounces.

Ol. resin extract. } 4 ounces.

Dissolve the extract in the spirit. Dose proportionate to the extract dissolved.

Emulsion of Cubebs.

Concentrated essence of cubebs, 4 ounces.

Mucilage of gum arabic, 4 ounces.

This emulsion mixes well with water, and will keep several days. The dose is a tea spoonful 3 or 4 times daily, mixed with a few spoonfuls of water. (*Soubeiran*, vol. ii. p. 49.)

Sp. 3. P. longum, long pepper. *Roxb. Fl. Ind.* i. p. 154.

Vern. Tipilie, *Tam.* Pipuloo, *Tel.* Pipilie, *Duk.* Pipel, *Hind.* Pippali, *Sans.* also Krishna. Dar filfil, *Arab.* Filfil Daraz, *Pers.*

Wild in India, along water-courses towards the Circar mountains, and much cultivated. The root is woody and perennial, stems numerous, creeping, pointed, round, branches bearing the fruit, erect, spike sessile, erect, stalked, cylindrical, imbricated, with five or more rows of small orbicular scales, spike of ripe fruit composed of firmly united 1-seeded drupes.

Root (Granthicka, *Sans.*) sliced and dried constitutes the *Pippula moola* of the native druggists, a substance much used as a stimulant remedy and spice.

The analysis of the fruits of the long pepper corresponds closely in results with those of the species first described.

Sp. 4. *P. trioicum.* Roxb. Fl. Ind. i. p. 154.

Vern. Mirial tiga, *Tel.*

Circar mountains, in shady places, with rich soil, fruit succulent, small, round, red, excessively pungent, an article of important commerce from Madras.

Sp. 5. *P. sylvaticum.* Roxb. Fl. Ind. i. p. 156.

N. W. Mountains of Bengal, *(Pahari pippul,)* used while green, and ripe also, as long pepper.

Sp. 6. *Piper Betle.* Roxb. Fl. Ind. i. p. 258. Bot. Mag. t. 3132. φυλλον μαλαβαθρον, *Diosc.*

Vern. Vettilei, *Tamul.* Pan, *Duk.* Tanbool, *Arab.* Barg tambool, *Pers.* Pan, *Hind.* Tamalap Akoo, *Tel.* Tambuli, *Sans.*

Cultivated all over India and the Malay countries, also in the West Indies.

Stems shrubby, much branched, running along the ground, or climbing to a great height, throwing out roots from the numerous joints; leaves alternate, deciduous or cordate, ovate, oblique at the base, acuminate, 4 to 7 inches long, glabrous, 5 to 7 nerved, nerves connected by transverse veins, the veins and nerves prominent beneath, petioles rounded, grooved on the upper side, while young having a pair of lanceolate stipules which are deciduous. Spikes opposite, the leaves peduncled, at first shorter than the leaf, slender, cylindrical, tapering, in fruit greatly enlarged, pendent, scales dense, peltate, stigma sessile, divided.

Leaf universally chewed in the East with lime and slices of the areca nut; a powerful stimulant to the salivary and digestive organs. The nut is sprinkled with lime, and each slice is wrapped in a leaf of the betle pepper.

Sp. 7. *P. methysticum.*

Ava pepper. A native of the Society, Friendly, and Sandwich islands, where it is called "Ava;" used in a tincture in chronic rheumatism, and in infusion as an intoxicating beverage, which is also deemed antisyphilitic. To cure venereal the patient drinks an infusion until he become drunk, after which copious perspiration ensues.

NAT. ORDER CXXVIII.—URTICEÆ.

This order, long considered as of insignificant interest in a medicinal light, is destined we believe to occupy a very prominent place in future systems of Materia Medica. It contains the well known hemp, *Cannabis sativa* and *indica*, which, as we shall point out in the sequel, supplies the physician with a powerful remedy in a disease long deemed beyond the resources of medicine, and of great benefit as a palliative, though not a cure for the most awful of all morbid affections to which mankind are exposed, namely, the effects of the bite of rabid animals.

Besides the hemp several other substances of value or interest occur in this order, which we are consequently led to study with some minuteness.

We may mention here the renowned Upas of Java, the hop of Europe, the demon nettles of Timor, the banyan and pipul of India, the mulberry, and the bread fruit tree, as instances of the important species of this order.

In the works of Feé, Lindley, and Soubeiran, the Urticeæ comprehend the figs and mulberries, which (with the bread fruit trees of Feé) are treated of separately by Royle, under the order *Artocarpeæ*. We follow the system of the former writers.

Essential Characters.

Apetalous dicotyledons, with definite erect ovula, an inferior calyx, distinct stipulæ, and an embryo with the radicle remote from the hilum.

Flowers monœcious or diœcious, scattered or clustered, calyx membranous, lobed, persistent; stamens definite, distinct, inserted into the base of the calyx, and opposite its lobes; anthers curved inwards in œstivation, curving backwards with elasticity when bursting, ovarium superior, simple, ovule solitary, erect, stigma simple. Fruit a simple indehiscent nut, surrounded either by the membranous or fleshy calyx. Embryo straight, curved or spiral, with or without albumen. Radicle superior, cotyledons lying face to face; trees, shrubs, or herbs; leaves alternate, with stipulæ, hispid or scabrous, often covered with pungent hairs. (*Lindley, Introd.* p. 931.)

The Artocarpeæ differ from the above characters in the inflorescence of the Urticeæ being panicled, in the ovulum being erect in the latter, and also in the presence of a milky juice. The whole are most extensivly distributed over tropical regions, and several find their way to temperate and cold climates.

Gen. 1.—Ficus.

Sp. 1. *F. Carica.* Common or edible fig.

Asia Minor, south of France, Piedmont; fruits (*Sycones*, Mirbel) grey, turbinate, of variable size and colour, according to cultivation; rounded and obtuse towards the summit, which is umbilicate, umbilicus orbicular, slightly prominent, closed before maturity, parenchyme succulent, fleshy, yellow or reddish, viscous, and sugar-like, containing a great quantity of seeds; inodorous, taste sweet, mild, and mucilaginous.

Figs are more important as an article of luxury than for alimentary or medicinal purposes.

Sp. 2. *F. indica.* Banyan tree.

Too well known to need description. The lac insect abounds on it, and the bark yields abundance of milky juice containing caoutchouc.

Sp. 3. *F. religiosa.* Pipul, bark deemed a good tonic; the lac insect also flourishes on this tree.

F. septica and *F. toxicaria* have an acrid and corrosive juice; *F. tinctoria* of the Society Isles gives a good yellow dye. The *Ficus elastica* of India (Sylhet and Assam especially) yields abundance of caoutchouc of the best quality. (*See* p. 560.)

Gen. 2.—Dorstenia.

Sp. D. Contrayerva.

Off. The roots.

Roots rather bitter, odour peculiar, an alleged antidote to poisons and snake bites, used as a tonic formerly, now obsolete.

Gen. 3.—Morus.

Sp. M. nigra. Mulberry.

A native of Persia or China, naturalized in India and many parts of Europe and America. The fruits contain mucilage, sugar, and tartaric acid. The bark is acrid and bitter, and was formerly considered purgative and vermifuge. The leaves are used for feeding silk worms. The *M. Papyrifera* (now Broussonetia) is used in China and Japan for the preparation of a paper. The inner bark is employed, the young branches being boiled in alkaline water to free them of epidermis, which is scraped off. It is then boiled to the consistence of a paste, which is moulded or fabricated on the plan described under the head of *Daphne*, (see *Thymeleæ*.)

GEN. 4.—URTICA.

Sp. U. dioica. Common nettle.

Europe, every where; leaves sting severely, causing an eruption very like that hence called Urticaria, or nettle rash. The expressed juice is an acrid poison; applied externally nettles have sometimes proved advantageous in paralysis and similar affections. The expressed juice has been given internally as an astringent. The stalks afford materials for cordage of great tenacity.

The *Urtica crenulata*, Roxb. which grows in the Calcutta Botanic Garden, stings so terribly that it has sometimes occasioned very formidable symptoms.

The *Daoun setan*, or demon nettle of Timor, is still more dangerous in its effects.

GEN. 5.—HUMULUS.

Sp. H. Lupulus. Hop.

A native of Europe, much cultivated in England, especially in Kent; lately by Capt. Kirke in Deyrah Dhoon.

The fruits (strobiles) are oval, elongated, composed of membranous scales, then persistent, soft, white, yellowish, supporting at their base two akenia, or round and black grains, surrounded by a granular powder of resinous properties. The strobiles of the wild hop are smaller, and destitute of this substance.

The odour is disagreeable and very strong, taste intensely bitter. Payen and Chevallier have analysed the resinous secretion, and detected *Lupuline*, resin, bitter matter, essential oil, silica, gum, malic acid, and salts of potash and lime, oxide of iron, and sulphur.

LUPULINE

occurs in transparent scales of yellowish white colour, slightly deliquescent, soluble in warm water, still at 212° this only takes up 0,005 of its weight. The solution is frothy. It has no action on test papers, is little acted on by acids or alkalies. It burns without smoke; inodorous, taste decidedly bitter.

To this principle it seems the medicinal virtues of the hop are attributable.

The preparations of hop are slightly narcotic and tonic, the odour and flavour of beer depend on its presence; an extract is much used as a tonic, and a pillow stuffed with the strobiles has been often known to induce sleep in restless patients. Lupuline in grain doses occasions giddiness, drowsiness, and symptoms of intoxication.

Many attempts have been made to substitute other bitter vegetables, such as gentian, quassia, &c. for the hop in the manufacture of malt liquors. The attempts have all failed, as none have ever imitated the delicate and indescribable aroma connected with the Hop bitter. The cultivation of the hop is a source of wealth and happiness to numerous districts in England, Germany, and France. It requires a rich strong soil, and warm seasons without wet. Mr. Royle states his opinion that it might be cultivated successfully in Nipal or the Dhoon, though he dreads that the rainy season would interfere much with the plant.

GEN. 6.—ANTIARIS.

Sp. A. toxicaria (Leschenault.) Upas.

Vern. Ipo toxicaria, *Pers.* A native of Java.

The juice of this tree is one of the most fearful poisons of the vegetable kingdom. The tree is often over 100 feet in height, its bark pale and smooth, its leaves oval, coriaceous, hairy, juice viscous, bitter, white or yellow, flowing abundantly from incisions, and concreting into a gummy resinous mass. The *Upas antiar* poison is prepared in an earthen vessel with this juice, which is mixed with the seed of the Capsicum frutescens, and various aromatics. This poison at first acts as a purgative and emetic, then as a narcotic, causing death by violent fits of tetanic convulsions. The *Upas-tieute* poison is prepared from a strychnos, and differs from this substance.

GEN. 7.—CANNABIS.*

Sp. Cannabis sativa or *C. Indica.* Hemp.

Vern. See the sequel.

Off. Resin and leaves.

The narcotic effects of hemp are popularly known in the south of Africa, South America, Turkey, Egypt, Asia Minor, India, and the adjacent territories of the Malays, Burmese, and Siamese. In all these countries hemp is used in various forms, by the dissipated and depraved, as the ready

* This article prepared for this work expressly has been published in a separate *brochure* dated 1839, in order to collect information on the subject.

agent of a pleasing intoxication. In the popular medicine of these nations, we find it extensively employed for a multitude of affections. But in western Europe its use either as a stimulant or as a remedy, is equally unknown. With the exception of the trial, as a frolic, of the Egyptian "Hasheesh," by a few youths in Marseilles, and of the clinical use of the wine of hemp by Hahneman, as shewn in a subsequent extract, we have been unable to trace any notice of the employment of this drug in Europe.

Much difference of opinion exists on the question, whether the hemp so abundant in Europe, even in high northern latitudes, is identical in specific characters with the plant of Asia Minor and India. The extraordinary symptoms produced by the latter depend on a resinous secretion with which it abounds, and which seems totally absent in the European kind. Still as the closest physical resemblance or even identity exists between both plants, difference of climate seems to us more than sufficient to account for the absence of the resinous secretion, and consequent want of narcotic power in that indigenous in colder countries.

In the subsequent article we first endeavour to present an adequate view of what has been recorded of the early history, the popular uses, and employment in medicine of this powerful and valuable substance; we then proceed to notice several experiments which we have instituted on animals, with the view to ascertain its effects on the healthy system; and, lastly, we submit an abstract of the clinical details of the treatment of several patients afflicted with hydrophobia, tetanus, and other convulsive disorders, in which a preparation of hemp was employed, with results, which seem to us to warrant our anticipating from its more extensive and impartial use no inconsiderable addition to the resources of the physician.

Botanical characters—Chemical Properties—Production.

Botanical Description.—Assuming with Roxburgh and Hamilton and other eminent writers that the *Cannabis sativa* and *indica* are identical, we find that the plant is diœcious, annual, about three feet high, covered over with a fine pubescence; the stem is erect, branched, bright green, angular; leaves alternate or opposite, on long weak petioles; digitate, scabrous, with linear, lanceolate, sharply serrated leaflets, tapering into a long smooth entire point; stipules subulate; clusters of flowers axillary with subulate bracts; males lax and drooping, branched and leafless at base; females erect, simple and leafy at the base. ♂ Calyx downy, five-parted, imbricated. Stamens five; anthers large and pendulous.

♀ Calyx covered with brown glands. Ovary roundish with pendulous ovule, and two long filiform glandular stigmas; achenium ovate, one-seeded.—*v. Lindley's Flora Medica*, p. 299.

The fibres of the stems are long, and extremely tenacious, so as to afford the best tissue for cordage, thus constituting the material for one of the most important branches of European manufactures.

The seed is simply albuminous and oily, and is devoid of all narcotic properties.

CHEMICAL PROPERTIES.—In certain seasons and in warm countries a resinous juice exudes and concretes on the leaves, slender stems, and flowers;—the mode of removing this juice will be subsequently detailed. Separated and in masses it constitutes the *Churrus** of Nipal and Hindostan, and to this, the type or basis of all the hemp preparations, are the powers of these drugs attributable.

The pure resin of the hemp is very soluble in alcohol and ether; partially soluble in alkaline, insoluble in acid solutions; when pure, of a blackish grey colour; hard at 90°; softens at higher temperatures, and fuses readily;—soluble in the fixed and in several volatile oils. Its odour is fragrant and narcotic; taste slightly warm, bitterish, and acrid.

The dried hemp plant which has flowered, and *from which the resin has not been removed*, is called *Gunjah*. It sells for twelve annas to one rupee the seer in the Calcutta bazars, and yields to alcohol twenty per 100 of resinous extract, composed of the resin (*Churrus*), and green colouring matter (*chlorophylle.*) Distilled with a large quantity of water, traces of essential oil pass over, and the distilled liquor has the powerful narcotic odour of the plant. The *Gunjah* is sold for smoking chiefly. The bundles of *Gunjah* are about two feet long and three inches in diameter, and contain twenty-four plants. The colour is dusky green—the odour agreeably narcotic—the whole plant resinous, and adhesive to the touch.

The larger leaves and capsules without the stalks, are called "*Bang, Subjee*, or *Sidhee*." They are used for making an intoxicating drink, for smoking, and in the conserve or confection termed *Majoon*. *Bang* is cheaper than *Gunjah*, and though less powerful, is sold at such a low price that for one pice enough can be purchased to intoxicate an "habituated" person.

According to Mr. McCann's notes, the *Gunjah* consumed

* For very fine specimens of *Churrus*, the Editor has to express his thanks to Dr. Campbell, late Assistant Resident at Nipal, also to Col. Stacy, now at Quetta.

in Bengal is chiefly brought from Mirzapúr and Ghazeepúr, being extensively cultivated near Gwalior and in Tirhoot. The natives cut the plant when in flower, allow it to dry for three days, and then lay it in bundles averaging one seer weight each, which are distributed to the licensed dealers. The best kinds are brought from Gwalior and Bhurtpore, and it is also cultivated, of good quality, in a few gardens round Calcutta. In Jessore, we are informed, the drug is produced of excellent quality, and to a very considerable extent of cultivation.

In Central India and the Saugor territory and in Nipal, *Churrus* is collected during the hot season in the following singular manner:—men clad in leathern dresses run through the hemp-fields brushing through the plant with all possible violence; the soft resin adheres to the leather, and is subsequently scraped off and kneaded into balls, which sell from five to six rupees the seer. A still finer kind, the *Momeea* or waxen *Churrus*, is collected by the hand in Nipal, and sells for nearly double the price of the ordinary kind. In Nipal, Dr. McKinnon informs us, the leathern attire is dispensed with, and the resin is gathered on the skins of naked coolies. In Persia, it is stated by Mirza Abdul Russac, that the *Churrus* is prepared by pressing the resinous plant on coarse cloths, and then scraping it from these and melting it in a pot with a little warm water. He considers the *Churrus* of Herat as the best and most powerful of all the varieties of the drug.

Popular uses.

The preparations of hemp are used for the purpose of intoxication as follows:—

Sidhee, *Subjee*, and *Bang* (synonymous) are used with water as a drink, which is thus prepared:—About three tola weight (540 troy grains) are well washed with cold water, then rubbed to powder, mixed with black pepper, cucumber, and melon seeds, sugar, half a pint of milk, and an equal quantity of water. This is considered sufficient to intoxicate an habituated person. Half the quantity is enough for a novice. This composition is chiefly used by the Mahomedans of the better classes.

Another recipe is as follows:—

The same quantity of *Sidhee* is washed and ground, mixed with black pepper, and a quart of cold water added. This is drank at one sitting. This is the favourite beverage of the Hindus who practice this vice, especially the Birjobassies and many of the Rajpootana soldiery.

From either of these beverages intoxication will ensue in half an hour. Almost invariably the inebriation is of the most cheerful kind, causing the person to sing and dance, to eat food with great relish, and to seek aphrodisiac enjoyments. In persons of a quarrelsome disposition it occasions, as might be expected, an exasperation of their natural tendency. The intoxication lasts about three hours, when sleep supervenes. No nausea or sickness of stomach succeeds, nor are the bowels at all affected; next day there is slight giddiness and vascularity of the eyes, but no other symptom worth recording.

Gunjah is used for smoking alone—one rupee weight, (180 grains) and a little dried tobacco are rubbed together in the palm of the hand with a few drops of water. This suffices for three persons. A little tobacco is placed in the pipe first, then a layer of the prepared *Gunjah*, then more tobacco, and the fire above all.

Four or five persons usually join in this debauch. The hookah is passed round, and each person takes a single draught. Intoxication ensues almost instantly; and from one draught to the unaccustomed, within half an hour; and after four or five inspirations to those more practised in the vice. The effects differ from those occasioned by the *Sidhee*. Heaviness, laziness, and agreeable reveries ensue, but the person can be readily roused, and is able to discharge routine occupations, such as pulling the punkah, waiting at table, &c.

The *Majoon*, or hemp confection, is a compound of sugar, butter, flour, milk, and *Sidhee* or *Bang*. The process has been repeatedly performed before us by Ameer, the proprietor of a celebrated place of resort for hemp devotees in Calcutta, and who is considered the best artist in his profession. Four ounces of *Sidhee* and an equal quantity of *ghee* are placed in an earthen or well-tinned vessel, a pint of water added, and the whole warmed over a charcoal fire. The mixture is constantly stirred until the water all boils away, which is known by the crackling noise of the melted butter on the sides of the vessel; the mixture is then removed from the fire, squeezed through cloth while hot—by which an oleaginous solution of the active principles and colouring matter of the hemp is obtained—and the leaves, fibres, &c., remaining on the cloth are thrown away.

The green oily solution soon concretes into a buttery mass, and is then well washed by the hand with soft water so long as the water becomes coloured. The colouring matter and an extractive substance are thus removed, and a very pale green mass, of the consistence of simple ointment, remains. The washings are thrown away;—Ameer says that these are intoxicating, and produce constriction of the throat, great pain, and very disagreeable and dangerous symptoms.

The operator then takes two pounds of sugar, and adding a little water, places it in a pipkin over the fire. When the sugar dissolves and froths, two ounces of milk are added; a thick scum rises and is removed—more milk and a little water are added from time to time, and the boiling continued about an hour, the solution being carefully stirred until it becomes an adhesive clear syrup, ready to solidify on a cold surface; four ounces of tyre (new milk dried before the sun) in fine powder are now stirred in, and lastly the prepared butter of hemp is introduced, brisk stirring being continued for a few minutes. A few drops of utter of roses are then quickly sprinkled in, and the mixture poured from the pipkin on a flat cold dish or slab. The mass concretes immediately into a thin cake, which is divided into small lozenge-shaped pieces. A seer thus prepared sells for four rupees: one drachm by weight will intoxicate a beginner; three drachms one experienced in its use. The taste is sweet, and the odour very agreeable.

Ameer states that there are seven or eight *Majoon* makers in Calcutta;—that sometimes by special order of customers he introduces stramonium seeds, but never nux-vomica;—that all classes of persons, including the lower Portuguese, or "Kala Feringhees," and especially their females, consume the drug;—that it is most fascinating in its effects, producing extatic happiness, a persuasion of high rank, a sensation of flying, voracious appetite, and intense aphrodisiac desire. He denies that its continued use leads to madness, impotence, or to the numerous evil consequences described by the Arabic and Persian physicians. Although we disbelieve Ameer's statements on this point, his description of the immediate effects of *Majoon* is strictly and accurately correct.

Most carnivorous animals eat it greedily, and very soon experience its narcotic effects, becoming ludicrously drunk, but seldom suffering any worse consequences.

Historical details—Notices of Hemp, and its popular uses, by the Sanscrit, Arabic, and Persian writers.

The preceding notice suffices to explain the subsequent historical and medicinal details. We premise the historical, in order to shew the exact state of our knowledge of the subject, when we attempted its investigation.

Although the most eminent of the Arabic and Persian authors concur in referring the origin of the practice of hemp intoxication to the natives of Hindoostan, it is remarkable that few traces can be detected of the prevalence of the vice at any early period in India.

The Pandit Moodoosudun Gooptu finds that the "Rajniguntu," a standard treatise on Materia Medica, which he estimates vaguely at 600 years date, gives a clear account of this agent. Its synonymes are "*Bijoya*," "*Ujoya*," and "*Joya*,"—names which mean, promoters of success; "*Brijputta*," or the strengthener, or the strong-leaved; "*Chapola*," the causer of a reeling gait; "*Ununda*," or the laughter-moving; "*Hursini*," the exciter of sexual desire. Its effects on man are described as excitant, heating, astringent. It is added, that it "destroys phlegm, expels flatulence, induces costiveness, sharpens the memory, increases eloquence, excites the appetite, and acts as a general tonic."

The "Rajbulubha," a Sanscrit treatise of rather later date, alludes to the use of hemp in gonorrhœa, and repeats the statements of the "Rajniguntu." In the Hindu Tantra, a religious treatise, teaching peculiar and mystical formulæ and rites for the worship of the deities, it is said, moreover, that *Sidhee* is more intoxicating than the wine.

In the celebrated "Susruta," which is perhaps the most ancient of all Hindu medical works, it is written, that persons labouring under catarrh should, with other remedies, use internally the *Bijoya* or *Sidhee*. The effects, however, are not described.

The learned Kamalakantha Vidyalanka has traced a notice of hemp in the fifth chapter of *Menu*, where Brahmins are prohibited to use the following substances—*Palandoo* or onions, *Gunjara* or *Gunjah*, and such condiments as have strong and pungent scents.

The Arabic and Persian writers are however far more voluminous and precise in their accounts of these fascinating preparations. In the first vol. of De Sacy's "Crestomathie Arabe" we find an extremely interesting summary of the writings of Takim Eddin Makrizi on this subject. Lane has noticed it too with his usual ability in his admirable work "the Modern Egyptians." From these two sources, the MS. notes of the Syed Keramut Ali and Mr. DaCosta, and a curious paper communicated by our friend Mirza Abdul Russac, a very intelligent Persian physician, the following epitome is compiled.

Makrizi treats of the hemp in his glowing description of the celebrated Canton de la Timbaliere, or ancient pleasure grounds, in the vicinity of Cairo. This quarter, after many vicissitudes, is now a heap of ruins. In it was situated a cultivated valley named Djoneina, which we are informed was the theatre of all conceivable abominations. It was famous above all for the sale of the *Hasheeha*, which is still greedily consumed by the dregs of the populace, and from the consumption of which sprung the excesses which led to the name of "Assassin" being given to the Saracens in the Holy Wars. The history of the drug the author treats of thus:—The oldest work in which hemp is noticed is a treatise by Hassan, who states that in the year 658, M. E. the Sheikh Djafar Shirazi, a monk of the order of Haider, learned from his master the history of the discovery of hemp. Haider, the chief of ascetics and self-chasteners, lived in rigid privation on a mountain between Nishabor and Rama, where he established a monastery of Fakirs. Ten years he had spent in this retreat without leaving it for a moment, till one burning summer's day when he departed alone to the fields. On his return an air of joy and gaiety was imprinted on his countenance; he received the visits of his brethren, and encouraged their conversation. On being questioned, he stated that struck by the aspect of a plant which danced in the heat as if with joy, while all the rest of the vegetable creation was torpid, he had gathered and eaten of its leaves. He led his companions to the spot,—all ate and all were similarly excited. A tincture of the hemp leaf in wine or spirit seems to have been the favourite formula in which the Sheikh Haider indulged himself. An Arab poet sings of Haider's *emerald* cup—an evident allusion to the rich green colour of the tincture of the drug. The Sheikh survived the discovery ten years, and subsisted chiefly on this herb, and on his death his disciples by his desire planted it in an arbour round his tomb. From this saintly sepulchre the knowledge of the effects of hemp is stated to have spread into Khorasan. In Chaldea it was unknown until 728 M. E. during the reign of the Khalif Mostansir Billah: the kings of Ormus and Bahrein then introduced it into Chaldea, Syria, Egypt, and Turkey.

In Khorasan, however, it seems that the date of the use of hemp is considered to be far prior to Haider's era. Biraslan, an Indian pilgrim, the contemporary of Cosröes,* is believed to have introduced and diffused the custom through

* By this term is probably meant the first of the Sassanian dynasty, to whom the epithet "of Khusrow," or Cosröes, equivalent to Káiser, Cæsar, or Czar, has been applied in many generations. This dynasty endured from A. D. 202 to A. D. 636—*Vide note* 50 *to Lane's translation of the Arabian Nights*, *vol.* ii. p. 226.

Khorasan and Yemen. In proof of the great antiquity of the practice, certain passages in the works of Hippocrates may be cited, in which some of its properties are clearly described—but the difficulty of deciding whether the passages be spurious or genuine, renders the fact of little value. Dioscorides (lib. ii. cap. 169,) describes hemp, but merely notices the emollient properties of its seeds—its intoxicating effects must consequently be regarded as unknown to the Greeks prior to his era, which is generally agreed to be about the second century of the Christian epoch, and somewhat subsequent to the lifetime of Pliny.

In the narrative of Makrizi we also learn that oxymel and acids are the most powerful antidotes to the effects of this narcotic; next to these, emetics, cold bathing, and sleep; and we are further told that it possesses diuretic, astringent, and especially aphrodisiac properties. Ibn Beitar was the first to record its tendency to produce mental derangement, and he even states that it occasionally proves fatal.

In 780 M. E. very severe ordinances were passed in Egypt against the practice: the Djoneina garden was rooted up, and all those convicted of the use of the drug were subjected to the extraction of their teeth; but in 799 M.E. the custom re-established itself with more than original vigour. Makrizi draws an expressive picture of the evils this vice then inflicted on its votaries—"As its consequence, general corruption of sentiments and manners ensued, modesty disappeared, every base and evil passion was openly indulged in, and nobility of external form alone remained to these infatuated beings."

Medicinal properties assigned to Hemp by the ancient Arabian and Persian writers, and by modern European authors.

In the preceding notice of Makrizi's writings on this subject we have confined ourselves chiefly to historical details, excluding descriptions of supposed medicinal effects. The Mukzun-ul-Udwieh and the Persian MS. in our possession, inform us as to the properties which the ancient physicians attributed to this powerful narcotic.

In Mr. DaCosta's MS. version of the chapter on Hemp in the Mukzun-ul-Udwieh, *Churrus*, we are informed, if smoked through a pipe causes torpor and intoxication, and often proves fatal to the smoker. Three kinds are noticed, the *garden*, *wild*, and *mountain*, of which the last is deemed the strongest;—the seeds are called *sheadana* or *shaldaneh* in Persia. These are said to be "a compound of opposite qualities, cold and dry in the third degree, that is to say, stimulant and sedative, imparting at first a gentle reviving heat, and then a considerable refrigerant effect."

The contrary qualities of the plant, its stimulant and sedative effects, are prominently dwelt on. "They at first exhilarate the spirits, cause cheerfulness, give colour to the complexion, bring on intoxication, excite the imagination into the most rapturous ideas, produce thirst, increase appetite, excite concupiscence. Afterwards the sedative effects begin to preside, the spirits sink, the vision darkens and weakens; and madness, melancholy, fearfulness, dropsy, and such like distempers, are the sequel—while the seminal secretions dry up. These effects are increased by sweets, and combated by acids."

The author of the Mukzun-ul-Udwieh further informs us—"The leaves make a good snuff for deterging the brain; the juice of the leaves applied to the head as a wash, removes dandriff and vermin; drops of the juice thrown into the ear allay pain and destroy worms or insects. It checks diarrhœa, is useful in gonorrhœa, restrains seminal secretions, and is diuretic. The bark has a similar effect."

"The powder is recommended as an external application to fresh wounds and sores, and for causing granulations; a poultice of the boiled root and leaves for discussing inflammations and cure of erysipelas, and for allaying neuralgic pains. The dried leaves bruised and spread on a castor oil leaf cure hydrocele and swelled testes. The *dose* internally is one *direm*, or 48 grains. The antidotes are emetics, cow's milk, hot water, and sorrel wine."

Alluding to its popular uses, the author dwells on the eventual evil consequences of the indulgence; weakness of the digestive organs first ensues, followed by flatulency, indigestion, swelling of the limbs and face, change of complexion, diminution of sexual vigour, loss of teeth, heaviness, cowardice, depraved and wicked ideas, scepticism in religious tenets;—licentiousness and ungodliness are also enumerated in the catalogue of deplorable results.

The medicinal properties of hemp, in various forms, are the subject of some interesting notes by Mirza Abdul Russac. "It produces a ravenous appetite and constipation, arrests the secretions except that of the liver, excites wild imagining, a sensation of ascending, forgetfulness of all that happens during its use, and such mental exaltation, that *the beholders attribute it to supernatural inspiration.*"

Mirza Abdul considers hemp to be a powerful exciter of the flow of bile, and relates cases of its efficacy in restoring appetite—of its utility as an external application as a poultice with milk, in relieving hæmorrhoids—and internally in gonorrhœa, to the extent of a quarter drachm of *bangh*. He states also that the habitual smokers of *Gunjah* generally die of diseases of the lungs, dropsy, and anasarca—"so do the eaters of *Majoon* and smokers of *Sidhee*, but at a later period. The inexperienced on first taking it are often senseless for a day, some go mad, others are known to die."

In the 35th chapter of the 5th volume of Rumphius' Herbarium Amboinense, p. 208, Ed. Amsterd. A. D. 1695, we find a long and very good account of this drug, illustrated by two excellent plates. The subjoined is an epitome of Rumphius' article.

Rumphius first describes botanically the male and female hemp plants, of which he gives two admirable drawings. He assigns the upper provinces of India as its *habitat*, and states it to be cultivated in Java and Amboyna. He then notices very briefly the exciting effects ascribed to the leaf, and to mixtures thereof with spices, camphor, and opium. He alludes doubtingly to its alleged aphrodisiac powers, and states that the kind of mental excitement it produces depends on the temperament of the consumer. He quotes a passage from Galen, lib. i. (*de aliment, facult*) in which it is asserted that in that great writer's time it was customary to give hemp seed to the guests at banquets, as a promoter of hilarity and enjoyment. Rumphius adds, that the Mahomedans in his neighbourhood frequently sought for the male plant from his garden to be given to persons afflicted with virulent gonorrhœa or with asthma, and the affection which is popularly called "stitches in the side." He tells us, moreover, that the powdered leaves check diarrhœa, are stomachic, cure the malady named *pitao*, and moderate excessive secretion of bile. He mentions the use of hemp smoke as an enema in strangulated hernia, and of the leaves as an antidote to poisoning by orpiment. Lastly, he notices in the two subsequent chapters varieties of hemp which he terms the *Gunjah sativa* and *Gunjah agrestis*.

In the *Hortus Malabaricus*, Rheede's article on the Hemp is a mere outline of Rumphius' statements.

Among modern European writers the only information we could trace on the medicinal use of Hemp *in Europe*, is in the recent work of Nees v. Esenbeck, from which the following is an extract kindly supplied by Dr. Wallich :—

"The fresh herb of the hemp has a very powerful and unpleasant narcotic smell, and is used in the East in combination with opium, in the preparation of intoxicating potions, &c. It is probable that the *nepenthe* of the ancients was prepared from the leaves of this plant. Many physicians, Hahnemann among them, prescribe the vinous extract in various nervous disorders, where opium and hyoscyamus used to be employed, being less heating and devoid of bitterness."*

No information as to the medicinal effects of hemp exists in the standard works on Materia Medica, to which we have access. Soubeiran, Feé, Merat, and De Lens in their admirable dictionary; Chevallier and Richard, Roques (Phytographie Medicale); Ratier and Henry (Pharmacopeé Française); and the Dictionnaire des Sciences Medicales—are all equally silent on the subject.

In the *Journal de Pharmacie*, the most complete Magazine in existence on all pharmaceutical subjects, we find hemp noticed in several volumes. In the Bulletin de Pharmacie t. v. A. 1810, p. 400, we find it briefly described by M. Rouyer, apothecary to Napoleon, and member of the Egyptian scientific commission, in a paper on the popular remedies of Egypt. With the leaves and tops, he tells us, collected before ripening, the Egyptians prepare a conserve, which serves as the base of the *berch*, the *diasmouk*, and the *bernaouy*. Hemp leaves reduced to powder and incorporated with honey, or stirred with water, constitute the *berch* of the poor classes.

The same work also (Bulletin, vol. i. p. 523, A. D. 1809,) contains a very brief notice on the intoxicating preparations of hemp, read by M. De Sacy before the Institute of France in July, 1809. M. De Sacy's subsequent analysis of Makrizi, of which we have given an outline, is however much richer in details than the article in the Bulletin.

In *Ainslie's Materia Indica*, 2nd vol. we find three notices of the plant and its preparations.

At page 39 "Banghie," (*Tamul*) with the Persian and Hindee synonymes of "Beng" and "Subjee," is described as an intoxicating liquor prepared with the leaves of the *Gunjah*, or hemp plant.

Under the head *Gunjah*, Ainslie gives numerous synonymes, and tells us that the leaves are sometimes prescribed in cases of diarrhœa; and in conjunction with turmeric, onions, and warm gingilie oil are made into an unction for painful protruded piles. Dr. Ainslie also gives a brief view of the popular uses and botanical peculiarities of the plant.

* *Handbuch der medicinisch-pharmaceutischen Botanik, von Dr. Th. Fr. Nees von Esenbeck and Dr. Carl Ebermaier, vol.* i. *p.* 338.

Majoon, lastly, is described by Dr. Ainslie, page 176, as a preparation of sugar, milk, ghee, poppy seeds, the seeds of the datura, powder of nux-vomica, and sugar. The true *Majoon*, however, as prepared in Bengal, contains neither datura nor nux-vomica. We have already described the process by which it has been manufactured before us.*

Experiments by the Editor—inferences as to the action of the drug on animals and man.

Such was the amount of preliminary information before us, by which we were guided in our subsequent attempts to gain more accurate knowledge of the action, powers, and possible medicinal applications of this extraordinary agent.

There was sufficient to shew that hemp possessed in small doses an extraordinary power of stimulating the digestive organs, exciting the cerebral system, of acting also on the generative apparatus. Larger doses, again, were shewn by the historical statements to induce insensibility, or to act as a powerful sedative. The influence of the drug in allaying pain was equally manifest in all the memoirs referred to. As to the evil sequelæ so unanimously dwelt on by all writers, these did not appear to us so numerous, so immediate, or so formidable, as many which may be clearly traced to over-indulgence in other powerful stimulants or narcotics, viz. alcohol, opium, or tobacco.

The dose in which the hemp preparations might be administered, constituted of course one of the first objects of inquiry. Ibn Beitar had mentioned a *direm*, or 48 grains of *Churrus*, but this dose seemed to us so enormous, that we deemed it expedient to proceed with much smaller quantities. How fortunate was this caution, the sequel will sufficiently denote.

An extensive series of experiments on animals was in the first place undertaken, among which the following may be cited:—

Expt. 1.—Ten grains of Nipalese *Churrus*, dissolved in spirit were given to a middling sized dog. In half an hour he became stupid and sleepy, dozing at intervals, starting up, wagging his tail as if extremely contented, he ate some food greedily, on being called to he staggered to and fro, and his face assumed a look of utter and helpless drunkenness. These symptoms lasted about two hours, and then

* Royle in his "*Illustrations*," p. 334, gives a very brief notice of the synonymes and epithets of the hemp resin, and he mentions also its intoxicating properties.

gradually passed away; in six hours he was perfectly well and lively.

Expt. 2.—One drachm of *Majoon* was given to a small sized dog, he ate it with great delight, and in twenty minutes was ridiculously drunk; in four hours his symptoms passed away, also without harm.

Expts. 3, 4, & 5.—Three kids had ten grains each of the alcoholic extract of *Gunjah.* In one no effect was produced; in the second there was much heaviness, and some inability to move; in the third a marked alteration of countenance was conspicuous, but no further effect.

Expt. 6.—Twenty grains were given, dissolved in a little spirit, to a dog of very small size. In a quarter of an hour he was intoxicated, in half an hour he had great difficulty of movement; in an hour he had lost all power over the hinder extremities, which were rather stiff but flexible; sensibility did not seem to be impaired, and the circulation was natural. He readily acknowledged calls by an attempt to rise up. In four hours he was quite well.

In none of these or several other experiments was there the least indication of pain, or any degree of convulsive movement observed.

It seems needless to dwell on the details of each experiment; suffice it to say that they led to one remarkable result—That while carnivorous animals and fish, dogs, cats, swine, vultures, crows, and adjutants, invariably and speedily exhibited the intoxicating influence of the drug, the graminivorous, such as the horse, deer, monkey, goat, sheep, and cow, experienced but trivial effects from any dose we administered.

Encouraged by these results, no hesitation could be felt as to the perfect safety of giving the resin of hemp an extensive trial in the cases in which its apparent powers promised the greatest degree of utility.

Cases of Rheumatism treated by Hemp.

The first cases selected were two of acute rheumatism, and one of that disease in the chronic form. In the two former but little relief had been derived from a fair trial of antiphlogistic measures, and Dover's powder with antimonials—In the last case, sarsaparilla at first, and subsequently the Hemidesmus Indicus with warm baths had been tried without advantage.

On the 6th November, 1838, one grain of the resin of Hemp was administered in solution, at 2 P. M. to each of these three patients.

At 4 P. M. it was reported that one was becoming very talkative, was singing songs, calling loudly for an extra supply of food, and declaring himself in perfect health. The other two patients remained unaffected.

At 6 P. M. received a report to the same effect, but stating that the first patient was now falling asleep.

At 8 P. M.—alarmed by an emergent note from Nobinchunder Mitter, the clinical clerk on duty, describing the patient's symptoms as very peculiar and formidable; went to the Hospital without delay, and found him lying on his cot quite insensible, but breathing with perfect regularity, his pulse and skin natural, and the pupils freely contractile on the approach of light.

On examining the other patients—found one asleep, the third awake, intelligent, and free from any symptoms of intoxication or alarm.

Returning then to the first, an emetic was directed to be prepared, and while waiting for it, on lifting up the patient's arm, the professional reader will judge of our astonishment, when we found that it remained in the posture in which we placed it. It required but a very brief examination of the limbs to find that the patient had by the influence of this narcotic been thrown into that strange and most extraordinary of all nervous conditions, into that state which so few have seen, and the existence of which so many still discredit—the genuine *catalepsy* of the nosologist.

To return to our patient, we raised him to a sitting posture, and placed his arms and limbs in every imaginable attitude. A waxen figure could not be more pliant or more stationary in each position, no matter how contrary to the natural influence of gravity on the part.

To all impressions he was meanwhile almost insensible; he made no sign of understanding questions, and could not be aroused. A sinapism to the epigastrium caused no evidence of pain. The pharynx and its coadjutor muscles acted freely in the deglutition of the stimulant remedies which we thought it advisable to administer, although the manifest cataleptic state had freed us altogether of the anxiety under which we before laboured.

The second patient had meanwhile been roused by the noise in the ward, and seemed vastly amused at the strange aspect of the statue-like attitudes in which the first patient had been placed, when on a sudden he uttered a loud peal of laughter, and exclaimed that four spirits were springing with his bed into the air. In vain we attempted to pacify him; his laughter became momentarily more and more incontrollable. We now observed that the limbs were rather rigid, and in a few minutes more his arms or legs could be bent, and would remain in any desired position. A strong stimulant drink was immediately given, and a sinapism applied. Of the latter he made no complaint, but his intoxication led him to such noisy exclamations, that we had to remove him to a separate room; here he soon became tranquil, his limbs in less than an hour gained their natural condition, and in two hours he said he was perfectly well and very hungry.

The first patient continued cataleptic till 1 A. M., when consciousness and voluntary motion quickly returned, and by 2 A.M. he was exactly in the same state as the second patient.

The third man experienced no effect whatever, and on further inquiry it was found that he was habituated to the use of *Gunjah* in the pipe.

On the following day we found with much pleasure that both the individuals above-mentioned were not only uninjured by the narcotic, but much relieved of their rheumatism ; they were discharged quite cured in three days after.

The fourth case of trial was an old muscular cooly, a rheumatic malingerer, and to him half a grain of hemp resin was given in a little spirit. The first day's report will suffice for all.—In two hours the old gentleman became talkative and musical, told several stories, and sang songs to a circle of highly delighted auditors, ate the dinners of two persons subscribed for him in the ward, sought also for other luxuries we can scarcely venture to allude to, and finally fell soundly asleep, and so continued till the following morning. On the noon-day visit, he expressed himself free from headache or any other unpleasant sequel, and begged hard for a repetition of the medicine; in this he was indulged for a few days, and then discharged.

In several cases of acute and chronic rheumatism admitted about this time, half-grain doses of the resin were given, with closely analogous effects ;—alleviation of pain in most —remarkable increase of appetite in all—unequivocal aphrodisia, and great mental cheerfulness. The disposition developed was uniform in all, and in none was headache or sickness of stomach a sequel of the excitement.

Case of Hydrophobia.

The following case is given as originally published in the Editor's Essay on this subject.

" On the 22nd November at 8 A.M. a note in English was handed to me by my servant, entreating my assistance for the Hakim Abdullah, then at my gate, who had been bitten by a rabid dog three weeks before, and who feared that the miserable consequences of the bite already had commenced. I found the poor man in a carriage ; he was perfectly composed, though quite convinced of the desperate nature of his case. He told me that the evening before, on passing near a tank he started in alarm, and since then was unable to swallow liquid. His eye was restless, suspicious, and wild, his features anxious, his pulse 125, the skin bedewed with cold moisture ; he stated nevertheless that he wished for food, and felt well;—a small red and painful cicatrix existed on the left fore-arm.

"He was immediately removed to the Hospital, where I accompanied him. By his own desire water was brought in a metallic vessel, which he grasped and brought near his lips; —never can I forget the indescribable horrors of the paroxysm which ensued. It abated in about three minutes, and morbid thirst still goading the unhappy man, he besought his servant to apply a moistened cloth to his lips. Intelligent and brave, he determinately awaited the contact of the cloth, and for a few seconds, though in appalling agony, permitted some drops to trickle on his tongue,—but then ensued a second struggle, which, with a due share of the callousness of my profession, I could not stand by to contemplate.

"Two grains of hemp resin in a soft pillular mass were ordered every hour ; after the third dose he stated that he felt commencing intoxication—he now chatted cheerfully on his case, and displayed great intelligence and experience in the treatment of the very disease with which he was visited. He talked calmly of drinking, but said it was in vain to try—but he could suck an orange ; this was brought to him, and he succeeded in swallowing the juice without any difficulty.

"The hemp was continued till the sixth dose, when he fell asleep, and had some rest. Early the ensuing morning, however, Mr. Siddons, my assistant, was called up to him, and found him in a state of tumultuous agony and excitement ; tortured by thirst he attempted to drink,—but I will spare the reader the details of the horrors which ensued.

"The hemp was again repeated, and again by the third dose the cheering alleviation of the previous day was witnessed. He ate a piece of sugar-cane, and again swallowed the juice—he partook freely of some moistened rice, and permitted a purgative enema to be administered. His pulse was nearly natural, the skin natural in every respect. His countenance was happy. On *one* subject only was he incoherent, and even here was manifested the powerful and peculiar influence of the narcotic. He spoke in raptures of the inmates of his *zenana*, and his anxiety to be with them. We ascertained however that he had no such establishment.

"Four days thus passed away, the doses of hemp being continued. When he fell asleep, on waking the paroxysms returned, but were again almost immediately assuaged as at first. Meanwhile purgative enemata were employed, and he partook freely of solid food, and once drank water without the least suffering. But about 3 P. M. of the fifth day he sunk into profound stupor, the breathing slightly stertorous; in this state he continued, and without further struggle death terminated his sufferings at 4 A. M. on the 27th November.

"Reviewing the preceding summary of this interesting case, it seems evident that at least one advantage was gained from the use of the remedy—the awful malady was stripped of its horrors;—if not less fatal than before, it was reduced to less than the scale of suffering which precedes death from most ordinary diseases. It must be remembered too, that in this the first case ever so treated, I possessed no data to guide me as to the dose or manner of administration of the drug. The remarkable cases of tetanus detailed in the sequel, throw light on these important points, and will lead in future cases to the unhesitating administration of much larger quantities than at first I ventured to employ. I am not however rash enough to indulge the hope which involuntarily forces itself upon me, that we will ever from this narcotic derive an effectual remedy, for even a solitary case of this disease—but next to cure, the physician will perhaps esteem the means which enable him 'to strew the path to the tomb with flowers,' and to divest of its *specific* terrors the most dreadful malady to which mankind is exposed."

While the preceding case was under treatment, and exciting the utmost interest in the school, several pupils commenced experiments on themselves, to ascertain the effects of the drug. In all, the state of the pulse was noted before taking a dose, and subsequently the effects were observed by two pupils of much intelligence. The result of several trials was, that in as small doses as the quarter of a grain, the pulse was increased in fullness and frequency; the surface of the body glowed; the appetite became extraordinary; vivid ideas crowded the mind; unusual loquacity occurred;

and with scarcely any exception great aphrodisia was experienced.

In one pupil, Dinonath Dhur, a retiring lad of excellent habits, ten drops of the tincture, equal to a quarter of a grain of the resin, induced in twenty minutes the most amusing effects.

A shout of loud and prolonged laughter ushered in the symptoms, and a transitory state of cataleptic rigidity occurred for two or three minutes. Summoned to witness the effects, we found him enacting the part of a Raja giving orders to his courtiers; he could recognize none of his fellow students or acquaintances; all to his mind seemed as altered as his own condition; he spoke of many years having passed since his student's days; described his teachers and friends with a piquancy which a dramatist would envy; detailed the adventures of an imaginary series of years, his travels, his attainment of wealth and power. He entered on discussions on religious, scientific, and political topics, with astonishing eloquence, and disclosed an extent of knowledge, reading, and a ready apposite wit, which those who knew him best were altogether unprepared for. For three hours and upwards he maintained the character he at first assumed, and with a degree of ease and dignity perfectly becoming his high situation. A scene more interesting it would be difficult to imagine. It terminated nearly as abruptly as it commenced, and no headache, sickness, or other unpleasant symptom followed the innocent excess.

Dr. Goodeve and more than thirty students were present at this occurrence.

In the symptoms above described, we are unavoidably led to trace a close resemblance to the effects produced by the reputed inspiration of the Delphic Oracles—perhaps it would not be very erroneous to conclude, that it was referable to the same kind of excitement.

Use in Cholera.

An epidemic cholera prevailing at this period, two of the students administered the tincture of hemp in several cases of that disease, and cures were daily reported by its alleged efficacy. Dr. Goodeve was thus led to try it in several cases, and his report was in the highest degree favorable. The diarrhœa was in most instances checked, and the stimulating effects of the drug clearly manifested. The Durwan of the College, an athletic Rajpoot, was attacked, and came under our treatment after he had been ill seven hours; he was pulseless, cold, and in a state of imminent danger, the characteristic evacuations streaming from him without effort—half a grain of the hemp resin was given, and in twenty minutes the pulse returned, the skin became warm, the purging ceased, and he fell asleep. In an hour he was cataleptic, and continued so for several hours. In the morning he was perfectly well and at his duty as usual.

It is but fair to state, however, that the character of the epidemic was not at the time malignant. We admit the cases to be inconclusive, but we conceive them to be promising, and that they deserve the due attention of practitioners.*

Use in Tetanus.

The first case of this disease treated by hemp was that of Ramjan Khan, æt: 30, admitted to the College Hospital on the 13th December 1838, for a sloughing ulcer on the back of the left hand. Five days previously a native empiric had applied a red hot *gool* (the mixture of charcoal and tobacco used in the hookah) to the back of the left wrist, as a remedy for chronic dysentery and spleen. The patient's brother was similarly cauterized on the same day. In both sloughing took place down to the tendons. Symptoms of tetanus occurred on the 24th December. The brother who had refused to avail himself of European aid, had been seized with tetanus at his own home four days previously, and died after three days illness. On the 26th of December spasms set in, and recurred at intervals of a few minutes; the muscles of the abdomen, neck, and jaws, became firmly and permanently contracted. Large doses of opium with calomel having been administered for some hours, without the least alleviation of symptoms, and his case having on consultation been pronounced completely hopeless, we obtained Mr. Egerton's permission to subject the poor man to the trial of the hemp resin. Two grains were first given at 2½ P. M., dissolved in a little spirit. In half an hour the patient felt

* Since this passage was written in 1839, the tincture of hemp has been used in a great number of cases, both European and Native, in the Hospital of the Medical College. We know no remedy equal to it, as a general and steady stimulant when given to Europeans, in the dose of half a drachm, during the *tractable* stage of this disease. We have known the pulse and heat return, and the purging checked by a single dose. It allays vomiting much more certainly than the opium preparations, and is not more likely than these to lead to cerebral congestion on the cessation of the cholera symptoms. The cheering effect on the patient's spirits is not the least benefit the remedy confers. Of course in every serious epidemic, especially at the commencement, many cases will occur, which seem, as Majendie expressed it, "to begin by death," and in which all remedies are alike ineffectual. In native cases, much less advantage was obtained, a circumstance which without doubt depends on the class of patients we had to treat; being almost universally *gunjah* smokers by long habit.—EDITOR.

giddy, at 5 P. M. his eyes were closed, he was sleepy, and expressed himself much intoxicated.

He slept at intervals during the night, but on waking had convulsive attacks.

On the 27th, two grains were given every third hour, (a purgative enema was also administered, which operated three times) the stiffness of the muscles became much less towards evening, but the spasms returned at intervals as before. Pulse and skin natural.

28th.—Improved; is lethargic but intelligent. Spasms occasionally recur, but at much longer intervals, and in less severity.

29th.—Dose of hemp increased to three grains every second hour. Symptoms moderating.

30th.—Much intoxicated, continues to improve.

1st January, 1839.—A hemp cataplasm applied to the ulcer, and internal use of remedy continued; towards evening was much improved; spasms trivial, no permanent rigidity; had passed two *dysenteric stools.*

2nd.—*Morning report.* Has passed a good night, and seems much better. Hemp continued. *Evening report.* Doing remarkably well.

3rd, 4th, and 5th.—Continues to improve. Hemp resin in two grain doses every fifth hour.

6th.—5 P. M. Feverish, skin hot, pulse quick, all tetanic symptoms gone, passing mucous and bloody stools; leeches to abdomen, a starch and opium enema with three grains of acetate of lead, every second hour; tepid sponging to the body. Hemp omitted.

7th.—6 A. M. Still feverish, stools frequent, mucous; abdomen tender on pressure. No appetite. The ulcer sloughy, ragged, and offensive. Opium and acetate of lead continued. Abdomen leeched. Sore dressed with water. At noon there was slight rigidity of abdominal muscles. Hemp resumed. At 3 P. M. became intoxicated and hungry, ulcer extremely dry, foul, and abominably fœtid—towards evening rigidity ceased. Hemp discontinued.

From this day the tetanus may be considered to have ceased altogether, but the dysenteric symptoms continued, despite of the use of opium and acetate of lead; the ulcer too proved utterly intractable. Some improvement in the dysenteric symptoms occurred from the 10th to the 15th, when natural stools were passed. He seemed gaining strength, but the wound was in no wise improved, the slough on the contrary threatened to spread, and two metacarpal bones lay loose in the centre of the sore; on consultation it was agreed to amputate the arm, but to this the patient peremptorily objected. The mortification now spread rapidly, and he died of exhaustion on the night of the 23rd January.

An unprejudiced review of the preceding details exhibits the sedative powers of the remedy in the most favorable light; and although the patient died, it must be remembered that it was of a different disease, over which it is not presumed that the hemp possessed the least power.

The *second* case was that of Chunoo Syce, (treated by Mr. O'Brien at the Native Hospital,) in whom tetanus supervened on the 11th December, after an injury from the kick of a horse. After an ineffectual trial of turpentine and castor oil in large doses, two grain doses of hemp resin were given on the 26th November. He consumed in all 134 grains of the resin, and left the Hospital cured on the 28th December.

Third case, Huroo, a female, æt: 25, admitted to the Native Hospital on 16th December, had tetanus for the three previous days, the sequel of a cut on the left elbow received a fortnight before. Symptoms violent on admission. Turpentine and castor oil given repeatedly without effect; on the 16th and 17th, three grains of hemp resin were given at bed-time. On the morning of the 18th she was found in a state of complete catalepsy, and remained so until evening, when she became sensible, and a tetanic paroxysm recurred. Hemp resumed, and continued in two grain doses every fourth hour. From this time till the third hour tetanic symptoms returned. She subsequently took a grain twice daily till the 8th of February, when she left the Hospital apparently quite well.

Mr. O'Brien has since used the hemp resin in five cases, of which four were admitted in a perfectly hopeless state. He employed the remedy in *ten grain doses* dissolved in spirit. The effect he describes as almost immediate relaxation of the muscles, and interruption of the convulsive tendency. Of Mr. O'Brien's seven cases, four have recovered.

In the Police Hospital of Calcutta, the late Dr. Bain has used the remedy in three cases of traumatic tetanus, of these one has died and two recovered.

A very remarkable case has recently occurred in the practice of Mr. Richard O'Shaughnessy of Calcutta. The patient was a Jew, æt: 30, attacked with tetanus during the progress of a sloughing sore of the scrotum, the sequel of a neglected hydrocele. Three grain doses were used every second hour, with the effect of inducing intoxication and suspending the symptoms. The patient has recovered perfectly, and now enjoys excellent health.

The preceding facts are offered to the professional reader with unfeigned diffidence, as to the inferences we feel disposed to derive from their consideration. They seem to us unequivocally to shew, that when given boldly and in large doses, the resin of hemp is capable in many cases of arresting effectually the progress of this formidable disease.*

The facts are such at least as justify the hope that the virtues of the drug may be widely and severely tested in the multitudes of these appalling cases which present themselves in all Indian Hospitals.

Case of Infantile Convulsions.

The subjoined details are given as originally published:—

"A very interesting case of this disease has recently occurred in my private practice; the particulars of which I have the permission of the family to insert in this essay.

"A female infant, forty days old, the child of Mr. and Mrs. J. L. of Calcutta, on the 10th September had a slight attack of convulsions, which recurred chiefly at night for about a fortnight, and for which the usual purgatives—warm baths and a few doses of calomel and chalk—were given without effect. On the 23rd the convulsive paroxysms became very severe, and two leeches were applied to the head. Leeches, purgatives, and opiates were alternately resorted to, and without the slightest benefit, up to the 30th of September.

"On that day the attacks were almost unceasing, and amounted to regular tetanic paroxysms. The child had

* While correcting this proof for the press, Mr. Raleigh, the able Professor of Surgery in the Medical College, has favoured us with the details of six cases of tetanus, three idiopathic, and three excited by wounds or injuries. In all, the hemp resin was freely given; but all proved fatal. Mr. Raleigh also states, that in his experience, tetanus is frequently cured by active purgatives, and other ordinary remedial measures.

The Editor's observation during two years, leads him to the conclusion, that the use of hemp is so *universal* among the lower classes of the natives of Bengal, that it is only in a small proportion of cases, among adult males especially, that its use will be found of the least advantage. In two of Mr. Raleigh's cases the patients denied being addicted to the habit; but we know that denial of the vice is as common as the habit itself. Females and children, therefore, afford the fairest subjects for trial of the remedy. Of the four cases Mr. O'Brien treated successfully, three were females. Messrs. Hughes and Templer, the skilful Veterinary Surgeons in Calcutta, have used the hemp resin in five cases of horses suffering from tetanus, and of these three have recovered. Dr. Sawyers has cured a pony under the same circumstances.

Drs. Esdaile and Macrae have used the hemp with success, the former in a case of tetanus, the latter in one of convulsions from neuralgia of the testis, which had resisted every other remedy.—In the Medical Gazette for December, a case of tetanus is reported by Mr. Lewis in which the hemp was used with the effect of great relief to the symptoms.—*Editor*.

moreover completely lost appetite, and was emaciating rapidly.*

"I had by this time exhausted all the usual methods of treatment, and the child was apparently in a sinking state.

"Under these circumstances I stated to the parents the results of the experiments I had made with the hemp, and my conviction that it would relieve their infant, if relief could possibly be obtained.

"They gladly consented to the trial, and a single drop of the spirituous tincture, equal to the one-twentieth part of a grain in weight, was placed on the child's tongue at 10 P. M. No immediate effect was perceptible, and in an hour and a half two drops more were given. The infant fell asleep in a few minutes, and slept soundly till 4 P. M. when she awoke, screamed for food, *took the breast freely*, and fell asleep again. At 9 A. M., 1st October, I found the child fast asleep, but easily roused; the pulse, countenance, and skin perfectly natural. In this drowsy state she continued for four days, totally free from convulsive symptoms in any form. During this time the bowels were frequently spontaneously relieved, and the appetite returned to the natural degree.

"October 4th. At 1 A. M. convulsions returned, and continued at intervals during the day;—five drop doses of the tincture were given hourly. Up to midnight there were thirty fits, and forty-four drops of the tincture of hemp were ineffectually given.

"October 5th. Paroxysms continued during the night. At 11 A. M. it was found that the tincture in use during the preceding days had been kept by the servant in a small bottle with a paper stopper; that the spirit had evaporated, and the whole of the resin settled on the sides of the phial. The infant had in fact been taking drops of "water" during the preceding day.

"A new preparation was given in three drop doses during the 5th and 6th, and increased to eight drops with the effect of diminishing the violence, though not of preventing the return of the paroxysm.

"On the 7th, I met Dr. Nicolson in consultation, and despairing of a cure from the hemp, it was agreed to intermit its use, to apply a mustard poultice to the epigastrium, and to give a dose of castor oil and turpentine. The child, however, rapidly became worse, and at 2 P. M. a tetanic spasm set in which lasted without intermission till 6½ P. M. A cold bath was given without solution of the spasm—the hemp

* The nurse, I should have mentioned, was changed early in the illness, and change of air resorted to on the river, but in vain.

was therefore again resorted to, and a dose of 30 drops, equal to 1½ grains of the resin, given at once.

"Immediately after this dose was given the limbs relaxed, the little patient fell fast asleep, and so continued for thirteen hours. While asleep she was evidently under the narcotic influence of the drug.

"On the 8th October, at 4 A. M. there was a severe fit, and from this hour to 10 at night twenty-five fits occurred, and 130 drops of the tincture were given in 30 drop doses, equal to 15 grains of the resin. It was now manifestly a struggle between the disease and the remedy, but at 10 P. M. she was again narcotised, and from that hour no fit returned.

"On the three following days there was considerable griping, and on administering large doses of almond oil, several small dark green lumps of the hemp resin were voided, which gave effectual relief. The child is now (17th December) in the enjoyment of robust health, and has regained her natural plump and happy appearance.

"In reviewing this case, several very remarkable circumstances present themselves. At first we find three drops, or one-twentieth of a grain, causing profound narcotism, subsequently we find 130 drops daily required to produce the same effect. The severity of the symptoms doubtless must be taken chiefly into account, in endeavouring to explain this circumstance. It was too soon for habit to gain ascendancy over the narcotic powers of the drug. Should the disease ever recur, it will be a matter of much interest to notice the quantity of the tincture requisite to afford relief. The reader will remember, that this infant was but sixty days old when 130 drops were given in one day, of the same preparation of which ten drops had intoxicated the student Dinonath Dhur, who took the drug for experiment. 130 drops are equal again to 15 grains of the resin, one grain of which occasioned profound trance (or catalepsy) in two men labouring under rheumatism.

Use in Delirium Tremens.

We have given the tincture of hemp a very extensive trial in this disease, and have had much reason to be gratified with its effects. In action it resembles opium and wine, but is much more certain than these remedies. In the cases in which the opium treatment is applicable, hemp will be found far more effectual. The changed state of mind it produces is truly wonderful. From the appalling terror which generally predominates, the patient soon passes into a stage of cheerful and often boisterous mirth, and sinks into a happy sleep. Of course there are many cases in which this or any other narcotic should not be used, and like all other powerful remedies its usefulness must depend on the discrimination with which it is employed.

Insanity occasioned by continued Hemp Inebriation.

Before quitting this subject, it is desirable to notice the singular form of insanity which the incautious use of the hemp preparations often occasions, especially among young men who try it for the first time. Several such cases have presented themselves to our notice. They are as peculiar as the "delirium tremens," which succeeds the prolonged abuse of spirituous liquors, but are quite distinct from any other species of madness with which we are acquainted.

This state is at once recognized by the strange balancing gait of the patient, a constant rubbing of the hands, perpetual giggling, and a propensity to caress and chafe the feet of all by-standers, of whatever rank. The eye wears an expression of cunning and merriment which can scarcely be mistaken. In a few cases, the patients are violent; in many, highly aphrodisiac; in all that we have seen, voraciously hungry. There is no increased heat or frequency of circulation, or any appearance of inflammation or congestion, and the skin and general functions are in a natural state.

A blister to the nape of the neck, leeches to the temples, and nauseating doses of tartar emetic with saline purgatives have rapidly dispelled the symptoms in all the cases we have met with, and have restored the patient to perfect health.

Doses, &c.—In *Tetanus*, a drachm of the tincture every half hour until the paroxysms cease, or catalepsy is induced. In *Hydrophobia* we would recommend the resin in soft pills, to the extent of ten to twenty grains to be chewed by the patient, and repeated according to the effect. In *Cholera*, 30 drops of the tincture every half hour will be often found to check the vomiting and purging, and bring back warmth to the surface. Our experience would lead us to prefer *small* doses of the remedy in order to excite, rather than narcotise, the patient.

The *resinous extract* is prepared by boiling the rich, adhesive tops of the dried *gunjah* in spirit (Sp. gr. 835.) until all the resin is dissolved. The tincture thus obtained is evaporated to dryness in a vessel placed over a pot of boiling water. The extract softens at a gentle heat, and can be made into pills without any addition.

The *tincture* is prepared by dissolving the extract in proof spirit. (See *Pharmacopœia.*)

NAT. ORDER CXXIX.—ULMACEÆ.

Bark of several species slightly bitter and mucilaginous, used as a diuretic, demulcent, and mild tonic. One species is officinal in the British Pharmacopœiæ, but nearly obsolete.

NAT. ORDER CXXX.—JUGLANDEÆ.

This order is formed of superb forest trees, which abound in all the temperate regions of Europe and Asia. The *Juglans regia*, or walnut, may be deemed the type of the whole family. It is common in the Himalayas, and in the valleys of Cashmere and Nipal.

GEN.—JUGLANS.

Sp. Juglans regia. Καρυα βασιλιχα, *Diosc.*
Vern. Fruit, Akrot, Charmughz, *Hind.* and *Pers.*
Too well known to need description.
The pericarp contains tannic and gallic acid in abundance.
The nut is emulsive, and very rich in a valuable drying oil.

OIL OF WALNUTS.

This oil is yellow, of light smell, acrid if expressed while hot, dries rapidly by exposure to the air, and is consequently much used in painting and varnishing.

The sap of the walnut tree is very rich in sugar. By tapping the upper part of the trunk with an iron tube half an inch in diameter and inserted 3 inches deep, the juice flows copiously. To prevent fermentation, it must be immediately boiled down. 100 lbs of sap give 2½ lbs raw sugar.

The bark of the root is stated to be rubefacient, the inner bark of the stem emetic. These reputed properties demand investigation.

NAT. ORDER CXXXI.—AMENTACEÆ.

This order contains many species of great economical importance, and some of medicinal interest.

The barks are generally astringent and bitter. In the willows, the bitter principle, *salicine*, is crystalline, and possessed of decided febrifuge properties. In the poplars, a white crystalline and sweet tasted substance, *populine*, exists in much abundance.

The fruits of the Amentaceæ are dry, but the seeds have fleshy, oily, and amylaceous cotyledons; some are acrid, containing bitter or astringent matter. The nuts of the hazel, beech, some species of oak and chesnut, are pleasant and nutritious. Wax is afforded by the fruits of the genus *Myrica;* many of the genera yield resin; *liquidambar* and *tacamahaca* resin are also products of species of this order.

GEN. 1.—SALIX,* *Willows.*

Sp. Salix alba, &c. White willow, a tall tree, a native of Europe.

Most species of willow yield the principle *salicine*, discovered by Leroux. The bark contains green fatty matter, yellow bitter colouring matter, tannic acid, resinous extract, gum, and magnesian salts.

SALICINE.

Salicine occurs in small rectangular plates with bevelled edges; it is inodorous, very bitter, melts at 204 without losing its water of crystallization; 100 parts of tepid water dissolve 6 parts, boiling water dissolves it freely. It is also soluble in alcohol and dilute acids; the concentrated sulphuric acid reddens it. It does not form salts, and contains no nitrogen.

The best process for the preparation of Salicine is that given by Nees Von Esenbeck. He boils the bark (that of *S. Helix* is the best) in water, adds to the liquid slaked lime, which precipitates the tannic acid, filters and evaporates to a syrup, adds alcohol to precipitate the gum, decants, and by evaporation obtains impure salicine. Redissolved in boiling water and filtered while hot, pure crystals are procured.

As a febrifuge salicine is used in doses of from 15 to 30 grains daily; there is much difference of opinion as to its efficacy.

We have carefully examined the *Salix tetrasperma*, the only willow found in lower Bengal, but could not detect in it any trace of salicine.

The Salix babylonica and aegyptiaca, (Khilaf bhulkee, *Arab.* Bed mooshk, *Pers.*) occur in gardens in Upper India. Salix Lindleyana, or dwarf willow, occurs at 12,000 to 13,000 feet on the Himalayas—S. hirta and rotundifolia in Kunawur;

* A distinct natural order, *Salicaceæ* in Lindley's Work.

a kind of manna, *bed kisht*, is said to be collected from the willows in Khorasan. *Royle.*

GEN. 2.—QUERCUS.

Sp. 1. *Q. Robur.* Oak.

A noble timber tree, a native of Europe.

Bark very astringent, and used in infusion, as the basis of an injection in mucous diarrhœa, and in discharges from the vagina. The kernels of the fruit, *acorns*, contain oil, resin, gum, tannic acid, bitter extract, starch, fibre, &c. Roasted and given in infusion, they are esteemed a valuable tonic and nutritive remedy. In Turkey they are buried for some time in the earth, by which the bitterness is destroyed. They are then dried and toasted. Their powder with sugar and aromatics constitutes the "*palamoud*" of the Turks, and "*racahout*" of the Arabs, an alimentary substance readily digestible, and very much esteemed.

The powdered bark is called *tan*, from its extensive application, and great consumption by the tanners.

Sp. 2. *Q. Ballota.*

Probably that described in Persian works as *Shah bulloot* and *Buloot ul mulk.* Ημερις, *Theophr.*

A native of Spain and Greece.

Fruits (glands) oval, elongated, having at the base a cupula with very slender scales, strongly imbricated and downy, kernels inodorous, of agreeable taste, like that of the chesnut. They contain no tannic acid or bitter principle; in several countries they are deemed a pleasant article of food, and thus we may perhaps explain the ancient traditions regarding the "acorn" constituting the food of the first wild tribes of the human race. The acorns of *Q. incana* are sold in the bazars as a medicine, under the name of *Bulloot.*

Sp. 3. *Q. Suber.* Cork tree.

Φελλος *Theophrast.*

Sp. 4. *C. coccifera*, or Kermes tree.

An insect called *Coccus* inhabits this tree, and is used for dyeing scarlet.

Sp. 5. *Q. infectoria.* Gallnut oak.

Vern. Galls. Majoophul, *Hind.*

Asia Minor, Armenia, and Kurdistan, a shrub 4 to 6 feet high. This tree when punctured by a *cyneps* allows an astringent juice to exude, which becomes the *gall nuts* of commerce.

GALLS.

Galls vary in size from half an inch to an inch in diameter. They contain large but variable proportions of tannic and gallic acid, on which their uses in the arts and in medicine depend.

Powdered galls are sometimes given in 3 to 10 grain doses in diarrhœa; an infusion is employed as an astringent injection in chronic discharges from the rectum or vagina. An ointment is prepared from the powder, which is of very great utility as an application to piles.

Sp. 6. *Q. tinctoria.* Dyer's oak. Quercitron.

A native of North America. The cellular part of the bark gives a yellow dye. Wool is dyed yellow when boiled in water with an equal weight of alumn and quercitron bark.

GEN. 3.—CASTANEA.

Sp. C. vulgaris. Common chesnut.

Fruits (nuts) thorny, containing 2 or 3 oval hemispherical chesnuts, brown, shining, smooth, subquadrangular, with an oblong white stain; substance firm, white, and lobed, inodorous, taste sweetish.

Chesnuts contain starch, gluten, and sugar. The envelopes are very astringent.

Sugar was successfully manufactured in France from these nuts during Napoleon's continental system. Chesnuts in some countries constitute a considerable part of the general food of the inhabitants. In Europe generally, they are a favourite article when roasted before the fire.

The *Castanea indica* of our eastern and northern mountains, yields an edible nut called *Nikari.* (Royle, p. 345.)

GEN. 4.—FAGUS.

F. sylvatica. Beech.

Fruit the size of a very small nut, exactly triangular, smooth, brown, marked with three longitudinal streaks, obtuse towards its base, which presents a triangular spot, summit sharp with a downy point, capsule coriaceous and membranous, internally smooth, one-celled, trivalved, nut white, streaked longitudinally, covered with a brown tender tunic, substance firm white, unequally lobed. Inodorous, taste weak and sweet. The envelopes are astringent. The almond contains fixed oil with starch in large proportion.

The oil is sweet, yellowish, does not congeal, spoils very slowly, and is of agreeable flavour. It is chiefly prepared in the forest of Compeigne in France.

GEN. 5.—CORYLUS.*

Sp. Coryllus Avellana. (Hazel.)

Abundant in the Himalayas, nuts *Bindick* and *Finduck* in bazars.

Fruits (nuts) grouped in clusters together, enveloped in a persistent, irregularly laciniated calyx, nut oval, compressed, smooth, furrowed, with a large spot at the base, subquadrangular, shell bony, sub-bivalved, one-celled, almond oval acute, white, easily cloven in two portions, covered with 1-2 dry, ash-coloured, rather rough tunics (episperm), parenchyme white, fleshy, brittle, rendering the saliva milky. Inodorous, taste sweet and agreeable. The almond becomes rancid very quickly.

By expression the kernel yields a very agreeable oil, nearly in the proportion of half its weight.

The wood of the hazel was the material of the divining rods of the magicians and snake enchanters, who even in modern times have had their believers in Europe.

GEN. 6.—BETULA.

Of little importance in a medicinal view. The white birch yields a bark which the Kamschatdales chop up with the eggs of the sturgeon, and use as their ordinary food. The sap is acid, and an agreeable beverage, and may be kept for years without undergoing fermentation. There are numerous other economical uses to which the products of this valuable tree are applied.

In Nipal the bark of the *Betula Bhojpattra* is used as a substitute for writing paper, and for wrapping hooka snakes.

NAT. ORDER CXXXII.—MYRICEÆ.

Ligneous aromatic plants with alternate leaves, charged with resinous points. Flowers amentaceous, wanting both calyx and corolla. The bark and root are astringent. From this order we obtain two balsams—the liquid styrax and liquidambar, both of which contain benzoic acid.

* Natural order *Corylaceæ* in Lindley.

Gen. 1.—Liquidambar.

This, according to Blume, is a distinct order, which he calls *Balsamifluæ*. It is formed of large trees with alternate leaves. There is a species in Assam, admirably described and figured by Mr. Griffith, in *Asiat. Res.* vol. xix, under the name of *Sedgwickia cerasifolia*, Wall. et Griff. (Liquidambar cerasifolia, Wall.) We are not aware that it yields any balsam.

Sp. L. styraciflua. Mexico and N. America.

Trunk 40 feet in height, sustaining a pyramidal head, leaves alternate or fascioled, petiolar, palmate, with 5 to 7 lobes, elongated and toothed, green and viscous. Flowers male and female, collected in globular clusters, fruit capsular, sunk in the cells of a common receptacle. From the bark we obtain the —

Liquidambar Balsam.

This substance is at first liquid, transparent, yellow, rather consistent; its odour is strong, and resembles that of liquid styrax; taste very aromatic and acrid. By long keeping it dries into a deep brown resin. It contains benzoic acid.

Guibourt describes two species of liquidambar: the first is that above noticed; the second resembles a soft pitch or turpentine, is opaque, whitish, of sweet and aromatic odour, and contains so much benzoic acid, that it often crystallizes on the surface of the mass.

All these balsams are obtained either by spontaneous exudation, by incision into the bark, or decoction of the bark, leaves, and branches.

When of the purest kind, it is dry, transparent and nearly white, and is then supposed to constitute the white Peruvian balsam of the druggists. In all its states it is used to mix with the common Peruvian balsam.

Liquid Styrax.

Soft, of the consistence of honey, tenacious, viscous, of greenish brown and grey colour, odour strong and heavy, taste aromatic, but not acrid, much adulterated with fragments of bark and earth, entirely soluble in alcohol. It hardens in the air, and absorbs oxygen. By distillation it affords an acidulous water, having the odour of benzoic acid, also a hot, limpid, and colourless oil; a solid coloured oil; benzoic acid, &c. Boiled with alcohol it deposits crystals on cooling.

There is still much difference of opinion regarding the origin of liquid styrax. Several writers attribute it to the

Liquidambar styraciflua. Guibourt assigns it to the *Liquidambar orientale.* Feé considers liquidambar and styrax to be identical, and doubts their oriental origin. Soubeiran deems the origin of styrax to be altogether unknown.

M. l'Heritier and several other authorities strongly recommend styrax as a most agreeable and efficient substitute for Balsam of Copaiba. Soubeiran gives some excellent formulæ for the administration of this substance.

Gen. 2.—Myrica.

Sp. 1. *M. Gale.*

Syn. Chamælagnus, *Pliny.* Belgium, North America.

The fruits are covered with a fatty, granular, pulverulent substance, extracted for various economical purposes. A similar substance is obtained from the *Myrica cerifera,* and several other species. The wax is separated by placing the fruits in boiling water. The liquefied wax rises to the surface, and is removed by spoons. It is converted into candles, which diffuse an agreeable odour, but give only a feeble light.

The *Myrica cordifolia* of the Cape is used for similar purposes.

Sp. 2. *Myrica sapida.* Wall. Tentam. Nipal. t. 45.

Vern. Kuephul, *Hind.*

Himalayas from the Sutlege to Nipal, fruit agreeably flavoured. The same, or a nearly allied species, is found in China and Japan.

The bark (Kuephul) is aromatic and stimulant, and a favourite native medicine.

Roxburgh's *Myrica integrifolia.* Fl. Ind. iii. p. 765, from our N.E. frontier, seems to be different; its fruit is acid and used for pickling.

Gen. 3.—Putranjiva.

Sp. P. Roxburghii. Wall. Tentam. p. 61. Nageia Putranjiva, *Roxb. Fl. Ind.* iii. p. 766.

Coromandel, Patna, Monghir hills, and from Sylhet to the Kheree jungle.

The Sanscrit name is compounded of *pootra,* a son; and *jeeva,* life. The Hindoostani name, *jeeapootra,* is similarly derived. The nuts are strung by parents round the necks of their children, to keep them in health. *Roxb.*

NAT. ORDER CXXXIII.—CONIFERÆ.

This very numerous and valuable order comprises trees of the greatest existing dimensions, and ligneous vegetables of the proportions of shrubs. The leaves are straight, narrow, pale-green, pointed, and fasciculated, the flowers are monœcious, the fruits are termed cones or catkins.

All parts of these plants are gorged with a turpentine or proper juice. This abounds especially in the bark, and also in the wood. The leaves are sometimes acid and astringent; the fruits afford turpentine very copiously; when the fruit is baccate, it is aromatic at the same time.

In a few instances the turpentine is associated with an acrid deleterious principle, as in sabine and the yew.

Feé divides the family into the groups of the pines, yews, and cypresses, an arrangement which is very convenient to the pharmaceutical student.

Tribe I—Abietinæ, or Pines.

The products of this extensive tribe are very uniform. Feé treats of it in a peculiar and very clear classification.

GEN.—PINUS.

Sp. 1. *P. longifolia.* Himalayas.

Vern. Cheer, sullah, surul, thausa.

Entrance to Nipal in the Kheree Pass, along Touse and Jumna rivers, at elevations of 5,000 and 6,000 feet.

Produce, gunda biroza, birje or cherkegond. Birozehtur, *Pers.* same name also given to Indian olibanum.

Sp. 2. *P. excelsa,* Wall. Pl. Rar. t. 201.

Narambetty, Nipal, Simla, Bootan.

Vern. *Kuel* of Sirmoor and Gurhwal, resembles the Weymouth pine, and is remarkable for its drooping branches.

Sp. 3. *P.* (*or Cedrus*) *Deodara,* leaves and twigs used in native medicine.

Vern. Kelon; the most celebrated of the Himalayan pines, noticed by Avicenna, found in Nipal, Kemaon, Kashmere, at 7,000 to 12,000 feet.

Prod. A turpentine called *Kelon ka tel,* used as a stimulant to foul ulcers.

Sp. 4. *Pinus Gerardiana.*
Vern. Neoza, chilgoza of Elphinstone, the seeds form one of the principal articles of subsistence in Kunawur.

Sp. 5. *P. sylvestris*, wild or Russian pine, native of the mountains of Europe.
Products, tenacious resin, tar, and pitch, excellent wood for packing cases and fuel; inner bark light and cork-like, contains a mucilaginous principle of a nutritive kind.
The *pinus rubra*, red or Scotch pine, is the nearest British substitute for this species.

Sp. 6. *P. maritima*, Sea-coast pine.
Products, Bourdeaux turpentine, tar, pitch, lamp-black, galipot, excellent wood; similar products are yielded by the P. australis and several others.

Sp. 7. *P. Mugho, torch pine of* Dauphiny.—Affords the products above mentioned, and Hungarian balsam.

Sp. 8. *P. Cembra.* Dauphiny, Piedmont, &c. The products are Carpathian balsam, &c. the kernels of the fruit are eatable and pleasant; expressed oil readily becomes rancid.

Sp. 9. *P. Pinea*, cultivated pine. Cones ovoid, four inches long, requiring three years to ripen, kernels oblong, rather angular, very white, inodorous, of sweet oily flavour.
The recent oil is pleasant to the taste.

Sp. 10. *P. balsamea.* Canada.
Produce, Canadian balsam, or false balm of Gilead.
Another Canadian pine is called in English the spruce hemlock.

Sp. 11. *P. picea*, common fir.
Products, Strasburg turpentine, common turpentine, lamp-black, Burgundy pitch. Bark astringent, leaves used in the North of Europe in a kind of beer; seeds yield lamp oil; the wood is especially useful for ship-building and masts.
Products, Venice or Briançon turpentine, essence of turpentine, resin, excellent wood for building and fuel, and little liable to decay.
Feé also enumerates the following species:—
P. Strobus, Weymouth pine.
Common in Canada, where it is of great value.
P. nigra, or black pine of the Ohio.

P. orientalis, or Levant fir, yields "pine tears" and a resin.

P. Cedrus, or cedar of Lebanon, yields a peculiar resin, and gives a manna-like substance; seed resinous and acrid.

P. or *Dombeya Araucaria*, one of the giants of the vegetable kingdom, attaining often 220 feet altitude.

PHARMACEUTICAL AND ECONOMICAL PRODUCTS.

These are resin, oil of turpentine, pitch and tar. These are called in native books of Materia Medica, Aluk zifh-rutub, zifh-yabis, kutran, and rateeanuj, the last synonymous with colophony.

Turpentine.

A proper juice contained in all parts of these trees, thick, viscous, shining, rather transparent, colour ranging from white to yellow or amber, odour strong and penetrating, taste bitter and acrid. It thickens by age by losing essential oil and absorbing oxygen from the air.

Turpentines are composed of resin and essential oil, separable by heat. The oil taken internally, gives an odour of violets to the urine.

Turpentines are of various kinds.

First sort. Larch turpentine, Brigantine or Venetian turpentine, product of the *P. larix.*

Usually liquid, transparent, of greenish colour, instantaneously solidified by the third of its weight of caustic soda, odour strong, not disagreeable, taste hot, bitter, and acrid.

"Venice" turpentine is an improper term for this juice, which does not come from Italy, and is chiefly the produce of the Alps of Dauphiny and the Jura. It is obtained by making augur holes in the trees in the spring season, when the sap is most abundant. In felling trees, large deposits of turpentine are often found.

This turpentine is easily purified by filtration through leather.

Second sort. "Strasburg turpentine."

Product of *Pinus picea*, or *Abies pectinata.*

Usually fluid, transparent, or slightly milky, odour strong and heavy, taste acrid, and very bitter. It is collected by puncturing the buds at the summit of the trees. It furnishes one-fourth its weight of essential oil. It is purified by filtration through pieces of the bark and the leaves of the tree itself. After purification, it is clearer and thinner than the preceding species.

These turpentines enter into a multiplicity of Pharmaceutical preparations, and are much used in the arts for paints and varnishes.

Third sort. Common Bordeaux, or Pine turpentine.

Product of *Pinus maritima, sylvestris*, and others.

Whitish, turbid, consistent, separating by rest into two portions, gives one-fifth of essential oil, odour unpleasant, taste acrid and nauseous. Collected by large incisions in the trunk of the tree. It flows from May to September, and is called *Galipot.*

Fir or pine " tears" are a concrete turpentine, which flows spontaneously from the ends of the branches. It is very clear, white, transparent, and is rare and costly.

Fourth sort. Boston turpentine, product of *P. Australis.*

Little different from preceding species in its physical characters, contains 17-100ths of essential oil. The odour is pleasant, taste somewhat bitter. It makes a liquid soap or liniment with soda.

Fifth sort. American turpentine, product of *Pinus strobus,* now unknown in commerce.

Sixth sort. Balsamic turpentine, product of *P. balsamæa.*

First variety. Liquid or rather soft, tenacious, white, forms a consistent soap with soda, and dissolves with difficulty in alcohol, odour aromatic and agreeable, taste bitter, but not acrid. Transudes through pores in the bark of the tree.

Second variety. Nearly colourless and transparent, of middling tenacity, sweet smell like that of Mecca balsam, bitter taste. This turpentine is obtained from the sacs or utricles found on the *Pinus balsamea;* these are crushed, and the juice which gushes forth is received in bottles and closed up hermetically. It is in Canada and in the adjacent territory of Maine that this balsam is collected; not more than 250 to 300 bottles are obtained annually and are mostly sold as " Balsam of Gilead."

Seventh sort. Dombeya turpentine.

Product of Norfolk Island pine, *P. Araucaria.* Glutinous and milk white, odour strong, taste acrid and bitter, of little value, as it is easily decomposed by heat.

With the preceding Feé includes dammar turpentine; this however is not the produce of a pine, but of *Shorea robusta,* see DIPTEROCARPI.

Eighth sort. Dammar turpentine.

Transparent, at first soft and viscous, but quickly concretes into an extremely hard resin. Regarding this M. Feé makes the strange observation, that dammar is of no use even in its native countries, owing to its excessive hardness.

Ninth sort. Trailegon turpentine.

But little known, the produce of Bogota.

We have now to examine the products of the turpentines, viz. their resins and essential oil. These are either naturally produced or the result of distillation by artificial heat.

Essence (or *volatile oil*) of Turpentine.

Very fluid, limpid, transparent and light, sp. gr. 792, boils at 313° Fahr. odour sharp and penetrating. Taste acrid and burning. By long keeping unites with oxygen, becomes yellow, loses its odour, and thickens. The pure oil is composed, according to Blanchet and Sell, of carbon 88.54, hydrogen 11.52.

It is very slightly soluble in water, freely in alcohol and ether, dissolves sulphur, and inflames by contact with nitric acid. When pure it unites with a watery solution of potassa, forming the compound called "*Starkey's soap.*" Turpentine deposits crystals on keeping.

Medicinal uses.—Diuretic, in 1ʒ doses, but apt to produce strangury, and inflammation of the kidneys—purgative in doses of half an ounce to ℥i. In this quantity it is almost an infallible remedy for tape-worm, which one or two doses usually expel dead. In dropsies and obstinate constipation, turpentine is often prescribed; in the latter case it is usually combined with castor oil. Oil of turpentine once enjoyed high celebrity as a specific in malignant puerperal fever. The practice was introduced by Dr. Brennan of Dublin, but has fallen into disuse of late years.

As an external stimulant, oil of turpentine forms the base of a very useful and cheap *liniment*, for which consult the Pharmacopœia.

Resins of Turpentine.

A. *Resins obtained without fire.*

1. Galipot.

In large opaque crusts, yellowish white, of slight hardness, mixed with impurities, such as fragments of bark and earth; odour that of turpentine, taste bitter.

Galipot is the residue of the turpentine, which has lost

its volatile oil by spontaneous evaporation. When purified, it is called Burgundy pitch, which is used in what is called the "warm plaster." Galipot in tears is called "false incense," being used as such in the churches of the districts in which the tree prevails.

2. Cedar Resin.

Transparent, friable, in granular masses or in stalactites. Odour aromatic, taste bitter, rare in commerce, an ingredient in the embalming mixtures of the Egyptians.

3. White Dammar.

In fragments of variable size, marked with reddish streaks, transparent, amber-like, brittle, with brilliant fracture, very inflammable, inodorous, and tasteless.

This resin flows from the *P. dammara*, which grows on the lofty mountains of Amboyna. It hangs from the branches, and resembles stalactites, the pieces being sometimes as large as the hand, and 4 to 8 inches long; some pieces are like *animi* resin.

The dammar of the Bengal bazars is usually the produce of the *Shorea robusta*.

Resins obtained by heat.

4. Colophony Resin.

Solid, glassy, transparent, brittle, friable, colour deep in shade according to the degree of heat to which it was subjected. Inodorous until rubbed, tasteless.

Colophony was formerly brought from Colophon, a town in Ionia. It is now prepared in Merecourt, a small town in the Vosges.

5. Yellow Resin.

Yellow, brittle, opaque, with glassy fracture, softens under the fingers, odour while cold feeble, on burning very powerful. The result of the distillation of a turpentine which has been heated with water—much employed in the arts, and in Pharmacy used for ointments and plasters.

6. Black Pitch.

Of fine black colour, smooth, brittle while cool, readily softened by the heat of the hands, odour strong and peculiar, taste faintly bitter. It is obtained by burning the straw through which the Galipot is purified, as well as the splinters of wood cut from the trees to facilitate the flow of the turpentines. All these materials are heaped up and set fire to at top. The resin melted and soiled by a little carbon is conducted into a cistern filled with water. In this it separates into a half solid matter, which must be gathered together to form the black pitch, and into a substance which swims at the top, and is called "*pitch oil*," or "*pisselaion*."

7. Tar.

Liquid or half liquid, tenacious, black, composed of resin, empyreumatic oil, and acetic acid; odour strong and disagreeable, taste bitter and very nauseous. It is prepared by the close distillation of the turpentine woods. Tar is very complex; besides the substances above enumerated, it has recently been proved to contain creasote, eupione, paraffine, and other principles.

Tar is chiefly employed for marine uses. Tar water has been until lately a celebrated remedy in the treatment of some chronic diseases of the lungs.

Non-Resinous Products of the Pines.

A. *Natural.*

1. Briancon Manna.

In the form of little white, round, yellow, rather glutinous grains, having faintly the odour and taste of turpentine. It forms on the larch trees in June and July before sunrise. It is purgative, and is rare in commerce.

2. The larch also affords a gum called *Orenburg gum*, which is dry, brittle, of reddish colour, totally soluble in water, of very slightly resinous taste and smell. Its history is very uncertain.

B. *Artificial.*

3. Smoke Black.

Colour black, with a bluish tint, of great lightness, adheres to the fingers, retaining a little of the oil of pitch, odour disagreeable, slightly empyreumatic; tasteless after calcination.

Smoke black is prepared by the combustion of different resinous bodies, especially of pitch. This substance is burned in large pans under a dome or chimney, within which cloths are suspended to which the soot becomes attached. This species of carbon is employed only in the arts, in the manufacture of printer's ink, of blacking for shoes, &c.

Tribe II—Cupressineæ.

Trees of moderate stature. Their essential oil is of very powerful odour, and is sometimes accompanied by an acrid and deleterious principle.

Gen. 1.—Juniperus.

Sp. 1. *J. Lycia.* Europe and Africa.

The stem is of middling height, with thin branches covered with very small oval leaves, rather fleshy, opposite, in sets of three, applied on the surfaces of the branches and imbricated, male and female flowers on the same or on different trees. Fruits exceeding the size of a pea, slow in ripening, containing nine oval and irregular seeds.

African incense is commonly attributed to this tree.

African Incense—Olibanum.

See *Boswellia thurifera*, p. 283.

In the form of tears or almonds; the tears are oblong, or rounded, of variable size, citron or reddish colour, rather solid, of waxy and dull fracture, softening in the mouth. The almonds are reddish, soften under the fingers, mixed with impurities and remnants of bark, the odour like that of the pine resins or tacamahaca, taste aromatic and slightly acrid. When long kept, this incense is often found to contain regular crystals of carbonate of lime.

What is termed "incense manna," consists of little round grains of equal size, supposed to have more decided properties than the incense itself.

Much difference of opinion exists regarding African olibanum; it is the Indian kind which is known to proceed from the *Boswellia thurifera.* M. Feé regards it as very likely that the African product will be found to owe its origin to a species of the same family. He adduces strong evidence in support of his opinion, that this olibanum is the produce of one of the Terebinthaceæ, and not of the Coniferous family.

Sp. 2. *J. communis.*—Common juniper.

Dry and barren hills of Europe; found by Captain Webb on Netee Pass, called *bilhara*, *pudma*, and *pumaroa;* and by Mr. Inglis in Kunawur—3 to 6 feet high, forming a dense, diffuse, irregular bush, occasionally tree-like, and attaining an elevation of 20 feet; bark brownish red, leaves verticillate, in threes, linear, acute, stiff, sharp, smooth, pale green or whitish, flowers axillary, solitary, almost sessile, supported on a scaly peduncle.

The berries are solitary, shortly peduncled, the size of a small pea, globular, smooth, shining, marked with three furrows, having a roundish spot towards the top; beneath this pericarp is a spongy succulent pulp of rust colour, within which are nestled three seeds, plane on one side, and convex on the other.

Odour of the leaves agreeable and balsamic, of the berries also agreeable, taste of the leaves resinous, rather bitter; of the berries sweet, aromatic, slightly saccharine, hot, and rather bitter.

The berries (*Abhul* and *Hoober*,) in bazars are considered diuretic and emmenagogue; brought from the Himalayas and Cabul. *Arkonus* and *baratee* are assigned as Greek names. *Royle*, p. 352.

The berries alone are now employed in medicine; these contain sugar, mucilage, and a little essential oil. The oil is white or yellowish, light, very liquid, of hot and acrid juniper taste, and very strong smell; the extract of the berries is called a "Rob." The oil is prepared on the large scale in Holland, and is often adulterated with turpentine.

The chief consumption of juniper berries is, however, for the flavouring of the spirit called *gin*. Besides its stimulating and narcotic properties, *gin* is also acknowledged to be a powerful diuretic.

Juniperus excelsa is, according to Royle, the Himalayan cedar.

Sp. 3. J. Oxycedrus. The wood of this tree distilled in a retort gives an empyreumatic oil, called by the French *Huile de Cade*.

This oil is liquid, brown, oily, and inflammable. Its odour is resinous, tar-like, but still more disagreeable, taste acrid and even caustic.

It is much used in France in veterinary medicine, and is deemed vermifuge when rubbed on the epigastrium.

Sp. 4. Juniperus Sabina.—Savine.

South of France, the Alps in warm valleys; trunk straight, with ascending or very branching branches, divided in threes, provided with small, oval, pointed leaves, applied to the branches so as to appear imbricated, berries lateral, rounded, 3-seeded, of bluish black colour at maturity, odour fœtid, fatiguing, and very strong. Taste bitter and disagreeable.

Oil of Savine.

Colour white or yellowish, odour strongly that of savine, taste resinous and burning.

To this oil the plant owes its properties. The leaves are powerfully excitant, are employed in powder to some ulcers, and enter into an ointment for keeping up a suppuration from blistered surfaces. The plant is said to be powerfully emmenagogue, and is often used for the purpose of producing abortion.

Gen. 2.—Thuya.

*Sp. T. articulata,** Africa, Barbary.

Of middling height, sometimes reaching 15—20 feet; according to Schoust this tree produces the vernix, or sandarac.

Sandarac.

In round or elongated tears, whitish or pale citron yellow, brilliant, transparent and limpid, brittle under the teeth, burns with a clear flame, soluble in alcohol, and difficultly so in turpentine, odour agreeable on burning. Taste resinous and slightly balsamic, used in varnishes, and its powder to prevent ink from spreading through unglazed or eroded paper.

In Sweden a sandarac is sold, which is certainly supplied by one of the junipers of that country; indeed M. Feé assures us that the common junipers secrete a similar resin, he therefore considers its reference to the Thuya as extremely doubtful.

Gen.—Cupressus. Cypress.

C. sempervirens, Evergreen cypress, *Suroo* and *Shujrudal hueyat*, or the tree of life; berries and leaves popularly deemed a panacea for all diseases.

C. pendula, Drooping cypress, *Goa cedar*.

South of Europe, fruits formerly deemed astringent, and much used in medicine, now obsolete. The oriental physicians used to send their patients labouring under lung diseases to breathe the air of Candia, where the cypress was abundant, in the persuasion that the emanations were particularly wholesome.

* Now called *Callitrix quadrivalvis*. Zoos of the Arabs; in north of Africa called *Arar*.

Tribe III—Taxineæ. Yews.

These present but little interest to the therapeutist.

NAT. ORDER CXXXIV.—NYMPHAEACEÆ.

There has been some difference of opinion as to the place in classification which this order should occupy—whether among the Monocotyledonous or Dicotyledonous division. It is now generally admitted to belong to the latter, in which it ought to have come in a preceding part of this work, next after Fumarieæ, p. 185. The species are aquatic, often creeping in a horizontal direction, and attached to the earth by numerous fibres. The leaves are displayed on the surface of the water. The flowers are very large and polypetalous.

The leaves are mucilaginous, the roots of many amylaceous, of some astringent and bitter; the flowers of several are very aromatic—those of the *Lotus* were long considered sedative and narcotic, till accurate experiment shewed the opinion to be unfounded.

The genus NUPHAR prevails chiefly in Europe and America, and the root of *N. lutea* is held to be slightly poisonous. The *Nymphea alba* and *odorata* have astringent and slightly narcotic roots.

The *Euryale ferox (Syn.* Anneslea spinosa, Roxb. *Vern.* Makana, *Beng.)* is found in lakes and ponds in lower Bengal, also at Chittagong, Tippera, &c. The floating leaves are from one to four feet in diameter, slightly prickly above, very much so and purple below, with very projecting veins anastomosing with each other. Petals violet blue, berry the size of an orange, swelled irregularly, containing about 20 seeds enveloped in a fleshy rose-coloured arillus *(Lindley.)* The seeds are farinaceous, and are a favourite article of diet among the natives. They are deemed powerful tonics by the Hindoos.

NAT. ORDER CXXXV.—CYCADEÆ.

GEN.—CYCAS.

Sp. 1. *C. revoluta.*

A native of Japan; a kind of sago is said to be obtained from the cellular substance. The whole plant yields a copious mucilage, which hardens into a transparent gum.

Sp. 2. *C. circinalis.* Chiefly occurs on the Moluccas; said to yield a sago, also a gum like tragacanth.

The genus *Zamia,* which is chiefly West Indian in its distribution, is the source of some of the best *arrow-root* of commerce.

PART VI.

THE VEGETABLE MATERIA MEDICA ARRANGED ACCORDING TO THE NATURAL SYSTEM.

Class II.

Monocotyledoneæ, or Endogeneæ.

This great division of phanerogamous plants differs essentially from the others, in having its seeds homogeneous instead of being divided into two lobes. Like the Dicotyledones they have a radicle and plumula, but with this difference—that in the former the two cotyledons separate to give passage to the rudimentary organs, while in the Monocotyledons the episperm splits to permit these to protrude.

The great tendency of the Dicotyledons is to become woody trees; of the Monocotyledons to remain in the herbaceous state. The latter are of soft consistence, of great flexibility, of loose and porous texture. Their stems are bundles of fibres, or vessels placed in the midst of a very abundant cellular tissue. Their surface is siliceous, their leaves have *parallel* fibres. The floral system is of the utmost simplicity, the flowers having but a single envelope.

The Dicotyledons, on the contrary, are of solid consistence, of firm structure, and close texture. The stems possess a medullary canal, and a vascular apparatus, having a double direction. The leaves are supplied with reticulated nerves. The floral system is usually complex, a calyx being often present as well as a corolla.

The arborescent Monocotyledons differ altogether from the Dicotyledons. But before tracing out the comparison, it is desirable to notice that botanists are not yet agreed regarding the limits between stems and roots. The *stipe* is cylindrical, and formed of woody fillets enveloped in cellular tissue. The vascular apparatus elongates itself vertically, the diameter is fixed from the first age of the plant; it seldom branches; does not endure grafting; and only bears leaves at its summit. The leaves are not deciduous, but dry up for the want of nutritive juices. Broken off by the winds the base alone remains, and marks the rings of the apparent trunk. The woody fillets produce a new leaf-bud, and in this the life of the vegetable resides, the tree being destroyed by the removal of the bud. The stipe is accordingly nothing but the channel which bears the nutritive juices from the earth to the summit of the plant.

The trunk of the Dicotyledons is entirely different, its shape is conical; it is formed of cellular tissue placed in the centre of the woody layers; the vascular apparatus has a double direction, at first towards the summit, secondarily from the centre to the circumference; the leaves, persistent or deciduous, spring along the branches and twigs; the buds scattered over the plant shew the equal subdivision of its vital forces; grafting is practised with success; increase in size takes place superiorly by the elongation of the concentric layers, and diametrically by their multiplication, and thus the age of the plant may be determined.

NAT. ORDER I.—AROIDEÆ.

In temperate climates all these plants are herbaceous, but in tropical latitudes they become shrubby or arborescent. The tropical arums have alternate leaves, large, entire, lobed or digitate, often coriaceous, and with sheathing petioles. The spadices are axillary, lateral, or radical, and very much developed. At the time of flowering their temperature increases very remarkably. All contain an acrid principle, volatile and soluble in water, and separable by washing from the fecula with which it is combined. The leaves are excessively irritating to the taste, and in some species possess blistering properties.

GEN. 1.—ARUM.

Sp. 1. ***Arum maculatum,*** Common arum. Wake robin.

Syn. Arum vulgare, Lamarck. Europe.

Roots tubercular, size of a pigeon's egg, covered with a thin, membranous, oval tunic, externally white, here and there fibrous, with thick fibres; the elongated and roundish tubercles are hard, and half-transparent when dried, the parenchyme white, fleshy, and succulent, inodorous, taste at first scarcely perceptible, then smarting and pungent to an excessive degree, especially when the plant is recent; powder whitish; by long keeping they become insipid, brittle, and friable, and soil the fingers like chalk.

The juice of the arum root turns syrup of violets green, and is coagulated by acids. The active principle is volatile, and dissipated by age or by roasting; being soluble in water it is removable from the fecula, which then becomes an alimentary substance of much value. It is met in commerce under the name of Portland sago, from the place where it is manufactured.

Sp. 2. *A. triphyllum*, Linn. Dragon's root.
Syn. Arisæma atrorubens, *Blume.*
A native of North America; when the acrid principle is volatilized the rhizoma yields a fine fecula like arrow-root.

Sp. 3. *A. Serpentaria*, v. *Dracunculus*, South of France.
Roots tuberous, large, parenchyme white, taste acrid, inodorous. Owing to the spots on the bark, which resemble a snake's skin, this shrub has received its specific name, and been recommended also as a remedy for the bites of venomous reptiles.

Sp. 4. *A. Colocasia.* Egyptian ginger.
Syn. Colocasia esculenta. Native of Crete, Syria, Egypt.
Vern. Kuchoo, *Beng.*
Roots large, tuberous, white internally, containing fecula in great abundance, cultivated in India, Egypt, Greece, and America.
The tubers of this arum are the chief food of the inhabitants in a great part of Egypt, and are also much used in Bengal.

Sp. 5. *A. orixense.* Roxb. Fl. Ind. iii. p. 504.
Syn. Typhonium trilobatum. *Blume.*
Vern. Ghetkol, Ghet kuchoo, *Beng.*
Various parts of India, tubers the size of a small egg, exceedingly acrid while fresh, and used as a counter-irritant in poultices, also as an application in snake bites. They are likewise given inwardly in doses of from 20 to 30 grains. Roxburgh describes this arum as a most powerful stimulant in proper hands.

Gen. 2.—Homalomena.

Sp. H. aromatica.
Syn. Calla aromatica. Roxb. Fl. Ind. iii. p. 513.
Vern. Kuchoo gundubee, *Beng.*
A native of Chittagong, tubers covered with the dried sheaths of the leaves, with long white fibres proceeding from every part.
When cut they exhale an aromatic scent like ginger. As a stimulant it is highly esteemed in India. (*Roxb.*)

Gen. 3.—Pothos.

Sp. P. officinalis. Roxb. Fl. Ind. i. p. 431.
Syn. Scindapsus officinalis.
Vern. Vushira, *Sans.* Guj-pipul, *Beng.*

A large creeper, the fruit cut in thin transverse slices is the *guj-pippul* of the bazars, and highly esteemed as a stimulant tonic.

NAT. ORDER II.—ACORACEÆ.

Plants of aquatic habits, and resembling rushes and the Cyperaceæ. Their properties are due to an essential oil.

Sp. A. Calamus. Sweet flag. *Ακοροv.* Diosc.
Vern. Buch, *Hind.* Vach, *Sans.* Sufed Buch, *Beng.*

A native of Amboyna, Ceylon, Nipal, Khaseea hills, Malabar, Bourbon, &c.

Root cylindrical, slightly compressed, branched, size of the finger, or larger, bent, and covered with brown scales with numerous thread-like, whitish fibres. When dry it occurs in the shops in longitudinal pieces, wrinkled and marked with projecting points, parenchyme somewhat starchy, brittle, and solid; a transverse section shews a multitude of pores red without, and whitish within.

The whole plant is aromatic, but the root alone preserves the flavour on drying. Taste rather bitter, but stimulant and spicy. By Tromsdorf's analysis it contains reddish yellow volatile oil, resin, extractive, gummy resinous matter, muriate and phosphate of potassa, inuline, and fibre. It is a favourite medicine among the Hindoos as a stimulant in flatulency and similar states.

The *A. verus* differs much from our article, and has been attributed erroneously to the Gentiana Chirayta. The *Calamus aromaticus* of the ancients is referred by Royle to the *Andropogon Calamus aromaticus.*

NAT. ORDER III.—PANDANEÆ.

The stem of the Pandaneæ is rather low, and differs but little from that of the palms. The leaves are disposed in a terminal crown, from the centre of which proceeds the spadix covered with flowers. The fruits form in the aggregate a mass as in the ananas. The prevailing principle in the fruit is starch; a very pervading perfume is exhaled from the flowers of the *Pandanus odoratissmus* (keora), from which a distilled water is prepared in the bazars. Its properties are gently stimulant and diaphoretic.

NAT. ORDER IV.—TYPHACEÆ.

Aquatic, smooth plants with creeping roots; the stem is simple without knots, straight, cylindrical, and leafy; leaves straight, flowers terminal. No plant of this order furnishes any medicinal product of the least value.

NAT. ORDER V.—CYPERACEÆ.

This order has a triangular stem very rarely cylindrical, and without knots; leaves sessile and sheathing; roots fibrous, rarely tuberous, sometimes fleshy. The plants may in fact be called the grasses of the river side.

The medicinal properties of the roots are due to the presence of mucilage, sugar, oil, and a slightly bitter and aromatic principle. A very brief notice of one or two species will suffice.

GEN. 1.—CYPERUS.

Sp. 1. *C. longus.* Κυπειρον. Europe.

Roots (rhizomes) blackish, rather woody, tenacious, cylindrical, branched, knee-like, marked with numerous rings, covered with a reddish and streaked bark, smooth, often divided into scales; substance reddish, odour agreeable, faintly ginger-like: taste bitter, balsamic, tenacious, pungent, slightly astringent; powder blackish brown. The odour is communicated to water, though no essential oil is obtained on distillation.

Uses—tonic, diaphoretic, or diuretic.

The *Cyp. juncifolius* (Nagur mootha, *Beng.*) is employed as a diaphoretic and diuretic in India. Its roots are fibrous.

Sp. 2. *C. rotundus,* (round.)

Vern. Mootha. *Beng.*

Roots (rhizomes) in ovoid bulbs, the size of a pigeon's egg, united by a long woody tracing radicle, of leafy texture; substance white, friable, and spongy, odour sweet, slightly aromatic, taste bitter, resinous, and balsamic, especially when the root is dry.

Its properties are the same as those of the preceding species.

Sp. 3. *C. esculentus*, Esculent cyperus.

Roots (rhizomes) composed of thin fibrils, to the extremities of which are attached round or oblong bulbs, externally brown, white within, substance white, tender, and farinaceous, odour slightly camphorate, taste sweet and agreeable, rather saccharine and mucilaginous. The bulbs on analysis afford starch, fixed oil, sugar, albumen, gum, salts of malic and tannic acid, and oxide of iron. The dry root contains one-sixth its weight of oil of beautiful golden colour, nut-like smell, slightly camphorate taste, sp. gr. 0.918; it deposits stearine by rest, and in its general properties resembles the other fixed oils.

The toasted roots have been used as a substitute for coffee, and yield a preparation resembling chocolate. The cultivation of the plant deserves attention for its considerable alimentary value.

Sp. 4. *C. geminatus*, (twin) Ainslie.

Bulbous roots eaten in India, flavour resembles that of sago.

The *papyrus* of the Egyptians belongs to this genus, and is still called *babier* in Syria. It is about 15 feet high; the exterior tunic of the stems cut in bands, and pressed, formed the paper of ancient Egypt and Europe; the leaves, which are several feet long, served for the same purpose, but were of inferior quality. This paper is but little liable to decay. Pliny, for instance, relates that the book of the laws of Numa Pompilius was found in Rome in a high state of preservation, after having been buried nearly six centuries in the earth.

Gen. 2.—Carex.

Herbs in tufts, sometimes creeping, fleshy, simple, and triangular, rarely cylindrical, inflorescence terminal.

Sp. C. arenaria.

German sarsaparilla, a native of sandy coasts, &c. in Europe.

Roots (rhizomes) long, knotty, cylindrical, blackish, the size of a goose quill, garnished with verticillate filaments, emitting thin fibres; substance white internally, odour slightly aromatic, tasteless, or of somewhat camphor-like flavour.

These roots differ from the true sarsaparilla—1. in the difficulty experienced in separating the woody from the cortical part; 2. in the size of the woody part; 3. in the difficulty of splitting this; 4. the ease with which it may be bruised; and, 5. by the different odour of the decoctions. The decoction of carex does not froth.

These roots afford starch 16, watery extract 20, alcoholic extract 10 per 100. The watery extract is of sweetish taste at first, afterwards slightly astringent. The alcoholic extract is rather bitter, and in odour is like guaiacum resin.

Numerous experiments made in Germany tend to prove that this root possesses all the properties of sarsaparilla. The plant is carefully propagated over the dikes of Holland, where its interlacing roots bind the sand together, and thus protect the country from fatal inundations of the sea.

NAT. ORDER VI.—GRAMINEÆ, or *Grasses*.

The grasses are lance-shaped herbs, generally with hollow stems, (though in a few these are solid and very large) marked with irregular knots, from each of which proceeds a sheathing leaf. The leaves are linear or lanceolate, of uniform green colour, sometimes sarmentaceous, sometimes villous. The roots are fibrous, and more or less branched, and must not be confounded with the creeping stems erroneously called roots, or with the bulbs which form an essential and integrant part of the stems (culms); and which like the culms spring from the plumule. The flowers are hermaphrodite, rarely unisexual, or sterile by abortion, number of stamina indeterminate, the majority having three. The fruit is a caryopsis, naked or covered. The embryo is small, and attached to the base of a farinaceous perisperm of larger size. The grasses are generally erect, a few are climbers, and they are all destitute of true thorns.

They are the most numerous and useful plants of the earth. They are provided with three radicles, as if to secure their extensive propagation. It would be superfluous to enter here on an exposition, such as that M. Feé indulges in, of the importance of this order to civilized society.

The external similarity of the grasses is fully confirmed by their chemical composition. The leaves contain a notable quantity of green starch, with mucilage and traces of sugar. The flower-bearing culms and subterranean stems are more saccharine than the leaves, and contain starch, especially in the large species, and in those subterranean stems which have a compact tissue.

The seeds of the grasses contain a farinaceous substance; mixed with the remnants of the envelope this constitutes *the flour* as we receive it from the mill. *Chaff* is the pericarp previously removed by thrashing and winnowing, and has many medicinal and economical uses.

Chemical analysis shews the farina of these grains to consist of gluten, starch, sugar, mucilage, and albumen, principles we have already described—*see page* 72.

There are certain principles which seem peculiar to the grasses, and to particular species of the family. Such for example are hordein (in barley) oryzine (in rice) and zeine (in maize). In the *Schœnanthi* there exists an aromatic principle resembling myrrh. Benzoic acid has also been found in the culm of many species. Lastly, in the *lolium temulentum* or darnel, the only poisonous species known, there is an acrid and volatile matter capable of causing symptoms of intoxication in small doses, and in larger quantities fatal in its effects.

By incineration we find in the ashes, oxide of iron and of manganese, alumina, the carbonates of lime and magnesia, and silica which is the most abundant of all; the large quantity of the latter principle accounts for the slow decomposition of seeds and grasses under water, for their superior qualities as materials for thatching, for the use of their ashes in polishing woods and marble, &c. &c.

The medicinal properties of the Gramineæ are closely connected with their alimentary uses.

The pericarp of the cereal grains (bran) is demulcent in wheat, slightly astringent in barley. The gruels prepared from oats and pearl barley are nutritive, and excellent articles of diet for invalids and convalescents.

Cereal Grains.

The cereal grains are those which are the object of a continuous culture for food.

The seeds of all the Gramineæ, those of the darnel alone excepted, are capable by cultivation of becoming alimentary. The value of grains generally speaking is directly as the size of the caryopsis, and inversely as the thickness of the pericarp. When the grain abounds in perisperm it is heavy, when the envelope is thick the grain is, on the contrary, light, thus:—

100 seeds of wheat weighed,	...	4,50. grs.
100 .... barley,	....	3,85.
100 .... rye,	....	2,60.
100 .... oats,	....	2,50.

The chemical composition of the grain influences materially the quality of the resulting bread. If the gluten be absent no fermentation takes place in the dough, if the gluten be in excess the bread is heavy and acid. Wheat flour may be considered the type of all that is suitable for alimentary purposes, and in the degree of deviation from this standard consists the inferiority of the other grains.

Several diseases infest the cereal grains, generally altering the perisperm, sometimes destroying it altogether; all these maladies are produced by minute cryptogamic plants (mushrooms), of which the three following are the most frequent:—

1. *Caries, (uredo caries,)* attacks wheat, usually spares the pericarp, but changes the perisperm into a black fœtid powder. The component globules are devoid of pellicles. The disease is highly contagious.

2. *Carbon or smut, (Uredo segetum)* occurs under the epidermis, is composed of spherical globules, attacks all the cereal grains indiscriminately, and resembles black dust.

3. *Ergot or spur*, (*Sclerotium clavus*,*) is elongated in form, black externally, white and horny within, exceedingly deleterious in its properties, if long taken; in large doses acts specially on the womb.

But little is known as to the native country of the cereal grains. Michaud states that he has seen wheat growing wild on Mount Atlas. Sicily has, but on insufficient grounds, claimed the honour. Pallas saw wild wheat between the Don and the Volga, but in all these cases the production of a few scattered plants is fairly accounted for on the grounds of the seeds having been transported thither by birds, or with the stores of wandering merchants or commissariat trains. Feé inclines to the belief that the ocean now covers the primitive country of corn, and refers to the catastrophes which formed the straights of Gibraltar, submerged the Atlantis of the ancient geographers, and caused America to spring from the waves, as proofs that we may easily account for our not discovering the native soil of the cereal grains.

* The *Ergotætia abortifaciens* of Pereira,—for this most important substance, see the art. *Fungi*—division *Cryptogamia*.

Without cultivation all the cereals speedily degenerate, as is said to be the case with oats at the Cape of Good Hope.

Gen. 1.—Triticum. D. C.

Sp. T. sativum. Wheat.

Vern. Gioon, Gom, *Beng. Hind.*

More than twenty varieties are described.

Seeds yellowish, oval, gibbous, obtuse at both ends, about two lines long, glabrous, bark convex, marked with a scar towards the summit, and with a longitudinal furrow, margins oval beneath, base downy; flour white, heavy, rather yellowish; starch friable, very white, in an adherent powder, or irregular hexagonal prisms; when compressed between the fingers emits a peculiar sound.

Gluten 12·5 per 100, bran 25 to 33 per 100, according to the varieties. Besides these principles, there are found gum, sugar, and vegetable albumen.

It is needless to mention the innumerable uses of wheat.

Gen. 2.—Secale.

Sp. S. cereale. Rye.

Τιφη, Theophrastus.

Seeds grey, conical, two lines long, acute, glabrous, back convex, marked with a longitudinal furrow, base obtuse, keeled, an oval scar towards the point, surface slightly folded. Flour white, nearly insipid, viscous, nutritive, gluten 9·48, bran 25·35, per 100.

According to Emhoff's analysis, rye flour contains albumen 3·27, gluten 9·48, mucilage 11·09, starch 61·09, sugar 3·27, bran 6·38—loss 5·42.

Rye thrives in poor soils where wheat cannot be cultivated. The bread is more compact than that of wheat flour, is of brown colour and sweetish taste, dries slowly; one part of rye with four of wheat flour afford an excellent and very wholesome bread.

Armenia, Crete, and the banks of the Volga, have been successively pointed out as the native districts of the rye, but on very inadequate evidence.

Gen. 3.—Hordeum.

Sp. H. vulgare v. *hexastichon.* Barley. Κριθη λευκη, Homer's Odyssey.

Vern. Jow, *Hind.*

Seeds oval, oblong, alternated at both sides, smooth, straw coloured, rather angular, with one longitudinal furrow, terminated at the summit by a linear crest; parenchyme white and farinaceous; gluten 3 per 100; starch 32 per 100, greyish, does not resound under the fingers; bran 18·75 per 100. Besides the usual constituents barley flour contains about 1 per 100 of oil.

The composition of barley before and after germination has been examined successfully by Proust, who has published the following tabular view of his results:—

Before germination.		*After germination.*
Yellow resin	1	1
Gum	4	15
Sugar	5	15
Gluten	3	1
Starch	32	56
Hordeine	55	12
Total	100	100

Hordeine.

A yellowish, insipid, inodorous dust, heavier than water, insoluble in water and alcohol, decomposable by the sulphuric and nitric acids into carbonic, oxalic, and acetic acid. According to Thenard, it is most closely allied to *lignine*, and Proust considers that it is probably converted into starch during the act of vegetation.

Barley being a cheaper crop than corn, is much used in Europe for the manufacture of beers and spirits; the strong and empyreumatic flavour of corn spirit is owing to a volatile oil with which it is impregnated.

Beer.—This beverage may be prepared with wheat, rye, maize, &c. The corn is first caused to germinate so as to develope sugar at the expence of the starch, the germination is then abruptly checked by turning and heating in a kiln.

When dried and ground a mash or infusion is prepared, this is allowed to ferment till alcohol is formed; the fermented liquor is then strained, and a sufficient quantity of the strobiles of the hop, *(humulus lupulus)* is added, to impart a bitter flavour.

According to the original temperature of the mash, the duration of the fermentation, and the proportion of sugar and hops, we procure pale ale, table beer, and porter. The last liquid is nearly black, and much stronger than beer. The following extract from Brande shews the proportion of spirit by measure in each kind, compared with other alcoholic liquors:—

	Alcohol per 100.
Table Beer.	1.28
Pale Ale.	6.87
Porter.	4.20
Sherry.	19.17
Port Wine.	22.96
Claret,	15.10
Brandy. / Rum. / Whiskey. (Proof.)	50.00

Beer and porter are stimulant, narcotic, and tonic, and in the hands of a skilful practitioner constitute admirable remedies for the treatment of persons convalescent from fevers, scurvy, and many other severe maladies.

In the French Codex beer is employed as a solvent for cinchona, and for the tops of spruce pine and the *raifort sauvage*, or *scurvy grass*. In Germany the medicinal substance is added during the fermentation, in France after the completion of that process.

Beers are very apt to run into the acetous fermentation, and are then exceedingly detrimental to the patients for whom good beer would prove most beneficial. In India an excellent article may be made during the cold season, and by careful corking will last in good order for a year; instead of the hop, chiretta, colombo, or better still, the *coptis* (mishme) *teeta* may be employed for medicinal purposes.

Medicinal preparations of Barley.

1. *Entire seeds* in decoction—slightly bitter, tonic, and astringent.

2. *Cleaned barley*, imperfectly deprived of the pericarp is employed in some French pharmaceutical preparations of little value.

3. *Pearl barley*, rounded and polished by a mill, entirely free from pericarp, is very much used as an article of diet for invalids.

4. *Barley flour*, much used in poultices in European Hospitals.

5. *Malt*, (seeds after previous germination) is incapable of being kept longer than one year. In the north of Europe it is much given in decoction in diseases of the lungs.

6. *Barley starch*, precisely the same as the other starches in its medicinal properties.

7. *Barley sugar*, syrup made with an infusion of barley boiled down to fusion, and tinged with saffron.

8. *Yeast* (Cerevisia).—The scum or sediment which forms during the fermentation of malt, and other saccharine substances. It is composed of minute cryptogamic vegetables. It is given internally as a stimulant in low fevers—dose two table spoonsful every third hour. It is also used as a poultice to gangrenous sores.

Gen. 4.—Avena. Oats.

About forty species of oats are known to botanists; the agriculturist only cultivates three.

Sp. A. sativa. Βρωμος and Βρομος.
Cultivated in Bengal.

Seeds cylindrical, unguiculate, covered with a black or white envelope, smooth, furrowed, or angular, grain naked, villous, pale grey, bearded at the summit, parenchyme snow-white, farinaceous. Taste sweetish, insipid, mucilaginous. Gluten according to Davy, 6 per 100; Vogel and Kesselmeyer deny its containing any of this principle. According to Vogel's analysis oatmeal is composed of (in 100 parts) starch 59, albumen 4·30, sugar and bitter principle 8·20, gum 2·50, fatty oil 2, fibrous matter 24. The pericarp yields an aromatic principle resembling vanilla in its perfume.

Groats or cutlings are the bruised oat seeds freed of the pericarp. They are much used for preparing gruel for invalids; *porridge*, an excellent article of hospital diet, is made by stirring groats or oatmeal into boiling water until the mixture thickens. It is eaten with milk, butter, or sugar.

Oats grow spontaneously in Sicily near Marsama, where barley also occurs, and have been found by Anson in the island of Juan Fernandez.

Gen. 5.—Oryza. Rice.

Two species only known, the Oryza latifolia (broad-leaved), and Oriza sativa (cultivated); of the latter there are numerous varieties.

Sp. O. sativa. Οριζον.
Vern. Dhan, Chawl, *Hind. Beng.*

Seeds when barked 1—3 lines long, white, nearly transparent, cylindrical, linear, furrowed, obtuse at both ends, brittle. Flour very white, friable, insipid, dry, inodorous and tasteless, very soft, and swelling much when cooked; gluten none.

According to Vogel's analysis rice contains in 100 parts, starch 96, sugar 1, fatty oil 1·5, albumen 0·2.

The absence of gluten prevents] the conversion of rice into bread, but it may be employed for preparing a kind of beer, and a spirit termed arrack. In Europe rice is considered astringent, and with milk is a favourite kind of food for persons labouring under chronic diarrhœa or other dysenteric affections.

GEN. 6.—MAYS OR ZEA.

Sp. Zea Mays. Maize.

Vern. Mokka, *Beng.* Bhotta, *Hind.*

A native of South America, Hindostan, &c. cultivated extensively in Europe.

Seeds rounded, crustaceous at the surface, smooth, naked, shining, of gilded, white, or purplish shades, disposed in a dense cylindrical spike, arranged in longitudinal ranks, and as if inlaid on the central axis or receptacle, parenchyme white and farinaceous. Inodorous, insipid, gluten 0, bran 3·25 per 100; flour slightly yellowish, 96·75 per 100. A substance named *Zeine* has also been separated by Bizio, and other chemists have confirmed his results.

Zeine is soft, malleable, elastic like gluten, solid when cold, colour golden-yellow, taste and smell peculiar, transparent in thin leaves, inflames at a taper, sp. gr. 1·0347, insoluble in cold water, softened but not dissolved by hot water, slightly by ether, soluble in alcohol and the oils, and is converted into a butter-like matter by nitric acid.

The uses of Indian corn for alimentary purposes are too well known to need description here. The flour makes an excellent cataplasm.

The stalks of the plant contain a considerable quantity of sugar, which has been economically manufactured in the crystalline state in several of the South American provinces.

GEN. 7.—HOLCUS.

All this genus are natives of the ancient continent. The seeds are large, but smaller than those of maize.

Sp. 1. *Holcus sorghum.*

Syn. Andropogon Sorghum.

Vern. Joar, *Beng. Hind.*

A native of India, and cultivated in Peru, and in Europe; seeds very hard, rounded, very variable, sometimes entirely smooth, insipid, parenchyme farinaceous; but little different from maize in chemical composition. The stalks afford sugar, but in less quantity than the next species.

Sp. 2. ***Holcus saccharatus.***

Syn. Andropogon saccharatus, *Roxb.*

A native of Caffraria.

Stalks thick, and full of a sugary medulla. Professor Arduino, (*Journ. Botanique*, iii. 198,) gives an account of his experiments on the extraction of sugar from this species. They were extremely satisfactory.

Sp. 3. ***Holcus spicatus.***

Syn. Penicillaria spicata, *Willd.*

Douranelle, *Egypt.* Couz-couz, *Africa.* Cambon, *Tamul.* East Indies, cultivated in Europe.

Seeds ovoid, obtuse, rounded at the top, contracted at the base, of bluish-grey with a yellow point to their attachment, fixed on a long spike, very close, and thinning from the base to the summit.

Gen. 8.—Panicum.

Sp. 1. ***Panicum miliaceum***, Millet.

Κεγρος, Hesiod. Diosc. Hippoc.

India, cultivated in Europe, seeds oval, slightly compressed, brilliant, about a line in length, bark or envelope blackish, brown or fair parenchyme, white, of sweet taste. Alimentary, but the pericarp is very difficultly separated from the grain; chiefly used in a kind of gruel or bouillie.

Sp. 2. ***P. italicum.***

Syn. Setaria italica, *Kunth.*

Vern. Kungoo, *Beng.*

India, cultivated in Europe. Seeds small, roundish, straw-coloured, pericarp brittle, with a round and partially pellucid grain, alimentary, but gives a heavy disagreeable bread.

Gen. 9.—Festuca.

Sp. F. fluitans, Glyceria fluitans, *Brown.* Τιφη, Theopr. Αγροςις ποταμιος, Diosc.

Poland manna, &c. Europe, New Holland, striped seeds small, yellowish white, parenchyme farinaceous, sweet and mucilaginous.

These succeed best in very wet districts.

Gen. 10.—Lolium, Darnel.

Sp. L. temulentum (intoxicating darnel.) Αιρα, Theoph. θυαρος *Dioscor*, Ζιζανιον of some authors, Ηρα, modern Greek.

Seeds small, convex, completely covered by the pericarp, furrowed longitudinally. Taste acrid and disagreeable. It grows in cultivated fields, and abounds especially after rainy seasons. The seeds when ground with the cereal grains render bread poisonous, producing vomiting, drunkenness, and giddiness.

The deleterious properties are strongest in the immature seed. Parmentier, a high authority on these subjects, affirms that the ripe seed is but slightly injurious.

Gen. 11.—Saccharum.

Fifteen to sixteen species constitute this genus, one only is of real importance—the true sugar-cane.

Sp. S. officinarum. Sugar-cane.

Καλαμος Αραβικος or ινδικος Diosc.

Vern. Ookh, *Beng.* Uch, *Hind.*

India, cultivated in West Indies, Spain, Sicily, &c.

Culms cylindrical, marked in spaces by knots or large and swollen joints, inodorous, medulla abundant, juicy, and saccharine.

Products.

1. *Raw-sugar,* cassouade, *gour;* variable in purity, contains molasses; crystalline, in considerable masses.

2. *Molasses,* uncrystallizable sugar, liquid, thick, of deep colour, strong smell, about 1½ per 100 of the whole produce of the cane.

3. *Rum,* the alcoholic liquid obtained by the fermentation of molasses.

4. *Refined-sugar,* muscovado, or gour refined so as afford a sugar of very white colour; solid, hard, friable, brilliant in some parts, scarcely diaphanous, sonorous, phosphorescent by friction in the dark. Sp. gr. 1570; soluble in water, insoluble in alcohol and the ethers, converted by nitric acid into oxalic and malic acids.

Loaf sugar is the product of the evaporation of the syrup of refined sugar; *candy* is crystallized sugar; the crystals are four-sided, with dihedral or sometimes trihedral summits.

Sugar has been adulterated with that of milk, with starch, with sulphate of zinc, &c. &c.

Sugar is much used in pharmacy, especially to correct the taste of nauseous medicines. Syrups, pastiles, conserves, electuaries, are preparations of this kind.

Gen. 12—Andropogon.

Sp. 1. *A. Schoenanthus*, Lemon grass.

Syn. Σχοινου ανθος Hippocrates.

Vern. Gunda Bena, *Beng.* Gund bel, *Hind.*

A native of Arabia, cultivated in India, Ceylon, and the Moluccas.

The culms are straight, cylindrical, slightly striated, pointed below, leaves linear, finely striated, glabrous, spikelets in pairs.

The odour is aromatic and rose-like, taste bitterish; by Vauquelin's analysis it afforded resinous matter resembling myrrh, a colouring substance, free acid, volatile oil, salts of lime, oxide of iron, and ligneous fibre.

The leaves of this species are used in India as a kind of tea, and are deemed tonic and slightly stimulant.

Sp. 2. *A. Iwaranchusa.*

Vern. Roosa, *Hind.*

A native of the low hills at the base of the Himalayas, also found at Asseerghur, and in Malwah, generally; root perennial, culm three to six feet high, filled with a spongy substance.

This plant has long been supposed to yield the celebrated "grass oil" of Nemaur, but Royle denies the correctness of this opinion, and refers the oil to a species he terms the *A. Calamus aromaticus;* the oil is used as a stimulant internally and externally, much in the same manner as oil of cajeput.

Grass Oil of Nemaur.

(Roosa-ke-tel, *Hind.*)

This valuable oil was first brought to the notice of the profession by Dr. Maxwell in 1824, and was further described by Dr. Forsyth in 1826.

The oil is obtained from the grass by distillation; 250 to 300 small bundles of the grass are placed in a boiler, covered with water, and distilled. About a seer of oil is obtained in the receiver. Dr. Forsyth describes it as volatile, extremely pungent, of light straw colour, very transparent, with a peculiar rich and agreeable odour.

Dr. Forsyth adds, that it is very highly esteemed by the wealthy natives for the cure of rheumatism, especially that of the chronic kind; two drachms of the diluted oil are rubbed over the pained part in the heat of the sun or before a fire twice daily. It causes a strong sensation of heat or pricking, lasting for two hours or longer. The natives also regard it as an efficacious remedy in slight colds. They anoint the soles of the feet with the oil, and it is stated that slight diaphoresis is thus produced. (See *Trans. Med.* and *Phys. Soc.* iii. p. 216.)

NAT. ORDER VII.—PALMÆ, *the Palms.*

This is probably the most remarkable order in tropical vegetation. Their products are numerous, and of inestimable local value. Sago, sugar, toddy, butter, wax, oil, and catechu are afforded by different individuals; no true poison exists in the order, but the fruits of the *Caryota urens* are of an acrid taste.

GEN. 1.—SAGUS, *Sago palms.*

Sp. 1. *S. lævis.* Sago tree.
Vern. Rambiya, *Malay.*

Sumatra and the Moluccas. The stem is as thick as that of the cocoa-nut tree, which is from 15 to 20 years in attaining maturity.

The soft cellular part of the trunk yields the well known and valuable—

SAGO. (Sagoo, *Beng.* Sabudāna, *Hind.*)

Sago is amylaceous, occurs in partially rounded grains of ash-white colour, smooth, hard, the size of a mustard seed. Sometimes of reddish grey colour; elastic, and difficultly powdered, inodorous, tasteless, little altered by time, insoluble in cold water, by long boiling in water it swells and gelatinizes, but the jelly is not uniform.

To prepare the sago the tree is felled, cut into billets, cleft, and the cellular matter extracted, and diffused through water. The mixture is decanted, and when the fecula subsides this is dried before the sun. Rumphius states that the natives of the Moluccas granulate the paste while drying, by forcing it through perforated plates; these grains are then sun-dried and slightly toasted, which gives them a reddish tinge. Feé throws doubt on this statement, and considers the state of the sago of commerce to prove that no toasting was performed.

One tree eight years of age will, it is asserted, afford from three to four hundred pounds of sago.

Sp. 2. *S. farinifera.* (Roxb. Fl. Ind. iii. p. 624.)

Also yields sago, but of inferior quality.

The *Cycades* and *Zamiæ* also produce this substance.

Sago is chiefly used in India and Europe as a light and agreeable article of diet for children and invalids.

GEN. 2.—CEROXYLON. *Wax palms.*

Sp. Ceroxylon andicola.

A native of the Peruvian Andes, of immense height, often attaining 250 feet in elevation; from fissures in the trunk there flows spontaneously a kind of grey waxy substance, containing two-thirds of resin and one-third of wax identical with that formed by the bee. Melted with a little suet this wax makes excellent tapers.

GEN. 3.—PHŒNIX. *Date palms.*

Sp. P. dactylifera, Date tree.

Vern. Kajur, *Hind.*

A native of Arabia, cultivated in Spain, Italy, and the south of France.

The fruits are cylindrical, drupe 12 to 18 lines long, covered with a thin, smooth, deep brown pellicle, enclosing a rich pulp and bony nut. The pulp is nearly inodorous, the taste sweet, mucilaginous, and agreeable. From the abundance of sugar the date fruit contains, its juice readily undergoes the alcoholic fermentation.

A single tree often affords in Arabia from 100 to 200 lbs. of fruit.

The sap of the Bengal date tree, Phœnix sylvestris, Roxb. is also very saccharine, and is much employed for the manufacture of sugar.

GEN. 4.—ELAIS, *Oil palms.*

Sp. E. guineensis.

A native of Africa and America, supposed to afford the palm oil of commerce, but this is really a mixture of various oily products of this order.

The Elais oil is obtained by expression from the pericarp and the substance of the fruit.

PALM OIL.

This substance occurs in commerce in masses of a soapy consistence, yellowish colour, liquefying at 96° Fahr., of slightly violet odour, becoming rancid by keeping.

Cocoanut oil which solidifies at the same degree is often in Europe substituted for the Elais oil, being tinged yellow with turmeric, and scented by orris root.

The true oil is soluble in alcohol and ether, and contains, according to Henry, 31 *stearine* and 69 *elaine* per cent.

The concrete palm oil is much esteemed in Europe for the preparation of perfumed unguents of various kinds.

GEN. 5.—COCOS, *Cocoanut palms.*

Sp. C. nucifera, the Cocoanut tree.

The products of this invaluable tree are too well known to need description in these pages.

GEN. 6.—ARECA, *Catechu, or Betelnut palms.*

Sp. Areca Catechu.

Vern. Soopäri, *Beng. Hind.*

A native of the Eastern Islands, cultivated in Bengal.

The fruit (a nut) is yellow, oval, the size of an egg, enclosing an oily kernel like a nutmeg, conical, rounded, pointed and marked with white and reddish veins; inodorous, but of very astringent taste.

By Morin's analysis the areca nut contains tannic and gallic acids in large proportion, acetate of ammonia, red matter, concrete oil, volatile oil, gum, acetate of lime, fibrous and saline matter.

The areca nut is one of the constituents of the famous masticatory, the *betel* of the East. Pān, the leaf of the piper betel, and shell lime, are mixed with slices of the nut, and chewed together. The lime gives a deep orange or red colour to the colouring matter of the nut, and thus dyes the lips and tongue in the peculiar manner so common among the natives of India.

GEN. 7.—CALAMUS.

Sp. C. Draco. Dragon's blood plant.

Vern. The resin, Damoolukwain, *Hind.*

A native of the Indian archipelago. The fruits are fleshy, red, astringent, and yield the resin called *Dragon's blood.*

This substance has been already noticed at page 297.

It is of much more importance in the arts than in medicine, being chiefly used as an ingredient in varnishes and paints.

In commerce it occurs in powder, grains, masses, drops the size of an olive, and in sticks enveloped in the leaf of the talipot palm.

Dragon's blood softens in hot water, alcohol nearly dissolves it, and the residue is reddish white. It stains marble, especially if the stone be heated. It is soluble in oils, and by nitric acid is converted into artificial tannic acid. It contains a small proportion of benzoic acid, which probably gives it slightly stimulating properties.

Dragon's blood is obtained either from the surface of the fruit, by incision in the stem, by natural exudation from various parts of the plant, or by exposing the fruits to steam and collecting the softened resin which exudes. An inferior kind is procured by boiling the fruits.

The *Dracæna Draco* of Linnæus, affords a similar secretion. A tree of this kind at Teneriffe measures 17 feet in diameter, and is on strong reasons estimated to be 1500 years old.

NAT. ORDER VIII.—SMILACEÆ.

Climbing thorny plants, sometimes of very large size, dioïceous; starch and a slightly bitter principle are the most remarkable constituents, and two peculiar principles, *Smilacine* and *Parigline*, are described as occurring in some species.

The roots of the *S. Sarsaparilla* have long been celebrated in medicine in the treatment of chronic or secondary syphilis, in scrofula, and in convalescence from severe acute diseases.

Gen.—Smilax. (*Sarsaparilla plants.*)

The sarsaparilla root of commerce is afforded by several species, chiefly South American. Pereira specifies the following:—

Smilax officinalis,..	New Granada.	Product, Honduras sarsaparilla.
——— medica, ..	Mexican Andes.	——— Vera Cruz sarsaparilla.
——— syphilitica,	Brazils.	——— Brazilian sarsaparilla.
——— sarsaparilla,	Virginia.	Not proved to yield the drug.

Lindley mentions many others, to some of which we shall subsequently allude.

The roots of the species above mentioned are several feet long, wrinkled, rather fibrous, red, brown, or greyish, of mucilaginous, and rather acrid taste, and slightly earth-like smell.

The cellular tissue is red in the Jamaica drug, white in the other varieties; the Jamaica article is considered the best, and according to Pereira those of deepest orange colour are to be preferred, and the more acrid and nauseous the taste the better. A great quantity of *beard* or root fibres, Pereira adds, is deemed a good test.

The Jamaica sarsaparilla is folded into bundles about half a yard long and five inches broad; the powder is pale brown, and contains starch. The extract is soluble in cold water; three parts of root yield one of extract. The Brazilian sarsaparilla is in larger bundles. Those from Lima average nine inches in diameter. It yields about a quarter of its weight of watery extract.

The latest analysis of sarsaparilla is that by Thubæuf (1834). He detected a crystalline substance, *salsaparine*, resins, colouring matter, fibre, starch, fixed aromatic oil, wax, and the muriate and nitrate of potash. Berzelius states that 100 lbs. of the root yield about an ounce of volatile oil.

Salsaparine.

Thubæuf's experiments shew that this is identical with the Smilacine and Parigline of previous writers. It is obtained in crystals by acting on a strong tincture of sarsaparilla by animal charcoal till the colour is destroyed; crystals form as the solution cools. Salsaparine is colourless, inodorous, and nearly tasteless when anhydrous, soluble with frothing in hot water, the solution being of bitter acrid taste; also soluble in alcohol, ether, and oils; does not form salts with acids, is coloured successively red, violet, and yellow, by strong sulphuric acid. In all its properties in fact it is almost identical with saponine or esculic acid.

Salsaparine in doses of nine grains causes a feeling of weight at the stomach, with nausea. It is no doubt the active principle of the root.

In 1838 there were imported into England 121,888 lbs. of sarsaparilla.

Medical effects, &c.—Notwithstanding the immense consumption of sarsaparilla, there is still much doubt as to the kind or amount of action which it exercises on the human system. All agree that it acts as a diaphoretic or diuretic. The only effect of very large doses is to produce nausea, vomiting, and loss of appetite. The majority of practitioners esteem it as a powerful, though gradual, alterative and tonic, especially in the treatment of secondary syphilis and cutaneous diseases.

It is sometimes given alone in infusion or decoction, but it is more generally combined with sassafras, mezereon, and guaicum, all stimulating diaphoretics. It is also often prescribed with small doses of blue pill, with nitric acid, and with quassia, gentian, or chiretta. In chronic rheumatism we have seen it employed with benefit, especially when given with Dover's powder in full doses.

For doses and mode of preparation, see in the Pharmacopœia the articles infusion, decoction, syrup, extract, and fluid extract.

Sp. 1. *Smilax China.*

Vern. The roots. Shookchina, *Beng.* Chob Chinee, *Hind.*

Wild in China; the rhizome is hard, large, woody, knotty, brown or blackish externally, white in substance.

The root is one of the China roots of the Bazars, it is much, and we believe advantageously employed as a substitute for sarsaparilla. It is largely imported into Calcutta from the Eastward, and much employed by native practitioners.

Of several species of smilax described by Roxburgh and other writers on Indian Botany, the two following seem the most deserving of attention.

Sp. 2. *S. glabra.*

Vern. Gotee shook China, *Beng.*

A native of Sylhet and the adjacent country. A climber with a large tuberous rhizome. The stem and branches are thornless, leaves lanceolate, pointed, pale green beneath. Flowers umbellate, axillary, sessile, and solitary. The root is identical in appearance with the China root of commerce.

Sp. 3. *S. lanceæfolia.* Eastern Bengal.

Vern. Hurria shook China, *Beng.*

Much resembles the former, the leaves are lance-shaped and three-nerved, umbels stalked.

Together with these we may notice, *S. Roxburghiana*, *Vern.* Koomaree shook China, and *S. oxyphylla*, *Vern.* Chotee or small koomaree. *S. rigida* and *ferox*, are Nipalese species. *S. elegans* extends to the Deyra Doon, and *S. maculata* is found in Nepal, Kemaon, and Missouree. *S. prolifera* occurs very generally, and *S. Villandia* on the Morung hills. (*Royle*).

Mr. Royle also mentions a root sold in the bazars under the name *Aoshba mugrabee.* This is translated sarsaparilla in Dictionaries, and the root much resembles that drug. Its origin is unknown.

Roxburgh states that the natives use the roots of the *S. glabra* in venereal and leprous ulcers, and that they also employ the *S. lanceæfolia* very extensively for the same purpose, and in the treatment of rheumatism.

Both these species deserve attentive examination. It seems however that the Ununtamol (*Hemidesmus indicus*) is likely to supersede all the varieties of sarsaparilla not only in Indian but in European practice.

NAT. ORDER IX.—DIOSCOREÆ. (*Yams.*)

Climbing and sarmentaceous plants, with alternate or sometimes opposite leaves.

The roots are large, tuberous, and very rich in nutritive fecula, hence they are much used as articles of diet. None have any medicinal properties.

NAT. ORDER X.—ALISMACEÆ.

Only remarkable for containing the *A. Plantago,* or water plantain. This insignificant plant some years ago obtained great notoriety as an alleged specific in hydrophobia. It has now fallen into deserved neglect.

NAT. ORDER XI.—MUSACEÆ.

The true plantain family—remarkable for the value of its fruit, but yielding no medicinal substance.

NAT. ORDER XII.—MARANTACEÆ.

Some species are of much celebrity as the chief sources of *arrow root;* a fecula obtained by washing the crushed or rasped root. In the W. Indies arrow root is obtained from the Maranta arundinacea, Allongia, and nobilis, also from the *Canna glauca,* called "*tous les mois.*" In the East Indies arrow root is prepared chiefly from *M. arundinacea,* also from *M. ramosissima,* a Sylhet species.

The stems of *M. dichotoma* yield the beautiful *sital pati* mats of Calcutta.

Arrow root may be regarded as a perfectly pure starch. It is sometimes adulterated with potatoe starch, but the fraud is detected by the microscope; the particles of potatoe starch are large, and marked with concentric lines. The name of arrow root is derived from the West Indians, who used it as an application to wounds from poisoned arrows.

NAT. ORDER XIII.—SCITAMINEÆ, OR ZINGIBERACEÆ.

[The Gingers.]

These plants have herbaceous stems with alternate leaves sheathing the stems. They chiefly abound in India, and thrive best in moist situations. The roots of nearly all the species are odoriferous, and contain an essential oil and resin, to which their stimulating properties are due. In some the roots are fleshy, and abound in fecula from which arrow root is prepared, sometimes again, as in the turmeric, this fecula is associated with a colouring principle, and is used in painting and dyeing.

No poisonous species is known.

Gen. 1.—Zingiber.

Sp. 1. *Z. officinale.* Narrow-leaved ginger.
Syn. Amomum Zingiber, *Linn.*
Vern. Adrak, Ada. *Beng.* and *Hind.*
Off. Roots.

The recent root is tuberous, ash-white externally, rugose, digitate, rampant, fleshy, yellowish interiorly, and covered with thin pellicles; when dried it is in fragments of about two inches long, branched, rather dichotomous, compressed at both sides, knotty, smooth, grey or ashy with oval knots, covered by a wrinkled epidermis, parenchyma white, with ready fracture, and rather resinous appearance.

The odour is penetrating, taste acrid, pungent, hot, aromatic. The powder is grey. Ginger is readily the prey of insects, to prevent which it is sometimes steeped in cream of lime or in a ley of wood ashes.

The *black* and *white* ginger of the shops are said to differ only in the latter having the epidermis scraped off.

Recent writers however state that the roots are obtained from different species. The powder of the best white ginger of Jamaica is of a pale yellow or straw colour.

On analysis the best ginger yields volatile oil, soft acrid resin, resin insoluble in ether or oils, gum, starch, woody fibre, organic extract, acetic acid, acetate of potash, sulphur, earthy salts, and oxide of iron.

The *volatile oil* is pale yellow, lighter than water, taste acrid and hot.

The *resin* is obtained by first treating the powdered root with water, and then with ether. The resin is yellowish, soft, aromatic, and hot to the taste.

Ginger is a very useful aromatic stimulant, principally used as a spice, but also an ingredient in some valuable pharmaceutical preparations. In infusion, tincture, or syrup, it is much employed internally, and ginger powder made into a paste with warm water gives a very useful counter-irritant application.

Sp. 2. *Z. Zerumbet.**

Syn. Amomum zerumbet.

Vern. Butch, mahaburee Butch, *Hind.* and *Beng.*

Found in the woods about Calcutta; the taste of the root resembles that of ginger, but is bitter as well as aromatic. It is not used in medicine by European practitioners.

Sp. 3. *Z. Cassumunar* (*yellow* zedoary).

Vern. Bun ada, *Hind* and *Beng.*

Rhizoma much larger than that of common ginger, smell camphor-like, taste hot and bitterish (*Roxb. Fl. Ind.* vol. i. p. 49.) Now very little used.

Gen. 2.—Curcuma.

Sp. 1. *C. Zerumbet.*

Vern. Kuchoora, Shoothee, *Hind.* and *Beng.* (*Roxb. Fl. Ind.* i. p. 20.)

A native of the East Indies, found at Chittagong, stemless, roots palmate and tuberous, pale yellow internally, smell pleasant and camphor-like, taste aromatic and bitterish.

This is the *long zedoary* of pharmacy.

* Erroneously called *round zedoary* by many writers.

Sp. 2. *C. zedoaria.*

Vern. Bun-huldi, *Beng.* Judwar, *Arab.* Roxb. i. p. 23.

A native of Bengal and China.

This is the *round zedoary,* all kinds of which resemble gingers in their medicinal qualities, but are inferior to it in strength and agreeableness of flavour.

Sp. 3. *C. rubescens.* Roxb. i. p. 28.

Vern. Tikor, *Beng.*

A native of Bengal; the root is highly aromatic, but its chief use is for the preparation of *tikor*—a very fine fecula, like arrow root. This in Travancore constitutes an important article of food.

Sp. 4. *C. leucorrhiza.* Roxb. i. p. 30.

Vern. Tikor, *Hind.* and *Beng.*

Common in Behar; horizontal tubers long and straight, colour very pale yellow—the tubers yield abundance of fine nutritious fecula.

Sp. 5. *C. longa.* Turmeric.

Vern. Huldi, *Beng.* Roxb. Fl. Ind. i. p. 33.

Tubers deep orange inside, bitter, and aromatic. The colouring matter of the dried root is bright yellow, soluble in alcohol and water, and changed to a deep red by alkalies. White paper dyed by an alcoholic tincture of turmeric is a very sensitive test for alkalies.

Sp. 6. *C. angustifolia.*

Vern. Tikor, *Hind.* Roxb. i. p. 31.

Common in India; the roots are used in the Benares district for the manufacture of arrow root.

Sp. 7. *C. Amada,* "Mango ginger."

Vern. Amada, *Beng.* Roxb. i. p. 33.

Also a native of Bengal. The name of mango-ginger is given to this root from its peculiar smell while fresh. It is a gentle stimulant, but now only used as an article for seasoning food.

Gen. 3.—Kæmpferia.

Sp. 1. *K. Galanga.*

Vern. Chundra moola, *Beng.* Roxb. i. p. 15.

Common all over India. Rhizoma fleshy, tuberous, with fleshy fibres; the roots are agreeably fragrant, and of warm bitterish aromatic taste. Notwithstanding its specific name, it is not the source of the true *galanga* root of the druggists, a drug now known to be the produce of the *Alpinia galanga.*

Sp. 2. *K. rotunda.*
Vern. Booi Champa, *Beng.* Roxb. i. p. 16.
This species is cultivated all over India, and was long considered to produce the *Zedoaries.* Feé still refers them to it. But Lindley, with most other writers of authority, states that this article is the root of the *Curcuma zedoaria.*

Gen. 4.—Amomum.

Sp. 1. *A. Cardamomum.* Roxb. Fl. Ind. i. p. 37.
Vern. Elachi, *Beng.*
Java, Sumatra, and mountainous parts of India. Rhizome like that of ginger; the capsules are sessile, globular, small, seeds roundish, angular, dotted, brown, very aromatic. This seems to be the round or cluster cardamom of the shops. It has not been analyzed.

Sp. 2. *A. angustifolium.* Roxb. Fl. Ind. i. 39.
A native of Madagascar, cultivated in the Mauritius; the fruit is the *greater cardamoms* of the old writers.

A. maximum, according to Pereira, yields the *great winged* cardamoms, referred by Lindley to *Elettaria.*

Sp. 3. *A. aromaticum.* Roxb. Fl. Ind. i. p. 45.
Vern. Morung elachi, *Hind.*
Chittagong, and the East of Bengal.
The capsule is ovate, the size of a nutmeg, 3-valved, 3-celled, seeds several in each cell, all similar in shape and properties to the true cardamoms.

A. dealbatum, is the *Burra elachi* of Sylhet.

Sp. 4. *A. Grana Paradisi.* Paradise grains, Malaguetta pepper.
A native of the coast of Guinea near Sierra Leone. Capsule 1½ inch long, ½ an inch in diameter, oblong, somewhat triangular, beaked, of dark reddish brown colour, hairy, powerfully aromatic. The seeds are of bright golden brown colour, excessively hot, acrid, and aromatic. The *A. grandi-*

fiorum of the same locality yields seeds of very different and camphor-like flavour.

Malaguetta pepper is the favourite spice of the natives of the Guinea coast, and largely imported into England as a fraudulent ingredient in beer, wines, and vinegar.

Gen. 5.—Elettaria.

Sp. 1. *E. Cardamomum.* True, or Malabar, or lesser cardamom.

Syn. Alpinia Cardamomum. *Roscoe*, and *Roxb. Fl. Ind.* i. 70.

Vern. Chotee-elachee, and Guzeratee-elachee, *Hind.*

A native of the mountains of Malabar and Canara; there is also a long capsuled variety, the capsule is oval, 3-sided, size of a small nutmeg, 3-celled, 3-valved, seeds numerous, blackish, very agreeably aromatic and pungent. They are much used as a spice, and as a stimulant remedy. (See the *compound tincture* in the Pharmacopœia.) 100 parts of the fruit yield 74 seeds, 26 of coats. According to Tromsdorff, they contain essential oil 4.6, fixed oil 10.4, malate of potash, fecula, yellow colouring matter, woody fibre, and other unimportant ingredients. The *fixed oil* is somewhat like castor oil, the *volatile oil* is of sp. gr. 0.943, insoluble in solution of potash, it is the source of the aromatic quality of the seeds.

Sp. 2. *E. Cardamomum medium.*

Syn. Alpinia card. med. *Roxb.* i. 74.

Vern. Dokeswa of Sylhet. Burra-elachee, *Hind.*

Capsules on long pedicels, ovate, oblong, 1½ inches long, nearly one in diameter, rather triangular, 1-*winged*, 3-celled, many-seeded, seeds grooved at one side. Lindley supposes this to be the *Cardamomum medium* of writers on pharmacy. Pereira considers it likely that the *wild cardamoms* of Calcutta are identical with these fruits. One hundred parts of the fruit yield 70 seeds and 30 tunics. One pound gives four scruples of volatile oil, of whitish colour, and thick consistence.

Sp. 3. *E. Cardamomum zeylanicum.* Pereira.

The produce of Quilon and Matura, the fruits are analogous to the Malabar cardamom in all their properties.

Gen. 6.—Alpinia.

Sp. A. Galanga. Roxb. Fl. Ind. i. p. 59.

Vern. Koolinjan, *Hind.*

A native of Sumatra, cultivated in the Indian archipelago; tubers slightly aromatic and bitter, the root-stock more so, pungent, acrid, and aromatic. They constitute the true galanga roots of the druggists, and are used for the same purposes as ginger.

Gen. 7.—Hedychium.

Sp. H. spicatum.

Vern. The root is called *secr, ruttee, kupoor kuchree;* the plant, *sidhuoul, Hind.*

The root is fragrant, warm, and aromatic. Royle, to whom is due the merit of tracing the true source of the root, thinks it may probably be the *ritte,* or *lesser galangal* of Ainslie.

Putchuk Root.

This root forms a rather important export from Calcutta. It is brought from Lahore, where it is called *koot,* and is sold in the Bengal bazars under the name of kooth, kust, and koshta; one kind is called *koosht tulkh,* or the bitter; another *koosht shereen,* the sweet or mild; the latter is of light yellow colour and pleasant smell. Mr. Royle supposes it to be identical with the Indian orris root, but this is called *beg banopsha,* and is imported from the Red sea. It appears to us to be in every respect identical with the true orris root.

Putchuk is of unknown origin; though usually referred to *Costus arabicus* or *speciosus;* the roots of the latter are quite insipid and inodorous. The putchuk is chiefly exported to China, where it is used as incense. Mr. Royle inclines to the opinion that it is in reality the produce of an umbelliferous plant; specimens have been seen by Mr. Beckett of Allyghur having hollow stems. (*Royle,* p. 360.)

NAT. ORDER XIV.—ORCHIDEÆ.

This is a very large order, and distinguished by several extraordinary peculiarities in its inflorescence, the groups of petals frequently resembling insects or birds. The *vanilla* and *orchis* are the most remarkable genera, the former yielding an exquisite perfume and aromatic, the latter the *salep* of the druggist.

SALEP. (Salep misree, *Hind.*)

The tubers of the *Orchis mascula* receive this name in works on pharmacy. They are compressed, ovoid, rather transparent, and composed chiefly of bassorine, soluble gum, and starch. Royle states that one drachm of the powdered root requires 60 drachms of boiling water to effect its solution; two drachms afford a sufficient meal for an invalid; good salep carefully prepared is in truth one of the best articles of diet a convalescent can use.

In India the salep of Cashmere is reckoned the best, and is obtained chiefly at the Hurdwar fair from the Cashmere merchants. Lindley and Royle consider the plant which produces this salep to be an *Eulophia*, not an *Orchis*.

This substance, from the peculiar shape of the tubera, has gained immense, but most unmerited celebrity as an aphrodisiac remedy. The same circumstance has given the plant its name both in the Greek and Arabic languages.

GEN.—VANILLA.*

Sp. V. aromatica. Vanilla plant.

The fruit is a pod-like capsule, the thickness of an adjutant's quill, a little compressed, reddish brown colour, 8 to 10 inches long, wrinkled transversely, unilocular, truncated at the summit, and contracted at the base. Parenchyme fleshy, coriaceous, rather unctuous, full of soft black paste, containing very small, black, roundish, brilliant seeds.

The odour is sweet, and resembles that of balsam of Peru, taste aromatic, hot, sweetish. To reduce the dried paste to fine powder it must be mixed with sugar.

Vanilla pulp contains a large quantity of essential oil and benzoic acid. The pericarp is nearly inodorous; vanilla is one of the most esteemed of all aromatics. The plant grows spontaneously on the banks of the Orinoco, in Venezuela, the Andes, and other South American territories. It thrives best in very hot but well shaded and irrigated localities. It has been lately introduced into the Calcutta Garden by Lord Auckland, but as yet has produced no fruit.

The fruits are gathered before perfect maturity, dried in the shade, and dipped in some fixed oil to prevent the dissipation of the volatile oil they contain.

Feé states that a kind of vanilla is brought from Hindostan, but in this he has evidently been misinformed; species

* Nat. Order, *Vanillaceæ* in Lindley.

of the plant occur at Singapore and Penang, but they are not known to yield this valuable article.

On the continent of Europe vanilla is much esteemed as an ingredient in some stimulating and tonic remedies.

NAT. ORDER XV.—IRIDACEÆ.

This order is remarkable for containing the saffron (*Crocus sativus*) and the *iris*, more than one species of which affords the Orris root of commerce. Of these we shall give a brief notice, their properties being but of trivial importance in a medicinal point of view.

Gen. 1.—Crocus.

Sp. C. sativus, Saffron.

Vern. Zafran, *Hind.*

A native of Asia Minor, naturalized in England, France, and many other parts of Europe—cultivated in Persia and Cashmere.

The saffron of commerce consists of the dried stigmata of the flower. These are picked out, dried on paper either in a kiln or by the sun. If compressed into cakes it is accordingly called *cake* saffron; *hay* saffron is what is usually met with.

The *hay* saffron consists of the stigmas, each about an inch and a half long, brown-red, the upper part flattened, widened, and cleft; the lower, hair-like and yellowish. The odour is fragrant, taste bitter but agreeable. Saffron tinges the saliva yellow. Mr. Pereira informs us that one grain of good saffron contains the stigmata and styles of nine flowers, so that one ounce of saffron is equal to 4,320 flowers.

Cake saffron as now met with contains none of the real article, being prepared from the florets of the safflower (see *Carthamus*) made into a paste with gum water.

According to the latest analysis (Aschoff's) saffron affords on analysis volatile oil 1·4, wax 4, polychroite 52, gum 10·4 fibre 19, water 10, balsamic matter 2.

The *volatile oil* is yellow, heavier than water, acrid, bitter, solidifies and whitens by long keeping, the white solid being lighter than water.

Polychroite, so called from its numerous changes of colour when subjected to chemical re-agents (πολυς many, χροα colour) is obtained by making a watery extract of saffron, and then an alcoholic tincture from the extract. It is of a bright red colour, bitter, inodorous, soluble in hot water, alcohol, and oils, slightly in ether; sulphuric acid turns it blue and lilac, nitric acid deep green, but the colour is not permanent.

Saffron is possessed of but trivial power in the system, either in health or disease, although it was once considered an energetic stimulant. It was also deemed emmenagogue and narcotic, useful in suppressions of the biliary secretion, in promoting the eruption in exanthematous diseases, in asthma, hysteria, and gout. Modern trials have shewn the total inefficacy of the drug, and it is now only used as a colouring principle and an ingredient in several culinary preparations.

Gen. 2.—Iris.

Sp. Iris florentina. Florentine iris.

A native of Italy and Asia Minor. The roots are the *orris root* of European shops. This article contains volatile acrid resin, astringent matter, gum, extractive, starch, and woody fibre; in full doses it is emetic and purgative. Peas turned from the wood are used in issues to support suppuration. Reduced to powder it is a favourite ingredient in hair and tooth powder. Excellent orris root is procurable in the Calcutta bazars under the name of *Begbanopsha.* Mr. Royle under this head very confidently refers the *putchuk* of commerce to this article. A species of iris is cultivated in India. Its roots are used in the same manner as those of the Florentine kind.

NAT. ORDER XVI.—AMARYLLIDEÆ.

This is a very extensive and interesting order, containing several emetics, purgatives, and diuretics.

Gen. 1.—Crinum.

Sp. A. asiaticum, variety *toxicarium.*

Vern. Sookh durson, Burra kanoor, *Beng.*

Bulb with a terminal, stoloniferous, fusiform portion issuing from the crown of the bulb descending deep into the mud or earth; from the last-mentioned portion proceed the ramous fibrous roots. Stem 0. Leaves radical, equally disposed on every side, linear, concave (so much so that a section forms nearly a perfect semicircle); margins smooth; length from 1 to 3 feet, and where broadest, little more than ¾ of an inch. Scapes generally shorter than the longer leaves, a little compressed, smooth, often coloured. Umbels with from 6 to 16 flowers. Spathe

2-leaved, with filiform bracts amongst the flowers. Flowers large, white, subsessile, fragrant during the night. Tube cylindrical, from 4 to 6 inches long, coloured, or pale-green, according to exposure, smooth. Divisions of the limb linear-lanceolate, equally disposed; margins waved a little; a recurved process at the apex of each. Filaments equally disposed, ascending, upper half coloured; anthers linear, incumbent. Ovary inferior; style as long as the stamens, declinate; stigma simple. Fruit membranaceous, subglobose, containing in one cell 1 or 2 rugose, bulb-like seeds, and although the flowers are subsessile, the capsules are on short stalks. *Roxb.*

The fusiform portion of the bulb, the bulb itself, and the colourless and sheathing bases of the leaves are of somewhat narcotic heavy odour, are readily dried in the stove, and reducible to powder after dessication.

From two to four drachms of the recent root or stem, bruised into a paste, and this squeezed through cloth, afford a juice which proves emetic after a few minutes; in smaller quantities it is nauseant and diaphoretic; we have never known it to occasion any untoward symptom.

The dried sliced roots are also an efficient emetic, but require to be given in double the dose of the recent article.

The natives use the bruised leaves with castor oil as a cataplasm to whitlows, and the juice is dropped into the ears in ear-ache.

We were induced to subject this article to trial by Dr. Horsfield's account of its emetic virtues in Java; we administered it in several cases, and found it to act as a certain and mild emetic in the doses we have already mentioned.

The extract, whether watery or alcoholic, is very uncertain in its action.

As this variety of Crinum is common in Bengal, and often cultivated in gardens, it is calculated to prove a very valuable addition to the native Materia Medica. It is indeed the only indigenous and abundant emetic plant we have had experience of, which acts without producing griping, purging, or other distressing symptoms. In the form of syrup it may probably be found to retain the active principles of the recent plant. The tincture of the fresh plant does not succeed, doubtless in consequence of the large quantity of spirit counteracting the emetic effect, by its stimulating energy.

GEN. 2.—BRUNSVIGIA.

Sp. B. toxicaria.

Syn. Amaryllis disticha, *Linn.*

A native of the Cape of Good Hope. The viscid juice of the bulbs is a powerful poison, and used by the Bushmen on their arrows.

Gen. 3.—Narcissus.

Several species of this genus are known to possess considerable power as emetics and cathartics.

The dried bulbs of the *Narcissus poëticus* of Europe are given in doses of 5—10 grains as a nauseant, and 30 grains as an emetic. The extract has been much used in hooping cough, in 2 to 3 grain doses. In large doses (2 to 3 drachms) it is a powerful poison.

The Narcissus tazetta is used in India, it is said with the same effect; we have not been able to test its virtues.

Gen. 4.—Agave.

Introduced by the Portuguese into India, the most common species being the *A. vivipara*, Bans-keora, *Hind.* The *A. americana* yields abundance of a saccharine and mucilaginous sap, which readily ferments and forms an alcoholic liquor. This is the favourite beverage of the Spaniards in Mexico, and is powerfully intoxicating. Its smell is said to resemble that of putrid meat.

NAT. ORDER XVII.—MELANTHACEÆ.

This order is celebrated for containing the Sabadilla and Colchicum, from which the powerful acrid and narcotic *veratria* is obtained.

Although the genera occur in India, none have yet been found to possess the active properties of the Colchicum or Veratrum of Europe.

Gen. 1.—Veratrum.

Sp. 1. *V. viride*, green Veratrum.

A common plant in the swamps of the United States; the roots are acrid, emetic, and stimulant, subsequently sedative.

Sp. 2. *V. album*. White hellebore.

A native of the south of Europe and the Caucasus. The rhizoma is rather horizontal, blackish externally, white internally.

The root is very acrid, occasioning inflammation wherever it touches; emetic in doses of two grains, in large quantities a virulent acrid and narcotic poison. It is rarely given internally, but the powder is occasionally made into an ointment in some obstinate cutaneous diseases, and for the destruction of vermin.

Sp. 3. V. Sabadilla.

A native of South America and the West Indies, affords one kind of the *Cevadilla* or *Sabadilla seeds* of commerce, from which *veratria* is prepared. We shall notice this principle and its effects when we have enumerated the other species in which it is found.

Gen. 2.—Helonias.

Sp. H. officinalis.

Syn. Veratrum officinale, *Asagrea* of Lindley.

A native of the Mexican Andes; bulbous. This also yields a kind of sabadilla seed. There is some doubt as to the genus to which the plant should be referred. *H. frigida,* also a native of Mexico, is very poisonous. The *H. Erythrosperma* of the United States is used for destroying flies. *H. dioica* affords a root used in tincture as a bitter tonic, in infusion as a vermifuge.

Gen. 3.—Colchicum.

Sp. C. autumnale. Meadow saffron.

A native of many parts of England and Europe. The cormus, or bulb-like root is ovate and large. The leaves dark green, very smooth, obtuse, more than a foot long, 1½ inch broad. Flowers several, radical, leafless, bright purple, with a long white tube appearing without the leaves in the autumn, capsules 3, distinct, though forming together one oblong elliptic fruit with intermediate fissures, seeds whitish, polished. (*Lindley.*)

The dried cormi and seeds are used for several pharmaceutical preparations, as well as for the preparation of veratria. If gathered after the flowers shoot the cormi are nearly inert, a circumstance which fully explains the conflicting statements made regarding their medicinal powers.

Sabadilla.

This important drug consists of the follicular fruits of the plants above specified, especially the *Helonias officinalis;* stalks and flowers are mixed with the samples.

The follicles are about ½ an inch long, and a line in diameter, of pale brown or reddish grey colour. Three follicles compose the fruit, adhering together at the base, open above, and each follicle containing two or three seeds. These are two or three lines long, curved, pointed, blackish brown, slightly winged, inodorous, but of bitter, acrid taste.

The seeds contain *cevadic acid*, a fixed oil, *veratria*, two kinds of resin, a principle called *sabadillina*, and a gum resin, differing from the latter only in containing one atom more water.

The seeds are powerfully acrid and narcotic; the tincture applied to the skin causes after some days the appearance of a slight eruption. Dr. Turnbull states, that rubbed over the region of the heart it has been known to reduce the strength and quickness of the pulse. He has given the alcoholic extract internally in minute doses in rheumatism and neuralgia. This practice is not likely to be much imitated. The chief, if not the only, use of this seed is for the preparation of veratria.

Veratria and Sabadillina.

To prepare veratria a tincture of bruised sabadilla seed is evaporated to an extract, this is boiled in water acidulated with sulphuric acid, and the solution concentrated by a gentle heat. The residue is neutralized by magnesia, pressed, washed, and dried. The dry matter is treated with spirit, this distilled; the residue, which is impure veratria, is purified by solution in dilute sulphuric acid, and precipitation by ammonia.

We have to notice another process in the Pharmacopœia. By that now described, one pound of sabadilla seed yields a drachm of impure veratria.

This contains *sabadillina*, a substance analogous to, but much weaker, than pure veratria.

Pure veratria is a whitish powder, devoid of odour, acrid and causing numbness and tingling when placed on the tongue, fusible at 240, slightly soluble in ether, readily in alcohol, alkaline in reaction; but its salts are difficultly crystallizable. Veratria is intensely reddened by sulphuric acid. The smallest quantity applied to the nostrils causes violent sneezing, and the tincture rubbed on the skin also causes heat and tingling.

According to Couerbe, veratria contains carbon 34, hydrogen 22, nitrogen 1, oxygen 6 equivalents = to 288.

Uses—similiar to those of aconitina, to which it is inferior in efficacy, at least in the local treatment of neuralgia. It has been used internally in gout, rheumatism, dropsy, and many other diseases. Its effects are stimulating, diuretic, occasionally cathartic, but generally constipating. The therapeutic results of the trials were altogether uncertain. The dose was one-sixth of a grain thrice daily, given in pills with crumb of bread, extract of Hyosciamus, or liquorice powder.

COLCHICINE.

The best analysis of Colchicum is by Pelletier and Caventou. They found fatty matter, volatile acid, supergallate of veratria, yellow colouring matter, gum, starch, lignin, and ashes. Geiger and Hesse have lately described a new principle, which they term *colchicine*. This is crystalline, alkaline, and bitter, and is prepared by the same manipulation as that directed for veratria under the preceding head. It is coloured blue by nitric acid, brown by sulphuric acid, and it does not excite sneezing; in all these properties it differs from veratria. It seems to be a very powerful, acrid, and narcotic poison.

It is however to the presence of veratria that colchicum chiefly owes its medicinal virtues.

In small doses, frequently repeated, colchicum tends to increase the secretions of the intestinal mucous membrane, the skin, liver, and kidneys. It frequently lowers the force of the circulation, but this is not an invariable effect. It occasionally acts as an anodyne, an effect especially observed in gout and rheumatism. In large doses colchicum and all its preparations prove poisonous, under symptoms of violent irritation and inflammation of the alimentary canal, with slight disturbance of the nervous symptoms.

Most authorities now admit the great efficacy of colchicum in alleviating paroxysms of gout. It seems to be most successful when it acts as a purgative. In acute cases, and patients of full habits, the use of this remedy should follow venesection. Sir Charles Scudamore recommends a draught of 15 to 20 grs. magnesia, and one to two drachms of sulphate of magnesia, with one to two drachms of the vinegar of colchicum. The whole to be given with any aromatic water and a little syrup or extract of liquorice.

As to the use of colchicum in rheumatism there is great difference of opinion; our own experience leads us to believe that in the common forms of rheumatism affecting the natives of India it is a very efficient remedy when given in the manner Scudamore recommends. In rheumatic gout Mr. Wigan recommends eight grains of the powder to be given every hour till copious purging, vomiting, or sweating is occasioned. We do not feel warranted in advising any repetition of this practice. If the drug be of good quality such doses in inexperienced hands are more likely to prove poisonous than beneficial.

In some cases of dropsy the diuretic effects of colchicum have led to considerable relief. It has also been used in inflammatory diseases, and in ardent fevers, as an auxiliary to venesection, and cathartics.

Lastly, in hysteria, chorea, and similar affections of the nervous system, it has been tried with very doubtful results.

The chief preparations of colchicum are the powder of the cormus and of the seeds; the tincture and wine of the seeds; wine and vinegar of the seeds or cormus; there are also an acetic extract, watery extract, and oxymel, all of which are described in the Pharmacopœia.

The Hermodactyl.

In the medicine shops of India generally, there are sold two varieties of a bulb called *soorinjan*, one the *S. tulk*, or bitter, the other *S. shereen*, or mild; both are identical with the Hermodactyls of the ancient Arabian and Greek writers. Their origin is unknown, but they are doubtless referable to some species of colchicum. The *tasteless* variety is about one inch long and the same in breadth, heart-shaped, rather flattened, grooved at one side, convex at the other. They are not wrinkled, and are easily broken and form a white powder. The *bitter* kind is smaller, and has a striped appearance. Pereira describes one of Mr. Royle's specimens as yellowish, somewhat transparent, horny, and striped lengthwise.

No satisfactory experiments, whether chemical or clinical, have been yet made with this article. In some trials we made with an acetous tincture of the *soorinjan tulk* we were led to believe it possessed of all the virtues of the dried colchicum of Europe. It certainly deserves careful and extensive examination.

NAT. ORDER XVIII.—LILIACEÆ.

This order is of much interest to the physician, containing the squill, aloe, and other important articles.

Gen. 1.—Erythronium.

Lindley describes one species, the *E. americanum*, the fresh root of which is emetic in the dose of 25 grains.

The *E. indicum* of Ainslie is now referred to the genus Ledebourea.

Gen. 2.—Aletris.

The *A. farinosa* of the United States is described by Bigelow as a bitter of great intensity. It is used as a tonic. In large doses it tends to act as an emetic.

Gen. 3.—Scilla.

Sp. 1. *S. maritima.* Squill.

A native of the Mediterranean coast. The bulb is rounded, ovate, sometimes very large, with pale green or reddish cuticle.

Squill contains an active principle, *Scillitin*, to which its acridity is due.

The dried bulb is white, acrid, bitter to the taste, yields its active principles to water or alcohol; applied while recent to the skin the sliced bulb causes irritation and blistering.

Taken internally in small doses the preparations of squill are nauseant, diaphoretic, or diuretic; in large doses emetic. They are chiefly used in chronic catarrh, asthma, croup, and hooping cough, also as a stimulant diuretic in dropsical cases. Squill is frequently combined with digitalis, and with mild mercurial preparations, especially the blue pill and calomel.

The principal preparations are the tincture, and vinegar.

The dose of the powder is as a nauseant, one to three grains; as an emetic, ten grains to half a drachm. It is but seldom used for the latter purpose.

Sp. 2. *S. Pancration.*

Supposed to be the Pancration of Dioscorides; the bulb is much smaller than in the preceding species. The effects are said to be similar, but milder, it occurs at Malta, Cadiz, and other Mediterranean localities.

Sp. 3. *S. indica.*

Called *Iskeel*, by the native gardeners.

Occurs on the sea-shores of the Indian Peninsula; the bulb is round, white, the size of an orange; leaves numerous, radical, sub-bifarious, ensiform, nearly flat, smooth on both sides, six to eighteen inches long. When in blossom the plant is entirely destitute of leaves; scape erect, round, smooth, naked, including the raceme from two to three feet long. Raceme very long, erect, flowers remote, long-pedicelled, drooping. *Roxb. Fl. Ind.* i. 147. Roxburgh states that the bulb is quite as nauseous and bitter as that of *S. maritima.*

We have examined the bulbs of this plant, obtained through the kindness of Dr. Jackson. They were inodorous, nearly tasteless, and devoid of any medicinal properties. Possibly this may have proceeded from their having been collected from an unfavourable locality, or at the improper season.

Few plants are so much influenced by climate and circumstances as the squill, instances being known on the Spanish coast of its being quite inert in one locality, while as active as usual but at the distance of a few miles.

Gen. 4.—Ledebouria.

Sp. L. hyacinthina.

Syn. Erythronium indicum.

A native of Bundlecund and Hydrabad. Martius and Ainslie describe the bulbs as a substitute for squill, and the latter writer informs us they are used in cases of strangury and fever in horses.

Through the kindness of Dr. Key, of Bolaram, we procured an ample supply of these bulbs. We found them to be slightly acrid and bitter, but although given in double and treble the usual quantity in which squill is employed they did not in any case produce the marked effects which squill occasions. The bulbs we used had not flowered that season. From our trials it would appear that this article holds out but little prospect of its ever being usefully employed in medicine.

Gen. 5.—Allium.

This genus contains the onion, ***Allium Cepa***, and the garlic, ***A. sativum.***

The raw bulb of the garlic is acrid and irritating, taken internally in small quantities by persons unaccustomed to its use it is stimulant, diuretic, and perhaps expectorant. According to Gassicourt's analysis 1406 parts of garlic contain mucilage 520, albumen 37, fibrous matter 48, water 801; there is also an acrid, yellow, very pungent volatile oil by which the irritating effects are occasioned. The recent bulb of the *onion*, according to Fourcroy and Vauquelin, contains white oil combined with sulphur, gluten, incrystallizable sugar, mucilage, phosphoric and acetic acid, and citrate of lime; the juice mixed with water and yeast ferments readily, and will yield nearly one-third its weight of spirit.

The bruised onion is sometimes used as a cataplasm. It is a stimulant diuretic; the juice mixed with sugar is sometimes given to children and old persons in non-inflammatory coughs and asthma.

Gen. 6.—Dracaena.

Sp. D. Draco.

A native of the Canary islands, where it attains enormous magnitude. A variety of the red resin called "Dragon's blood" is obtained from all parts of the tree by incisions or from natural fissures. (See *Pterocarpus.*)

Gen. 7.—Aloe.

Most of the species of this genus yield a bitter juice, which hardens into the drug called aloes. The quality of the product is apparently more dependent on soil, climate, and preparation, than on specific differences in the plant. Barbadoes, the Cape of Good Hope, and Socotra afford the mass of the aloes found in commerce, but it has occasionally been prepared from different species in Spain, France, and India.

We shall first enumerate the most remarkable species which produce the drug, and then treat of the varieties of this substance.

Sp. 1. *Aloe vulgaris*, common aloe.

Syn. A. barbadensis. A. perfoliata.

A native of the East Indies, now cultivated in many tropical and hot countries. The leaves are armed with spines, and are a little mottled; flowers yellow.

This species yields the *Barbadoes aloes* of commerce, by some called *Hepatic* aloes.

Sp. 2. *A. socotorina.* Socotorine aloe.

A native of the island of Socotra, leaves minutely serrated, flowers scarlet at the base, pale in the middle, green at the point.

Yields Socotorine aloes, also the true *hepatic* and *Mocha* aloes.

Sp. 3. *A. spicata.*

A native of the interior of the Cape of Good Hope, leaves distantly toothed, with a few white spots, the flowers filled with purplish honey.

Sp. 4. *A. indica.* Royle.

A species with reddish flowers, common in dry situations in the North-west of India, probably the source of some of the common aloes (*musabhir*) of the bazars.

Produces Cape aloes, and the coarse variety called the fœtid, *caballine*, or horse aloes.

Aloes. Mushābhir, *Hind.*

This valuable drug differs considerably in appearance and properties, generally according to the mode of preparation. The best kind is obtained by making transverse incisions through the leaves, and allowing the juice to drop out. This is evaporated to dryness by a gentle heat. Dipping the leaves in hot water facilitates the flow of the juice.

By pressure large quantities of viscid mucilage are forced out, and mix with the proper bitter juice, which is proportionately deteriorated. The extract of a decoction of the leaves contains still more impurities.

In Socotora and Barbadoes the exudation process is resorted to, and the juice boiled down till a portion of the hot fused mass solidifies, and becomes brittle on being cooled. The Jamaica drug is a watery extract of the leaves.

Socotorine aloes is exported from Bombay. The colour is reddish brown. Its surface shining, structure transparent, fracture shelly, taste very bitter. The powder is of bright yellow colour; when burnt it evolves a very fragrant odour.

The *true hepatic* aloes, also exported from Bombay, and probably the produce also of the Socotorine aloe, differs from this kind in being opaque and olive-coloured.

Barbadoes aloes is what is commonly termed *hepatic.* It is exported in gourds, ranges in colour from dark brown or black to red or liver colour, fracture dull or glossy, odour disagreeable, and increased by breathing upon the surface, powder dull olive yellow.

Cape aloes is deep brown, shining, of greenish tint and resinous fracture, edges transparent and ruby coloured, powder greenish-yellow, odour strong.

The *fœtid* or *caballine aloes* is now no longer found in commerce.

We are indebted to Mr. Heddle of Bombay, for three specimens of aloes marked Socotorine, Kurachee, and Deckan.

That marked *Socotorine* is rich, brown, shining, soft, ductile, and adhesive at 82° Farht.; of strong and not disagreeable odour, wrapped up in and including leaves. It much resembles the best Bengal opium in general appearance. Water dissolves 82 parts per 100.

The *Kurachee aloes* is nearly black, opaque, rather vascular, structure of shelly fracture, faint smell, powder blackish, slightly adhesive to the touch. It is identical with the better kinds of Musabhir of the Bengal Bazars. Water dissolves only 52 per 100.

The *Deckan* specimen is deep brown, of earthy and slightly resinous fracture, and faint odour, powder brown. Soluble in water in proportion of 98 per 100.

The common *Bazar aloes* in Bengal is black, brittle, of semi-vitreous fracture, and too impure for medical use.

Chemical composition.

The most remarkable constituent is a bitter principle soluble in water, and of a partly saponaceous nature. It has been termed *aloesin*, and is in the proportion of 60 to 80 parts per 100. It contains nitrogen; is very little soluble in alcohol.

Aloes also yields a resin from 10 to 15 per 100. There is much discrepancy in the statements of writers regarding its properties.

There is also present a peculiar acid, the *aloetic*, which produces an olive brown colour with the persalts of iron. Its general properties are unknown.

Medicinal uses. Aloes is one of our most valuable remedies, being tonic, gently aperient, or purgative, according to the dose; some writers also deem it to be diuretic. In small doses it is tonic, promotes digestion, and is generally thought to increase the secretion of the liver. In large doses it proves purgative after several hours, (from eight to twenty-four), acting chiefly on the large intestines, and often occasioning considerable irritation of the rectum. It also stimulates the uterus and its appendages, and thus frequently increases or brings on the menstrual discharge. Socotorine aloes is generally, but very vaguely, supposed to have less of this tendency to occasion irritation of the rectum and uterus, than the Barbadoes variety of the drug.

From the above properties aloes is perhaps the most useful of all purgatives in habitual costiveness, loss of appetite, and dyspepsia, when these depend on a torpid state of the system, and when inflammation does not exist. In repressed hæmorrhoids, and to relieve the symptoms of cerebral congestion this state often occasions, aloes in full doses is the best remedy we can employ, after the more immediate symptoms are relieved by bleeding or leeching. From its special tendency to the rectum, aloes is often used for the expulsion of the *ascaris*, or thread worm, which chiefly infests that intestine.

In stricture of the rectum, inflammatory states of the intestinal tube, during pregnancy, and in persons liable to over profuse menstrual or hæmorrhoidal discharges, the use of aloes is highly improper.

Aloes is usually given in the form of pill, to the extent of from one to twenty grains, according to the effect desired.

The *compound aloetic pill*, containing gentian and oil of caraway, is a very useful preparation. Aloes is also given with asafœtida, myrrh, iron, guaiacum, canella, carbonate of potash, and other substances, according to the effect desired. There are also officinal, a purified extract, tincture, compound tincture, and wine, and we find aloes a constituent in several formulæ to which its name is not attached, for example, the *compound colocynth pill;* all these preparations are fully described in the Pharmacopœia.

Division II.

CRYTOGAMIA, OR FLOWERLESS PLANTS.

ORDER I.—ALGÆ.

(*Sea-weeds.*)

These are leafless, flowerless plants, usually growing in water; none are poisonous; some contain mucilage, gelatine, or a peculiar principle analogous to these; sugar is also frequently present; many are highly nutritious, of delicate flavour, and well adapted for the diet of invalids. Iodine exists in a considerable proportion in some of these plants, which before the discovery of that substance enjoyed celebrity in the treatment of scrofula. The *Fucus vesiculosus*, common sea-weed, or bladder-wrack, was used for this purpose by Dr. Russell in 1769; the whole plant bruised was rubbed on the affected parts, and he also gave the expressed juice internally. Iodine and its preparations have now altogether superseded the use of this article.

The *Chondrus crispus*, or Irish rock-moss (carrageen), is purplish white, and nearly transparent, with flat nerveless fronds. It swells up like tragacanth in water, and by boiling forms a light nutritious jelly, which differs in several respects from the ordinary vegetable principle of that name. It is an excellent demulcent remedy, but has no higher virtues.

The *Gigartina helminthochorton*, or Corsican moss, has enjoyed much celebrity as a vermifuge; what is sold under this name is a mixture of several marine vegetables and minute animals. It contains vegetable jelly, carbonate of lime, and traces of iron. Some consider it diuretic and diaphoretic; it has been vaunted as a remedy for cancer, but on very inadequate grounds.

The *Gigartina lichenoides*, or Ceylon moss, was first described under the name of *Fucus amylaceus* in a paper by the Editor of this work in 1834; the following extracts from the paper in question afford a summary of what is known respecting this valuable substance:—

The Gigartina Lichenoides, or Ceylon Moss.

"I beg leave to forward to you the results of the analysis you requested me to make of the vegetable substance you sent me, under the designation of an "*edible moss*," and which, as far as I can ascertain, has not been described by scientific writers. It is a very small and delicate fucus, of white colour, and flattened filiform shape. The longest of the separate individuals in the specimen I received, did not exceed two inches from the ciliary processes corresponding to the root, to the extremities of the ramifications, which were not very numerous or regular. I could not discover any organs of fructification, perhaps owing to the season of the year when the fucus was collected. As it is, however, my chief object at present to contribute to the chemical history of the substance in question, I shall not enter into its description more minutely, but I shall venture, for mere convenience of reference, to apply to it the provisional term of *Fucus amylaceus*, from its remarkable and important peculiarity of containing a large proportion of true starch.

"I proceed to describe the results of the analysis, and I shall subsequently offer a few very brief remarks on the relations the *Fucus amylaceus* bears tq other edible congenerous vegetables; I shall lastly point out the mode in which its alimentary ingredients may be made available in culinary preparations.

"*Analysis of the Fucus amylaceus.*

"Sec. A.

"1. Twenty grains of the fucus in its dry state were macerated for twenty-four hours in cold distilled water. A great increase of bulk was produced, the fucus still retaining its natural outline and proportions as if seen through a powerful magnifying lens: on pouring off the water, and removing all mechanically adherent moisture, the twenty grains were found to have imbibed of water fifty-four grains.

"2. The decanted fluid, A 1, was neutral to test paper; did not coagulate on boiling; had a strong saline, but no bitter taste; when evaporated to the consistence of a syrup it afforded a flocculent precipitate on the addition of alcohol.

"3. The precipitate, A 2, when collected and dried, weighed 0.80 grains; it was soluble in water, hot and cold; was precipitated by alcohol and subacetate of lead, and with all other re-agents gave the usual characters of gum.

"4. One half of the fluid from which the gum had been thus separated, A 2, when diluted with water, gave precipitates with the nitrates of silver and baryta, but not with oxalate of ammonia, tartaric acid, or chloride of platinum.

"5. The remaining half of the fluid, A 2, evaporated to dryness; and the residuum, calcined on platinum foil, gave a saline mass weighing 0.65 grains.

"From these experiments it is obvious that the fucus under examination differs from the Iceland moss in containing no bitter principle, that it holds in combination 4 per cent. of gum, and 6.50 per cent. of muriate and sulphate of soda.

"Sec. B.

"1. Ten grains of the fucus were cut into very minute shreds, and boiled for twenty-four hours in two ounces of distilled water, which was constantly renewed as evaporation required: when allowed to cool, the liquid gelatinized, the jelly being mixed with an abundance of undissolved shreddy masses.

"2. The jelly, B 1, re-dissolved by boiling, and filtered through muslin, was neutral to test papers; free from bitter taste; transparent and colourless: gave no precipitate with tincture of galls; with iodine gave a faint and very transitory blue tinge when cold; was very soluble in caustic potassa, from which it did not gelatinize; acetic acid added in excess to the alkaline solution, separated the jelly unchanged in the form of a clear coagulum.

"3. A particle of the insoluble residuum on the filter, B 2, when quite cold, was agitated with distilled water in a small glass tube, and iodine added; the particle became gradually blue, but the fluid was not affected: the contents of the tube were then boiled, allowed to cool, and more iodine added, with exactly the same effect—the starch remaining in the particle of fucus, and not being dissolved from it by the boiling water.

"4. The solid residue, B 2, weighing 3.50 grains, was boiled in alcohol; the alcoholic fluid separated and dissolved gave traces of wax.

"5. The same solid particles, B 2, thus freed of wax, were reduced to a very fine powder by diligent trituration: the powder was boiled in distilled water, the solution filtered and allowed to cool; iodine now struck with it an intensely blue colour; two grains of solid insoluble matter containing no starch were left on the filter in the experiment.

"6. These two grains were insoluble in water or alcohol, and with the strong alkalies and acids exhibited the characters of ligneous fibre. Incinerated, this gave a minute saline residuum, composed of sulphate and phosphate of lime and traces of iron.

"*Conclusions.*

"The preceding experiments shew that the fucus under examination is composed of vegetable jelly, nearly identical with the pectin of Braconnot (experiment B 1 and B 2), true starch (exp. B 2 and B 5), wax (exp. B 4), gum (exp. A 2 and A 3), sulphate and muriate of soda (exp. A 4), sulphate and phosphate of lime and traces of iron (exp. B 6), and lastly, ligneous fibre (exp. B 5 and B 6). The following ingredients existed in one hundred grains of the fucus:—

Vegetable jelly	54·50
True starch	15
Wax	a trace
Ligneous fibre	18
Gum	4
Sulphate and muriate of soda	6·50
Sulphate and phosphate of lime	1
Iron	a trace
	99
Assume the traces of wax, the iron, and loss, at	1
Total	100

"You are of course aware, that several individuals of the Lichen and Fucus families are possessed of valuable alimentary or medicinal properties; while some, such as the *Cetraria islandica*, or Iceland moss, combine both these virtues in a remarkable degree. The very disagreeable bitterness of the lichen, although removable, it is true, by immersion in an alkaline solution, must ever constitute a material obstacle to its general alimentary consumption. In one important particular, namely, in the proportion of true soluble starch, the Iceland moss is, moreover, far below the *Fucus amylaceus* in alimentary value. The same observations apply almost as aptly to the celebrated *Clandonia rangiferina*, or rein-deer moss, which is quite as bitter as the former. Among the *Fuci*, several very curious individuals are included; some of which are of known alimentary utility. One of the most singular of these is the *Gelidium corneum*, valuable from the immense quantity of soluble and nutritive pectin which it contains, and from its entering, according to the statement of Guibourt, into the formation of the edible swallow's nests of the Javanese highlands. The *Laminaria saccharina* is interesting from the fact of its containing sugar. It is highly esteemed in Japan, where it is extensively used as an article of diet; being first washed in cold rain water, and then boiled in milk or broth. Another, the *Durvillia edulis*, of Bory St. Vincent, is sold commonly as a vegetable for the table in the markets of Chili; but I believe it has never been subjected to chemical examination. In Great Britain, the *Chondrus crispus* has recently attracted much attention. This production abounds on the western coasts of Ireland, round the Orkneys, Hebrides, the Scilly Islands, &c. indeed every where, except on the limestone or chalk maritime districts; it enjoys high popular celebrity as a remedy in phthisis, and in Ireland it is but too well known as the occasional resource of a famishing population. By long decoction it affords a considerable quantity of a nutritious but nauseous jelly; the unpleasant flavour being chiefly owing to the very large proportion of sulphate of soda it contains. Starch, however, does not enter into its composition; so here this individual also yields in value to the *Fucus amylaceous*, which contains no bitter or unpleasant principle, no iodine, and but a very moderate proportion of sulphate of soda.

"From the preceding remarks the probable value of the *Fucus amylaceous* may be readily inferred. With regard to the best mode of rendering it available as an article of diet, I made several experiments, which I need not describe minutely, but the results of which afford some useful indications.

"In the first place, from the tendency of pectin or vegetable jelly to form insoluble compounds, with saline and earthy bases, it is necessary to steep this fucus for a few hours in cold rain water, as the first step in its preparation: this removes a large proportion, if not the entire, of the sulphate of soda, leaving all the gelatine and starch. It should then be dried by the sun's rays, and ground to a fine powder; I say ground, for cutting or pounding, however diligently or minutely performed, still leaves the amylaceous globules so mechanically protected and so closely involved in an external sheath of tough ligneous fibre, that scarcely a particle of the starch can be extracted by boiling, even though the decoction is prolonged for several hours. When ground, on the contrary, boiling for twenty-five minutes or half an hour dissolves all the starch and gelatine; the solution, while hot, should be passed through muslin or calico, and thus the ligneous fibre is removed: lastly, the strained fluid should be boiled down, till a drop placed on a cold surface gelatinizes sufficiently.

"With milk and sugar, and flavoured by lemon juice or sherry, this substance when prepared as I direct, would afford the invalid a pleasant article of diet, especially at sea, where other jellies or their materials cannot be so easily preserved."

Mr. Previté also gives the following directions for the preparation of this jelly.

"Put into an open stew-pan half an ounce (being the quantity contained in the cover of the canister) of the prepared moss, and a quart of boiling water. Boil briskly for twenty-five minutes, or until a spoonful of the liquid forms into a firm jelly within two or three minutes after it is taken from the pan. Flavour with wine, a little cinnamon, lemon or orange juice and peel, and sweeten according to taste. Boil the whole for five minutes, and pass it two or three times through a jelly bag or doubled muslin. Leave it *undisturbed*, and it will become a firm jelly in ten minutes. If it be required perfectly clear for table use, add the white of two eggs beaten up into a whip before the second boiling, and allow it to stand for a few minutes away from the fire, with some hot coals on the cover of the pan. When clear, pass it through the jelly bag, and leave it to congeal. Should the jelly be required particularly firm, add an ounce of the moss to the quart of water.

"The moulds best adapted for this jelly are of white earthenware, to which it adheres much less than to tin or copper. No heat is required to separate the jelly from the mould, but a little care is necessary in turning it out, on account of its brittleness, or want of elasticity. One pound of the prepared moss will make sixteen quarts of jelly."

Besides the above, there are many edible sea-weeds which need no special notice.

Almost all the plants of this order yield soda and iodine on incineration. Until very recently they were collected in large quantities, and burned for the sake of the soda yielded by the ashes; after separating the alkali iodine was obtained from the mother liquors. Although the trade in *kelp* (the local name of sea-weed soda) has been nearly annihilated by the plan for making soda from common salt, still sea-weed ashes constitute the sole source from which iodine is manufactured.

The green *Conferva* which floats on the Salt-water lake near Calcutta readily yields iodine. It should be dried, burned, the ashes packed in crucibles and heated to bright redness. The residue treated with water, on evaporation yields a saline mass of muriate and sulphate of soda, chloride of potassium, and iodide of potassium and sodium. Nearly all the salts may be separated from the iodides by crystallization. Mix the mother liquors with peroxide of manganese in a retort, add sulphuric acid, the iodine will be liberated, and can be condensed in a common receiver.

Mr. Royle informs us that the natives of the districts at the base of the Himalayas use in the treatment of goitre a dried leaf "brought from a great distance," and which they call *gillur ke putta*, or goitre leaf. It much resembled fragments of a common fucus.

ORDER II.—LICHENES.

Of the lichens several are nutritious, some bitter, some yield to ammoniacal solutions a variety of brilliant colours, and are much used as dye stuffs. They are perennials, spreading in the form of a crust over rocks, trees, or the surface of the earth.

The *Cetraria islandica*, or Iceland moss, is brownish or greyish white, inodorous, slightly bitter. It contains starchy matter 44.6, bitter principle 3.0, sugar 3.6, chlorophylle 1.6, extractive matter 7.0, gum 3.7, fibrin 36.72, salts of potash and lime 1.9.

The bitter principle, *cetrarin*, is white, very bitter, soluble in alcohol, difficultly so in water, is tinged blue by muriatic acid, and precipitates the salts of iron red.

Iceland moss is freed of the bitter matter by being steeped in water containing 1 in 300 parts of carbonate of potash. It is then well washed, after which it may be used in the same manner as the Ceylon moss; if the bitter matter be not removed it may be regarded as a tonic of moderate power, but most disagreeable flavour.

The *Rocella tinctoria* of the Canaries and Azores is the source of the *orchil* of the dyers. It contains brown resin, wax, glutinous matter, insoluble starch, yellow extractive, and yellowish brown gummy matter, soluble starch, tartrate and oxalate of lime and common salt. The brown resin exposed to the action of air and water of ammonia yields a purple colouring matter called *erythrin*.

The whole plant inclosed in a corked phial with a weak solution of ammonia, at a temperature not exceeding 130° gives a purple red solution.

The *Lecanora tartarea* is found on the rocks of Norway, Scotland, and other northern countries. It yields the valuable dye stuffs *cudbear* and *litmus*.

Cudbear is made by acting on this plant with ammonia; on the colour being produced the plant is made into a paste or powder.

The process for making *litmus* is still a secret; the lichen is said to be fermented with putrid urine. Litmus is sold in small light blue cakes containing carbonate of lime, and yielding their colouring matter to water and alcohol; acids redden the colour; alkalies restore it, and in excess change it green. The *litmus paper* so universally used as a test, and so useful in numerous chemical processes, is prepared by steeping unsized paper in a watery solution of this dye.

Chulchilhera Lichen of the Himalayas.

This is the *Borrera ashneh* of Royle; with ammonia it gives a reddish brown colouring matter, and is used accordingly as a dye stuff. We have examined this and several other Indian lichens, and repeated upon these the processes described under the heads of cudbear and litmus, but without success in the production of any valuable colour.

ORDER III.—FUNGI.

(The Mushrooms.)

This remarkable order contains several highly nutritious species, many destructive poisons, but scarcely any medicinal article. It is not certain whether the properties of the ergot of rye, which owes its existence to a fungus, depend on the fungus itself, or on the altered condition of the parts on which it is supported.

The principles termed *fungin*, *amanitin*, the boletic and fungic acid, mannite, and sugar, are found in different species of this order.

The common field mushroom, the morel (Kana kuchoo, *Hind.*) and truffle, are the species of this order most usually eaten. But several poisonous fungi so closely resemble the common mushroom, that the utmost caution is necessary in their use. No test whatever, whether botanical or chemical, can be relied on to distinguish the dangerous from the wholesome kinds. Special cultivation is the only sure mode of procuring the mushroom of invariably good quality.

The only products of this order used in medicine are the *ergot* and the *agaric* of the oak (*Polyporus igniarius*, or *boletus ig.*)—a spongy porous mass, once much used as a styptic.* Its action is solely mechanical, and the article is now very seldom used. *Amadou*, or German tinder, is a similar substance.

The poisonous mushrooms occasion symptoms of great irritation of the digestive organs, with disorder of the nervous functions. There is no antidote. Free vomiting must be had recourse to without delay, and then either stimulants or sedatives must be employed, according to the nature of the symptoms.

GEN.—ERGOTÆTIA.

Sp. Ergotætia abortifaciens. Ergot fungus.

ERGOT OF RYE, OR SPURRED RYE.

Syn. Secale cornutum.—Acinula clavus, (*Fries*). The growth of this substance is occasioned by the germination of the fungus called *Ergotætia abortifaciens*, in or upon the seed of rye corn.

* It is found in the Indian bazars under the name of *Agarikoon*.

Spurred rye, or ergot, occurs in grains averaging an inch in length, and one-tenth to one-eighth of an inch in breadth, curved, cylindrical, taste slightly acrid, odour (of large quantities) heavy and sickening, colour externally bluish brown or black, substance white, with a tinge of blue, texture brittle.

According to the recent investigations of Quekett, it appears satisfactorily proved that the ergot is a diseased condition of the rye grain, occasioned by a parasitical fungus.

The grains of many other *Gramineæ* become affected in the same manner, but it is uncertain whether the ergot thus produced possesses the same medicinal properties as the one now under notice. It is especially desirable to ascertain whether the rice and maize of India afford an ergot available in medicine.

The most recent analysis by Wigger and Chevallier shew the ergot of rye to contain—

Ergotin,	1·25
Peculiar fixed oil,	35·00
White crystallizable fat,	1·05
Cerin,	0·76
Fungin,	46·19
Vegetable ozmazome,	7·76
Peculiar saccharine matter,	1·55
Gummy extractive, with red colouring matter,	2·33
Albumen,	1·48
Superphosphate of potash,	4·42
Phosphate of lime with trace of iron,	0·29
Silica,	0·14
	102·20

Ergotin is a resinous substance insoluble in ether, dissolved by boiling alcohol, insoluble in water. It is brown, acrid, and poisonous. Whether this be the constituent which acts specifically on the uterus is still open to dispute. The oil is said to occasion the disease called *ergotism*, so frequently occasioned epidemically by the altered cereal grains, but which is distinct altogether from the special agency of this substance on the uterine system.

The general effects of ergot on the lower animals have been made the subject of extended experiment; general feebleness, partial paralysis, dilatation of the pupil, vomiting, and death have been caused by half an ounce swallowed by a dog; very large quantities however have been eaten by unimpregnated cows, sheep, and goats, with perfect impunity.

Many experiments are still on record which prove that if the animal be pregnant, and the natural period of gestation nearly elapsed, the uterus will be thrown into contractions by the introduction of ergot into the stomach or rectum, and by its injection into the veins; Mr. Youatt's experience is perfectly decisive on this point.

In doses of half a drachm to two drachms, the utmost effects produced on the human male are slight disturbance of the stomach and bowels, giddiness, headache, and dilatation of the pupils; and if the ergot be taken for a long period in small quantities the disease already alluded to. This assumes two forms, the *gangrenous*, and *convulsive*. For a description of both these states, we must refer to Christison's *Treatise on Poisons*, 3d ed. p. 833.

In the female the effects on the uterine system in the gravid state are special and conspicuous. In ten to twenty minutes after the administration of an infusion of ½ a drachm, if labour has already commenced, the uterus is thrown into the most powerful and almost permanent contractions, which may even produce the rupture of the organ if the fœtus be not expelled.

These effects will ensue in nine-tenths of the cases in which it is employed. We may mention in proof of their entire independence on the "imagination" of the patient, that we have witnessed the effects described within ten minutes after its administration to an insensible patient.

The use of the ergot has been asserted to be fatal to the child. The results of several hundred cases have fully disproved this opinion.

Although there is still much difference of opinion respecting the power of ergot to induce premature labour at *early* periods of gestation, the majority of practitioners describe it as capable of doing so; our own experience supports this opinion. Even in the unimpregnated uterus small doses of ergot display an unequivocal tendency to cause contractile pains, to increase or bring on the menstrual secretion, or to reduce its excess when this proceeds from an atonic state of the organ.

Uses. Ergot has been employed by regular practitioners of medicine only since 1807, and has had to encounter the opposition of many of the leading practitioners of obstetric medicine. Among others, Dr. Hamilton, the celebrated Edinburgh professor, rendered himself conspicuous by the ridicule he cast upon the practice. His name, and influence as the teacher of a large class of midwifery students, has thus checked the introduction of a remedy which has providentially still won its way into general esteem, and has saved hundreds of mothers from a sudden and terrible death.

The ergot is chiefly given to increase the contractions of the womb in protracted labours occasioned by debility or fear, and independently of mechanical obstacles to the delivery of the child.

The proper period is when the child's head has passed the brim of the pelvis, or when the os uteri has been duly dilated. Should the outlet be too small, the os uteri preternaturally contracted, or tumors interfere in the passage, the ergot cannot be given. It is given also in hæmorrhages and convulsions during delivery, and to expedite the expulsion of the placenta, of clots, polypi, or hydatids.

Ergot is also given at early periods of gestation to produce abortion, in cases when the natural passages are too contracted to permit the delivery of a full grown child.

In leucorrhœa and gonorrhœa the ergot seems also to exercise considerable curative power.

Administration. The infusion is by far the best form. A drachm of bruised ergot is infused in four ounces of hot water, and allowed to stand till cold. For a woman in labour one-third or one-half of this to be given every half hour. The powder or tincture in small doses, corresponding to two to five grains thrice daily, seem preferable when ergot is to be used in menorrhagia, gonorrhœa, and leucorrhœa.

ORDER IV.—LYCOPODIACEÆ.

Lycopodium, or vegetable sulphur, is procured from a cryptogamic plant called the *club moss.* It consists of minute yellow particles, and is used principally to prevent the cohesion of pills, a portion being placed in the pill box; for this purpose magnesia is now preferred by most apothecaries.

ORDER V.—FILICES. (*Ferns*).

A few species of this order have been used in medicine. The root stock of the *Nephrodium filix mas*, or male fern, has been celebrated as an anthelmintic, and that of *Polypodium Caliguala* as a diaphoretic and diuretic; neither of these occur in India. The leaves of the ferns generally are mucilaginous, slightly astringent, and some rather aromatic. It is in a fixed oil that the vermifuge properties of the male fern reside ; thisarticle is the basis of Madame Nouffer's celebrated specific for the expulsion of tape worm, which she sold to Louis XVI. for 8000 rupees. It has now fallen into disuse in consequence of the far superior efficacy of the pomegranate root bark, and the essential oil of turpentine. The ethereal or alcoholic extracts of the fern, consisting chiefly of black oil, have lately been much given on the continent of Europe. The dose is half a drachm to one drachm, in the form of electuary, pills, or emulsion *(Pereira)*, and followed afterwards by a dose of castor oil.

Mr. Royle informs us that many of these articles are still used in medicine in India. The rhizomes, or dried leaves of *scolopendrium*, are sold under the altered name, *Iskoolikundrioon*. Those of Polypodium are called *bulookunboon*. The Asplenium radiatum, *morpunkhee*, or peacock's fan, is employed by the natives probably as an anthelmintic. The *Adiantum capillus veneris*, or Venus' hair, is indigenous in the Himalayas, where it is called *shuer-ul-jin*, or fairy's hair. *Moobarkha* and *hunsraj* are also applied to it, and like the European article it is given as an expectorant. In Europe it is the basis of the celebrated *Syrop de Capillaire*.

PART VII.

ARTICLES OF MATERIA MEDICA DERIVED FROM THE ANIMAL KINGDOM.

Under this head we shall give a sufficient summary of those facts regarding the drugs derived from the animal kingdom, which are really of importance to the medical student.

The Sponge.

Spongia officinalis, *Latin.* Mooabadul, *Hind.* Abermoordep, *Pers.* Isfenj, *Arab.*

There is still much doubt whether sponge is a vegetable or animal substance. Professor Grant places it in the animal class, *poriphera.* Other and able authorities consider it to be a vegetable intermediate between the Algæ and Fuci.

Sponge is a soft, elastic, porous, irregular-shaped substance, of yellow or brown colour; it occurs chiefly in the Red Sea and Mediterranean, and is collected by divers from the submerged rocks to which it adheres. It is while fresh covered with a gelatinous substance, which must be washed off to prevent putrefaction. According to Hatchett's analysis, dry sponge consists chiefly of gelatine and albumen.

From the readiness with which it absorbs fluids sponge is very extensively used in surgery.

Sponge tents are prepared by dipping sponge in melted wax, and pressing it till the wax hardens; a tent of this kind introduced into a wound or cavity enlarges as the wax softens. The practice is however nearly obsolete.

Burnt sponge consists of carbon, silica, common salt, sulphate of lime, *iodide of sodium* (2.1 parts in 660) *bromide of magnesia*, (7 parts), carbonate of lime, magnesia, protoxide of iron, and phosphate of lime. Heated with sulphuric acid it emits violet fumes of iodine. The burnt sponge was much used in the treatment of scrofula long before iodine was discovered, or its virtues known. Iodine and its preparations have now supplanted the sponge in medical practice.

The Leech.

Sanguisuga, or *Hirudo medicinalis:* nat. cl. Annulosa of Macleay.

βδελλα of the Greeks. Jonk, *Beng.* and *Hind.*

There are several species of leech, of which the following are the most remarkable:—

The *officinal* or green *leech* is of blackish green colour, with six reddish brown, longitudinal streaks.

The *English*, or *speckled leech*, has six stripes spotted with black, the belly is greenish-yellow, and spotted.

We are indebted to the Pundit Modhusoodun Gooptu for an account of the principal varieties of the animal used medicinally in Bengal.*

It is altogether unnecessary for us to enter into details regarding the anatomy and natural history of this animal. It will suffice to say that they are oviparous; the mouth is tri-radiate, having three sets of lips meeting in the centre. Within are three very muscular jaws, each armed with about sixty small and very sharp teeth, by which they cut into the skin by a saw-like movement.

Leeches are apt to suffer from ulcers, stricture, and also from a disease strongly resembling scurvy, from all which causes they occasionally perish in vast numbers.

In some parts of France and also in Bengal leeches are taken by men who go naked into the waters they inhabit, and

* The following note is taken from the *Susruta*, p. 40, vol. i.

There are twelve species of leeches, six are poisonous and six are not poisonous.

The description of the former species is as follows:—

Sp. 1. *Krista* is very black, and its head is large.

Sp. 2. *Karbura* is long, alternately contracted and dilated in its middle.

Sp. 3. *Alagurda* is covered with hair, its mouth is black, and body is thicker on both sides.

Sp. 4. *Indrandha* is marked by longitudinal lines of various tints on its back.

Sp. 5. *Samudrika* is yellowish black, and has different spots of various colours on its back.

Sp. 6. *Gochardana* is divided on its tail, its mouth is very narrow and pointed.

The following symptoms occur after their bites. Swelling of the part, accompanied with itching and burning pain, vomiting, dulness, and fainting.

The description of the latter species is as follows:—

Sp. 1. *Kapila* is red on the sides, shining, and green on the back.

Sp. 2. *Pingula* is slightly red and yellow, and having a round body.

Sp. 3. *Sunkumoochee* is liver-coloured, its mouth is long, sharp, and it sucks the blood very quickly.

Sp. 4. *Moosika* is like a rat in its colour and shape, and has a very bad smell.

Sp. 5. *Poonderikmookhee* is of a green colour, and having a flat mouth.

Sp. 6. *Saberika* has a shining green colour, is eighteen fingers in length, and used for animals, as for horses, &c.

The above mentioned leeches are found in Persia, Delhee, and Poonah, &c.

Those leeches which are produced and live in clean water are generally good, and those are poisonous which are found in water containing putrified animal matters.

The leeches should be kept in earthen water pots, or kulsees, partly filled with pure water and partly by mud.

Aquatic plants and powdered roots of water lily are given for their food, grass and leaves of the water lily for their bed.

Every second or third day their water and food are to be changed, and the water pot every week.

allow them to fasten on the skin. Liver baits are often used. Sometimes they are caught by fine nets or by the hand.

The leeches used in the Calcutta Hospitals are caught in tanks and jeels in the direction of Baraset by persons who allow them to fasten on the naked skin. They are to be procured at all seasons; but are occasionally scarce during the months of April and May, when the tanks dry up. The bazar price is two rupees per hundred. In the Upper Provinces a superior kind of leech is used, called the *Shakooabadee jonk*, caught in the tanks about *Shakoabad* in the Agra district. The Punjaubee leeches are the next best, and are procured in abundance about Pateealah in the Sirhind district. The Shakooabadee leech will generally bear three applications, and is the only description of leech that will do so. The animal is of a light olive green colour, and marked with two bright yellow stripes on the sides. The common wild leech of the Upper Provinces is called "Daubree;" but for Hospital purposes it is very inferior to those above mentioned. The average price of Shakooabadee leeches varies from three to four rupees per hundred. The Daubrees from eight annas to one rupee per hundred. *(Mr. Daly's notes.)*

In Europe leeches are kept in pans with a little soft water, the vessels being covered with canvas to admit the air. In Bengal they are placed in a common earthen vessel with moist clay.

The consumption of leeches is immense. In France since the promulgation of Broussais' doctrines, 100 millions are used annually.

The common leech used in the Bengal Hospitals averages 50 grains in weight, and draws from two to three fluid drachms of blood.

Pain, inflammation, and ulceration are not unfrequently the consequences of the bite. These effects are popularly attributed to the animal being poisonous, or its teeth being left in the bite. We believe the state of ill health of the patient to be the chief cause. In India the most distressing results have been witnessed from the neglected ulceration of these bites. In Ceylon and Assam especially such mischief is thus occasioned as to lend some confirmation to the idea of the poisoned nature of the wound.

In applying leeches, the part should be carefully cleaned and shaved; moistening the skin with a little milk and water, or sugared water will often induce the animal to bite when it seems otherwise disinclined to attempt it; salt, grease, and acid always prevent its biting. After it has gorged itself and dropped off, a little salt applied about the head acts as an emetic, and the animal being wiped with a soft towel, and placed in fresh water, will recover its vigour in a few days.

The bleeding from leech bites is sometimes, especially in children, so profuse as to occasion very dangerous symptoms, or even end fatally; compression, the application of a little cone of lint, or the spider's web, will commonly be found to arrest the bleeding; if these means fail, the lunar caustic scraped to a fine point should be tried, and will usually be found effectual. In very obstinate cases, touching the bite with a red hot needle, or applying a silk ligature, must be had recourse to.

Serious accidents are often occasioned by the swallowing of leeches. This is especially common in Egypt, Ceylon, and Assam, where they infest the wells and tanks in vast numbers, and are of such small size as to be scarcely perceptible. Hæmorrhage from the stomach and bowels, distressing pain and great weakness are the usual symptoms observed. The most effectual treatment consists in the administration of common salt or vinegar, which soon proves fatal to the animal, and a purgative or emetic will remove it. The convalescence is often very tedious, and the patient's sufferings severe.

Blistering Flies.

There are several kinds of fly which when applied to the skin cause great irritation, inflammation, and blistering. These symptoms are occasioned by an acrid principle called *Cantharidin*, contained in these insects. The ancients chiefly employed two species of *Mylabris*, one of which, the *Mylabris cichorei*, (vern. *telini*) has been used for ages, and is so at present by the native physicians of India and China.

The *Cantharis vesicatoria*, or Spanish blistering fly, is the species officinal in the British Pharmacopœiæ. Its colour is bright shining green or bluish, length about $\frac{3}{4}$ of an inch, breadth $\frac{1}{4}$th to $\frac{1}{3}$rd of an inch. It occurs in the South of Europe generally, especially in Italy and Spain, and is found occasionally in England.

The flies are killed by being dipped in hot vinegar and water, then dried, and kept in stoppered bottles, a few drops of very strong vinegar being introduced to prevent the attack of mites, by which the fly is soon destroyed if this precaution be not adopted.

Pereira informs us that it is a common practice among druggists to mix Euphorbium with the powder and plaster of these flies.

According to Robiquet's analysis, the *Cantharis vesicatoria* contains *Cantharidin*, green fixed oil soluble in alcohol, fatty matter insoluble in alcohol, other animal matters, acetic and uric acid, phosphate of lime and magnesia.

Cantharidin.

This is the active principle of all the blistering insects. It is prepared by concentrating an alcoholic tincture, from which it crystallizes; the crystals are to be purified by washing with cold alcohol, and then boiling with alcohol and animal charcoal.

It seems to resemble camphor in its chemical habits. It is soluble in boiling spirit, in ether and volatile oils, also in the concentrated mineral acids, potash, and soda. It is not affected by ammonia, and is insoluble in water or acetic acid, unless the other principles of the fly be present. It is stated to be composed of carbon 616.8, hydrogen 6.04, oxygen 32.33.

Cantharidin vesicates so severely that the 1-100th part of a grain has been known to cause extensive blistering. During its preparation the utmost caution is requisite. It is volatile at a moderate temperature, and its vapour is so acrid as to have frequently caused ophthalmia, blistering, and other distressing symptoms to persons employed in its preparation.

Applied to the skin the moistened powder of cantharides soon occasions heat, pain, redness or blackness, swelling, and effusion of fluid between the epidermis and true skin. This fluid contains 6 per 100 of albumen, 93 of water, and traces of various salts, the same as those found in the serum of the blood.

The inflammation thus produced sometimes proceeds to severe ulceration and gangrene. In some persons a blister occasions great febrile excitement, and in many there is pain and irritation of the genital and urinary organs, difficulty of passing water, much anxiety, and distress. These symptoms are termed *strangury*. Some writers assert that applying fine tissue paper or muslin between the blister and the skin prevents this distressing effect; but our own experience is opposed to the common belief of the efficacy of this practice.

Taken internally in poisonous doses cantharides produce the most violent inflammation, and such torture as cannot be described. Heat, excitement, pain, and inflammation of the sexual organs, disturbed intellect, convulsions, and other symptoms of disorder of the nervous system are among the effects observed.

The use of cantharides is chiefly external. The powdered fly in plaster or ointment, the tincture, and the acetous tincture, are the preparations usually employed; these are separately noticed in the Pharmacopœia.

Internally cantharides have been given (minute doses of the tincture especially) in dropsy, diabetes, paralysis of the bladder, in impotence, amennorhœa, and in obstinate gonorrhea. But little benefit is derivable in any of these cases, except the last, from this very dangerous remedy, which other and safer substances will not more certainly induce. Cantharides are popularly considered a certain aphrodisiac. Pereira however well observes, that a quantity sufficient to excite the sexual feelings is enough to endanger the patient's life.

When given internally the usual dose of the powdered cantharides is one to two grains in the form of a pill.

For the preparation and application of blisters, see the Pharmacopœia.

In cases of poisoning by cantharides—emetics, the stomach pump, mucilaginous or albuminous drinks, such as milk, or the white of eggs diffused through water, should be at once resorted to; bleeding, leeches, and purgatives will also be required; castor oil is by many deemed objectionable from its solvent power over cantharides; opium, and the warm bath will be found beneficial. In the strangury so often observed, these are our best remedies.

The preceding remarks apply, with but little modification, to the blistering flies of India. These are chiefly the Mylabris or Meloe cichorii, the Cantharis gigas, and the Cantharis violacea.

The *Meloe*, or *Mylabris cichorii* (Telini, *Hind.*) is common in the neighbourhood of Dacca, in the Hydrabad country, and numerous other localities. We have received fine specimens of the Dacca fly from Colonel Stacy, and of that of Hydrabad from Dr. Key. Dr. Hunter has published a good account of this article in the 5th vol. of the *Transactions of the Asiatic Society*, p. 216.

The insect is about an inch long, and ⅓rd broad; the elytra or wing coverts are marked with six cross stripes of deep blue and russet brown.

The *Buprestis* of ancient writers is met with in the bazars under the name of the golden fly (*sunamuki.*) The *Cantharis violacea* is often mixed with specimens of *Meloe* in the bazars.

The telini fly if procured before the mites have commenced its destruction, yields on an average one-third more of cantharidin than the *Spanish fly* of the European shops. The blue fly is of uncertain strength; the Buprestis, in all the specimens we obtained, was quite inert.

A species of Meloe called the *M. trianthema*, from its being usually found on the plant named *Trianthema decandra* (biscopra, *Hind.*) is described by Dr. Fleming.

A tincture, acetous tincture, plaster, and ointment of the Meloe cichorii are described in our Pharmacopœia. Some prejudice exists against the article on account of its alleged excessive severity of action. This is solely owing to the presence of a greater quantity of *cantharidin* than that contained in the common fly. Diluting the tincture, and adding to the proportion of lard and wax in the plaster and ointment, perfectly assimilate the action of the indigenous and the imported insects.

Cochineal Insect.

Coccus cacti, (ord. Hemiptera.)

This celebrated insect, a native of Mexico and India, is the source of a most lucrative commerce between South America and Europe. It was once supposed to possess valuable medicinal properties, but this idea is now abandoned. Its sole consumption at present is as a dye stuff for scarlet and crimson colours, and in the manufacture of lake and carmine. The favourite food of the insect is the *Cactus coccinellifer*, now cultivated in the Botanical Garden of Calcutta.

The Bee.

Apis mellifica (*ord.* Hymenoptera.)

Bramara, *Sans.*

This valuable insect yields us honey and wax. We cannot dwell upon its history, which nevertheless is full of interest to the general student.

Honey.

Vern. Madhu, *Sans.* Shahid, *Pers.* Ussel Ulnehl, *Arab.* Teyni, *Tel.*

Honey is a vegetable product, and occurs chiefly in the nectaries of various flowers. The bee collects it and brings it to the hive to store it up for the food of the community.

Honey consists essentially of sugar, with variable proportions of gum, wax, and aromatic and colouring principles. It is nutritive and slightly laxative. In some localities it is poisonous, owing to the deleterious nature of the plants from which it is collected.

Honey forms the basis of several very popular medicinal preparations. Beyond acting as very agreeable demulcents, these have no remedial virtue. Combined with vinegar, honey forms the *oxymel* of the Pharmacopœia, which is given in doses of from a drachm to an ounce as an expectorant and demulcent.

Wax.

Cera, *Latin.* Siktha, *Sans.* Shuma, *Arab.* Moom, *Pers.* and *Hind.*

For some of the properties of wax, refer to page 75. Two kinds occur in commerce—the yellow, and white or bleached wax.

Wax is secreted by the bee, and used in the construction of the comb; several insects of other families also secrete this principle. It is the product moreover of many members of the vegetable kingdom.

To extract the wax the comb is pressed, then dipped in hot water, the wax skimmed off, and cast in moulds. In this state it is yellow, of peculiar smell, sp. gr. 960 to 965., sometimes adulterated with suet, pease-meal, or dammer. The resin may be dissolved out by cold alcohol, which does not dissolve the wax, the meal by the action of boiling water, which on cooling will be coloured blue by tincture of iodine. Yellow wax is bleached by being melted, rolled into thin strips, and then exposed for some weeks to the action of the sun and air.

Wax was formerly employed internally as a demulcent and emollient, but is never prescribed at present. It constitutes the basis of simple plaster, cerate, and liniment, and is used in many similar preparations, as subsequently explained.

Isinglass, or Icthyocolla.

Isinglass is the commercial term for the swimming or air-bag of the sturgeon, *Accipenser sturio,* and of some other fishes. The article is valued for the large quantity of pure *gelatine* it affords.

The sturgeon fishery is chiefly carried on in the Caspian and Black Seas, and their tributary rivers. Isinglass is prepared in America from the *Labrus squeteague;* the intestines of the Cod, *Morrhua vulgaris;* and in Calcutta from the *Polynemus Sele.* Sulea, *Beng.*

The air-bag, or sound, is a bag containing air, usually communicating with the œsophagus, or stomach. The air-bag is cut open, dried by exposure to the air, and the inner coating detached. According to the form in which it is prepared it is termed leaf, staple, ribbon, or book isinglass. The best staple from the Volga and the Caspian sells in London for 13*s*. 6*d*. the pound. The Brazil and American *ribbon* brings but 4*s*. the lb. We are not aware of the details of the manufacture, or the market price of the article which Dr. M'Clelland and Mr. Speed have prepared in Calcutta.

Isinglass should be white, inodorous, and completely soluble in hot water. It consists almost entirely of the animal principle—gelatine. This is soluble in water, insoluble in alcohol, ether, the oils, or muriatic acid; it is an abundant constituent of many animal tissues, forming 33 per 100 of the bones of the human adult. It is highly nutritious, being composed of carbon, hydrogen, oxygen, nitrogen. It forms an insoluble precipitate with tannic acid; this is the substance formed in the tanning of hides by the action of the tannic acid of the astringent matter on the gelatine of the skin.

Gelatine is much used in the arts as a size and cement, also for clarifying wines, syrups, &c. A coarse kind called *size* is prepared from clippings of parchment and skins; *glue* is made from the hoofs and tendons of various animals; the bones of the young calf are very rich in this principle, and the jelly prepared from these is a favourite article of luxury amongst Europeans. The putrefaction of the dead body does not alter the gelatine of the bones, and this may accordingly be removed by boiling under pressure in the apparatus called the "Digester," from the bones of animals dead even for several centuries. *Bone gelatine* is now used in many of the French Hospitals, as the chief ingredient of the diet soup.

Isinglass is very little used in medicine; in pharmacy it is employed as the basis of an excellent adhesive plaster. The black *court plaster* of the shops is prepared by brushing a solution of isinglass with a little tincture of benzoin over black sarcenet silk.

THE EGG OF THE DOMESTIC FOWL, *Gallus Domesticus*.

Unda, *Beng*. Ovum, *Latin*.

The white, yelk, and shell of the common egg are used in pharmacy.

The sp. gr. of the egg is 1.080 to 1.090; the shell consists of carbonate of lime 97, phosphate of lime and magnesia 1, animal matter and traces of sulphur and iron 2 per 100.

The white (glaire, or *albumen*) consists of a fine membranous matter forming cells, in which a liquid albumen is contained. The whole white contains water 85, albumen 12, mucus and salts 3 per 100. It is coagulated by heat, by acids, sulphuric ether, corrosive sublimate, prussiate of potash, &c.

The yelk (*vitellus*) is an emulsion of oily globules and crystallyzable fat, contained in a sac or bag. It consists of yellow oil and fat 28.75, albumen with phosphorus 17.47, water 53.8. The yellow oil is prepared by boiling the egg hard, removing the yelk, and acting on this by boiling alcohol, in which the oil is dissolved.

The white of egg is a valuable antidote in cases of poisoning by corrosive sublimate, sulphate of copper, and the corrosive poisons generally. The yelk is sometimes used as a convenient medium for forming an emulsion of the thick turpentines with water; these mixtures are used as enemata.

The egg shell calcined at a low red heat affords a very pure form of carbonate of lime.

Spermaceti.

Cetaceum, *Latin.*

A concrete, fatty substance, found in several parts of the body of the *Physeter macrocephalus*, a species of whale called also the great-headed cachalot.

The head is the chief repository of this secretion, especially a cavity in the upper jaw, in which it exists mixed with oil.

The spermaceti whale occurs in the Pacific, Indian, and Chinese seas.

The liquid first drawn from the head of the animal is a mixture of spermaceti and sperm oil; from this the solid matter is separated by filtration through bags, and subsequent compression. After this it is melted in water, skimmed, and re-melted with a little potash water, to remove the last traces of the oil; lastly, it is permitted to concrete slowly, during which it crystallizes in brilliant white masses.

Pure spermaceti is white, tasteless, inodorous, crystalline, insoluble in water, slightly soluble in boiling alcohol; it forms a soap with potash. It is composed of carbon 81.66, hydrogen 12.86, oxygen 5.47.

Spermaceti was once much used internally as a demulcent and emollient, especially in troublesome catarrhs and dysentery. It is at present employed solely as an external application, being an ingredient in numerous cerates and ointments.

AMBERGRIS. Shahbooi, *Pers.* Minumbir, *Tam.*

This is another product of the sperm whale; it is used as a perfume and stimulant aromatic, somewhat resembling musk. It is a greyish opaque solid, containing a peculiar fat, (ambreine), benzoic acid, and extractive matter. Its origin was long unknown; but it has lately been ascertained that ambergris is the hardened fæces of the animal above named.

MUSK. Mishk, *Hind.* and *Pers.*

This celebrated article is a concrete secretion contained in the follicles of the prepuce in the musk animal—*Moschus moschiferus.*

The sac is of oval form, flat, and smooth where it is in contact with the abdomen of the animal, convex below, 1¼ to 1¾ inch broad, 2 to 2½ inches long, ½ to ¾ inch deep. The sac consists of several parts—1. the hairy coat or skin, in which it will be noticed that the hairs are arranged circularly round the orifice; 2. the muscular coat, consisting of two layers of fibres which surround the sac, and between which the penis is situated; the urethra projects beyond the glands in this organ; 3. a fibrous coat; 4. a soft pearly membrane, lining the cells; 5. the inner lining of the sac, silvery white externally, yellow internally; 6. glands of a yellowish brown colour.

The sac in the adult animal contains from 1½ to 2 drachms of dry musk. In the recent and pure state the musk is a soft, reddish brown, granular mass, of strong, bitter, aromatic taste, and powerful peculiar odour. There are three kinds of musk—the Chinese, Russian, and Bokharian, the last but little known.

The *Chinese* musk is exported from Canton in small boxes containing about 25 sacs; each sac is covered with brownish yellow hair.

The average weight of the pod is 6 drs. and 12 grs.; of its contents 2 drs. 42 grs.

The *Russian* musk is inferior to the first variety, and is often marked by a very heavy and disagreeable odour.

The pods of musk are liable to many adulterations and imitations.

False sacs are made of the skin of the animal, in which is inserted a mixture of dried blood, ammonia, and a little musk. The spurious sac has no aperture, the hair is not disposed circularly, and there is no trace of the penis, which is found in every genuine pod. Of two pods purchased from a well-known dealer in Calcutta about two years since, one had the weight increased by several leaden shot introduced through the small natural opening.

Musk contains several fatty principles, gelatine, albumen, aromatic matter, ammonia, salts, &c. with about 45 per 100 of combined water. The aromatic principle has not been obtained in a separate state, and its properties are not fully known. It is one of the most pervading of all odours, and heightens the aroma of many other perfumes.

Medical uses. Musk is a powerful stimulant, and in large doses a narcotic. Its local action on the stomach is irritating; sometimes, but not commonly, it excites the sexual organs; very frequently it proves diuretic or diaphoretic. The urine and cutaneous secretion of persons taking musk are powerfully imbued with its odour, and after death the body generally, the brain, abdominal and thoracic viscera evince the same effect.

Musk has been used with advantage in some cases of hysteria, epilepsy, chorea, and many other spasmodic diseases, provided there be no organic disease, nor plethora in the system. It seems by the concurrent testimony of most writers that musk is an antispasmodic of great efficacy. It is used too in low fevers, in retrocedent gout, the collapse of delirium tremens, typhoid pneumonia, and similar cases, and with decided benefit. The dose of musk is from five to eight grains, with water, mucilage, or sugar. A mixture, and tincture, are described in the Pharmacopœia.

Hartshorn.

Cornu Cervinum, Latin.

The shavings of the horns of several species of deer have been long used as a source of gelatine, which they give out to boiling water. The decoction is therefore nutritious and demulcent.

These shavings are one of the ingredients used in preparing the antimonial powder of the Pharmacopœia.

When incinerated the hartshorn leaves 57.5 per 100 of phosphate of lime. Burned hartshorn was formerly used, reduced to fine powder, as an absorbent, and in the disease called ricketts. The practice has justly fallen into disuse.

Mutton Suet.

Sevum. Adeps ovillus. Beri ke churbee, *Hind.*

This is the fat from the vicinity of the kidneys of the sheep, *Ovis aries.* It is refined by melting at a gentle heat, and straining through cloth. It contains carbon 65, hydrogen 21.5, oxygen 13.5, and proximately is chiefly composed of the principles stearine and elaine. Its sole use in medicine is as an ingredient in ointments, cerates, and plasters.

Cow's Milk.

Lac, *Latin.* Doodh, *Hind. Beng.*

This has been already described at page 81.

We insert a table of the results of the analysis of several kinds of milk by MM. O. Henry and Chevallier.

Constituents.	Cow.	Ass.	Woman.	Goat.	Ewe.
Caseum, ...	4,48	1,82	1.52	4,02	4,50
Butter, ...	3,13	0,11	3,53	3,32	4,20
Sugar of milk, ...	4,77	6,08	6,50	5,28	5,00
Various salts, ...	0,60	0,34	0,45	0,58	0,68
Water, ...	87,02	91,65	87,98	86,80	85,62
Total.	100,00	100,00	100,00	100,00	100,00
Solid matter.	12,98	8,34	13,00	13,20	14,38

Hog's Lard.

Adeps suillus, *Latin.* Soor ke churbee, *Hind.*

This is the fat about the loins of the hog, *Sus scrofa.* It is purified by melting and straining. Its melting point is from 78° to 88°. Fahrt; inodorous and tasteless while fresh, readily grows rancid. Lard contains carbon 79.098, hydrogen 11.146, oxygen 97.56—proximately it consists of ealine 62, stearine and margarine 38 per 100. In the rancid state it contains the margaric and stearic acids, and a peculiar volatile acid.

In Europe hog's lard is much employed in ointments, but in India the strong prejudice against the article renders it desirable to exclude it as much as possible from all pharmaceutical preparations, substituting for it the "simple liniment."

Castor.

Castoreum, *Latin*. Goond beduster, *Pers*.

This is a concrete animal substance, formed in the preputial follicles of the beaver, *Castor fiber*.

Both male and female beavers have sacs which contain this substance. In the male each sac is composed of an external or cellular coat, inclosing muscular fibres; within there is a vascular coat covering a scaly glandular membrane; externally this membrane is shining and silvery, internally scaly and glandular. The castor is contained in this bag; while fresh it is liquid, yellow, and of strong odour.

The beaver inhabits North America chiefly. Two kinds of castor are known in commerce—American and Russian.

The American consists usually of two isolated sacs, wrinkled and connected by a ligament; the sacs are long and pear-shaped. Pereira states that the colour, and other external characters, are quite variable.

The article called by the English druggists "Hudson's Bay castor" is deemed the best kind now to be found.

The *Russian* castor has become so dear and scarce that it is no longer available.

Castor yields a pale yellow volatile oil, of acrid bitter taste; a fatty crystalline substance called *castorin*, obtained by boiling the castor in alcohol; a resinous matter of acid and bitter taste, and several other constituents of less importance.

Castor was once much relied on as an antispasmodic and a stimulant of the uterine system—dose ʒii in pills. A simple tincture and an ammoniated tincture are given in the British Pharmacopœiæ. In the present day it is seldom or never prescribed in any form.

Bezoar.

Zeher morah, *Duk.* and *Pers.* Faduj, *Arab.* Padzehr kani, *Pers.* Gorochana, *Sans.* There are several kinds of bezoar, all being concretions found in the gall-bladders or intestines of various animals. Some are prized for the fine yellow colouring matter in which they abound; others are celebrated in eastern works as remedies for snake bites, hydrophobia, &c. Bezoars are never used by European practitioners, and do not deserve the least confidence.

PART VIII.

MISCELLANEOUS INORGANIC SUBSTANCES.

Under this head we shall notice very succinctly a few remarkable substances, administered as medicines, or of use or interest in pharmacy, and which are either not prepared artificially, or must be made on too large a scale to admit of their manufacture by the apothecary—or for other reasons are not included in the Pharmacopœia.

Amber.

Karooba, *Pers.* Kepoor, *Hind.* Ambar, *Malay.* Kernulbehr, *Arab.*

Amber is found chiefly in Madagascar, Japan, and on the shores of the Baltic. In its appearance and physical properties it strongly resembles copal, which is often fraudulently sold as amber in the Indian bazars. When rubbed amber is highly electric. Its origin was long uncertain, but it is now universally supposed to be a vegetable resin, the product probably of a Pinus. When distilled it yields an empyreumatic oil, and an acid liquor still admitted in many Pharmacopœiæ, and prescribed in several spasmodic diseases. It scarcely, if at all, differs in its action from common naptha.

Amber is proximately composed of volatile oil, two resins, an acid termed the *succinic,* &c.

The acid is white, crystalline, soluble in water, and in boiling alcohol. The succinate of ammonia throws down a reddish precipitate from the persalts of iron, and on this account is much used as a test.

Bitumen and Petroleum.

Petroleum, Mittee ke tal, *Hind.* Neft, *Arab.*

We have been favoured by Capt. Halsted, of H. M. ship *Childers,* with several specimens of Petroleum collected by that officer in his recent survey of Cheduba, on the Arracan coast.

The specimens varied in colour and consistence, from perfectly transparent sherry red to nearly opaque tar-like brown. The specific gravity of the lightest specimen is 0.819 at 85° Fahrt. On distillation, a small quantity of soft unctuous matter remains.

This petroleum is nearly identical with that of Persia and Barbadoes. Besides true liquid naptha, it contains the newly discovered principles parraffine, and eupione, in considerable abundance.

Petroleum is a useful external application, especially in rheumatism. It stimulates the skin, and entering the circulation by imbibition proves diuretic or diaphoretic. Internally it has also been given as a warm stimulant and diuretic, especially in rheumatism and gonorrhœa, in doses of from twenty to thirty minims diffused through water, by mucilage or starch.

Asphaltum, or *black Bitumen*, (Zift-roomie, *Pers.*) is a deep black, pitch-like solid; hard, softens at 150°, and melts above that; highly inflammable, believed to be the result of the natural distillation of petroleum. It is produced in abundance in Barbadoes and Mesopotamia. It is a valuable lacquer for the protection of iron or tinned iron vessels. A lump rubbed over the heated metal coats it with a hard adhesive brilliant coat, which resists most of the common corrosive agents.

The naptha distilled from coal, in the manufacture of gas, when purified by redistillation is nearly the same in its most important properties as the distilled petroleum of Arracan.

As these liquids contain no oxygen, they are used for preserving potassium and sodium. They must be previously freed from water by brisk agitation with dry fragments of chloride of calcium, (muriate of lime.)

Bole Armenian.

Ghil Armenie, *Pers.* and *Hind.* Hejr Armenie, *Arab.*

This is a soft, yellowish red, unctuous earth, consisting of alumina, silica, magnesia, and oxide of iron. It is brought from the Persian Gulf, but it also occurs of fine quality in the Rajmahl hills, where it is termed *Geru mittee.*

Reduced to very fine powder it is used as an absorbent application sprinkled over ulcers or other raw surfaces. In many countries, Bengal and South America especially, this and other unctuous earths are eaten freely by pregnant women to allay the craving for food so common in that state. In times of scarcity it has been used by both sexes as a mechanical substitute for proper food.

TABASHIR.

Tabashir, *Arab. Pers.* and *Hind.* Banslochun, *Beng.* Tivakshera, *Sans.*

A siliceous concretion found in the joints of the female bamboo. It is bluish white, concrete, adhesive to the tongue, at a red heat fuses into a transparent glass. It is composed of silica 70, potash 30, per 100. The Persians deem it tonic and aphrodisiac. The Arabs suppose it to be astringent. From its composition we are warranted in supposing it to be entirely inert.

TALC.

Abraka, *Sans.* Tulk, *Pers.* and *Duk.* Ubruk, *Hind.*

Several varieties of this beautiful and useful mineral are found in India, especially in Behar. It readily splits into transparent, elastic flakes. It consists of nearly equal parts of silica and magnesia, and about 6 per 100 of lime.

Slips of talc afford the young chemist a very convenient substitute for platinum foil, in several experiments, especially on the effect of heat on organic bodies.

We subjoin a list of inorganic substances much used in the arts and in medicine, and usually sold as common market articles.

Substance	Common name	Reference
Acetate of Copper,	Verdigris, ..	*v.* See Pharmacopœia, preparations of copper.
Acetate of lead,	Sugar of lead, ...	*v.* Pharm. prep. of lead.
Acetic acid, ..	Vinegar, ...	*v.* Pharm. art. acids.
Acid, Arsenious,	Arsenic, ...	
——Hydrochloric or muriatic,	.. .. ..	
——Nitric, ...	Aquafortis, ..	
——Sulphuric, ..	Oil of vitriol,	
Alcohol, ...	Spirit of Wine,	*v.* Pharm. art. alcohol.
Alumn, ...	————	*v.* Pharm. prep. of potash.
Ammonia, muriate of	Sal ammoniac,	*v.* Pharm. prep. of ammonia.
————, Carbonate of, ..	Sal. volatile,	
Animal charcoal, ivory black, ..	————	.. *v.* Pharm. art. carbon.
Antimony, Sulphuret of	.. ..	*v.* Pharm. prep. of antimony.
———— Golden sulpht.	.. ..	
———— Glass of	.. ..	
———— Metallic	.. .. ..	

Argol, ... Crude cream of tartar, .. } *v.* Pharm. prep. of potash.
Arsenic, White oxide, ...
——— Yellow sulphuret, ..
——— Red sulphuret, ... } *v.* Pharm. prep. of arsenic.

Black salt or Bitlaban, .. } ... .*v.* Pharm. prep. of soda.
Baryta, Sulphate of, (imperial white,) .. .. .. } *v.* Pharm. article *tests*.
Barilla, Impure carbonate of soda, ..*v.* Pharm. prep. of soda.
Berlin or Prussian blue, ...*v.* Pharm. art. prussic acid.
Bismuth, nitrate of, pearl white, ..*v.* Pharm. art. bismuth.
Bittern of salt works, ...*v.* Pharm. prep. of magnesia.
Black lead, .. Plumbago. ..
Bleaching powder, or chloride of lime, ... } *v.* Pharm. prep. of lime.
Blende, ... zinc ore, ...*v.* Pharm. prep. zinc.
Blue vitriol, .. Sulphate of copper, .. } *v.* Pharm. prep. copper.
Borax, ...*v.* Pharm. prep. soda.

Calamine, .. zinc ore, ...*v.* Pharm. prep. zinc.
Carbonate of lime, chalk, ...*v.* Pharm. prep. lime.
——— lead, white lead, ..*v.* Pharm. prep. lead.
——— potash, ...*v.* Pharm. prep. potash.
——— soda, ...*v.* Pharm. prep. soda.
——— zinc, calamine, ...*v.* Pharm. prep. zinc.
Castile soap, ...*v.* Pharm. prep. soda.
Ceruse, ... white lead, ..*v.* Pharm. prep. lead.
Chalk, ...*v.* Pharm. prep. lime.
Chloride of lime, bleaching powder, *v.* Pharm. prep. lime.
Cinnabar.. .. vermilion, ..*v.* Pharm. prep. mercury.
Colcothar of vitriol .. .. } red oxide of iron, *v.* Pharm. prep. iron.
Copper, acetate of, verdigris, ...*v.* Pharm. prep. copper.
——— sulphate of, blue vitriol, ..*v.* Pharm. prep. copper.
Copperas, white, sulphate of zinc. ..*v.* Pharm. prep. zinc.
——— green, sulphate of iron, *v.* Pharm. prep. iron.
Corrosive Sublimate, ... } .. ..*v.* Pharm. prep. mercury.
Cream of tartar, ...*v.* Pharm. prep. potash.
Creasote, ... } *v.* Pharm. art. Empyreumatic oils.

Epsom salts, ..Sulphate of magnesia, .. } *v.* Pharm. prep. magnesia.

Ether, Sulphuric, ... } v. Pharm. art. ethers.
—— nitrous, spirits of, ... }
Extract, Goulard's, ... v. Pharm. prep. lead.

Fever powder, James' .. .. .. v. Pharm. prep. antimony.
Flake white, ... v. Pharm. prep. bismuth.
Flowers of sulphur, ... { v. Pharm. article Sulphuric acid.

Galena .. .. sulphuret of lead, v. Pharm. prep. lead.
Glauber's salt .. sulphate of soda, v. Pharm. prep. soda.
Golden sulphuret of antimony, .. v. Pharm. prep. antimony.
Graphite, or black lead, ... See "Crucibles," page 34.
Green vitriol, ... v. Pharm. prep. iron.

Hydriodate of potash, ... v. Pharm. prep. potash.

Iodine, ... v. p. 62, and Pharm. art. iodine.
Iron, black oxide of, ferroprussiate of, peroxide, sulphate of, } .. .. v. Pharm. prep. iron.

James' powder, ... v. Pharm. prep. antimony.

Kelp, ... v. Pharm. prep. soda.
Kermes' mineral, ... v. Pharm. prep. antimony.

Labarraque's soda liquid, ... v. Pharm. prep. soda.
Lead, acetate of, Sugar of lead, } v. Pharm. prep. lead.
—— carbonate of, White lead, .. }
Lime, burnt, ..
—— Carbonate of, Chalk, ... }
—— Chlorite of, Bleaching powder, ... } v. Pharm. prep. lime.
—— Hydrate of, fresh slaked, }
—— Water, .. }
Litharge, ... v. Pharm. prep. lead.
Lunar caustic, ... v. Pharm. prep. silver.

Magnesia, Calcined, ... }
———— Carbonate of, ... } v. Pharm. prep. magnesia.
———— Sulphate of, ... }
———— Madras, ... }

Article	Synonym	Reference
Manganese, Peroxide of,		v. Pharm. art. chlorine.
Marble,	————	v. Pharm. prep. lime.
Massicot,	————	v. Pharm. prep. lead.
Mercury,		v. Pharm. prep. mercury.
——— Corrosive sublimate,		v. Pharm. prep. mercury.
——— Mild muriate, calomel,		v. Pharm. prep. mercury.
——— Red oxide of,		v. Pharm. prep. mercury.
——— Sulphuret of,		v. Pharm. prep. mercury.
——— ——— Black,		v. Pharm. prep. mercury.
——— ——— Red,		v. Pharm. prep. mercury.
——— ——— Native,		v. Pharm. prep. mercury.
——— Native oxide of,		v. Pharm. prep. mercury.
——— Yellow sulphate,		v. Pharm. prep. mercury.
Minium,	Red lead,	v. Pharm. prep. lead.
Muriate of ammonia,	Sal ammoniac,	v. Pharm. prep. ammonia.
——— Soda,	Common salt, Rock salt,	v. Pharm. prep. soda.
——— Mercury, mild,	Calomel,	v. Pharm. prep. mercury.
Mercury, Corrosive,	Cor. sublimate,	v. Pharm. prep. mercury.
Muriatic acid,	————	v. Pharm. art. acid.
Naptha,	————	v. Petroleum, page 692.
Nitrate of Silver,	Lunar caustic,	v. Pharm. prep. silver.
——— Potash,	Saltpetre, nitre,	v. Pharm. prep. potash.
——— Soda,		v. Pharm. prep. soda.
——— Sweet spirits of,		v. Pharm. art. ethers.
Nitric acid,		v. Pharm. art. acids.
Nitro-muriatic acid,		v. Pharm. art. acids.
Oil of vitriol,		v. Pharm. art. acids.
Orpiment,	Yellow sulphuret of arsenic,	v. Pharm. art. arsenic.
Oxalate of potash,	"Salt of lemons"	v. Pharm. prep. potash.
Oyster shells, prepared,		v. Pharm. prep. of lime.
Pearl ash,		v. Pharm. prep potash.
Petroleum,		See page 692.
Phosphate of soda,		v. Pharm. prep. soda.
——— of lime,		v. Pharm. prep. lime.
Phosphorus,		See page 62.
Potash, pyrolignate of,		v. Pharm. prep. potash.
——— bin-oxalate of,		v. Pharm. prep. potash.
——— bi-carbonate of,		v. Pharm. prep. potash.
——— bi-tartrate of,		v. Pharm. prep. potash.
——— Carbonate of,		v. Pharm. prep. potash.

4 U

Potash, Caustic, ...	
—— Prussiate of, ...	
—— Hydriodate of, ...	
—— Nitrate of, ...	v. Pharm. prep. potash.
—— Chlorate of, ...	
—— Soap, ...	
—— Sub-carbonate of, ..	
—— Sulphuret of, ...	
Powder, antimonial, ...	..v. Pharm, prep. antimony.
Prussian blue, ...	...v. Pharm. prep. iron.
Prussiate of Potash, ...	..v. Pharm. prep. potash.
Realgar, ...	..v. Pharm. art. arsenic.
Red precipitate of Mercury,	..v. Pharm. prep. mercury.
Rochelle salt, ... ——	..v. Pharm. prep. soda.
Sal Ammoniac,... Muriate of ammonia,	v. Pharm. prep. ammonia.
— Prunell, .. Fused nitre,	...v. Pharm. prep. potash.
— Gemma, ... Rock salt.	..v. Pharm. prep. soda.
Salt, Common, ...	v. Pharm. prep. soda.
—— Rock, ...	
—— Bitter purging, ...	..v. Pharm. prep. magnesia.
—— Black, ...	..v. Pharm. prep. soda,
—— Epsom, ...	..v. Pharm. prep. magnesia.
—— Glauber, ...	..v. Pharm. prep. soda.
—— of sorrel, ...	..v. Pharm. prep. potash.
—— Rock, ...	
—— Tasteless, ...	v. Pharm. prep. soda.
—— Rochelle, ...	
Saltpetre, ...	...v. Pharm. prep. potash.
Salts, smelling or volatile, ..	..v. Pharm. prep. ammonia.
Soap, white, ...	
—— Castile, ...	
—— Hard.	v. Pharm. prep. potash. and soda.
—— Soft, ...	
—— Yellow	
Seidlitz powders, ...	..v. Pharm. prep. soda.
Shells, ...	.. See page 83.
Silver, nitrate of,..	..v. Pharm. prep. silver.
Soda, Carbonate of, ...	
—— Borate of—borax, ...	
—— Chloride of, . ..	
—— Phosphate of, ...	
—— Muriate of, ...	v. Pharm. prep. soda.
—— Sulphate of, ...	
—— Water	
—— Powders, ...	
Soft soap, ...	..v. Pharm. prep. potash.
Sponge, ...	..See page 678.

Sulphate of Copper, ...	...v. Pharm. prep. Copper.
——— Iron, ...	..——— Iron.
——— Zinc, ...	..——— Zinc.
——— Soda, ...	..——— Soda.
——— Potash, ...	..——— Potash.
——— Magnesia, ...	..——— Magnesia.
——— Baryta, ...	..——— Baryta.
Sulphur, ...	} v. p. 61, & Pharm. art. acid.
——— Roll, ...	
——— Washed, ...	
——— Liver of	..v. Pharm. prep. Potash.
Sulphuric acid, ...	..———art. Acids.
——— ether, ...	..——— Ethers.
Talc, ...	..See page 694.
Tar, ...	..See page 618.
Tartar, ...	} v. Pharm. prep. Potash.
——— Cream of	
——— Soluble, ...	
——— Emetic, ...	..——— Antimony.
Tartaric acid, ...	..——— Acids.
Tartarized antimony, ...	..——— Antimony.
Tin, ...	..——— Tin.
Tincal, or crude borax, ...	..——— Soda.
Tutty.	..——— Zinc.
Verdigris, ...	..——— Copper.
Vermillion, sulphate of mercury,	..——— Mercury.
Vinegar, ...	} ——— art. Acids.
——— Aromatic, ...	
Vitriol, blue, ...	..———prep. Copper.
——— green, ...	..——— Iron.
——— white, ...	..——— Zinc.
——— oil of, ...	..——— Acids.
Volatile alkali, ...	..——— Ammonia.
Water, factitious mineral, &c...	..——— Mineral waters.
Wines, ...	..See page 251.
Zinc, carbonate of, ...	} v. Pharm. prep. Zinc.
—— sulphate of	

THE

BENGAL DISPENSATORY

AND

PHARMACOPŒIA.

Appendix.

No. 1.—*Report and Correspondence on the Manufacture of an improved Pottery from Indian Clays.*

To G. A. Bushby, Esq.

Secretary to the Government.

Gen. Dept.

Sir,—I have the honor to forward a report on the inquiries and experiments on Native Clays and Pottery, which I have conducted during the past six months, and which I have much pleasure in stating have been more successful than I expected.

Specimens are also forwarded of the Clays and articles of Ware described.

I have the honor to be, Sir,

Your most obedient servant,

W. B. O'Shaughnessy, M. D.

Assistant Surgeon, Chemical Examiner.

Calcutta, 10*th December*, 1840.

REPORT ON NATIVE POTTERY.

In December 1839, a communication was received from the Medical Board by the Materia Medica Committee, forwarding a despatch from the Honorable the Court of Directors, regarding the heavy expences of supplying the common Earthenware from Europe, and directing an attempt to be made to procure an efficient substitute in India.

From Court of Directors to Military Department, No. 48 of 1839.

The Board in forwarding this communication expressed their desire, that the general improvement of Native Pottery should be considered the chief end in any experiments which might be undertaken.

The Committee in reply forwarded the following Memorandum, which I had drawn up for their consideration, and in which the circumstances are pointed out to be attended to at the commencement of the inquiries :—

Copy of Memorandum.

"I have the pleasure to circulate for your perusal, the annexed letter from the Medical Board, together with an extract from a despatch from the Honorable the Court of Directors, relative to the attempt to substitute Indian Earthenware for the European article in the department of our Medical Stores.

"We must all regard as a matter of much importance, any attempt to introduce among the natives of India, the improved and admirable processes which European science has devised for the manufacture of Earthenware of every variety. There are circumstances, it is true, in the religion and habits of the great mass of the natives, which so long as they continue Hindus, will prevent their using vessels of any but the very coarsest and cheapest kind. Still the comparative few who will certainly consume the improved article, and the demand which the spread of chemical knowledge must soon rapidly create, afford sufficient inducement to the attempt now under consideration.

"The materials for the manufacture of even the best Porcelain are stated on indisputable authority* to be abundant, and accessible in the range of low Hills between Rajmahal and Colgong. The clay of disintegrated granite, felspar, quartz, flint, soapstone, and potstone, all these minerals are found in inexhaustible profusion. According to Dr. Buchanan's statements, the quarries are already open, and sufficiently near the Ganges, to permit the raw material to be cheaply brought to Calcutta.

"It will give me the utmost pleasure to superintend the very important experiment of attempting to manufacture good articles of Pottery from the materials I have described. A furnace should be built in some convenient situation, (perhaps considering my avocations, the College grounds may be preferred,) and a suitable (fire-brick) boiler and mixing vats erected. I cannot form an accurate estimate of the probable cost; but from my experience in building furnaces in India, I would suppose 1,500 to 2,000 rupees would cover the entire expense.

"The materials for a sufficiently conclusive experiment, including the glazing process, could not at the maximum cost more than 1,000 rupees.

"It would, however, be desirable in the first instance, that the proper authorities in Bhagulpore and Rajmahal should be directed to institute inquiries as to the exact state, site, and precise proximity to water carriage of the "Khari" quarries, and as to the rate at which the material can be conveyed to Calcutta. A sufficient quantity of good flint is available in the ballast yards of the Presidency for the purpose of experiment, while the quartz quarries of the Colgong Hills are under exploration.

"In the immediate neighbourhood of Calcutta the potters are numerous and expert. They are willing, moreover, as I have learned by personal inquiry, to adopt any new and cheap process they may be taught. Three or four of these people might be employed to commence the experiment.

"With reference to Mr. Assistant Surgeon Jeffreys' experiments, I am in possession of no accurate information. The great ingenuity and perseverance for which that gentleman was distinguished, render it very probable, that he did succeed.

* Dr. Buchanan Hamilton's *Statistics of Behar.*

Indeed the chief difficulty in this, and all such trials, seems to be the general dependence thereof, on private resources at the first starting.

"In offering to undertake the management of the experiment in question, I beg it to be understood, that I possess no practical knowledge of the manipulations of the art. But having access to good authorities on the subject, and being most anxious that the attempt should succeed, I will direct and watch over it to the best of my ability, should the Government resolve on carrying the proposition into effect."

2d December, 1839. W. B. O'SHAUGHNESSY.

The Medical Board immediately submitted this Memorandum to Government, and on the 17th February 1840, again addressed the Materia Medica Committee, forwarding the orders of Government for the commencement of the experiments suggested above.

On receipt of the Board's despatch, active measures were taken to obtain specimens of clays from various parts of India, and the adjacent countries.—Before proceeding to further details, I should here premise a few remarks on the existing common Pottery of Bengal.

No. 1. Common clay.
2. Do. fused at redness.

The common native Pottery of Bengal is formed of a clay, containing so much oxide of iron and carbonate of lime, that the vessels melt into a slag at a temperature little above that of redness.

Specimen No. 2.
a, Clay.
b, Do. heated.

Deposits of a black stiff clay, containing much vegetable matter occur in many districts, vessels made from which sustain a higher temperature without fusion; but crack and warp so much, as to be of very little use.

Specimen No. 3. Mr. Piddington's Serampore "glazed" ware.

Of true glazes for ordinary ware, the native potter may be said to be entirely ignorant. In many districts, mixtures are used of clays of very fine texture, easily reduced to powder, which are applied with care as a paint, and then heated till they adhere closely; *but without fusion.* This operation is rather painting than glazing, and though it renders vessels impermeable to fluids for a few operations, it is but a very inadequate substitute for the true vitreous coating.—The "varnish" in question may be scratched through by the point of a pin.

In none of the native furnaces which Buchanan described, (See the Vol. on Behar) or which I have myself examined, is there such a disposition or arrangement as would admit even of the most fusible lead glaze being successfully employed. The Pottery being burned in direct contact with the fuel, the oxide of lead would necessarily be reduced to the metallic state, and no glazing could be performed.

My object in commencing these experiments was, in the first place, in conformity with the wishes of the Honorable the Court of Directors, to procure common and cheap vessels, combining the following properties:—

1. Mechanical strength.
2. Infusibility at high temperatures.
3. Lightness of colour.

* The marginal notes refer to the specimens which accompanied this Report.

4. Impermeability to water, oil, and ordinary culinary liquids.

5. A cheap glazing, free from lead or any other deleterious substance, and capable of resisting corrosive chemical fluids at high boiling points, and under long continued heat.

The first step towards succeeding in these objects was the procural of suitable clays;—these should combine—

A. Ductility under the lathe.

B. Infusibility.

C. Regularity of contraction, &c. in heating.

D. Burning to a pale colour.

On reference to Buchanan's admirable work, descriptions were found of clays occurring in the Rajmahal and Bhagulpore hills, and in the neighbourhood of Patna, which seemed to promise the qualities desired.

A strict search in the Museum of the Asiatic Society only led to the finding of one promising clay marked "Cherra-poonji," evidently a felspathic earth, proceeding from decomposed granite.

Letters were accordingly addressed to the under-named gentlemen, soliciting their co-operation in procuring supplies of clay for examination on a large and practical scale, and setting forth the local and general benefits which must accrue from the successful prosecution of this inquiry.

Mr. Oman, indigo planter, Colgong; Dr. Leckie, civil surgeon, Bhagulpore; Mr. W. B. Johnson, opium department, Patna; Dr. Davenport, civil surgeon, Cherra; Lieut. Braddock, gunpowder agent, Madras; Mr. Jas. Colquhoun; Mr. Blundell, commissioner of the Tenasserim provinces, Moulmain; Messrs. Lackersteen and Co. Calcutta. The last parties were addressed with reference to the clays of Moulmain and Singapore, in consequence of information I had received of the existence of white clays in great abundance, and in situations of ready accessibility at both these localities.

By the replies received from all the gentlemen addressed, and copies of which are appended, the Government will observe the zeal, interest, and liberality with which the subject was taken up.

Specimen 4. On the 10th May, Mr. Oman forwarded a specimen of white clay, ***Khari***, obtained from the Modiram Hill, one mile from his residence. He described the quarry as extensive, the clay procurable in any quantities, the quarry about a mile from the river, *never worked; and almost unknown to the natives of the place.*

Specimens 5, 6. Mr. Oman also forwarded two other specimens. 1. Geria Mittee, [coarse steatite.] 2. Saboon Mittee, a dark brown clay, strongly resembling "*fuller's earth,*" occurring on the same hill, and used by the natives as a substitute for soap.

On the 19th May, Mr. Oman despatched 28 maunds of the white earth, *Khari*, and 11½ maunds of the brown clay; the consignments reached Calcutta safely in 18 days.

Dr. Leckie's Specimens. Dr. Leckie, of Bhagulpore, was kind enough to forward specimens:—

1. Kullee, identical with, and from the same locality, as Mr. Oman's *khari.*

2. A similar clay from the Rajmahal district.

3. Ditto, locality uncertain, a bazar specimen.
4. Gohurthapulla, *steatite.*
5. The same as 4.
6. Coarse ditto.

Of the specimens sent by Dr. Leckie, as will be subsequently explained, Nos. 1 and 2 were alone deemed of practical value; but as these were sent in large quantities by Mr. Oman, there was no further need for having recourse to Dr. Leckie's willing and ever ready aid.

Mr. Davenport's Specimens.

Mr. Davenport sent four specimens. No. 1 and 3, which promised to be the best, were marked "not abundant." No. 2 was identical with the black clay of Bengal. No. 4. decomposed granite, strongly impregnated with iron. Mr. Davenport considered that the cost of the clays sent to Calcutta, during the rainy season, would be eight annas the maund; but he stated that the scarcity of coolies would render it necessary to use Government cattle for the procural of the clay to any extent.

Mr. W. Johnson's Specimens.

Mr. Johnson of Patna wrote as follows, in despatching the clays marked 8, 9, and which had been described by Buchanan in his account of the Statistics of Behar :—

Extract from Mr. Johnson's *Letter.*

"Agreeable to your request, I have despatched by Dawk and by Banghy, specimens of the clay. It is procurable at Phatuah, on the south side of the river. There is an excellent clay procurable at Peerpointee; also a good clay at Behar, and at Allygunge Sewar, near Chuprah, of which I will try and procure specimens for you. I have given directions to the sirdar of the third fleet to take you a basket of the first mentioned clay, the cost of which is very trifling; the boat hire and landing would be about 12 or 13 rupees per 100 maunds."

A notice of the quality of this clay occurs in another place. It has proved of little or no value.

Rhotas clay Specimens.

Mr. Piddington, of Calcutta, having supplied me with a specimen of clay from Rhotas on the Soane, and informed me that it was used by Messrs. Boyd and Co. in considerable quantities in their sugar establishment, I addressed that firm for a supply, which they very kindly and promptly furnished. The clay contains 7 per 100 of chalk. Samples are given of the clay in the raw state, and after it has been exposed to intense heat, which causes a partial fusion and spongyness of its texture.

Mr. Blundell's reply to my letter reached me late in July, and accompanying it were four bags of clay from Moulmein and Mergui. I subjoin an extract from Mr. Blundell's letter :—

"The quantity (of all specimens) appears to be unlimited, and easy of access, being generally the stratum of low hills; the expense of collection very trifling, of conveyance to Calcutta about 20 rupees the ton. The earth is not used by the Natives for their potteries, and is only resorted to by the soldiers as pipe clay."

The clays were all white, free from lime or iron.—No. 1, very sandy or micaceous. No. 2 extremely soft and ductile—all very refractory, and burning of a white colour; but the ware cracked irregularly, and was devoid of cohesion when fired. No. 1 and 3 resembled very closely the *Khari* of Colgong.

The late Lieutenant Braddock of Madras, on the 20th August, forwarded seven specimens of clay and pottery, with the subjoined remarks :—

Lieut. Braddock's Madras Specimens.

"I have the pleasure to acknowledge yours of the 6th instant, requesting specimens of the earths and clays about Madras, I have herewith the pleasure to send you some. We have no great variety.

"No. 1.—A fire clay from Sreepermeter, about twenty-eight miles from Madras.

"No 2.—Variety of ditto.

"No. 3.—Crucible clay from Yerra Mootoopollam, about 15 miles from Madras.

"No. 4 —Variety of ditto.

"No. 5.—Clay used at Madras for the common pottery of the bazar.

"No. 6.—A broken piece of a vessel made of ditto.

"No. 7.—A broken piece of a vessel said to be made at Arcot.

"I shall make further inquiries about Pottery clays ; but I am of opinion that these varieties include all that are in use here. If I should get any further specimens, or any further information that might be useful to you, I will let you know."

In a subsequent letter, Lieut. Braddock added,

"I have herewith the pleasure to send you a specimen of earth said to be obtained at about 60 miles from Madras. It is brought that distance, and made here into white goglets, (vessels for water) ; but different (probably) from the piece of white pottery I sent you, *i. e.* this clay is probably different from the clay of which that piece of pottery was made. Of this, however, you will be able to judge by analysis."

Of these clays, Nos. 1 and 2 correspond closely with the Colgong khari. Nos. 3 and 4 with the Patna Phatuah, and No. 5 with the common clay of Bengal.

Of the two specimens of pottery, the red is inferior in appearance and texture to the common Bengal ware ; the whiter kind is strong, and shews plainly, that if properly prepared and heated, the clay of which it is composed, would give a very superior article of ware.

In October 1840, Captain Halsted of her H. M's. brig *Childers*, kindly favoured me with several specimens, some from Mergui, which were almost identical with Mr. Blundell's ; but there was one from Singapore by far the most valuable of any I had before met with.

Singapore Specimens.

This clay is white externally, mottled red within, contains large nodules perfectly white, is smooth and unctuous to the touch, readily forms a fine paste with water, is ductile and plastic on the lathe, perfectly refractory in the fire. The white parts yield a strong close white biscuit. The whole clay ground together gives a biscuit of a pale yellow colour, hard enough to strike sparks from steel, and without glazing quite impermeable to water.

Trials of the Clays.

Reserving further details regarding these clays for another report, I proceed to notice the steps I took to subject them to a fair working trial.

An expert native potter, Bonomallee Paul, was engaged on a salary of twenty rupees per mensem. He was encouraged to use the common implements of his trade, as far as concerned the preparation of materials and their mechanical construction. I adopted this plan in preference to the use of any expensive apparatus, from the conviction, that improvements in this art (as in others) to be generally diffused through the country, must be of that kind, which involves no great outlay of funds, and as much as possible interwoven with methods and contrivances with which the people are familiar.

The potter's wheel is of the simplest kind, and has been perfectly described by Buchanan. I shall not repeat what he has said—suffice it to say, that a horizontal fly wheel, the frame of wood, the rim heavily laden with clay, two to three feet in diameter, weight sixty to eighty lbs. is put in motion by the potter's hand, assisted by a stick; once set spinning, it revolves for from five or seven minutes with a perfectly steady and nearly *true* motion. The mass of clay to be moulded is placed on the centre of the wheel, and the potter squats before it on the ground.

This machine has doubtless several defects; but it answered my purpose perfectly. My object was but to test the qualities of the clays, and to construct small vessels. Any favourable inference in favour of a ware prepared on such a wheel, would leave no room to doubt the result on adopting the European form of apparatus.

Furnace.

The native furnace is simply an excavation in the ground, of variable depth, in which the ware is placed layer by layer, with dry reeds, straw, &c. and all are burnt together. This rude system must of course give way to the European method, for the construction of all the superior kinds of vessels.

A biscuit furnace of which I forward a plan and section, was erected in the laboratory yard. It consists of a cylindrical dome, five feet in internal diameter, seven feet ten inches in internal height—four fire-places are disposed at equal distances all round, each fire-place is twenty-four inches deep to the grate, two feet six inches square area, and opens by a flue under the floor of the cylinder.

The fire-places and cylinders are lined with fire-brick. An entrance was left for the arrangement of the ware. This entrance is walled up on each experiment. The top of the dome opens by an aperture eighteen inches square into a horizontal flue, leading to one of the laboratory chimnies, thirty-five feet in height.

The expense of this furnace was Co.'s Rs. 650.

The temperature attainable was that of a white heat of iron, by the combustion of ten maunds of Burdwan coal and six of wood. It was sufficient to fuse all common glazes, and to bake ware to the consistence and hardness of striking fire from steel. It was scarcely sufficient, however, for the porcelainous fusion of any of the earths under experiment.

For this purpose, I have hitherto been compelled to employ the common draught furnace of the laboratory, burning the trial pieces in muffles or saggars. I have now, however, completed a glazing furnace on the same plan as that already described, but the dome being of much smaller dimensions. In this my future experiments on glazes and enamels will be conducted.

Analysis of the Clays.

The experiments under this head, were performed by Nobin Chunder Paul, one of the past Students of the Medical College, and an expert and careful operator.

A qualitative analysis was first made in each instance to ascertain the presence or absence of lime, magnesia, or iron; subsequently a certain portion of the clay was carefully subjected to the action of the gaseous hydrofluoric acid, and the loss of silicia ascertained. As these experiments will form the subject of a separate paper, I shall reserve the results to which they led for description in that document. The analysis indeed was comparatively of remote interest, as we had to investigate exclusively, in this stage of our inquiries, the *mechanical* properties of the several clays we obtained. Much more speedy and practically useful results were always obtained from the preparation of a few cups of thin ware, from each of the clays under trial, than from the nicest analysis. This has still, however, a high degree of interest, when we consider the ultimate perfection of our processes, and the adoption of the ornamental branches of the art; and it will accordingly receive full attention as we proceed.

Practical Trials of the Colgong Khari.

N. B.—The remarks under this head apply also to the Moulmein clays, Nos. 1, 3, 4,—the Mergui No. 2,—the Madras, Nos. 1 and 2—the Bhagulpore, Nos. 1, 2, 3,—and the Cherra, No. 1.

These clays occur in shapeless blocks, white, harsh to the touch, free from smell, absorb water with a loud hissing sound, and fall to pieces in slate-like layers. The moistened pieces are easily reduced to pulp under water. This operation was performed in our experiments by the hand, and by beating with a wooden pestle in a stone mortar. The creamy liquid was strained through calico, and thus all pebbly, coarse, micaceous and sandy particles were removed.

A paste of this clay was worked with difficulty on the lathe, being but little plastic or tenacious; on burning, the trial vessels prepared from it cracked and fell to pieces. The colour after baking was a pure white or pale pink tinge.

Such clays are evidently unfit by themselves for the manufacture of earthenware. Specimens. *They afford an admirable natural substitute for the ground flints of the English stoneware manufacture;* but they require a more ductile material to be mixed with them.

Experiments with the Colgong "Saboon Mittee," or Fuller's Earth.

This earth is brown, easily reducible to pulp, very ductile and tenacious, exceedingly refractory, but burns to a deep brick colour. It gave good vessels as far as density and tenacity were concerned; but they were liable to crack, and of a dirty disagreeable colour.

Mixtures of both the preceding Clays.

The potter having reported, that a very small portion of the saboon mittee mixed with the khari, gave this the proper tenacity for the lathe, the following mixtures were made up for firing in the biscuit oven:—

Khari.	Parts.		Parts Saboon Mattee.
No. 1	16	......	0
2	16	......	1
3	16	......	2
4	16	......	3
5	16	......	4
6	16	......	5
7	16	......	6
8	16	......	7
9	16	......	8
10	16	......	9
11	16	......	10
12	16	......	11
13	16	......	12
14	16	......	13
15	16	......	14
16	16	......	15
17	16	......	16

The mixtures were modelled into cylindrical vessels all of the same size, and after drying for an equal time, were heated together in the biscuit furnace. The following are the results obtained:—

No. 1 (Km. 16, S,m. 0). Fell to pieces, fragments white, crumbling to powder on pressure.

No. 2 [Km. 16, S,m. 1] White, much cracked, brittle, very soft.

No. 3 [Km. 16, S,m. 2] But little different from No. 2.

No. 4 [Km. 16, S,m. 3] White, dense, very slightly cracked, soft, but little cohesive.

No. 5 [Km. 16, S,m. 4] Faint tinge of pink, texture smooth, dense, and strong; no cracking, very hard where heat was greatest and at the edges.

No. 6	[Km. 16, S,m. 5]	But little different from No. 4.
7	[Km. 16, S,m. 6]	
8	[Km. 16, S,m. 7]	
9	[Km. 16, S,m. 8]	
10	[Km. 16, S,m. 9]	Colour pink, texture close and strong.
11	[Km. 16, S,m. 10]	
12	[Km. 16, S,m. 11]	Yellowish red, hard, strong and light.
13	[Km. 16, S,m. 12]	
14	[Km. 16, S,m. 13]	Deeper and closer than two last Nos.
15	[Km. 16, S,m. 14]	
16	[Km. 16, S,m. 15]	Brick red, hard, dense, light and strong.
17	[Km. 16, S,m. 16]	

From these and many similar experiments, it was evident that in the mixtures of the two Colgong clays, Khari 4, Saboon 1, we have the materials for the manufacture of stoneware and of all culinary and chemical utensils, in which a pure white colour is not a desideratum, and strength, hardness, density and infusibility are the qualities required.

The colour of the ware producible from these mixtures, is buff to pale pink.

Of this ware in biscuit very beautiful vases, coolers, water goglets, and bottle holders may be constructed. I have kept such articles for three months in water, without their texture being injured.

Lastly; for crucibles, fire-bricks, and fire-cement, these materials cannot be surpassed, and they thus afford the native and local manufacturer cheap substitutes for articles which have hitherto been imported from Europe at an extravagant outlay. Fire-bricks on an average cost in Calcutta ten rupees the hundred. With these clays, as good bricks can be made and sold at a fair profit for 2 rupees 8 annas the hundred.

Specimens forwarded of bricks & tile.

Rotas Clay.

This earth, from the large quantity of carbonate of lime it contains, is unfit for ordinary pottery; but when very intensely heated, it yields a beautiful buff porcelain. I reserve it for further experiments on the superior kinds of ware in the second furnace now finished.

Moulmein Clay.

2, 3, and 4, of Mr. Blundell's specimens may be substituted in every way, for the Colgong Khari. No. 3, gives ductility to the paste; but the vessels I have yet made with this mixture, have cracked in the firing. I hope in subsequent trials to be enabled to remedy this evil.

Madras Clays.

Of these 1 and 2 correspond to the Khari of Colgong. None are plastic enough for the lathe; but with a fourth part of the "fuller's earth" of Colgong, they will make excellent common ware.

Singapore Clays.

By far the best clay I have met with, is that given me by Captain Halsted, and which he procured at Singapore.

It occurs, as I am informed, close to the beach, and the Messrs. Lackersteen of Calcutta inform me, it can be brought to Calcutta for six annas the maund.

This clay is found in thick strata. The detached masses are of a pink tint, broken into they contain nodules of perfectly white earth. They absorb water eagerly, and yield an exceedingly soft, ductile, and tenacious paste.

On firing, this clay is found to resist a temperature sufficient to fuse English blue pots. The vessels made from the coarsest parts of this clay are strong, hard, of a beautiful and rich crimson colour. The *picked* clay gives a snow-white biscuit; unpicked and simply worked up as it is dug, it gives a light yellow stoneware of the very best kind, as far as density, hardness, strength, lightness, and colour are concerned.

Specimen.

Trials of several Glazes.

In noticing this subject, I beg leave to refer again to a previous paragraph, in which I have described the qualities of what I would consider to be a good glaze.

To glaze the common Kedgeree-ware of Bengal, I look upon as a vain attempt. It is so fusible itself, that no glaze but one containing an unusually large proportion of lead could be employed at all. Such vessels must prove detrimental to health, and useless in chemical operations.

My first attempts at producing a glaze free from lead, were made with the sajee mittee, or soda clay of Bengal. This well-known mineral contains about 50 per 100 of carbonate of soda with alumina, sand, carbonate of lime, and oxide of iron. On being heated nearly to whiteness, it fuses, effervesces and runs into a green glass. By increasing the proportion of sand, a good bottle glass is obtained, which though green in mass, is transparent and colourless in thin pellicles.

By reducing the mineral to very fine powder, and mixing the powder with weak gum-water, the Colgong biscuit-ware is readily made to take on a uniform coating of the material, either by immersing the vessels in the mixture, or applying this with a brush. The glaze readily fused; but to my regret, I found after numerous and tedious trials, that its rate of contraction on cooling differed so much from that of the clays employed, that it invariably cracked and peeled off, despite of the most careful annealing of the ware.

I have much pleasure, however, in reporting, that I have still succeeded fully in my object, and have obtained a glaze, combining all the qualities I desired. The glaze has never been used before; at least it is not mentioned in any work or essay on pottery to which I have access.

New Glaze—the Borate of Lime.

After failing with the soda earth, I next turned my attention to *borax*, (the bi-borate of soda,) and the compounds of boracic acid, with earthy and metallic bases.

I accordingly prepared specimens of the borates of lime, magnesia, alumina, lead, iron, tin, &c. Thin pieces of biscuit-ware, four inches long by two broad and one-eighth thick, were made of the Colgong clay mixture, 4 K. 1 S. and the several borates tried on these in a furnace capable of melting cast iron, and regulated by a register in the usual way.

Borax alone fused, glaze irregular and blistering.

Borate of Lead, fused, glaze regular, but cracked on cooling.

Ditto of Magnesia, infusible.

Ditto of Alumina, ditto.

Ditto of Lime, fused, glaze smooth, uniform, did not crack.

These were the results of several trials, and the superiority of the borate of lime was so manifest, that my attention was thence directed to ascertaining its applicability on a larger scale.

I find that it is most easily applied to our new biscuit, by mixing the powdered borate into a thin cream with weak solution of the common bazar gum. This mixture is applied with a brush, and the ware is then exposed to the sun, or kiln-dried.

To fuse this glaze, requires a somewhat higher temperature than that needed for the preparation of the biscuit. The glaze being, when properly prepared, transparent and colourless, it leaves the vessel of its natural tint, and as lustrous as the best English ware. I submit herewith a specimen of the glaze applied on a stone-

Specimen. ware paste. The specimen in question has been boiled for two hours in the strongest sulphuric acid, and for the same period in nitric and muriatic acids, and yet it has not suffered in the least degree. These qualities render it of extreme value for the manufacture of vessels for the operations in chemistry and in the arts, in which corrosive liquids are concerned.

The lime solution is prepared by dissolving shell lime in bazar vinegar, till a neutral liquid is obtained, and boiling this down to the consistence of a thin syrup. In working a pottery, the impure pyroligneous acid would be employed and prepared on the spot. In a subsequent paper, I will shew how this may be made a source of considerable profit to the potter.

The solution of borax is made by dissolving 1 lb. of sohaga, (bazar borax,) in 12 quarts of warm rain water, and straining through clear gunny cloth. This solution is to be added to the lime solution, in portions of a pint at a time, so long as any precipitate occurs.

The milky fluid is next to be thrown on a calico strainer. The solid matter which is already finely pulverulent, should be washed with cold rain water, again strained through calico, and dried for use.

The minute quantity of this article required for the glazing of a vessel, renders its expense scarcely worth calculation.

By the preceding experiments, I conceive that I have fulfilled the task I was set, in ascertaining the feasibility of introducing into India the manufacture of superior articles of common pottery, for culinary and chemical purposes—and for the packing and conveyance of medical stores. The materials requisite have been found in accessible sites; their cheapness and abundance shewn; their *mechanical* properties investigated; and the practical circumstances studied, essential for the commencement of the manufacture by the common potters of the country. It remains for me, in future experiments, to attempt the production of the finer and more ornamental kinds of articles, and to study the fitness of our ware to receive coloured glazes, gilding, &c. after the European and Chinese methods. This, however, I look upon as a matter of very secondary importance, contrasted with the results already gained.

It is necessary too to observe, that all the specimens I have had made up, have been either hand-made, or turned on the native potter's wheel. They consequently want the finish which machinery can alone impart. The density of structure too is much less than it would be in a large factory, where *great quantities* of materials could be stored for *long periods*. The influence of these two circumstances in causing the better union of the clays and compactness of the work, is well known to potters in all countries. I may thence reasonably conclude, that, if in my experiments on *pounds* weight, and performed as soon as the materials could be mixed, we succeeded in producing a ware impermeable to liquids, and hard enough to strike fire from steel, large and long continued operations must materially improve all these good qualities.

I have lastly to represent respectfully, that in these and similar experiments, I can only engage to point out to Government and to individuals, how a certain manufacture may be undertaken. I cannot offer, for example, to supply from my own small furnaces any portion of the ware the public stores may require. I can only shew others how to make it, and then leave them to commence the manufacture themselves.

A very trifling capital will suffice to start a small pottery. Of the 600 rupees charged for the College furnace, 260 were for English fire-brick. Now this item would be reduced to one-fourth by making bricks of the Colgong materials. The clay may be brought to Calcutta, in large quantities, for six annas the maund.

The expense of two furnaces, biscuit and glazing, with chimnies, sufficient for the commencement of a considerable trade, I estimate at 1,000 rupees.

I leave it to others to consider whether it would be expedient to have a separate factory to give the supply needed by Government. I would in preference recommend that a contract be offered to the Native potter I have taught, and a small sum of money lent him on adequate security to encourage him to commence. He is intelligent, honest, and of good character in his trade.

I should not conclude this Report without prominently stating, that I have seen a fragment of excellent salt glazed stoneware, bearing the stamp "Futteygurh," and which I am informed, was manufactured by Mr. Jeffreys, late of our Medical Establishment. I have been unable to procure any information as to the materials this gentleman used, the processes he employed, or the expense of the vessels. The manufacture has been abandoned since Mr Jeffreys' departure from India.

W. B. O'Shaughnessy, M. D.

Medical College, 15*th December*, 1840.

Catalogue of Specimens of Native Clays, Pottery, and Fire-Brick, submitted to Government with the Report.

1. *a.* Common Bengal potter's clay.

1. *b.* Ditto, fused at a red heat.

2. Another Bengal clay, more infusible than No. 1; but at a full red heat it swells and cracks, as seen in the specimens.

3. A specimen of a ware made at Serampore, and having a varnish, (not a glaze,) to render it impermeable to fluids, presented by Mr. Piddington, with a memorandum of the native process.

4. Colgong white clay, (Khari.) This constitutes the body of the new stoneware proposed in the Report.—It is a perfect substitute for the ground flint of European stoneware.

5. The same clay, after being subjected to a fierce white heat for several hours.

6. Colgong *soap clay*, "fuller's earth (Saboon Mittee)."—This constitutes a fourth part of the new ware.

7. *Khari* clay from Bhagulpore, identical with No. 4.

8. *Steatite* from Bhagulpore.

9. *Geru muttee*, a silicious clay from Bhagulpore, very refractory in the fire, and makes good coarse ware with a fourth part of Colgong soap earth.

10. A clay resulting from decomposed granite, obtained from Cherra Punji. Though of little value, it shews the probability of much superior clays being found in the same locality.

11. A clay from Cherra Punji, described in Dr. Davenport's letter, "as not abundant," of very good quality.

12. *Phatua clay*, from the bank of the Ganges, described by Buchanan ; gives a good common ware, but is very easily fusible.

13. Clay from Rhotas Gurh, contains 8 per 100 carbonate of lime, and is very fusible. Will afford a useful material for the manufacture of porcelain.

14. The same clay, softened at a full red heat.

15. *Borate of lime*, the substance recommended in the Report as a glaze for the new stoneware.

16.
17.
18.
19.
20. } Clays from Moulmein, described in the Report.

21.
22. } Identical with the Colgong khari.
23. A good crucible clay.
24. The same as khari.
(21–24) } *Madras Specimens.*

25. Common Madras potter's clay.

26. Common pottery of Madras.

27. Finer pottery from Arcot.

28. Singapore clay.

29. A small cup of stoneware, made of three parts Colgong *khari* and one part Colgong *soap earth*, glazed outside with *borate of lime*. This specimen has been heated to the melting point of cast iron ; is hard enough to strike fire from steel, and has been boiled for two hours in nitric acid to prove the stability of the glaze.

30. A lighter kind of stoneware, of similar composition.

31. A cup made of the Colgong soap clay, fired at a white heat, colour brick red. This ware would make excellent saggars or cases for the firing of fine pottery, porcelain, &c.

32. Singapore clay, a cup fired at a white heat. This clay gives a very beautiful pink biscuit.

33. A cup of the red clay of Bhagulpore, fired at a white heat.

34. A cup of Singapore clay, from which the coarser red pieces had been picked out—perfectly white.

35. A cup of Cherra Punji clay of the same properties as No. 32.

36. A cup of *Phatua clay*, fired at a red heat.

37. Cup of common black clay, exposed to a low red heat.

38. Fragments of stoneware made of Colgong clays, glazed by *salt* after the English method.

39. A jar of biscuit stoneware, made of Colgong clays.

40.
41. } Porous biscuit-ware of same materials.

42.
43. } A tile and two bricks made of same materials. See Captain Wilson's report.
44.

45. Ditto ditto.

These specimens have been exposed to the fiercest heat of a powerful draught furnace, which melted down blue pots and American fire-bricks. They have been hastily and roughly made up; but are in every respect equal to the best English fire-brick, and can be prepared at three rupees the hundred. The English brick costs (average) ten rupees.

W. B. O'S.

Calcutta, December 22, 1841.

Mr. Piddington's Memorandum, to accompany a set of Specimens of Varnish Earths.

1. In establishing an extensive Sugar Refinery, I was desirous of avoiding the heavy expense of English sugar moulds, and the draining pots on which they stand. I knew that common native pottery had been extensively tried by others, and that it would not stand the penetrating effect of the sugar when poured, as it is, boiling hot into the moulds, and left for weeks during the claying process.

2. My attention was naturally directed to the native sugar-boilers' and sweet-meat-makers' pans, called *kolas*. These I knew were used for boiling sugar, and frying mixtures of sugar and ghee, (which must require a very high boiling point,) for weeks together, and many times a day; and I found that their destruction was always owing to cracks by heat; but that their varnish resisted every thing to the last. It was clear that this was the varnish I wanted, and I succeeded at last in obtaining it, and, by employing men as varnishers separately from the potters, in making sugar moulds, which though not so strong, would with care almost rival English ones at eighteen rupees per hundred. For those of the largest sized loaves, holding a maund and a half of syrup, I proceed to describe the earths and the process used.

3. I shall first mention, that the pottery was of the common red kind, sold in all the bazars, and made from the silt of the banks of the river; but the best *kolas* are made at Kulna, a little above Sooksaugor, on the Burdwan side. I know these are highly preferred and even carried into Jessore. I should mention that the oven is the common old-fashioned semi-elliptic one, open in front and at the top, such as is used for burning tiles in Europe and in India. The pottery is burnt at one firing only, being varnished when put into the kiln.

4. There are two kinds of earth used, of which specimen No. 1 is called *belutti*. It is a coarse siliceous ochry yellow earth, with veins and patches of a siliceous aluminous earth interspersed through it. When washed, it leaves a residuum of small gravel, mostly siliceous, with a little felspar. The best sort is found at eight or nine coss from Kulna; but I have lost the name of the village.

From this *belutti* is prepared only one of the three varnishes used, and it is also called when prepared, *belutti*. It is sold at Kulna at one and a half rupee per maund of raw earth, and two rupees per maund of prepared belutti. Fifteen days are required to prepare a quantity properly. No. 3 is sample of prepared belutti. No. 2 is the next sort of earth. It is called *ooporomee*, (or upper wash). It may be described as a strong brown tenacious or clayey loam. The best is found at a village called Monad, ten coss west of Chinsurah, and at Panchdowkie, eight coss S. W. of Kulna. The raw earth is sold at four annas the maund; but the *prepared ooporomee*, No. 4, is worth three rupees per maund. Three months are, they pretend, required for its proper preparation; and ten seers ooporomee are procured from each maund of the raw earth. There are also two other sorts of varnishing earth, prepared from this ooporomee, which are,

No. 5. *Gád*, or scum.—Though it is obtained at the bottom of the washing vessel, and No. 6, *Majaree*, (or middle sort.)

All these prepared specimens—belutti, ooporomee, gád, and majaree are obtained by washing, great care being taken to select the water of a very pure tank, no doubt to avoid saline mixtures, which would act as fluxes. The belutti when prepared, is a mixture of the yellow ochre and alumina in slightly variable proportions. The majaree and gád are the first settlings of the raw ooporomee when dissolved in water, and the ooporomee itself is the finer part, which remains suspended, and is separated by pouring off successive waters, when it slowly deposits.

The application of the Varnish Earths.—The ware being thoroughly sun-dried, is first smeared inside with the sort called gád, No. 5, which is diluted in water to the consistence of a thick cream. This smearing, for it is nothing else, is done by a rag. The ware is now again left to become thoroughly dry in the hot sun.

Upon the coat of the gád is smeared, in the same way, one of the prepared belutti, No. 3, and this is also allowed to dry. The ware now appears as if smeared over with a *thin* wash of yellow ochre, for it is not laid on to bring thickness.

Upon the belutti is again smeared a thin coat of the ooporomee, and by examining the sample of ware sent herewith, the effects of these smearings will be distinctly seen. It would appear, that the cream must not be too thin to disturb the coat below, nor too thick, nor thickly laid on, when I suppose it might run or peel off. The majaree is used in ordinary works in the place of the ooporomee, and it will be seen, that it is only a coarser variety of it.

I regret greatly that I had not time to examine these varnish earths; but I was much overloaded with work at the time, and have not been able to take them up since. A purely earthen varnish for common red ware, has always I think, been a desideratum. And in the hands of European chemists and potters, I have no doubt that this curious fact of the fusion of the varnish, by the aid of the carbonate of iron of the ochre, (which I take to be the flux of the mixture,) would be turned to account. I sent a set of these samples to the Society of Arts, and another to America, together with one to Mr. Jas. Prinsep; but by a singular fatality, all have been lost. At least I have heard nothing of them. The great value of this varnish seems to be its remarkable power of resisting long heat, and a very penetrating solution like that of sugar.

H. Piddington.

The fragment of a *kola* sent herewith, is of the best kind of them. The native *kola* is a small one from the bazar, and they say not of the best sort.

The process so clearly described by Mr. Piddington, is as good *a substitute for a glaze*, as could well be contrived. The coating is for a time quite impermeable, but it is so soft, that it may be scratched through with the point of a pin. I have not been able to melt mixtures in all proportions of the material Mr. Piddington had the kindness to send me, in a furnace which fuses the body of the ware itself into a pumice-like sponge.

Extracts from a subsequent Report.

Pottery.—The experiments on pottery have been persevered in, especially on the Singapore clays. Of these No 1 has afforded a beautifully white biscuit, which stands the fiercest heat without cracking.

I have also prepared several specimens of fire-bricks, and have the pleasure to append the report of Captain Wilson, of the Cossipore Foundry, and Major Forbes of the Calcutta Mint, on the trials made of the bricks at these establishments.

Information has been received, that the Colgong clay quarries are to be had for an annual rent of twenty-six rupees the year, and measures are now being taken, which will ensure a cheap source of supply of good glazed stoneware, fire-cement, crucibles, and fire-bricks, for the use of Government, and the public at large.

1st *May*, 1841. W. B. O'S.

Reports on New Fire Brick.

To W. B. O'Shaughnessy, M. D.
Chemical Examiner to Government.

Sir,—I have been favoured with the receipt of your letter of the 19th instant, with the specimen of fire-bricks made under your superintendence, and I beg to congratulate you on the perfect success of your experiment. I tried a portion of the brick yesterday, and it withstood the fiercest heat as well as the English, and they appear to me only to want a greater compression in the moulds, to render them equal to the best English fire-bricks.

The specimen you sent me on being cut through, shewed a want of solidity and compactness in the centre, which by the application of a more powerful pressure, could, I imagine, be easily remedied.

I have &c.
(Signed) A. Wilson, *Captain,*
Officiating Superintendent and Director of Foundry.

Cossipore, 22*d April*, 1841.

No. 30 *of* 1841-42.

To W. B. O'Shaughnessy, Esq. M. D.

Sir,—I have the honor to acknowledge the receipt of your letter of date the 19th ultimo, forwarding a specimen of fire-brick, prepared under your superintendence, from materials obtained at Colgong, and having had it subjected to trial, you will perceive by the accompanying Report, that although not quite equal in quality to Stourbridge fire-brick, it has been concluded that its inferiority is mainly, if not alone, attributable to the comparatively imperfect mixture of the substances of which it is composed.

I have the honor to be, Sir,
Your most obedient servant,
(Signed) W. N. Forbes, *Mint Master*.

Calcutta Mint, *the* 15*th May*, 1841.

10*th May*, 1841.

Made a trial on fire-brick sent to the Mint by Dr. O'Shaughnessy, and said to be prepared from materials raised near the river at Colgong, and consisting of 3 parts of Colgong *khari clay*, and 1 part of fuller's earth, *saboon muttee*.

The brick was placed on its end in one of the Mint parting furnaces, with another, *Stourbridge* fire-brick, and fired on with coke to the greatest strength the draft would admit of, for five hours, and remained to cool down the next day. On examining the bricks on the following day, it was found that the Stourbridge brick was completely vitrified; but had not lost its figure. The Colgong brick was also vitrified, and had lost its figure on one side, it having run into holes; but on the other side, one of the original letters, which the brick was marked with, remained a very little disfigured. Previous to putting the brick into the fire, I observed that the materials composing it had not been well mixed, and which I think accounts for the irregular wasting that took place.

I think the Colgong fire-brick good, but inferior to the Stourbridge; but I think the Colgong fire-clay would answer in most cases where Stourbridge clay is used.

(Signed) J. Gilbert.

(A true Copy,)

W. N. Forbes, *Mint Master*.

Calcutta Mint, *the* 12*th May*, 1841.

No. II.—*Report on the Investigation of Cases of real and supposed Poisoning.*

In this paper there are given, *first*, a brief summary of each of the poison cases referred to me within the last twelve months; *secondly*, a general but minute description of the processes followed in their investigation; *thirdly*, an account of Marsh's remarkable process for the detection of arsenic, with an explanation of the fallacies to which it is liable, and the precautions necessary in its practice; *fourthly*, a description of an original process for the detection of the *lalchittra* (plumbago rosea), the root employed so extensively by the natives to cause abortion; *lastly*, the official reports are appended, containing the details of the cases of which a summary is given in the first section.

SECTION I.

SUMMARY OF CASES.

1st Case.

Cholera proving fatal under suspicious circumstances.

The first was a man named *Mahmood Alee*, who after a quarrel with a fellow servant, was suddenly taken ill, and died in eleven hours; the symptoms being vomiting, purging, cramps, and collapse.

The stomach and intestines shewed no marks of inflammation, but were coated with a creamy fluid. This was alkaline to test paper. Examined by the processes hereinafter described, there was no indication of any metallic poison. On destroying the intestines by nitric acid, evaporating the solution, and expelling the excess of acid, a large quantity of crystals of the nitrate of soda were formed.

These experiments sufficed to shew, that the changes in the blood and intestinal fluids, now well known to be occasioned by Cholera, had taken place in this case. The serous portion of the blood had passed into the intestinal tract, which caused the alkaline reaction on the test paper; and with the soda of the fluid, the nitric acid formed the crystals of nitrate of soda, obtained in such remarkable abundance.

On this evidence the Coroner's Jury returned a verdict of—*Died by Cholera;* which disease was at the time prevalent at Calcutta.

Case 2d.

Case of Capt. P. late Political Agent at M———d———

Suspected death by poison.

This was a case of very deep interest. On the 26th of June, 1840, I received by express a package, containing the stomach and intestines of Captain P., a distinguished officer, and the representative of government at a native court. Suspicions having arisen as to the cause of his death, it became desirable to subject the matter to minute investigation.

In the experiments performed in this case, I had the valuable aid of Dr. Thomson, a young chemist of great promise, recently arrived in India, the son of Dr. Thomson, Professor in the Glasgow University.

Referring for details as to the mode of examination to the processes hereinafter described, it suffices here to say, that not the least trace could be found of any of the deleterious substances which analysis enables us to detect.

Case 3.—Poisoning by Yellow Sulphuret of Arsenic.

Dr. Kean of Moorshedabad, in a communication, dated the 14th of July, sent a substance obtained from the stomach of a man supposed to have been poisoned.

The sulphuret of arsenic was detected by the method of examination subsequently detailed.

Case 4.—Poisoning of three Persons by Aconite.

On the — October, the Coroner of Calcutta ordered the examination of a liquid obtained from the stomach of one of three persons, who had suffered from severe and peculiar symptoms soon after their morning meal; one died in eleven hours, the others recovered.

Analysis gave no indication of the presence of any poisonous material. But from the following circumstances, I felt myself warranted in giving it as my opinion in evidence, that the deceased had been poisoned; and that the poison given was in all probability the *bish*, the root of the *aconitum ferox*.

All these persons suffered almost immediately after taking food. The symptoms in all were burning in the throat, numbness of the extremities, transient loss of sight, and giddiness. To this succeeded collapse, sinking of the pulse, and in one case death in eleven hours.

The food eaten was a prawn curry. Cholera was not epidemic at the time. While the symptoms were different from those of all ordinary diseases, they coincided closely with those I had witnessed as the effects of aconite, when given medicinally to man, or as a poison to animals. This aconite, moreover, is one of the best known of the native poisons, and is procurable in every bazar. In the opinion I gave on the inquest, the Police Surgeon, Dr. Maxton, fully agreed.

Case 5.—Poisoning of five Persons by White Arsenic.

On the 29th October, five persons were received into the Hospital of the Medical College, labouring under severe symptoms of gastric irritation; these symptoms supervened immediately after taking food eight hours before, (dhal and rice,) and they resembled strongly the usual effects of arsenic.

An emetic of sulphate of zinc was administered to each patient by the clinical pupil on duty. On the emetic operating, the vomitted matters were kept; but through an oversight, were all mixed together.

The remains of the food had meantime been sent to the College, and sealed up by Mr. Siddons, my assistant.

On analysis the ensuing day, a large quantity of white arsenic was found in the food, and this poison was also detected in the vomitted matters.

Case 6.—Attempt to Poison Major H———n's family.—Detection of Arsenic.

On the 21st October 1840, I received a note from Dr. Garden, forwarding the remains of a rice pudding, on the copper plate in which it had been cooked. Dr. Garden stated that this pudding had been served the evening before at Major H.'s table; that Mrs. H., her European servant, and metranee had eaten of it; that Major H. had tasted it, and that all had been immediately taken ill. A bitter taste was observed by the parties, and the pudding was said to be discoloured.

The pudding was removed from the copper plate by a bone knife. The plate was observed to be very slightly abraded. There was no unpleasant odour, or any other sign of decomposition in the pudding.

A portion, about three ounces, was agitated with distilled water, the solution concentrated, and the tests for copper applied, without the slightest evidence of this metal being present.

No arsenic could be detected, even by Marsh's process *in the watery solution.*

A small portion was now treated with strong and hot nitric acid till dissolved, the solution mixed with eight times its bulk of water, and then neutralized with carbonate of soda. A portion of this solution was introduced into Marsh's apparatus, and the presence of arsenic at once recognized and proved. These experiments, with others, denoted, that it was the sulphuret, not the common arsenic which was used, and proved that impregnation of the pudding with copper, was not the cause of the illness of the sufferers. I am inclined to believe, that the substance introduced was one of the compound native poisons, of which orpiment is an ingredient, and not the pure arsenical poison alone. The bitterness of taste, the proportionately small quantity of arsenic present, and the symptoms of giddiness and intoxication experienced in two of the cases, are my chief reasons for entertaining this opinion.

Case 7.—Supposed Abortion by Drugs.

This case was brought under investigation by Mr. Graham, officiating magistrate at Burdwan, at the desire of Dr. Cheek.

The substance for analysis was a bottle of the fluid found in the stomach and cavity of the abdomen. No trace of the plumbago, *(lalchittra,)* nor of any of the metallic poisons was detected. The generative organs, or the fluids therein found, should have been forwarded for analysis.

Case 8.—Supposed Poisoning by Arsenic.

Mr. Edgeworth, joint-magistrate of Seharunpore, forwarded a piece of bread, which was part of a meal, soon after which a man suffered violently, and died in four hours. The results of the analysis were negative. There was no detectible poison present.

Case 9.—Examination of suspected Powders—Detection of Copper, Red Arsenic, and Corrosive Sublimate.

On the 15th March, Dr. Esdaile forwarded three powders, suspected to be of a poisonous nature. On analysis, the 1st was found to be acetate of copper; the 2nd, a mixture of red arsenic, peroxide of iron and brick dust; the 3d, a mixture of calomel, corrosive sublimate, and brown vegetable matter.

Case 10.—Suspected Arsenic and Aconite.

Mr. Drummond, officiating magistrate of Behar, forwarded two bottles containing a mixture obtained from the stomach of a man, who died under symptoms of poisoning. Three persons had partaken of the poisoned food, and two recovered.

All were rendered insensible. Those who recovered stated, they had experienced intense burning pain and convulsions.

Arsenic and the Nipal poison, *dackra* or *bish*, (aconitum ferox,) were suspected; no arsenic was present. The aconite of course, if present, could not be detected.

Case 11.—Attempt to Poison by Arsenic—Poison detected.

This case came under my investigation by desire of the Calcutta Police on the 14th April. A cook in the family of the Rev. Mr. Wendauger attempted to get rid of the khansamah, by sending a present of fruit, syrup, powdered grain and milk. With the grain, there was white arsenic in a very large quantity.

Case 12.—Murder by Arsenic—Detection of the Poison in the remains of two individuals, after ten months' interment.

These are by far the most interesting cases which I have ever met with. The respectability of the individuals implicated; the extraordinary period which elapsed during which the bodies were exposed, without coffins, to the destroying influences of the heat and rains of Bengal; the curious changes which the poison underwent, and which it occasioned in the parts of the body which it preserved from ordinary decay—constitute an array of circumstances scarcely surpassed in medico-legal interest by any but those of the celebrated Laffarge trial.

As the case scarcely admits of being stated more briefly than in Mr. Latour's letters, I have to refer to the correspondence and report for the details.

SECTION II.

NOTES ON THE EXAMINATION OF SOLIDS OR LIQUIDS, SUSPECTED TO CONTAIN POISON.

The symptoms in each case or set of cases will afford, in most instances, a distinct clue to the class of poisons, one of which may have been used. Of these again, the circle is much narrowed by the circumstance, that several poisons familiarly known and used in Europe, are here either unknown altogether, or so little, as to be never employed.

Again, of the poisons to which the symptoms may point, there are a vast number which cannot be detected by chemical analysis. All animal and vegetable poisons fall under this rule, with the exception of opium, the *lalchittra* or Plumbago, (sp. Europea rosea and zeylanica,) the nux vomica, nut and bark, and the alkalies these contain—lastly, croton oil.

If the symptoms be those of narcotism, viz. deep sleep or insensibility and dilated pupil, and if the general circumstances point to poisoning rather than natural disease, the poisons indicated are *opium*, or its preparations ; *gunjah*, in some of its forms; *stramonium*, or the thorn apple (*datura*). The second case in its commencing stages is generally marked by laughing delirium, and when the narcotism is complete, the body is usually rigid, as if cataleptic. The third is pointed to by deep lethargic sleep and blindness, and this symptom in a majority of cases remains long after recovery. If the sufferer complains of an acrid taste, succeeded by numbness of the mouth and pharynx, numbness, prickling, or partial paralysis of the limbs, giddiness, and a feeling of intoxication, with vomiting and gastro-intestinal irritation, transient blindness, a very slight disturbance of the intellect, and stupor rather than insensibility, the *aconite* root, *(bish,)* is most likely to be the substance used.

Tetanic convulsions denote the effects of the *nux vomica* poisons as a class.

Violent vomiting and purging, cramps, and excruciating pain in the stomach and bowels, are indications of the *arsenical poisons*, or of *ruskapur*, (native corrosive sublimate), *euphorbium*, the *croton oil*, or seeds, (jumalgotha,) the bark of the root of the *lalchittra*, (plumbago.) Cases have taken place in Calcutta, in which sulphate of zinc, and sulphate of copper were the poisons used, and from which similar symptoms would proceed.

I beg it to be remembered, that my object here is to give but a few general hints, and that I do not profess to enter deeply on the subject. Nevertheless, the following Table will be found of some practical utility, by those as yet inexperienced in the chemical examination of these cases* :—

* Hydrocyanic acid, the mineral alkalies, and oxalic acid are omitted, as these poisons do not occur in the practice of medico-legal analysis in India.

Symptoms of,	Denote	Detectible by Analysis.	Not detectible by Analysis.
1. Narcotism. ..	Opium, ...	.... *	
	Gunjah, ...	....	.... *
	Spirits, ...	.... *	
With blindness. .. Narcotism. ..	Datura, ...	....	.... *
With gastric irritation, numbness, and partial blindness.	Aconite, ...	....	.... *
2. Tetannic spasms.	Nux Vomica Bark, Kuchila Mulung, and preparations.	*	
3. Vomiting, purging, cramps and inflammation of stomach and bowels.	Tartar Emetic, ...	*	
	Arsenic, (white or yellow,)	*	
	Corrosive Sublimate, ...	*	
	Euphorbium, ...	....	.... *
	Lalchittra, (Plumbago),	*	
	Copper Poisons, ...	*	
	Croton Oil, ...	*	
	The Mineral Acids, ...	*	
4. Colic and Constipation. ..	White Lead, ...	*	

From my experience in poison cases in India during seven years, I have no hesitation in stating it as my opinion, that in not more than a very trivial proportion of the cases which occur, is the poison one not included in this Table.

ANALYSIS.

Trial Experiments.

Class 1st.

If the symptoms point to the 1st class, our analysis must be directed to opium and spirits.

The smell will often aid us in detecting either. If alcohol be present, it will be almost certainly recognized by the odour. The material suspected should then be introduced into a retort, and distillation conducted over a water bath.

If alcohol, the product will be recognised by its odour and inflammability.

Should opium be suspected, the substance under examination should be evaporated on a water bath to dryness, then boiled with alcohol 835°, in the proportion of four oz. of the spirit to the ounce of solid matter. The tincture obtained should be strained through cloth, then filtered and evaporated on the water bath to dryness. Re-dissolve the extract in distilled water acidulated with muriatic acid,—filter. The alkaline bases, morphia and anarcotine, will be found in this liquid, in combination with muriatic acid.* Ammonia precipitates these alkalies as a whitish powder. Let this dry. Nitric acid strikes a deep red, the permuriate of iron a fine blue colour when dropped upon it.

Class 2d.

The process in this case is directed towards the detection of strychnine and brucine, the active ingredients of this class of poisons.

* If opium be present in any quantity exceeding ten grains.

Treat with alcohol as in the last case; but in testing any precipitate, instead of per-muriate of iron, use the proto-muriate of tin, this with brucine strikes a very fine violet colour. An infusion of nux vomica nut or bark, is turned red by nitric acid, and this simple test will give important corroborative evidence, in cases in which the tetanic paroxysms had been strongly marked.

Class 3d, and 4th.

Examine the solid matters carefully, and observe if any heavy white or yellow powder be seen to separate from the mass. Then wash with distilled water, frequently decanting; white or yellow powders will thus often subside. Test any fluid part with blue litmus paper; if it be very strongly reddened, the presence of the mineral acids may be suspected. Try whether the fluid causes effervescence when dropped on chalk, if it does, the evidence of the presence of a strong acid is much corroborated. The symptoms of the case will throw light upon the question. The strong acids invariably cause an insupportably acid and burning taste, followed quickly by corrosion and excoriation of the lips, mouth, and fauces. The acids, however, are so little used in India, that poisoning by them must be extremely rare, if it ever occurs. No case has fallen within my observation in seven years' experience.

Detection of the Mineral Acids.

Should, however, acids be indicated, neutralize with pure carbonate of soda, dilute with distilled water, filter and test as follows:—

To a portion of the liquid, add a solution of nitrate of baryta—if a copious precipitate takes place, which is not dissolved on adding nitric acid, it indicates *sulphuric acid.* Collect, dry, and weigh the precipitate; 118 grains of sulphate of baryta, correspond to forty grains of sulphuric acid.

It must be remembered, that the contents of the stomach and intestines are naturally acid, and sulphate of magnesia or soda may have been taken medicinally by the person, whose case we are investigating. As the elucidation of this difficulty depends altogether on general and on pathological evidence, I need notice it no further.

To a second portion of the liquid, add a solution of nitrate of silver; if a precipitate ensues, collect and dry it.

Ascertain if it be soluble in ammonia and the solution be precipitated by being acidulated with nitric acid. 144 grains of the precipitate after being heated nearly to redness, correspond to 36½ *muriatic acid.*

It must however be borne in mind, that muriatic acid is naturally present in the stomach, and that the muriate of soda of ordinary food will give this precipitate. I need not, however, dwell on the difficulties thus presented. Muriatic acid is very unlikely to be used as a poison in India, and if so used, the investigation presents so many difficulties, that none but an expert analyst could overcome them. It is not to such that these cursory remarks are addressed.

Nitric acid will always give evidence of its action by the yellow stains it causes almost immediately, and on every tissue with which it comes in contact. Neutralize the solution with carbonate of lime, note the degree of effervescence, evaporate to dryness on a water bath, heat the residue with alcohol at 900°—filter. This dissolves the nitrate of lime; evaporate as before. Introduce the residue into a very small retort and add its weight of sulphuric acid; distil; nitric acid is obtained, and if one drop be procured, we can readily identify it. A few copper filings thrown on it, causes lively effervescence and the escape of brown fumes of nitrous acid; and a particle of morphia placed on it, becomes of a vermillion color.

In all these experiments, it will be seen that we have employed as re-agents, only the following articles:—

Water.	Nitrate of silver.
Alcohol.	Morphia.
Ammonia.	Carbonate of lime.
Nitric acid.	Permuriate of iron.
Sulphuric acid.	Protomuriate of tin.

While the detectible poisons we are in search of are,

Compounds of antimony, copper, arsenic, mercury, lead, the lalchittra, and the croton oil.

Therefore all the liquids and products of the preceding experiments may be mixed apart for further examination, except the portion to which the permuriate of iron and protomuriate of tin had been added as tests. If the solid or fluid mixture be considerable in quantity, take a small portion, agitate with boiling distilled water, strain through cloth, then filter through paper, and when cool, try small separate portions by the following tests:—

Trial Tests for Metallic Poisons.

1. Ammoniaco-nitrate of silver.
2. Hydro-sulphuret of ammonia.
3. Hydriodate of potash.
4. Ammonia.
5. Ferro-prussiate of potash.
6. Proto-muriate of tin.
7. Ammoniaco-sulphate of copper.
8. A slip of polished iron.
9. A slip of gold, with an iron wire round it.

If *white arsenic* be present in solution,

No. 1 will give a yellow precipitate. }
No. 2 a yellow. .. .. .. } or traces of these effects.
No. 7 a green. .. .. .. }

If *copper* be present in solution,

No. 2 will give a black precipitate... .. }
No. 5 a brown; 4, a blue solution. .. .. } or traces of these effects.
Nos. 8 and 9, a coating of metallic copper. }

If *antimony* be present in solution, 2 gives an orange precipitate.

If *mercury* be present in solution, 6 will give a grey precipitate, 3 a yellow or red soluble in excess of the test, 2 a black precipitate, 9 a coating of metallic mercury.

If *Lead* be present in solution, 3 gives a yellow, 2 a black precipitate.

But arsenic may be present as *sulphuret*, and antimony, copper, or mercury in the insoluble state, and these tests give no indication whatever of the presence of the poison; a further process is therefore requisite. Acidulate the mixtures strongly with a concentrated solution of tartaric acid, and a little muriatic acid—boil and filter.—This dissolves the insoluble antimonial compounds, which may be present as poisons. Test the solution (previously evaporated to the consistence of thin syrup) with hydrosulphuret of ammonia. If *antimony* be present, an orange precipitate is formed.

If this test gives no indication, it remains to seek for arsenic in the insoluble form.

Mix all the solid matters and fluids with twice their bulk of the strongest nitric acid in a China vessel, and heat gently.

When all is dissolved, dilute with four times its volume of distilled water, neutralize with carbonate of soda, acidulate with acetic acid slightly, and filter through Nipal paper—divide into two portions.

With one portion repeat the trial tests already described.

With the second, have recourse to *Marsh's method* for the detection of arsenic. This admirable process cannot be too prominently brought to notice, and it needs, moreover, certain precautions not yet sufficiently attended to in the practice of forensic analysis.

MARSH'S PROCESS FOR ARSENIC.

Marsh's process consists essentially in causing hydrogen gas to be slowly liberated in contact with the arsenical substance, with which it combines. On burning the gas in a glass tube, a crust of metallic arsenic and of arsenious acid is deposited, and may be recognised by characters described in the sequel.

The following simple apparatus suffices to perform this process :—

Have the bottom of a quart bottle cut off by one of the native workmen who prepare shells and glass bangles, and who are found in all the bazars. To the neck of the bottle adjust a cork and a jet made of brass or sheet copper, provided with a stop cock, if this can be had, if not a little piece of wood with a conical hollow may be adapted as a stopple to the tube, and used from time to time to check the issue of the gas.

In this bottle, place a slip of *rolled zinc*, and then the cork being removed, introduce the whole into a jar half-full of dilute sulphuric acid, (strong acid one, water ten parts,) as soon as there is effervescence, stop the jet. The gas collecting within will displace the acid, and cause the liquid to ascend in the outer vessel—open the jet and allow the gas to escape. Repeat this twice or three times, in order to expel all the common air the inner jar contains, otherwise an explosion may occur on lighting the gas, as mixtures of hydrogen and common air detonate with extreme violence. By following the precautions above stated, no accident can occur.

Now inflame the gas. If the zinc be pure the flame is nearly invisible, does not fume, and is devoid of odour.

To study Marsh's process, and witness its extreme delicacy, it is now only necessary to remove the cork, and pour into the inner bottle two or three drops of the common watery solution of arsenic, known as "Fowler's Drops." On inflaming the gas, it will be seen that the flame has assumed a dull leaden colour, it evolves a white vapour, and emits a decided garlic smell.

Apply the flame, which must not be larger than a pea, to the inside of a glass tube open at each end, a crust of metallic nature and steel grey crystalline aspect is immediately deposited just above the flame; above the crust is a whitish deposit, and towards the top, drops of condensed watery vapour are formed.

If the tube be applied to the nostril, the garlic smell is extremely evident. If the metallic crust be heated over a spirit lamp flame, it is volatilized and dispersed.

If the crust be touched with a glass rod previously dipped in dilute nitric acid, then touched with a solution of nitrate of silver, and lastly the tube held over a phial of ammonia, the interior of the tube is soon covered with bright yellow flakes of the arsenite of silver.

In our search for arsenic, we first try this process by pouring a part of the fluid matter suspected into the interior jar, *after having previously burned a portion of the gas produced by the zinc alone. The common bazar zinc contains arsenic itself, and must never be used in these experiments.* New zinc must also be used in each distinct case, as zinc which has once detected arsenic, is apt to retain a trace of the poison.

The fluid matter often occasions inconvenient frothing in the jar. When this occurs, the gas will not burn. The best plan to prevent it, is by pouring a very thin layer of sweet oil on the fluid in the internal jar.

Application of Marsh's Process *to the Sulphurets of Arsenic.*

If the fluid part of the suspected mixture contain no arsenic, we have next to seek for it in the solid part. Here it may be in the state of the red or yellow sulphuret, neither of which compounds can be detected by Marsh's process, which will only succeed with the oxyacids and soluble oxysalts of this metal.

Boil the solid matter in a porcelain capsule with strong nitric acid in excess, when brown fumes cease to be disengaged on the addition of fresh acid, boil down to the consistence of a syrup. Dilute largely with distilled water, neutralize with carbonate of soda, and filter. If there has been the smallest conceivable quantity of arsenic in the solid matter, Marsh's process will now detect it in this solution, the nitric acid having converted the sulphuret of arsenic into arsenious or arsenic acid.

It is not necessary to use the whole of the fluid resulting from the nitric acid process in our search for arsenic. Two-thirds of the acid liquid may be reserved, neutralized without filtration, re-acidulated with a few drops of nitric acid, and tested for mercury by a slip of gold and iron wire; for copper, by ammonia, hydro-sulphuret of ammonia and prussiate of potash; for lead, by hydro-sulphuret of ammonia, and ioduret of potassium.

In using the latter test, it must be always applied to a neutral solution.

I may mention here, that a good substitute for litmus paper is made of white blotting paper, coloured by the blue juice of the flowers of the *Hibiscus rosa-sinensis*—shoe-flower, (Jaba, *Sans.*)—turmeric paper is best prepared with fine post paper, dyed by a tincture of turmeric root in proof spirit.

Fallacies in Marsh's Process.

1. Impurities of the zinc;—the mode of avoiding this, I have already pointed out.

2. Antimonial compounds also give a metallic crust with a white clouded stain. The subsequent test of nitrate of silver and ammonia, distinguishes these to the most inexperienced, while persons familiar with the appearances of arsenic cannot be deceived by the resemblance of the crusts separately.

3. Orfila has lately announced the discovery of arsenic in the bony parts of the human body in exceedingly small proportions; but still detectible by Marsh's method. I have used the whole of the stomach and intestines in Captain P.'s case, and the whole of the same viscera in case No. 1, without an atom of arsenic appearing—*and appear it must, had it been present.* Still Orfila's evidence should make us cautious; finding a mere trace while operating on *large quantities* will not suffice to satisfy a British jury or judge in the face of Orfila's discovery—though strange to say, his finding such a trace under such circumstances exactly, led to the condemnation of Madame Laffarge.

Lastly.—The sulphuric acid of commerce often contains arsenic; so does the nitric acid, also the peroxide of iron, so much used of late as an antidote. The analyst must therefore subject equal quantities of these re-agents separately to trial, in order to enable him to give a positive opinion.

To detect Corrosive Sublimate, Lalchittra, and Croton Oil.

Agitate the suspected solution with one-third its volume of sulphuric ether in a tall narrow glass vessel. When the ether has risen to the surface, remove by a small syphon to a capsule. Repeat this while the ether is coloured. Let the ethereal solutions evaporate spontaneously. If corrosive sublimate be present, crystals are deposited, which are soluble in water, give an orange precipitate with lime water, a carmine red with hydriodate of potash, and a stain of metallic mercury when placed on gold leaf moistened with dilute sulphuric acid, and touched with an iron wire.

If croton oil be present, the ethereal solution deposits the oil as it evaporates. This cannot be recognized by any further test than administration to a dog, in which two or three drops will soon cause violent purging.

If the ethereal solution contains the *lalchittra*, this is at once detected by the superb crimson colour it strikes with every alkaline solution; nay so delicate is it to these re-agents that a little calcined magnesia thrown into a solution containing traces of this substance, will in a few hours assume a delicate rosy hue.

Some years since, in investigating a case of alleged poisoning for the Calcutta Police, I observed that the filtering paper employed was stained at the edges of a fine red colour. The same phenomenon was observed on adding subacetate of lead in one of the trial tests. I was not then acquainted with the *lalchitra*, and could not trace the cause of these appearances; but their nature is now sufficiently evident.

I must mention prominently, however, that there are other yellow colouring matters, which with alkalies, present analogous appearances; but to any one who takes the trouble of comparing the effects in a series of experiments on such articles as turmeric, rhubarb, colombo root, the mishmee teeta, &c. no difficulty will arise in his decision if plumbago be present. Rhubarb perhaps approaches nearer than any other; but with caustic magnesia, rhubarb gives a yellowish brown, while plumbago gives a crimson sediment.

To illustrate the delicacy of this process, five grains of powdered plumbago were mixed with eight ounces of putrid blood and filth from the dissecting room; dilute sulphuric acid was added, and the mixture warmed and strained through cloth. A nearly colourless solution was obtained, this was treated with ether, and the ethereal solution separated; on mixing this with a weak solution of potash in water, the characteristic crimson colour at once appeared.

Preservation and Despatch of Suspected Matters.

Three objects should be carefully attended to in the despatch of all suspected matters;—the proof of identity; the impossibility of any interference during transit; and, thirdly, preservation from decomposition.

I have frequently received articles for analysis in bottles merely corked, in wooden boxes, secured by a few nails, &c. In more than one case the contents of bottles had partially escaped, or those of various parcels were mixed together.

It is obvious that it would be exceedingly difficult to convict any accused party on evidence given on the analysis of such articles.

Articles for analysis should be, whenever practicable, enclosed in glass bottles accurately corked, tied, and sealed with hard wax, and by the private seal of the surgeon or magistrate. Bottles should be enclosed in a thick layer of raw cotton, and all placed in tin and soldered up. When wooden boxes must be used, these should be sealed and taped at every opening, below as well as above.

All liquid and animal matters liable to decomposition should be put up in or mixed with the strongest spirit available. This effectually prevents decomposition, and without interfering with the subsequent analysis, thereby obviates many serious accidents. I have known two instances of bottles bursting, and the contents being totally lost in transit by the fermentation of their contents. In Major P's. case, one of the bottles exploded in the Laboratory with a loud report, and the contents were lost except a small portion.

Poison Cases—Extracts from Correspondence and Reports.

Supposed abortion by drugs.

To the Chemical Examiner, *Calcutta.*

Sir,—I have the honour to forward an extract from a letter addressed to me by Mr. Civil Assistant-Surgeon Cheek, and also the bottle of fluid therein alluded to, and shall feel obliged by your analizing the contents and favouring me with your opinion as to whether they contain any poisonous matter.

West Burdwan Jt. Magte. Office, T. W. Graham,
January 2, 1840. *Offg. Joint Magistrate.*

Extract from a letter from Mr. G. N. Cheek, Civil Assistant-Surgeon of Bancoorah, dated 30th December, 1840.

I cannot say if drugs had been given to procure abortion. I can say the vagina shewed none of the effects. I can say from the extensive adhesions, considerable inflammation had previously existed, particularly in the liver and stomach and omentum; from the dissection, I am of opinion the woman died from disease, not from drugs. However, as it is of great moment to detect if any poison has been given, I beg leave to send a bottle, containing part of the fluid found in the stomach and cavity of the abdomen, and trust you will please send it for examination, &c.

True Extract,
(Signed) T. W. Graham,
Offg. Joint Magistrate.

(For Result see page 720.)

Poisonous and suspected Powders.

To the Chemical Examiner, *Calcutta.*

Sir,—May I request you to be good enough to examine the accompanying Powders, and give me your opinion of their nature, for the information of the Magistrate.

(Signed) J. Esdaile.
Hooghly, March 15, 1841.

To Dr. Esdaile,
Civil Surgeon, &c. Hooghly.

Sir,—In reply to your letter of the 15th inst. I have the honour to inform you of the results of the analysis of the contents of the little parcels therewith forwarded.

No. 1. was of light blue colour, difficultly soluble in water, dissolved by strong sulphuric acid, emitting copious vapours of acetic acid;—solution diluted with water gave a copious precipitate of metallic copper on the introduction of a slip of zinc.

Result. Acetate of Copper.

No 2. Red, and confusedly crystalline. Heated on platinum foil to redness was volatilized with the exception of about one-third. The residue was partially dissolved by nitro-muriatic acid, still leaving an earthy reddish matter. The solution when diluted, was precipitated blue by prussiate of potash, and black by tincture of galls. Heated in a small glass tube a sublimate of two zones, one bright yellow, the second vivid red, was formed.

Heated with caustic potash in a small glass tube, a metallic crust was formed by sublimation.

A very small portion of the original powder was boiled with a few drops of nitric acid, the solution neutralized and introduced into Marsh's hydrogen apparatus. The hydrogen inflamed in glass tubes gave copious metallic crusts, which became vivid yellow when touched with ammoniaco-nitrate of silver.

Result. Peroxide of Iron.
Earthy matter, probably brick-dust.
Red Sulphuret of arsenic (Realgar.)

No. 3, *a brown powder*—burned away rapidly on platinum foil—mixed with water, a white heavy powder subsided. A portion of this powder was volatile in dense white fumes from platinum foil, insoluble in water; boiled with nitro-muriatic acid, the solution crystallized on cooling—the crystals were dissolved in water; solution precipitated red by potash, yellow and red by hydriodate of potash, gave a silvery metallic stain to gold leaf on being touched with iron wire.

Another portion of the powder was agitated with sulphuric ether in a long glass tube. The ethereal solution by spontaneous evaporation gave crystals presenting the characters above described.

The brown vegetable matter did not offer any special characters.

Result. Vegetable matter.
Calomel, } Probably powdered *Ruskapore*, a
Corrosive sublimate } native mixture of both.

Besides the above, No. 3 contained small particles of acetate of copper like No. 1.

In reporting these details I would feel obliged by your communicating to me any particulars as to the purpose to which the powders were applied, or under which these became the subject of inquiry.

(Signed) W. B. O'S.

CALCUTTA, *the* 15*th March*, 1841.

Poisoning by Sulphuret of Arsenic.

TO THE CHEMICAL EXAMINER, *Calcutta*.

Moorshedabad, 14*th July*, 1841.

MY DEAR SIR,—About a fortnight ago, the body of a man was sent to me with the view of ascertaining the cause of his death. On opening the body, I found the internal coat of the stomach inflamed, as if painted with vermillion, and corrugated towards the pylorus, like bundles of worms. The same symptoms of inflam-

* Two such.

matory action extended throughout the inner coat of the œsophagus, the duodenum, and small intestines, and they all contained a glairy gelatinous sort of matter of a yellowish tinge. The external coats were little if at all affected.

The eyes were very red, and the brain and its membranes highly vascular. Other viscera all natural except the lungs and pleura, which were highly inflamed. In the contents of the stomach I observed pieces of a substance like the root called by the natives "Meetah," and yellow particles, which are probably orpiment, also pieces of a substance of a darkish colour, and others (only a few) whitish and shining, the former probably an ore of arsenic, and the latter the white oxide.

The sulphuret being so little soluble was most abundant. I tried the fluid with ammoniated nitrate of silver and sulphate of copper, but from the presence of the gelatinous matter I suppose, the result was not satisfactory. I then mixed the matter (dried) with charcoal and subjected it to a red heat in a tobacco pipe, when I obtained an incrustation of a bluish metallic appearance; but so minute that I could not be sure that it gave out an alliaceous smell on burning, though I perceived it did.

I enclose for you some of the matter dried on filtering paper, just as it was taken from the stomach, and will feel obliged if you will test it, and let me know whether I am right in pronouncing it arsenic.

(Signed) A. KEAN.

Calcutta, 18*th July*, 1840.

MY DEAR SIR,—In reply to your letter received yesterday, I have to acquaint you, that on examining the yellow substance it enclosed, and which I received with the seal of the packet uninjured, I find it is chiefly composed of the yellow sulphuret of arsenic. I reduced it to the metallic state by Marsh's hydrogen process, and subsequently tested the metal in the usual way.

(Signed) W. B. O'S.

Attempt to Poison by Arsenic.

TO CAPTAIN BIRCH,
Superintendent of Police, Calcutta.

DEAR SIR,—I send you a man, who was several months my Cook. I found him often to be a thief as he made the Bazar, therefore I took a Khansamah some weeks ago, to the greatest dislike of the Cook. By this you may have a clearer insight in the following. This morning my Khansamah told me, that the Cook sent him something by the milk woman, to whom he sent; he wishes the Khansamah to eat this, but he would not eat it, when he would himself give it to him; the Khansamah heard this by the woman, who warnt him not to eat it. He therefore supposes that there is poison in it. I send the thing, which is supposed to be poisoned, and the Cook to you, that you may do as you find it the best.

MIRZAPORE, *the* 14*th April*, 1841. J. CH. WENDRAGET.

Result,—A large quantity of white arsenic was found in the dish.

W. B. O'S.

Suspected poisoning.—Death by Cholera.

Copy of Deposition before the Coroner in the case of Mahomed Ali.

29th October, 1840.

I received from Dr. Maxton a stomach, a piece of its lower or pyloric orifice, some liquid stated to have been contained in the stomach, and the small intestines, with the contents thereof, all stated to have been removed from the body of a man I saw lying dead in the Native Hospital on the 26th instant.

I have analysed the liquid of the stomach, the washings of the same organ, and the contents of the intestines. I have also analysed the whole substance of the small intestines, and have no hesitation in stating that no trace whatever of arsenic, antimony, mercury, copper, zinc, nor of any of the metallic poisons, existed in the substances examined. I saw no powder nor other vegetable irritating substance, nor any appearance of its action. I found on the mucous membrane of the small intestines, a pasty liquid mixed with albuminous flakes. I analysed it, and found it to agree in chemical composition with the matter voided by purging in the disease called Cholera, which matter is of a peculiar nature, and easily distinguished from ordinary evacuations.

I have also heard the symptoms of the illness of the deceased described by Mr. O'Brien. Assuming the description to be correct, I am opinion from it, and the facts above stated, and the appearance of the intestines, that the deceased died of Cholera. I wish to add too, that Cholera may prove fatal without the occurrence of any profuse evacuation from the bowels.

W. B. O'SHAUGHNESSY.

Bread supposed to be Poisoned.

TO THE CHEMICAL EXAMINER, *Calcutta.*

SIR,—I have the honour to transmit copies of correspondence noted in the margin, and to request that you will analyze the piece of bread herewith enclosed, and favour me with the result whether any poison is contained in it or not.

Joint Magistrate's letter to Civil Surgeon, No. 318, dated 18th November 1840.
Civil Surgeon's reply, dated the 19th ditto.
Joint Magistrate's letter, No. 323, dated 28th ditto.
Civil Surgeon's reply, dated 30th ditto.
Memorandum dated 1st December.
Officiating Magistrate's letter to Sessions Judge, No. 843, dated 23rd December, do.
Letter from Secretary to Government of Agra to Sessions Judge, No. 32, dated 7th January, 1841.

(Signed) M. P. EDGEWORTH,
Joint Magistrate.

MAGISTRATE'S OFFICE,
ZILLAH SEHARANPOOR,
The — January, 1841.

To G. W. Bacon, Esq.
Session Judge of Zillah Seharanpoor.

Sir,—I have the honour to enclose copies of communications from the Civil Surgeon, relative to a case of alleged poisoning.

2. As there appear strong grounds for presuming that the deceased Dassee, was poisoned, and as the body was burned without medical examination, it is of importance to ascertain whether the piece of bread preserved by his brother, contains poison or not; I therefore beg you will take such measures as may be necessary to procure its examination, &c.

(Signed) M. P. Edgeworth,
Officiating Magistrate.

No. 318.

To H. Falconer, Esq. *Civil Assistant Surgeon, Seharanpoor.*

Sir,—I have the honour to request that you will examine the accompanying piece of bread, the remains of a chapattee, which is said to have been the cause of the death of Dasi Bania, and to inform me whether you can find any trace of poisonous matter in it.

I have, &c.

(Signed) M. P. Edgeworth, *Joint Magistrate.*

To M. P. Edgeworth, Esq.
Joint Magistrate of Seharanpoor.

Sir,—In reply to your letter No. 318 of yesterday, I have the honour to inform you, that I have not the means of satisfactorily going through the very complicated chemical analysis, which would be required to determine the presence or otherwise of poisonous matter in the portion of chapattee sent to me, I therefore beg to return it, and in case of an analysis being required for the ends of justice, I would suggest your having the suspected matter sent on to Dr. O'Shaughnessy, Calcutta, through the Agra Government.

I have, &c.

(Signed) H. Falconer, M. D. *Civil Assistant Surgeon.*

Seharanpoor, 19*th November*, 1840.

No. 323.

To H. Falconer, Esq.
Civil Assistant Surgeon, Seharanpoor.

Sir,—With reference to the same case in which I sent you some bits of bread for analysis, I have now the honour to send two Hukeems, with a copy of their depositions before me, who attended the deceased; and shall be obliged if you will examine them yourself, and inform me, if from the symptoms they detail you can form any opinion, whether the deceased appears to have died from poison or disease.

MAGISTRATE'S OFFICE,
ZILLAH SEHARANPOOR,
The 28th November, 1840.

I have, &c.
(Signed) M. P. EDGEWORTH, *Joint Magistrate.*

To M. P. EDGEWORTH, ESQ.
Joint Magistrate, Seharanpoor.

SIR,—In reply to your letter No. 323, of the 28th instant, I have the honour to inform you that I have minutely examined the Hukeems Shibdial and Sewak Ram regarding the case of the late Dassee Bunneeah, inhabitant of Gungo, and I am of opinion that from their evidence there are the strongest presumptive grounds to support the belief, that the deceased died of poisoning by an active corrosive poison, such as arsenic, and not from a natural disease.

The Keyfeats sent with your letter are herewith returned.

I have, &c.
(Signed) H. FALCONER, M. D.
Civil Assistant Surgeon.

SEHARANPOOR, *30th November*, 1840.

Memorandum of the Evidences given by Shibdial, and Sewak Ram, Brahmin, Hakeems, regarding the case of Dassee Bunneeah, of Gungo.

Both deponents state that they were summoned about 9 or 10 o'clock at night to go and see Dassee; that on their arrival they found him insensible, with weak thready pulse; that he soon became cold, and they left him in a moribund state.

They aver, that so far as they could learn from his relations he was in excellent health up to about half an hour after sunset, when after eating his evening meal, consisting of wheat cakes and Arabee, he went out, and immediately felt unwell, and was brought back by the aid of other men, complaining of intense pain in his stomach, burning heat in his throat, great depression of strength, and general agony; that he had one bout of vomiting after a draught of water saturated with salt; he had no convulsions, nor discharge from the bowels; and died within three or four hours after his meal.

Spasmodic cholera is a most unlikely explanation of such a case; and I know of no other natural disease which could in the least account for it.

On the whole, I am of opinion that there are strong presumptive grounds for entertaining the belief that the deceased died from poisoning. The symptoms which he exhibited are exactly such as are observed to follow a large excessive dose of arsenic in certain cases.

(Signed) H. FALCONER, M. D.
Civil Assistant Surgeon.

SEHARANPOOR, *1st December*, 1840.

M. P. EDGEWORTH, Esq.

Joint Magistrate, Seharanpoor.

SIR,—I have the honour to report that I have examined and analysed the piece of bread which accompanied your letter, No. 15, of January 1841. The bread contains none of the poisons which can be detected by chemical analysis.

(Signed) W. B. O'S.

Poisoning probably by Aconite.

TO THE CHEMICAL EXAMINER, *Calcutta.*

Sir,—I have the honour to forward by this day's dawk, a box containing two bottles, the contents of which I request the favour of your subjecting to chemical analysis, for the purpose of ascertaining the presence of poison, and the nature thereof.

The circumstances of the case are briefly as follows:—Three men on their way from Bengal to the N. W. Provinces were joined on the road by a fourth individual, who accompanied them about two stages and took an opportunity of mixing poison of some description with some suttoo and goor, which he gave them to eat, or (which is more probable,) with some water which he gave them to mix with the above mentioned food at about noon of the 27th ultimo. One of the men who died from the effects of the poison, became insensible almost immediately, and died about 4 P. M.

The other two who had drunk less of the water, became also, after a short interval, insensible; but recovered through the application of remedies during the night, about twelve hours after taking the poison.

They describe their sensations as those of great heat and burning internally, accompanied with the most violent contortion of their limbs, and a feeling as if they were struggling under an exceedingly heavy load upon their shoulders.

The man who died, laid down almost immediately after taking the poison, and never again betrayed any symptoms of animation beyond slight respiration.

A copy of the certificate of the Civil Surgeon is annexed, from which you will see, that he suspects the presence of arsenic; but a vegetable poison called "Dakra," a root I believe imported from Nipal, is also much used in this part of the country, and it is not improbable may have been used on this occasion.

I beg the favour of your informing me, as soon as possible, of the result of your investigation, and giving me at the same time whatever information you may possess regarding the nature of the Dakra poison, with the best antidotes to be used in cases where it may have been given.

(Signed) EDMUND DRUMMOND,
Officiating Magistrate.

BEHAR MAGISTRACY, *Gyah, the 7th April,* 1841.

Civil Surgeon's Certificate.

Gyah, 28th March, 1841.

Examined the body of a man, (name unknown,) who is reported to have eaten suttoo with two other men, and shortly afterwards all three were taken ill with similar symptoms, and the deceased died about four hours after partaking of the food.

On opening the abdomen, found a considerable degree of inflammation generally of the intestines, and the stomach contained a quantity of undigested suttoo, its lining membrane was in a very highly inflamed state, and there was also some effusion of bloody fluid in the cavity of the abdomen. The above appearances I considered sufficient to account for death.

Having preserved the contents of the stomach, I next day gave a small portion to a chicken, which had the effect of making it apparently very uneasy during the day, and it died next morning about 20 hours after eating the suttoo. I also attempted some of the usual tests for arsenic, but my means of analysis were too imperfect to give any results; but from the circumstances attending the case as related to me, the simultaneous illness of the three men, and the highly inflamed state of the stomach of the deceased, I think there exist the strongest grounds for concluding, that some poisonous substance was mixed with the suttoo eaten by the three men; and should it appear necessary to ascertain the nature of the poison, I would beg to suggest, that the contents of the stomach (which I have preserved) be forwarded to the Government Chemical Examiner for analysis.

(Signed) J. B. Dickson,
Civil Assistant Surgeon.

(A true copy,)
Edmund Drummond, *Officiating Magistrate.*

Report.

To Edmund Drummond, Esq.
Officiating Magistrate, Behar.

Sir,—I have the honour to acquaint you that I have analysed the contents of the bottles described in your letter of the 7th instant. They contained no metallic poison, and from their putrefaction and state of admixture, no vegetable poison could be detected.

The poison you allude to, is the root of the Aconitum Ferox of Nipal. No antidote for it has yet been discovered, and it cannot be detected by chemical analysis, unless when used in much larger quantities than are sufficient to destroy life.

From the symptoms you describe, I am of opinion, that this aconite, together with the seeds of the stramonium, were the poisons used in the cases reported.

(Signed) W. B. O'S.

22d April, 1841.

No. 93.

Poisoning of two persons of rank. Discovery of ARSENIC *in the remains after burial for eight months.**

TO THE CHEMICAL EXAMINER,

Medical College, Calcutta.

SIR,—I have the honor to intimate, that in pursuance of orders received from the Session Judge of Bhaugulpoor, I have this day despatched by dâk banghy to your address two jars containing the remains of two individuals who died on the 27th of May last, from the effects of arsenic, as deposed in evidence.

2. The defendant, a woman of high connection, is now under trial on my commitment at Bhaugulpoor for wilful murder.

3. No medical examination having taken place at the time of the death, or on the arrival of the bodies at Monghyr (five days afterwards), and there being no chemical apparatus or any kind of laboratory in the Bhaugulpoor or Monghyr establishment, Mr. Williams has directed me to transmit their remains as exhumed in my presence, and selected by Dr. Macrae to you, with a request that under the circumstances above set forth, you will kindly undertake the investigation, and submit the results.

I have &c.,

(Signed) E. LATOUR,

Joint Magistrate.

MONGHYR FOUZDARRY ADAWLUT,

The 5*th February*, 1841.

Report.

TO E. LATOUR, ESQ.

Joint Magistrate, &c. Monghyr Fouzdarry Adawlut.

SIR,—The boxes, the despatch of which was announced by your letter of the 5th instant reached me on the 21st, and I this day proceeded to their examination.

2. The seals on both were in good preservation; the jar contained in No. 1 was entire, and its coverings and seals perfect; the jar No. 2 was broken, but its contents uninjured in any way.

3. The jar No. 1, contained a mass of bones, decomposed animal matter and earth, together weighing 4 lbs. 10 oz.; one mass which weighed 2 lbs. 10 oz. was found to consist of the lumbar vertebræ, sacrum, and the right side of the pelvis of a human male subject of small stature, but adult age. The rectum or straight intestine was in its natural position and in a state of preservation. Adjacent to it were masses of muscular and membranous fatty tissues, partially converted into a firm ammoniacal soap, or the substance usually termed *adipocire*. There was but little odour perceptible, and that quite different from that of ordinary putrid animal matter.

4. The jar No. 2 contained a mass of soft animal matter, chiefly converted into ammoniacal soap, but in which the stomach and portions of the intestines of an adult

* The bodies were buried without coffins, and exposed to the influence of the rains.

W. B. O'S.

human subject were easily traced. The membranous walls of the organs were in fact in so perfect a state of preservation, as to enable me distinctly to ascertain, that during life they had been the seat of violent inflammatory action.

Jar. No. 1.

On laying open the rectum intestine, its coats were found to be dyed throughout in several patches of an intensely vivid yellow colour, not removable by washing or friction. The intestine was devoid of smell and empty.

A small portion, about 2 drachms, of the yellow membrane was boiled in a porcelain capsule with 2 drachms of nitric acid till it was completely dissolved. The acid was then neutralized with ammonia and half of the resulting liquid *(a ×)* subjected to the action of hydrogen in Marsh's apparatus. By the burning of the hydrogen in glass tubes, several brilliant metallic crusts were obtained. These crusts were volatile by heat, evolved a powerful smell of garlic, and when touched with ammoniacal nitrate of silver, became of a vivid canary colour. Portions of the liquor *(a ×)* were also tested by the common method with ammoniaco-nitrate of silver *(a)* am-sulphate of copper *(b)*, and hydro-sulphuret of ammonia *(c)*, and gave characteristic yellow *(a)*, green *(b)*, and yellow precipitates *(c)*.

These experiments clearly prove the presence of yellow arsenic in the intestines of the deceased. They shew too that arsenic must have been taken or administered during life, and in a quantity more than sufficient to cause death.

There was no arsenic found in the earthy matter or in the adipocire.

It is not certain that it was the *yellow* arsenic which was given during life. It may have been the *white* arsenic, and that this was changed to *yellow* by the presence of sulphurretted hydrogen in the intestines immediately before or even after death.

Jar. No. 2.

At one end of the stomach a bright yellow patch was noticed. This was detached, the colour was found to pervade the whole structure of the part. On washing with water the colour was not removed, but the whole of the tissues of the part became distinct, and high vascularity, with destruction of the membrane by ulceration were perfectly evident.

A portion of the yellow membrane having been examined in the manner above specified, yielded abundant crusts of metallic arsenic.

The remains unemployed in these experiments and the arsenical products, have been carefully preserved under my seal, for further reference if required.

The zinc, acids, tests, apparatus, &c. employed in the above processes, were all simultaneously tried, and found to be entirely free from any arsenical ingredient.

I have, &c.

(Signed) W B. O'Shaughnessy, M. D.

Chemical Examiner to Government.

Medical College, *Calcutta, 23rd February,* 1841.

SECTION IV.

GENERAL TREATMENT OF POISONING.

The indications of treatment are,

1. To remove the poison from the stomach and alimentary canal.

2. To chemically neutralize the poison, or render it insoluble, and thereby prevent the absorption into the circulation of what cannot be at once removed.

3. If any absorption has taken place, to cause the poison to be excreated as soon as possible.

4. To obviate the local and remote effects the poison may have occasioned.

To meet the *first* object, we have recourse to the stomach pump, emetics, and purgatives.

For directions as to the use of the stomach pump, see p. 137—I should here remark, that in the case of poisoning by nux vomica or strychnine, the stomach pump cannot be employed. In an awful case of this kind I lately witnessed, every touch of the instrument on the patient's throat threw him into almost fatal convulsions. The stomach pump too is not invariably successful in removing the poison. There is in the museum of the Medical College, the stomach of a woman poisoned by white arsenic, in whom the pump had been ineffectually though skilfully used an hour after the poison was swallowed. The arsenic adhered so firmly to the mucous coat of the organ that none could be removed for analysis by washing, or even by the finger. Thus the employment of the stomach pump must never be allowed to supersede the use of other measures.

Emetics.—These remedies are especially useful in the treatment of poisoning by the *narcotics*, and chiefly in the cases of datura, spirit, opium, and aconite. The *acrid* poisons generally cause vomiting themselves. In India, however, compounds of acrid and narcotics are often employed, by which the vomiting is checked, while the poison is doing its work.

As a general rule, whenever narcotic symptoms preponderate, an emetic of a large desert spoonful of the best mustard flour uniformly diffused through a wine glass full water should be at once administered, and repeated after a quarter of an hour if not effectual.

The mustard emetic is of the utmost utility in poisoning by *opium* and *datura*. It is inferior to the next in the cases specified below.

Sulphate of Zinc.—Twenty to thirty grains dissolved in a wine glass full of water will generally cause copious vomiting almost immediately. The dose should be repeated in ten minutes, and the action of the emetic promoted by draughts of tepid water. This emetic is chiefly suitable to poisoning by spirit, aconite, gunjah, and the metallic poisons.

Tartar Emetic is to be avoided as much as possible in cases of poisoning. It is slower in action, and less certain in operation, than the sulphate of zinc, and it complicates the analysis by the introduction of antimony, which adds much to the difficulty the investigation presents, owing to the effect it produces in *Marsh's apparatus.*

In all cases whatever a mustard poultice should be applied at once to the pit of the stomach. This will often materially aid the action of the emetic. It also acts as a stimulant of great power in *narcotism*, and as a counter-irritant in acrid poisoning.

PURGATIVES.—Large doses of castor oil are best suited to the treatment of arsenical and mercurial poisoning.

Half an ounce to an ounce of sulphate of magnesia, or four ounces of infusion of senna, with turpentine two drachms, in an emulsion with the white of eggs, are far preferable for the narcotic poisons. Where aconite, opium, or datura have been administered, the *turpentine* enema is of great utility.

2.—To remove, neutralize, render insoluble, and prevent the absorption of poisons, *antidotes* are employed.

Antidotes are of two kinds, the chemical and therapeutical.*

To the general principles which regulate the operations of the counter-poisons, Dr. Christison alludes in these terms:—

"In the instance of internal poisoning, the great object of the physician is to administer an antidote or counter-poison. These antidotes are of two kinds. One kind takes away the deleterious qualities of the poison, before it comes within its sphere of action, by altering its chemical nature; the other controuls its poisonous action after it has begun, by exciting a contrary action in the system. In the early ages of medicineal most all antidotes were believed to be of the latter description, but in fact very few such antidotes are known.

"The chemical antidotes act in several ways, according to the mode of action of the poison for which they are given. If the poison is a pure corrosive, such as a mineral acid, it will be sufficient that the antidote destroy its corrosive quality; thus the addition of an alkali or earth will neutralize sulphuric acid, and destroy, or at least prodigiously lessen, its poisonous properties. In supplying this rule, care must be taken to choose an antidote which is either inert, or if poisonous, is like the poison for which it is given, a pure corrosive or local irritant, and one whose properties are reciprocally neutralized. If the poison, on the other band, besides possessing a local action, likewise acts remotely by an impression on the inner coat of the vessels, mere neutralization of its chemical properties is not sufficient; for we have seen above that such poisons act throughout all their chemical combinations which are soluble. Here, therefore, it is necessary that the chemical antidote render the poison insoluble or nearly so, and that not only in water, but likewise in the animal fluids, more particularly the juices of the stomach. The same quality is desirable even in the antidotes for the pure corrosives; for it often happens that in their soluble combinations these substances retain, some irritating, though not any corrosive power. When we try by the foregoing criterions many of the antidotes which have been proposed for various poisons, they will be found defective, as precise experiments have in recent times actually proved them to be."

The first group of poisons for which an antidote is required, is that of—

THE MINERAL ACIDS.

Of these Dr. Christison speaks as follows:—

"Since the mineral acids act entirely as local irritants, it may be inferred that

* The remarks on *antidotes* are chiefly taken from the Editor's *Manual of Chemistry*, 1st. Edition.

their poisonous effects will be prevented by neutralizing them. But in the applying that principle to the treatment, it is necessary to bear in mind their extremely rapid operation; for if much time is lost in seeking for an antidote, irreparable mischief may be caused before the remedy is taken. Should it be possible then to administer chalk or magnesia without delay, these are the antidotes which ought to be preferred. But if it will consume time to get them, then a solution of soap, an article more likely to be at hand, should be administered, and while it is in preparation the acid should be diluted by the free use of any mild fluid, milk, or oleaginous matters being preferred. The carbonates of the alkalies are by no means eligible antidotes, being themselves possessed of corrosive properties. After the proper antidote has been given to a sufficient extent, the use of diluents ought to be continued, as they render the vomiting more easy.

"The treatment of the supervening inflammation does not differ from that of ordinary inflammation of the stomach."

On this subject we may remark, that chalk is, for many reasons, the best remedy here, and it should never be forgotten, that it is always at hand in the ceiling and walls of every apartment. The first thing, then, to be done is, to break off a piece of plaster from the wall, grind it to coarse powder in the quickest manner, and administer it in suspension in water or milk. It must, however, be recollected, that in the case of the nitric and muriatic acids, the resulting compounds, the nitrate and muriate of lime, are themselves highly destructive to animal life; we should, therefore, as soon as possible, follow up the administration of the chalk by draughts of broth or milk containing the carbonate or phosphate of soda in solution; an insoluble carbonate or phosphate of lime is thus generated, and every trace of the poisonous agent is removed.

The corrosive effects of Iodine may be considerably alleviated by the immediate use of starch in its ordinary form, or in that of any amylaceous substance, as wheat, flour, potatoes, &c. An iodide of starch is thus formed, which may be extricated by vomiting more easily than the iodine itself, and which being rapidly converted into hydriodic acid in the alimentry canal, is eliminated quickly through the various excretory channels.

In poisoning by Chlorine taken in solution into the stomach, or by chloride of lime, the use of the bicarbonate of soda in water, seems to offer some encouragement, by converting the excess of chlorine into muriate of soda. No experiments, however, are yet recorded, to prove the efficiency of this treatment. The protosulphate of iron in drachm doses may be taken with advantage untill vomiting occurs.

Oxalic Acid, finds a certain antidote in the carbonate of lime or magnesia. It is to be remarked, however, that the oxalates, (which are nearly of equal virulence) are not thus decomposed. We therefore recommend, as an invaluable remedy in these cases, the *solution* of the bicarbonate of magnesia, invented by Dr. Murray, of Belfast, which precipitates the acid itself and all its soluble combinations.

Fixed Alkalies, for these we find two certain chemical remedies in acetic acid and oil; the latter appears to be preferable, as it combines the effect of a mechanical demulcent with its chemical virtue. It is almost needless to observe, that a soap is formed by the combination. In poisoning by Ammonia or its carbonates, acetic acid is preferable, as the ammoniacal soaps are of a very irritating nature.

A very important set of poisons comes next in order, viz. the SULPHURETS OF THE ALKALIES. These, it will be recollected, long held great reputation as antidotes themselves, but it has been of late satisfactorily established, that in such small doses as three drachms, they are capable of inducing fatal symptoms, depending, it is probable, on the rapid disengagement of sulphuretted hydrogen gas. Dr. Christison cites a case, according to the results of which it would appear, that the use of the chloride of lime or soda will effect a cure by decomposing the sulphuretted hydrogen as quickly as it is evolved,—the chlorine uniting with the hydrogen, and the sulphur being set free.

USE OF THE SULPHURETS AS ANTIDOTES.

Notwithstanding the decided proofs that recently-prepared sulphurets are themselves strong poisons, yet I think there is some reason to regret that in the revolutions of fashion, they should have nearly been discarded from the list of our chemical auxiliaries in the treatment of metallic poisoning. Besides their own poisonous energy, it has been alleged, that the insoluble compounds which they generate in all deleterious metallic solutions, are also poisonous themselves. The sulphuret of arsenic for example, is instanced as being an agent nearly as virulent as the arsenious acid.

I believe that this objection to the sulphurets is not founded on sufficiently comprehensive views of their various relations. In the first place, it is evident that the quantity of the sulphuret of potash, which would be fatal *per se*, would produce no bad effects if it encountered in the alimentary canal a metallic solution, of lead, bismuth, copper, silver, or tin, for example, with each of which it enters into combinations insoluble in the intestinal fluids. It is thus manifest, that if we are called to a case in which we are certain that half an ounce of the acetate of lead has been swallowed, we may safely administer the sulphuret of potash beyond the dose in which it would by itself prove fatal, inasmuch as all the sulphuretted hydrogen extricated from it, is quickly absorbed by the acetate of lead, and an insoluble sulphuret of that metal produced.

Secondly, it certainly is an error to suppose, that the metallic sulphurets are generally poisonous themselves. The source of this mistake is, we believe, to be traced to the ascertained fact, that the sulphuret of arsenic is beyond all doubt nearly as destructive as the arsenious acid, but this I am inclined to regard as the exception, not as the general rule; and it unquestionably depends on the solvent power which the gastric fluids are capable of exercising over this sulphuret, but which they do not exert in other instances. Thus Orfila has established, that half an ounce of the black sulphuret of mercury has no effect whatever on dogs. The red or orange sulphurets of antimony are also inert, compared with the other preparations of this metal. Dr. Duncan, of Edinburgh, was every year accustomed to prove this fact to his clinical pupils, by giving it in scruple doses twice or three times a day. We have ourselves given twice that quantity without any effect, beyond slight nausea, and it is probable that as much brick-dust would have been equally energetic. The case of Dr. Duffin, too, is fresh in the recollection of the profession; this gentleman having accidently taken a poisonous dose of tartar emetic, was successfully treated by Dr. Duncan with the sulphuret of potash. We had ourselves a precisely similar case in one of our own servants, who accidentally swallowed a solution of forty grains of tartar emetic; no vomiting had ensued for fifteen minutes when she was first seen; ten grains of the sulphuret of potash were administered every quarter of an hour till the sixth dose, when she vomited a large quantity of the red sulphuret of antimony, and in six hours was perfectly well.

The sulphuret of copper still more decidedly exemplifies the correctness of these opinions. Orfila gave a nounce of it to a dog, without any effect being produced. If long kept it becomes oxidated, it is true, but it will be remembered that the sulphuret of potash forms it at *once* in the stomach, where it is effectually beyond the reach of oxidation, at least for the short time it remains within that viscus.

The same observations apply with increased force to tin, zinc, bismuth, silver, gold, platinum, and lead. Not one of the sulphurets thus formed acts as a poison, and though the sulphuret of potash would it is true,.produce dangerous symptoms if given in large quantities to a person whose alimentary canal is free from those metals, yet if the metallic solution or compound be present, the noxious influence of both is counteracted, and a harmless compound results. For these several reasons I do not hesitate to recommend the sulphuret of potash as an effectual antidote to the preparations of copper, zinc, antimony, tin, lead, bismuth, mercury, platinum, and gold. It will be valuable, especially, in the numerous instances in which we are without any information respecting the actual poison which has been taken; and in cases where a mixture of different metallic poisons has been given, (and such an instance of atrocious cunning is on record,) it is our most comprehensive, if not our only auxiliary. It will seldom or never be necessary to employ more than a drachm or two of the sulphuret, which should be given in divided doses of ten grains in solution, repeated every ten minutes or quarter of an hour. The effects produced must be carefully watched, and nothing can justify the practitioner in leaving the patient while the antidote is employed.

I proceed to enumerate the several other antidotes which have acquired reputation in the treatment of poisoning by metallic preparations.

Albumen (the white of eggs) possesses undoubted efficacy in cases of poisoning by *corrosive sublimate*, which it reduces to the condition of calomel. In poisoning with the soluble salts of copper it exerts a somewhat similar but less decided action, for while in the former a protochloride is formed, a compound insoluble in the acids of the stomach, in the latter *an oxide* is produced, which is readily separated by weak acetic or muriatic acid from the coagulated albumen with which it is combined. Albumen is, however, of essential service in this, as in many other forms of poisoning, by mechanically enveloping the noxious substance, and causing it to be more readily ejected from the alimentary canal. With zinc, tin, bismuth, gold and silver, albumen acts in both ways thus specified, and it is especially useful in cases where the stomach-pump is applied: it does not cause any decomposition of the salts of lead, platinum, or arsenic, or tartar emetic, and is consequently less universal in its applications than the sulphuret of potash.

The Ferro-cyanate (or Prussiate) of Potash is another substance which exerts a very extended action over the metallic poisons, and which has not received from toxicologists in general the attention it deserves. For copper in all its forms it affords a perfect antidote. It likewise decomposes the soluble salts of mercury, lead, tin, antimony, silver, and gold, causing with them insoluble precipitates; but it does not decompose some of the more insoluble preparations of these metals, which are nevertheless capable of acting as destructive poisons. The ferro-cyanate of potash has itself no poisonous properties.

The Alkaline Carbonates once obtained general confidence as antidotes to the metallic poisons; they should however, never be resorted to, because all the precipitates which they occasion in metallic solutions are soluble in the gastric fluids and in several acids; and, moreover, their operation does not extend to the insoluble poisons. Thus, it we treat a patient who has taken the acetate of lead with the carbonate of soda, carbonate of lead is thrown down; this is still more deleterious than the acetate itself.

Of Vegetable Gluten it is sufficient to observe that its virtues are similar to, but weaker than those of albumen.

I have next to consider a few metallic poisons which have antidotes peculiar to themselves.

The soluble salts of Lead are thus effectually counteracted by the phosphate or sulphate of soda, which throws down a thoroughly insoluble phosphate or sulphate of lead. These antidotes, however, do not operate on the carbonate of lead, or on the yellow or red oxides of that metal.

The *soluble* Barytic salts are rendered innocent by the sulphates, which throw down an insoluble sulphate of baryta. The carbonate, however, is not interfered with by these re-agents.

Of the *antimonial* salts, Tartar Emetic is said to find an antidote in Peruvian bark, and some cases are recorded of the success of this remedy. It is, however rather inconsistent with the virtues of the bark in this respect, that many physicians are in the habit of prescribing tartar emetic in a decoction of bark without the antimonial action being at all impaired. I would, in every instance, prefer the sulphuret of potash.

For Arsenic, the *hydrated peroxide of iron* is becoming daily of more celebrity. Several cases of its successful administration have been published.

I proceed to the consideration of the few organic poisons which are asserted to possess antidotes peculiar to themselves.

The first in order of these is the Hydrocyanic or Prussic acid, for which ammonia and chlorine have been strenuously recommended. When we recollect, however, that Prussic acid is one of those poisons which retains its destructive power in all its soluble combinations, we cannot repose any confidence on ammonia *as a chemical antidote*, though we consider it of the utmost value as a powerful diffusible stimulant, by which the narcotism induced by the acid is opposed. The second remedy, chlorine, combines high chemical and physiological powers; by the first it decomposes the prussic acid, and prevents it doing further harm, while by its stimulating properties, it contributes to obviate the *effects* the poison has already induced. The best mode of using this antidote is by inhaling the vapour of its solution in water sufficiently diluted. The chloride of lime in solution may at the same time be taken into the stomach. It should not however be forgotten that insensibility will usually have occurred before medical assistance is obtained; in this case inhalation is impossible; we can only inject the solution of the chloride into the stomach. It would be easy, however, to contrive an apparatus by which artificial respiration might be carried on, and chlorine mingled with the air introduced.*

For Opium we possess no antidote of any effect. The alkaline carbonates have been recommended on the grounds of their precipitating morphia from its solutions. But the precipitate which they occasion is itself a poison of great energy.

The last class of poisons—the *nux-vomica* or *strychnine groupe*, for which we have reason to believe an antidote to exist, is thus alluded to by Dr. Christison:—

"Very lately M. *Donné* of Paris has stated that he has found iodine, bromine, and chlorine, to be antidotes for poisoning with the alkaloid of nux-vomica, as well as for the other vegetable alkaloids. Iodine, chlorine, and bromine, he says, form with the alkaloids compounds which are not deleterious,—two grains and a half of the iodide, bromide, and chloride of strychnia, having produced no effect on a dog. Animals which had taken one grain of strychnia, or two grains of veratria, did not sustain any harm, when tincture of iodine was administered immediately afterwards. But the delay of ten minutes in the administration of the antidote rendered it useless. In the compounds formed by these antidotes with the alkaloids, the latter are in a state of chemical union, and not decomposed. Sulphuric acid separates strychnia, for example, from its state of combination with chlorine, iodine, or bromine, and forms sulphate of strychnia, with its usual poisonous qualities. It remains to be proved that the same advantages will be derived from the administration of these antidotes in the instance of poisoning with the crude drug nux-vomica, as in poisoning with its alkaloid."

I have made numerous experiments at the Medical College on the administranion of iodine to animals poisoned by brucine, nux-vomica nut and bark, but in no instance was any good effect produced.

Third object.—If any absorption has taken place, to cause the absorbed matter to leave the system as soon as possible.

In 1829, I shewed by numerous experiments published in the "Lancet," and quoted by Dr. Christison in his admirable work, that *Iodine* appeared in the urine in a few minutes after its being taken into the stomach, and continued to be present in the urine for a long period after it ceased to be detectible in the alimentary canal.

M. Orfila has recently made the important discovery, that arsenic is similarly absorbed, and excreted by the urine chiefly. He has shewn that dogs dosed with arsenic, generally recover if treated by *diuretics*, and on the other hand, usually perish where other methods are had recourse to.

These important facts will doubtless be extended to many other poisons, and they deserve the closest attention of the practitioner.

Diuretic action in these cases is best promoted by small doses of the nitrate or acetate of potash, copious tepid drinks of water with any mucilaginous seed, (such as the Behcedana or Ispagool,) gentle exercise, with light clothing, in a cool apartment. The perspiration from the skin must be checked, in order to carry this mode of treatment fairly into effect.

* The best of all remedies is the cold affusion, and it should be used along with the antidote ust described.

In cases which are likely to become the subject of legal investigation, the urine should be preserved for analysis. Arsenic has been detected in this fluid several days after the administration of the poison, and the cessation of its urgent effects.

Digitalis and squill, though powerful diuretics, are not suited to these cases.

Fourth object.—To obviate the local and general effects the poison may have occasioned.

These are chiefly.—1. Inflammation and ulceration of the alimentary canal.—*Symptoms.*—Pain, vomiting, bloody stools, tenderness of the abdomen on pressure.

Treatment.—*Bleeding,* if the patient be robust, and after the poison has been removed, or rendered inactive. *Leeches* to the abdomen—mustard poultices. Blisters often exasperate the symptoms by causing strangury, and preventing the diuretic action so very desirable. Diluent drinks—Dover's powder in doses of five to ten grains thrice daily, gives much relief in the milder cases. After the poison has been removed, to combat dysenteric symptoms give acetate of lead three grains, opium one grain made into a pill with conserve of roses, every third hour. The diet should be on the lowest scale, and consist of sago, Ceylon moss, arrow-root or tapioca.

2. *Symptoms.*—Flushing or purple congestion of the face and neck, pupils usually contracted, pulse full and quick, breathing stertorous, insensibility, bowels torpid. The effects of congestion of blood on the brain.

Treatment.—After removal of poison, bleed if the patient be robust and young. Shave the head, apply ice or solution of muriate of ammonia, or sulphuric ether—leeches to the temples. Blister to the back of the neck, mustard poultice to the pit of the stomach—turpentine enema. After the immediate symptoms are relieved, a gentle course of mercurials is beneficial.

In opium poisoning it is strongly recommended by many to keep the patient moving about actively, either supported by assistants, or in a carriage. While cool and fresh air must be useful, fatigue ought certainly to be avoided as much as possible.

3. *Symptoms.*—Insensibility, dilated pupil, blindness, small weak pulse, coldness of extremities, natural respiration—usual effects of Datura.

Treatment.—Stomach pump, or sulphate of zinc emetic at first, affusion of cold water over the head and shoulders, *turpentine enema,* mustard poultice. Small doses of brandy and ammonia; subsequently blisters to the nape of the neck and free purging.

4. *Symptoms.*—As in No. 3, with slight twitchings; if insensibility be not complete, stupid incoherence; dilated pupil, indistinct vision, tenderness of abdomen—usual effects of Aconite.

Treatment.—Stomach pump or sulphate of zinc, mustard poultice, turpentine enema, leeches to epigastrium; subsequently saline purgatives.

5. *Symptoms.*—Insensibility interrupted by fits of laughing delirium, muscles often rigid—effects of Bang or Gunjah.

Treatment.—The same as No. 3.

6. *Symptoms.*—Tetanic spasms, body bent back and resting on the back of the head, the elbows, and heels.

Treatment.—Emetic of sulphate of zinc; two drops of croton oil in two ounces of mucilage. A turpentine enema. After free vomiting and purging, give extract of hemp two grains, and repeat this every half hour according to the effect produced.

The warm bath gives great relief. Avoid blisters and sinapisms, and keep the patient in a quiet, cool, and dark room.

The hemp is likely to prove of the utmost value in such cases. We have thus treated with success several dogs to which large doses of strychnine had been administered. The hemp subdues the convulsive tendency more effectually than any other narcotic.

7 *Symptoms.*—Violent colic—irregular convulsions, constipated bowels—usual effect of carbonate of lead.

Treatment.—After removal of poison, brisk purgatives of castor oil and turpentine—diluents,—mustard poultices. After free purging or vomiting, give Dover's powder in ten grain doses every third or fourth hour, according to the effects.* * *

APPENDIX No. 3.—MEAN TEMPERATURE.

We are indebted to Dr. Wise for the following valuable memorandum of the Mean Temperature of the year, deduced from morning observations made at Chinsurah during the year 1832. A register thermometer was employed, and it was placed under an open gate-way, out of the influence of the reflection of the sun.

	Month.	Quarter.	Yearly. Mean.
September,	83.17		
October,	80.94	78.97	
November,	72.84		
December,	66.00		
January,	64.81	67.54	
February,	71.73		
March,	81.14		77.08
April,	85.26	83.09	
May,	85.32		
June,	87.61		
July,	84.56	78.71	
August,	83.72		

APPENDIX No. 4.—ON THE CULTIVATION OF THE POPPY.

By Mr. W. B. Johnson of Patna.

The Poppy requires a good, rich, dark, soil, well prepared with manure, and divided off into small oblong plots, of about 6 × 4 feet for the convenience of weeding and patching. The sowings commence early in November. The day the seed is sown the land is well watered, and the next day, the ryot breaks all the lumps with his khoorpü. The plant soon shoots up, and when about 6 inches high, it is thinned and weeded; it is kept well watered until the capsules are nearly ripe, and the petals falling off; it then depends upon the state of the weather; if mild, the irrigation is continued; if strong winds, it is discontinued for fear of being blown down. As soon as the petals fall, or are pulled off, (for the purpose of making leaves for the envelope of the opium for the China market, of

*** *Sulphate of zinc poisoning.*—Several dangerous accidents have occurred in Calcutta within the last two years by the fraudulent substitution of Sulphate of zinc for Sulphate of magnesia (Epsom salts).—Give copious draughts of tepid water—twenty grains of carbonate of soda every half hour to the third or fourth dose, encouraging vomiting—sinapism to the pit of the stomach, subsequently castor oil and laudanum—occasional aperients for some days.

which each cake or ball consumes five chittacks of these leaves,) the bleeding or tapping commences, which is a wound made in the exterior surface of the capsule with 4 or 5 heartshaped lancets tied together with some thread ; it is generally (or ought to be) done in the hottest part of the day, that the juice as it exudes in the night, may be protected by the pellicle formed in the day ; the wound ought to be diagonal to prevent the juice from falling off in the night when the dews are heavy. A biggah of good land requires about 3 seers of seed, if not required to be resown, and yields to the ryot 15 seers of Opium. At the present price paid for it by the H. C. Co's. Rs. 3/10, this gives Co's. Rs. 4/56. Five maunds of seed at the average bazar rate of 25 seers per Rupee, bring eight Rupees. The leaves are also bought for filling up the boxes, (or rather chests,) in packing, at 4 annas per maund, and are called trash or *pate*. The petals are formed into masses and paid for at first quality 10 Rs. per maund—second ditto, at 7 Rupees—third ditto, at 5 Rupees—produce say 15 Rupees—so that the total value of a good biggah of Opium land is Co's. Rs. 80, with the stalks for fire wood, exclusive of other crops in the year.

The quantity of Opium paid for, from each district last year is as follows; viz.

Tirhoot, . . Factory maunds.	3507	13	15¼
Sarun, ...	5197	37	15¾
Champarun, ...	3931	26	11¾
Shahabad, ...	3881	21	1¼
Behar, ...	2610	13	10¼
Patna, ...	2400	36	60
Bhauglepore, ...	218	23	12¼
Monghyr, ...	812	12	5¾
Purneah, ...	360	20	5¾
Total, at 80 tola weight and 70 lowest consistence, maunds,	22,922	9	3¾

APPENDIX No. 5.—BRITISH-INDIAN WEIGHTS AND MEASURES.*

The unit of the British Indian ponderary system† is called the tola. It weighs 180 grains English Troy Weight. From it upwards, are derived the heavy weights, viz: *Chitak*, *Seer*, and *Mun* (or Maund);—and by its subdivision the small or jeweller's weights, called *mashas*, *ruttees*, and *dhans*.

The following scheme comprehends both of these in one series:

Mun.	Pusserree.	Seer.	Chitak.	Tola.	Masha.	Sutter.	Dhan.
1	8	40	640	3200	38400	307200	1228800
	1	5	80	400	4800	38400	153600
		1	16	80	960	7680	30720
			1	5	60	480	1920
				1	12	96	384
					1	8	32
						1	4

* From Prinsep's *Useful tables* and Rushton's *Bengal and Agra Gazetteer*.

† The advantages of this system are,—

1. That the maund formed from the modified weight would be precisely equal to 100 English troy pounds; and

2. That thirty-five seers would also be precisely equal to seventy-two pounds avoirdupois:—thus establishing a simple connection, void of fractions, between the two English metrical scales and that of India.

The *Mun* (or that weight to which it closely accords in value, and to which it is legally equivalent in the new scale) has been hitherto better known among Europeans by the name of *Bazar Maund*, but upon its general adoption, under regulation VII. 1833, for all transactions of the British Government, it should be denominated the BRITISH MAUND, (in Hindee *Ungrezee Mun*,) to distinguish it at once from all other weights in use throughout the country.

The *Pusseree* is, as its name denotes, a five-seer weight, and therefore should not form an integrant point of the scale; but as its use is very general, it has been introduced for the convenience of reference.

The *Seer* being the commonest weight in use in the retail business of the Bazar in India, and being liable according to the pernicious system hitherto prevalent, to vary in weight for every article sold, as well as for every market, is generally referred to the common unit in native mercantile dealings, as, 'the seer of so many *tolas*,' (or siccas, barees, takas, &c.) The standard or *bazar seer* being always 80 *tolas*.

The *Chitak* is the lowest denomination of the gross weights, and is commonly divided into halves and quarters, (called in Bengalee *kacha*;) thus marking the line between the two series, which are otherwise connected by the relation of the seer, &c. to the tola.

The *Tola* is chiefly used in the weighing of the precious metals and coin; all bullion at the mints is received in this denomination,

British Indian Weights.		English Troy Weights.					French Weights.
		lbs.	oz.	dwt.	grains.		grammes.
One MAUND, ...	=	100	0	0	0	=	37320.182
One SEER, ...	=	2	6	0	0	=	933.005
One CHITACK, ...	=	0	1	17	12	=	58.310
One TOLA, ...	=	0	0	7	12	=	11.662
One MASHA, ...	=	0	0	0	15	=	0.972
One RUTTEE, ...	=	0	0	0	1.875	=	0.122

Comparison with Troy weights.

For the conversion of English troy weights into those of India, the following scale will suffice, since the simplicity of their relation renders a more detailed table unnecessary.

Lb. Troy.	Ounce.	Penny-weight.	Grain.		TOLAS and Decimals.
1	12	240	5760	=	32 000
	1	20	480	=	2.6666 &c.
		1	24	=	0.1333 &c.
			1	=	0.0055 &c.

APPENDIX No. 6.—ON THE USE OF DANIELL'S HYGROMETER.

(From Daniell's Meteorological Observations.)

"Thus the Hygrometer marks with infallible precision the comparative degrees of moisture and dryness in the atmosphere, and by exhibiting them in degrees of the thermometer, refers them to a known standard of comparison, and speaks in a language which every body understands. But its observations may be made applicable to a much wider field of research, and adapted to still more important objects. By means of tables, we can find with the utmost accuracy and ease the positive weight of aqueous vapour diffused through any given portion of space, and its force or elasticity as measured by the column of mercury which it is capable of supporting: we discover at once the proportion of moisture in any space to the quantity which would be required to saturate it, or what has been termed the true natural scale of the hygrometer: we can calculate with perfect ease the specific gravity of any mixture of air and aqueous vapour: and we can measure the force and quantity of evaporation. Upon the *data* employed in the construction of the tables, it will be necessary that I should premise a few reflections.

"The second column of Table I. exhibits the force of aqueous vapour, in inches of mercury, at the temperature marked in the corresponding line of the first column.

"Upon these two *data*, namely, the force and temperature of the vapour, are chiefly founded the calculations which have furnished me with the series of the third column, which contains the weight in grains of a cubic foot of the vapour at the corresponding temperature and pressure. The method of computing it is as follows:—Steam at 212°, and under a pressure of 30 inches of mercury, is, as nearly as possible, 1700 times lighter than an equal bulk of water at its maximum of density; and a cubic foot of water, at the temperature of 40°, weighs, according to the accurate investigations of Dr. Rice, 437272 grains: the weight, therefore, of a cubic foot of steam at the above temperature and pressure is $\frac{437272}{1700}$, or 257.218 grains. Hence we may find the weight of an equal bulk of vapour of the same temperature under any other given pressure, suppose 0.560 inches for the volume being in inverse proportion to the pressure,

Ins.		Ins.		Grs.		Grs.
30	:	0.560	: :	257.218	:	4.801

the weight required.

"Having now obtained the weight of a cubic foot of vapour, at a pressure of 0.560 inches, and at a temperature of 212°, we may proceed to find its weight under the same pressure at any other temperature, suppose 60°. It has been fully established, that all aëriform bodies (vapours out of the contact of their respective fluids as well as gases,) expand $\frac{1}{480}$th part of their volume for every accession of temperature, equivalent to one degree of Fahrenheit's scale; therefore, reckoning a volume of gas at 32° as unity, its volume at 60° is to its volume at 212°, as $1+\frac{28}{486}$ is to $1+\frac{180}{480}$, or : : 1.0583 : 1.3749, and the density and weight being in inverse proportion to the volume,

Vol. at 60.		Vol. at 212.		Grs.		Grs.
1.0583	:	1.3749	: :	4.801	:	6.222

the weight of the cubic foot of vapour at the temperature of 60° and under a pressure of .560 inches.

"It has also been proved by Mr. Dalton, that as much vapour of determined temperature is formed in a given bulk of air as in a vacuum of equal space, therefore, the above result gives the weight of vapour which can exist in a cubic foot of air at the temperature of 60°. The fourth column of the table contains the proportionate expansion for the corresponding degrees.

TABLE

Shewing the Force, Weight, and Expansion of Aqueous Vapour, at different Temperatures, from 0° *to* 95°.

Temp.	Force.	Weight of a Cubic Foot.	Expansion.	Temp.	Force.	Weight of a Cubic Foot.	Expansion.
0	0.068	0.856	.9334	49	0.388	4.407	1.0354
1	0.071	0.892	.9355	50	0.400	4.535	1.0375
2	0.074	0.928	.9375	51	0.414	4.684	1.0395
3	0.077	0.963	.9396	52	0.428	4.832	1.0416
4	0.080	0 999	.9417	53	0.444	5.003	1.0437
5	0.083	1.034	.9438	54	0.460	5.173	1.0458
6	0.086	1.069	.9459	55	0.476	5.342	1.0479
7	0.089	1.104	.9480	56	0.492	5.511	1.0500
8	0.092	1.139	.9500	57	0.508	5.679	1.0520
9	0.095	1.173	.9521	58	0.526	5.868	1.0541
10	0.098	1.208	.9542	59	0.543	6.046	1.0562
11	0.103	1.254	.9563	60	0.560	6.222	1.0583
12	0.107	1.308	.9584	61	0.577	6.399	1.0604
13	0.111	1.359	.9605	62	0.594	6.575	1.0625
14	0.115	1.405	.9625	63	0.615	6.794	1.0645
15	0.119	1.451	.9646	64	0.636	7.013	1.0666
16	0.123	1.497	.9667	65	0.657	7.230	1.0687
17	0.127	1.541	.9688	66	0.678	7.447	1.0708
18	0.131	1.586	.9709	67	0.699	7.662	1.0729
19	0.135	1.631	.9730	68	0.722	7.899	1.0750
20	0.140	1.688	.9750	69	0.745	8.135	1.0770
21	0.146	1.757	.9771	70	0.770	8.392	1.0191
22	0.152	1.825	.9792	71	0.796	8.658	1.0812
23	0.158	1.893	.9813	72	0.822	8.924	1.0833
24	0.164	1.961	.9834	73	0.849	9.199	1.0854
25	0.170	2.028	.9855	74	0.877	9.484	1.0875
26	0.176	2.096	.9875	75	0.906	9.780	1.0895
27	0.182	2.163	.9896	76	0.936	10.107	1.0916
28	0.188	2.229	.9917	77	0.966	10.387	1.0937
29	0.194	2.295	.9938	78	0.997	10.699	1.0958
30	0.200	2.361	.9959	79	1.028	11.016	1.0979
31	0.208	2.451	.9980	80	1.060	11.333	1.1000
32	0.216	2.539	1.0000	81	1.093	11.665	1.1020
33	0.224	2.630	1.0020	82	1.127	12.005	1.1041
34	0.232	2.717	1.0041	83	1.162	12.354	1.1062
35	0.240	2.805	1.0062	84	1.198	12.713	1.1083
36	0.248	2.892	1.0083	85	1.235	13.081	1.1104
37	0.256	2.979	1.0104	86	1.273	13.458	1.1125
38	0.264	3.066	1.0125	87	1.312	13.877	1.1145
39	0.272	3.153	1.0145	88	1.351	14.230	1.1166
40	0.280	3.239	1.0166	89	1.390	14.613	1.1187
41	0.292	3.371	1.0187	90	1.430	15.005	1.1208
42	0.304	3.502	1.0208	91	1.470	15.432	1.1229
43	0.316	3.633	1.0229	92	1.510	15.786	1.1250
44	0.328	3.763	1.0250	93	1.551	16.186	1.1270
45	0.340	3.893	1.0270	94	1.593	16.593	1.1291
46	0.352	4.022	1.0291	95	1.636	17.009	1.1312
47	0.364	4.151	1.0312				
48	0.376	4.279	1.0333	212	30.000	257.218	1.3749

The manner of using the table, will perhaps be best understood from an example. Let the temperature of the atmosphere be 70°, and the point of condensation, as found by the hygrometer, 55°; the pressure of the vapour, under these circumstances, is immediately found opposite to the degree of its constituent heat 55° = 0.476. To find its weight, we proceed thus :—Supposing that the temperature of the air had not differed from that of the dew point, its weight would have been found upon the same line as its pressure = 5.342 grains. But its bulk is expanded by the excess of atmospheric heat, we must, therefore, seek in the fourth column for the degree of expansion at 55° = 1.0479, and at 70° = 1.0791, and apply the correction thus:

Bulk at 70°		Bulk at 55°		Grs.		Grs.
1.0791	:	1.0579	: :	5.342	:	5.175

which is the weight required.

"Again,—the dryness of the atmosphere, under the above conditions, may be conveniently expressed as 15°, in terms of the thermometric scale : but it may be desirable also to know what it would be upon the natural scale of the hygrometer. This is readily ascertained by dividing the elasticity of vapour at the temperature of the dew-point, by the elasticity at the temperature of the air: the quotient will express the proportion of moisture actually existing, to the quantity which would be required for saturation; for calling the term of saturation 1.000, as the elasticity of vapour at the temperature of the air is to the elasticity of vapour at the temperature of the dew-point, so is the term of saturation to the actual degree of moisture,—thus,

$$\frac{\text{Elas. at } 55^\circ\ .476}{\text{Elas. at } 70^\circ\ .770} = 618$$

The relation of this mode of expressing the degree of moisture to that of denoting the degree of dryness, by the thermometric scale, will be elucidated by selecting a different example. Let the temperature of the air be 47°, and the dew-point 32°; the dryness represented by the former expression will be 15°, as before, but by the latter the degree of moisture will be reduced to .593.

Thus, by two simple observations, and very easy calculations, we ascertain with precision, the following points of the utmost interest to meteorology.

Temperature of the air	70°
Dew-point	55°
Degree of dryness on the thermometric scale	15°
Degree of moisture on the hygrometric scale...	618
Elasticity of the vapour	.476 ins.
Weight of vapour in a cubic foot	5.175 grs.

APPENDIX No. 7.—DESCRIPTION OF THE GOLD BATTERY LATELY CONSTRUCTED AT THE MEDICAL COLLEGE OF CALCUTTA.*

We now arrive at the last and greatest step to perfection in this apparatus, by which the chief faults previously existing are remedied, and which, while it opens prospects of still greater success, at once places the galvanic battery among the

* From the Editor's *Notes of Lectures* on Galvanic Electricity.

most constant, portable, manageable, and powerful of all the instruments which science has given to mankind.

Mr. Grove, an English barrister, is the contriver of this most original and valuable apparatus. The elements consist of amalgamated zinc and platinum, separated from each other by porous earthenware cells. In contact with the platinum is placed the strongest nitric acid. In contact with the zinc, a mixture of one part sulphuric acid and ten parts water.

No action whatever occurs in this arrangement till the extreme plates are united by a conductor. Water is then decomposed as in all the other cases—and its hydrogen being transferred through the porous earthen cells to the platinum is there intercepted by the nitric acid with which it gradually forms water, thus diluting the acid.

The platinum undergoes no change whatever—the battery is perfectly constant in its action. Its powers are so enormous, that by the usual tests it has been proved that ten such couples, each four inches square are equal in power to more than thirty-eight times that surface of the best previous construction of zinc and copper.

On this principle, using (for local reasons merely) gold instead of platinum, I have prepared a battery of forty-eight couples, of which the following is an exact description :—

Each couple consists of two zinc cylinders and one gold cylinder, which with the porous earthenware vessel fit in a pint glass tumbler.

The gold cylinder is two inches broad, four deep, and is provided with a gold strap half an inch broad and three inches long. It is placed in the circular cell formed by the two concentric walls of the earthenware cylinder, and this is filled with the strongest nitric acid. In the centre is placed the small zinc, outside all the large zinc, and the straps belonging to these are bent in contact with each other, between them being placed the gold from the next cup, the contact being preserved by a little copper spring clasping the straps together like a finger and thumb. In contact with the zincs is poured the usual mixture of sulphuric acid and water.

In electric power this battery equals for equal surfaces those of Mr. Grove's platinum cells. The effects produced are given in detail. I should mention here however that I have found by recent experiment that well gilt porcelain produces exactly the same effect as gold, and I have accordingly sent orders to France for fifty cylinders gilt at both sides, and each exposing two superficial feet. I have also found that a mixture of two parts by weight of sulphuric acid to one of saltpetre gives as effective a liquid for the gold surface as the strongest nitric acid. These facts render the gold batteries in construction as cheap as those of copper, and in sustaining action much cheaper, inasmuch as the expense of the mixture I describe is not more than one-third of that of the solution of sulphate of copper.

The gold of the battery above described is worth about 500*l*.

APPENDIX No. 8.—ECONOMICAL OIL PRESS.*

(With Plate.)

We proceed to give a description of a most ingenious, cheap, and effective press, in which all the other mechanical powers are brought into operation; viz. the *wheel* and *axle, lever, wedge, inclined plane*, and *pulley*. It is one of the inventions of Mr. Ewings, a talented member of the London Mechanics' Institution, who obtained for it Dr. Fellowes's annual prize of ten pounds. This press, which is applicable to the packing of goods, pressing of juice from fruits, oil from seeds, or other purposes to which the screw-press is usually applied, consists of a frame-work, and two or more blocks or beams, between which the articles to be subjected to pressure are to be placed; and these vary in form, size, and material, according to the purposes for which they are intended. Mr. Ewings does not claim any novelty in the construction of these parts, but only in his method of producing the pressure, which is effected by bringing together the pieces that act on the articles to be pressed by wedges: these are forced in by levers (in the manner represented by the following figures 1 and 2), in both of which the same letters of reference represent similar parts. *a* is the base of the press furnished at each end with ratchet notches *bb*, which constitute the fulcrums of the levers *hh*; *c* is the top of the press, supported by the frames *dd*; and *ee* are the pieces acting on the goods, either downwards, upwards, or both, according as the pressure may be required; in *Fig.* 1 it is represented acting upwards; and in *Fig.* 2 it is represented acting both ways; *ffff* are friction rollers, between which the wedges *gg* are projected. A cord is fixed to a hook on the end of one of the levers, and passing over a pulley *k*, on the end of the other, is attached to a small drum *l*, which is furnished with a ratchet-wheel and pall, and is turned by a winch. We have seen other modifications of Mr. Ewings's press, but we have selected the above as best calculated to shew the principle of its action. Amongst the advantages of this press have been noticed the simplicity and economy of its construction, as it may be made by almost any person accustomed to handle carpenter's or smith's tools, of very cheap materials; and also the facility with which its power may be varied: it may be diminished or increased to any extent, simply by changing the form of the wedges; but the drawings exhibit its various applications and mode of operation so obviously as to preclude the necessity of further remarks.

APPENDIX No. 9.

DR. WIGHT'S FORMULA FOR THE PINEY VARNISH.†

The *Vateria Indica (Chloroxylon Dupada*, Buchanan and Ainslie, and Pinney marum of the Hindoos) produces a resin, resembling Copal, much finer than that procured from the other species natives of India, the finer specimens of which are as transparent as amber, and nearly colourless. It is procured by the very

* From Hebert's Cyclopædia, p. 338.

† Wight's Illustrations of Botany.

simple process of cutting a notch in the tree, sloping inwards and downwards. This is soon filled with the juice, which in a short time hardens by exposure to the air. When used as a varnish the usual practice is to apply the balsam before it has become hard: but when that is not procurable the resin melted by a slow heat and mixed with boiling linseed oil forms a varnish which answers equally well for most purposes.

As this varnish is of the finest description, the following formula for its preparation may prove useful to some who are unacquainted with the process. Into a new and perfectly clean earthen vessel (a chatty) put one part of the Piney dammer, in coarse powder, cover closely, and apply a *very gentle* heat until the whole is melted; then add about two parts of linseed oil, nearly boiling hot, and mix well with a wooden spatula. Should the varnish prove too thick it can at any time be reduced by the addition of more oil, or if required may be made thicker in the first instance.

It is essential to the success of the process that the Piney be melted in a covered vessel over a very slow fire, and the whole of it reduced to a fluid before the addition of the oil, which must, to ensure an equal mixture, be nearly boiling hot. This varnish is used for carriages and other fine furniture requiring to have their paint well protected, or to which it is desirable to impart a fine gloss.

A spirit varnish is prepared by reducing to powder about six parts of Piney and one of Camphor, and then adding hot alcohol sufficient to dissolve the mixed powder. Alcohol does not dissolve Piney without the aid of the Camphor, but once dissolved will retain it in solution.

The varnish thus prepared is employed for varnishing pictures, &c., but before being used requires to be gently heated to evaporate the Camphor, which otherwise will produce by its after evaporation a roughness and inequality on the surface of the picture, and spoil its appearance.

INDEX.

E.

H.

L.

N.

Q.

R.

U.

X.

Y.

Z.

Plate 1st

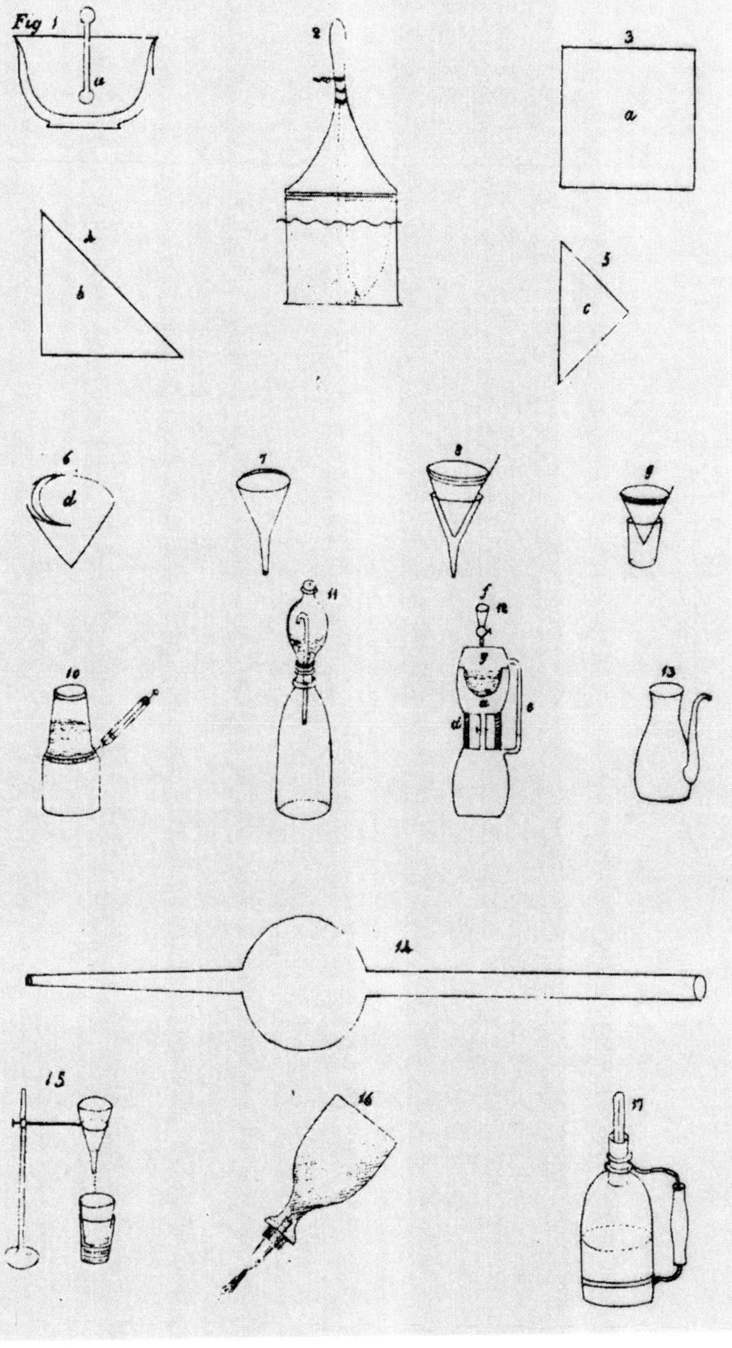

Plate 2nd

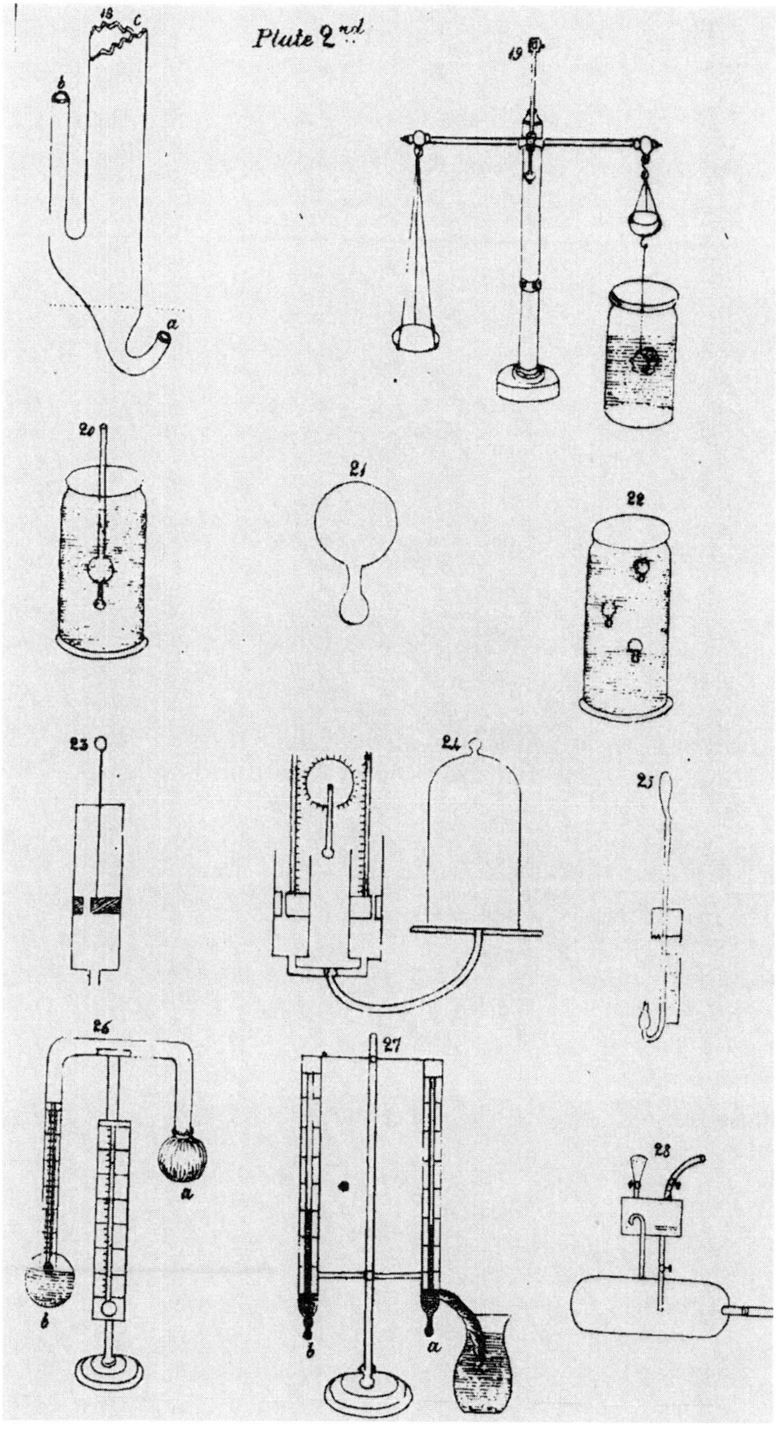

Plate 3rd

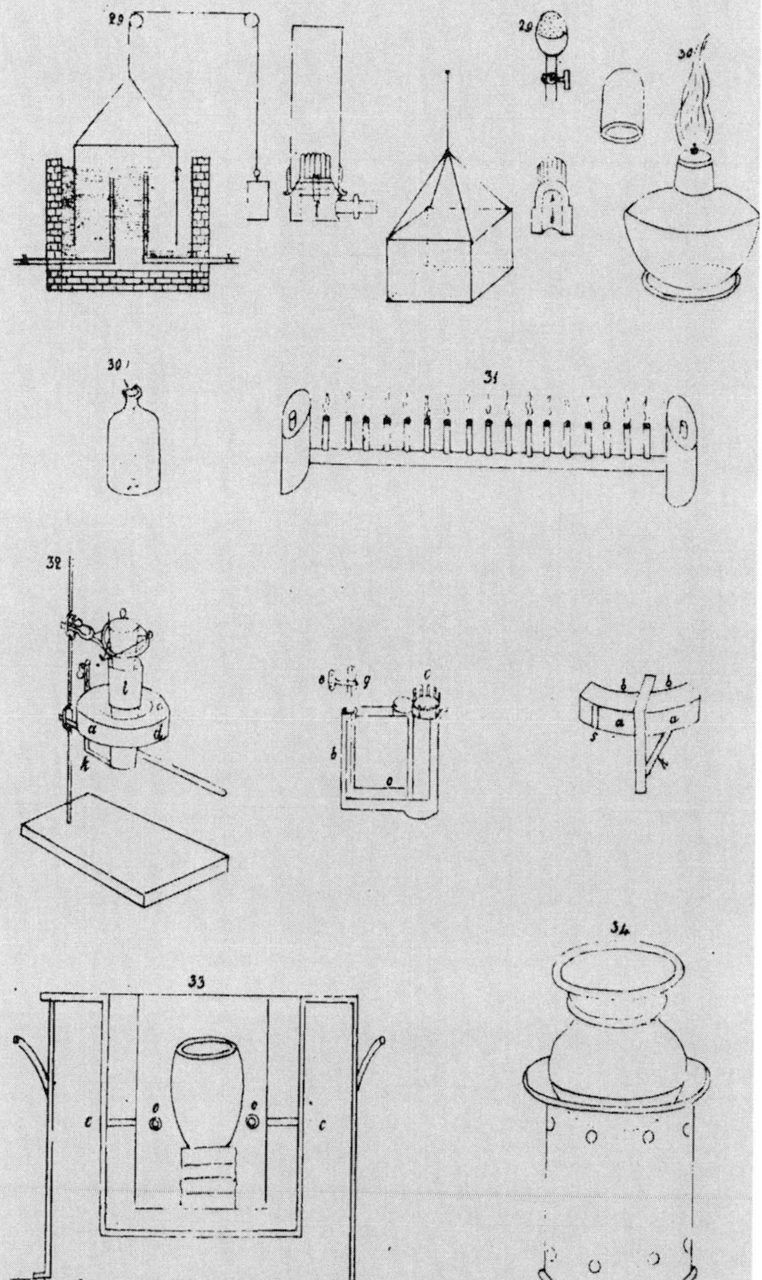

Plate 4th

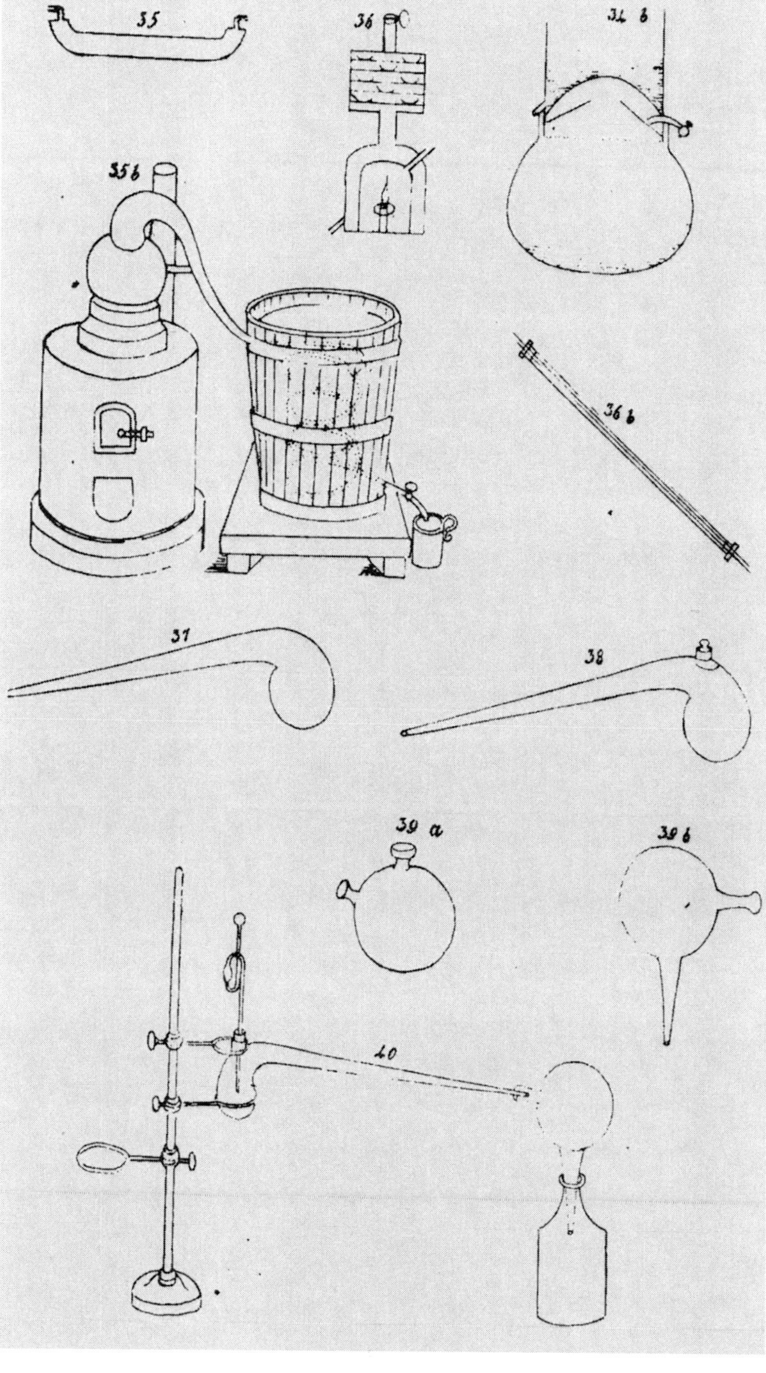

Plate 5th.

41

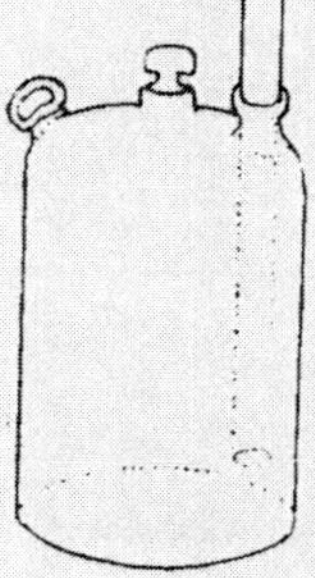

42

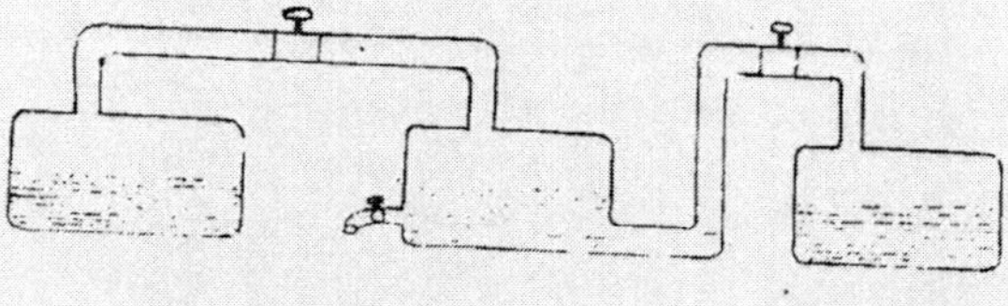

43

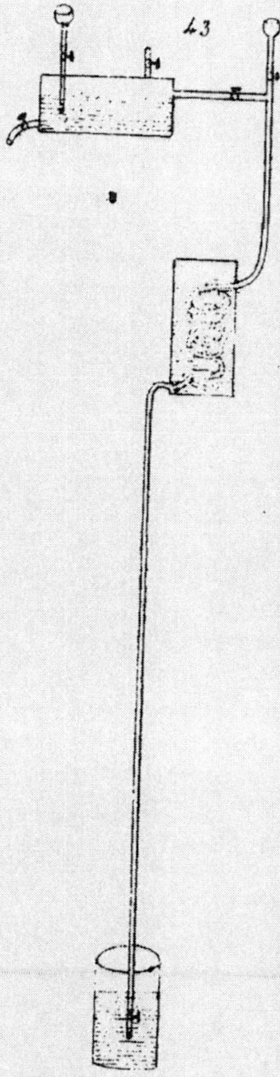

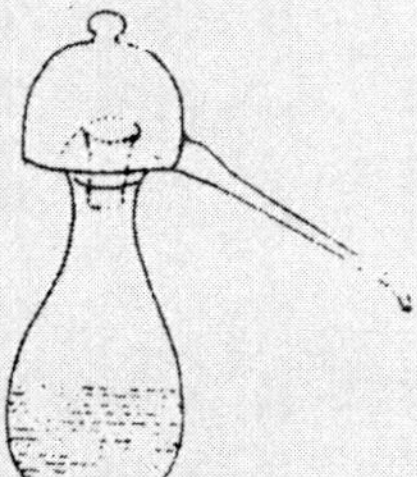

46

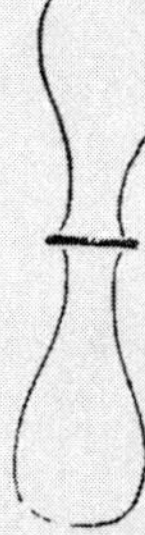

47

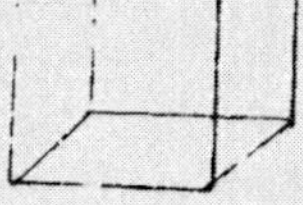

48

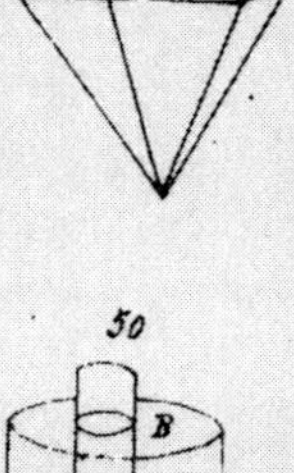

49

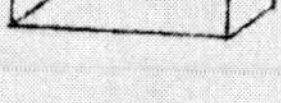

50

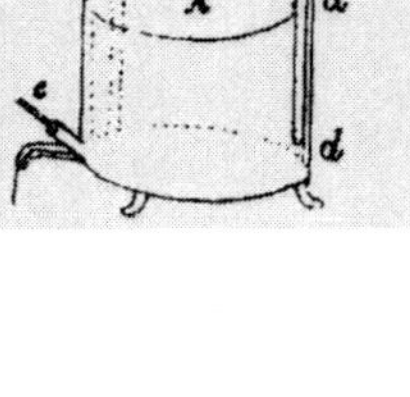

Plate 6

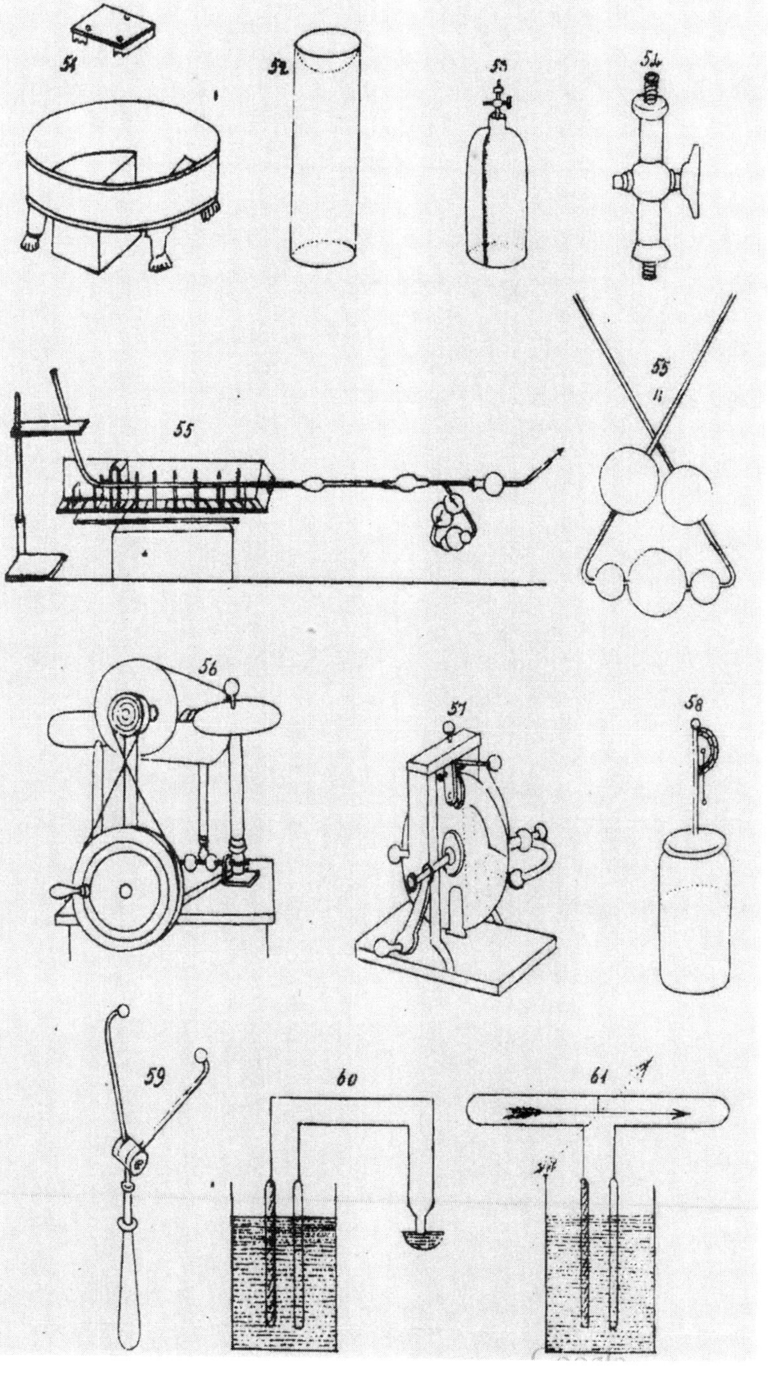

Plate 7

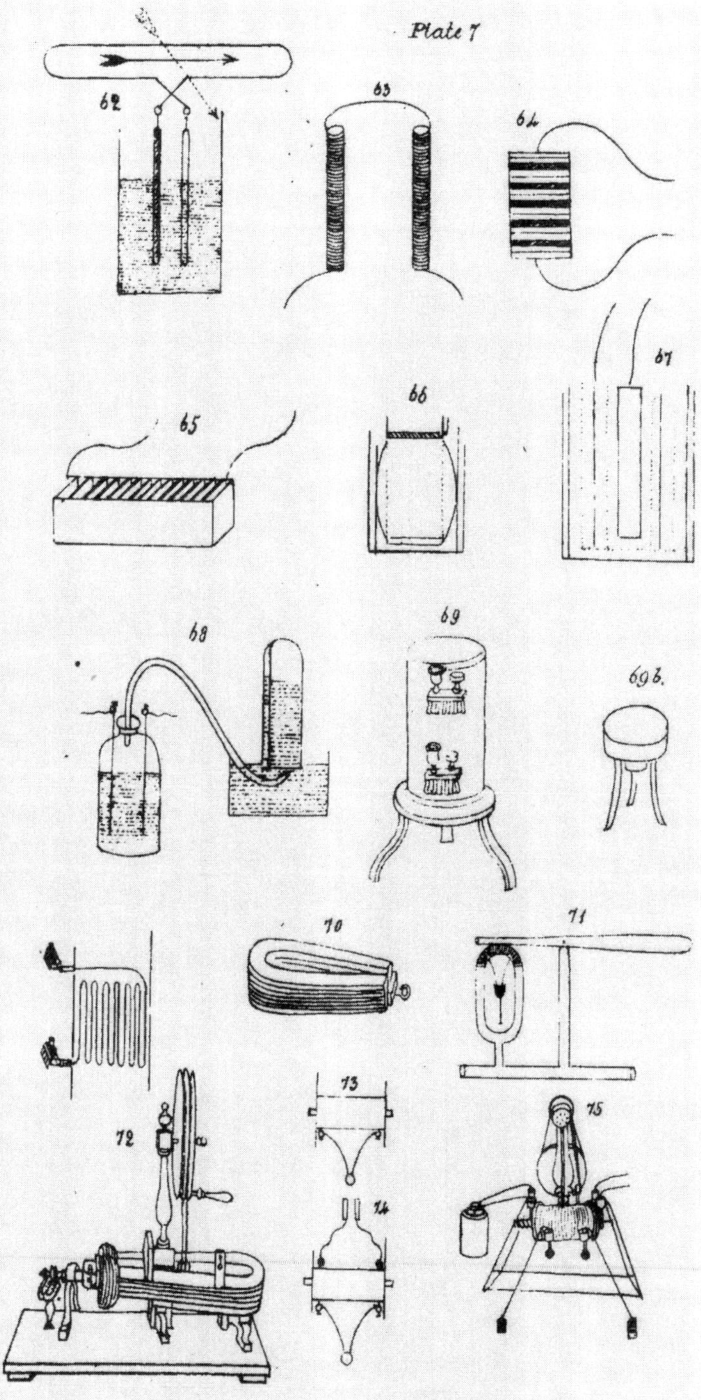

Plate 8.

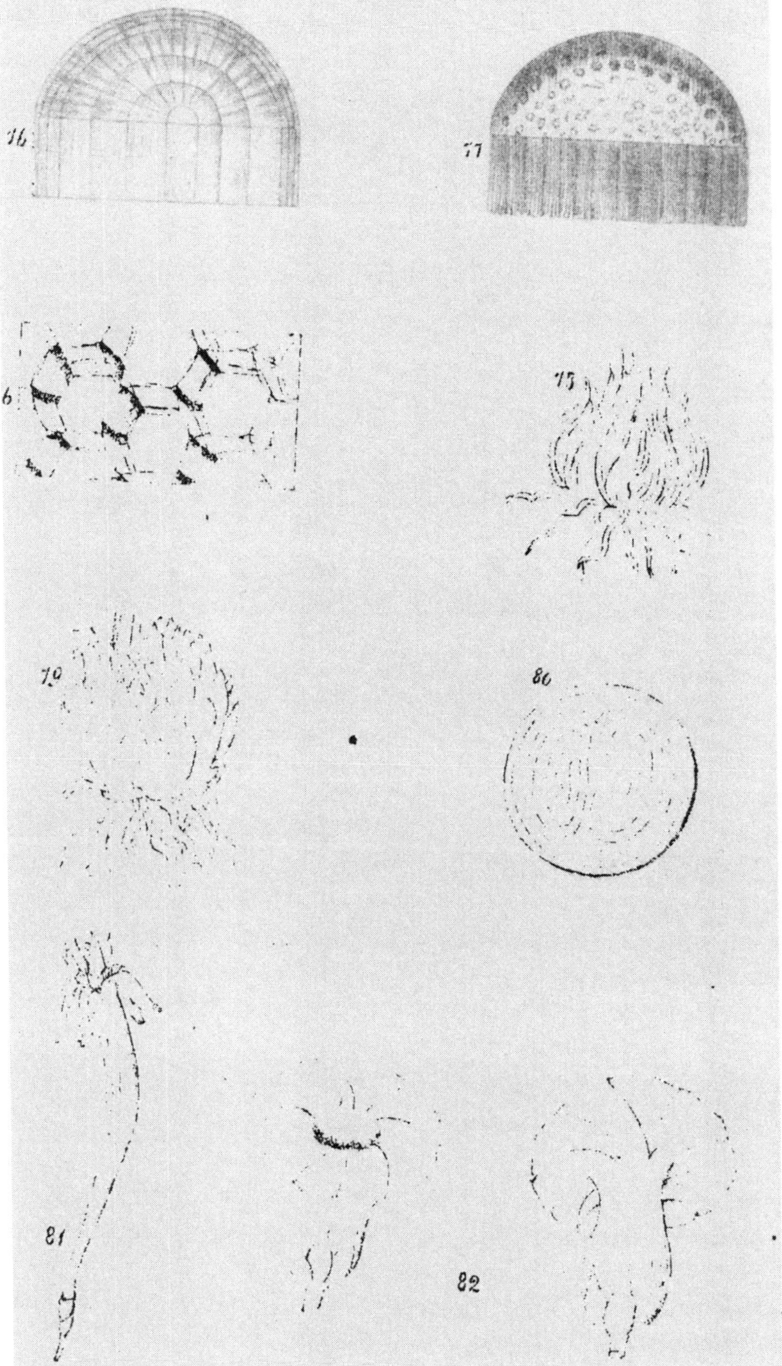

Plate 9.

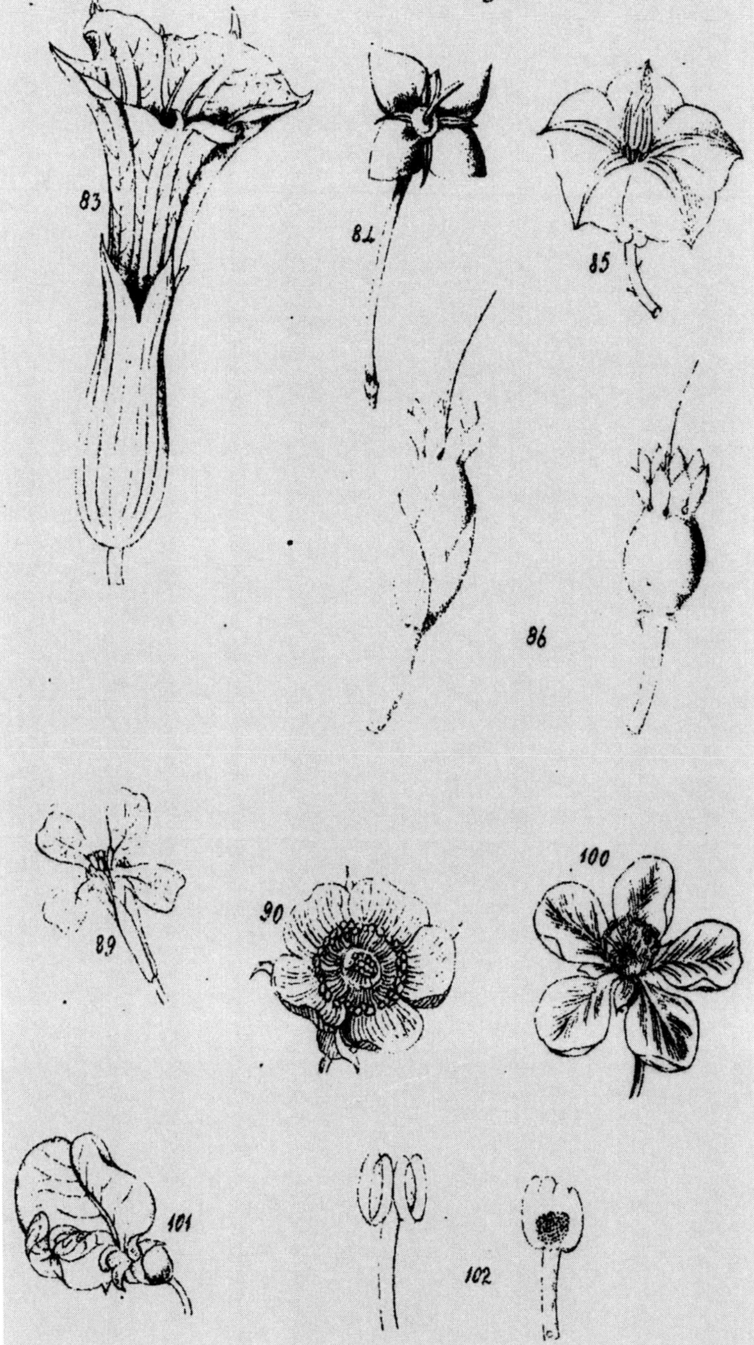